SURFACE DYSLEXIA
NEUROPSYCHOLOGICAL AND COGNITIVE
STUDIES OF PHONOLOGICAL READING

SURFACE DYSLEXIA

Neuropsychological and Cognitive
Studies of Phonological Reading

edited by
K. E. Patterson, J. C. Marshall, and M. Coltheart

WITHDRAWN

LAWRENCE ERLBAUM ASSOCIATES, PUBLISHERS
London   Hillsdale, New Jersey

Lawrence Erlbaum Associates Ltd., Publishers
Chancery House
319 City Road
London EC1V 1LJ

British Library Cataloguing in Publication Data

Surface dyslexia: neuropsychological and
  cognitive studies of phonological reading.
  1. Dyslexia — Diagnosis   2. Oral reading
  I. Patterson, K.E.   II. Marshall, John C.
  III. Coltheart, M.
  616.85'53075   RC394.W6

ISBN 0–83677–026–6

Typeset by Latimer Trend & Co. Ltd, Plymouth
Printed and bound by A. Wheaton & Co. Ltd., Exeter

Contents

V

List of Contributors

M.-F. Beauvois, Groupe de Recherche de Neuropsychologie, (INSERM U. 84), Hôpital de la Salpêtrière, 47 Boulevard de L'Hôpital, 75634 Paris, France.

D. Bub, Montreal Neurological Institute, 3801 University Street, Montreal, Quebec H3A 2B4, Canada.

A. Cancelliere, Department of Neurology, St. Joseph's Hospital, London, Ontario N6A 4U2, Canada.

D. Caplan, Montreal Neurological Institute, 3801 University Street, Montreal, Quebec H3A 2B4, Canada.

N. R. Carlson, Psychology Department, University of Massachusetts, Amherst, Massachusetts, U.S.A.

M. Coltheart, Department of Psychology, Birkbeck College, University of London, Malet Street, London WC1E 7HX, U.K.

J. Derouesné, Groupe de Recherche de Neuropsychologie, (INSERM U. 84), Hôpital de la Salpêtrière, 47 Boulevard de L'Hôpital, 75634 Paris, France.

U. Frith, MRC Cognitive Development Unit, 17 Gordon Street, London WC1H 0AH, U.K.

M.-C. Goldblum, Unité de Recherches Neuropsychologiques et Neuro-linguistiques (INSERM U. 111), 2ter Rue d'Alesia, 75014 Paris, France.

L. Henderson, Psychology Academic Group, School of Natural Sciences, Hatfield Polytechnic, P.O. Box 109, Hatfield, Herts. AL10 9AB, U.K.

P. Karanth,   All India Institute of Speech and Hearing, Manasa Gangothri, Mysore 570 006, India.

J. Kay,   Department of Speech, The University, St. Thomas Street, Newcastle-upon-Tyne NE1 7RU, U.K.

A. Kertesz,   Department of Neurology, St. Joseph's Hospital, London, Ontario N6A 4U2, Canada.

H. Kremin,   Unité de Recherches Neuropsychologiques et Neurolinguistiques (INSERM U. 111), 2ter Rue d'Alesia, 75014 Paris, France.

A. J. Marcel,   MRC Applied Psychology Unit, 15 Chaucer Road, Cambridge CB2 2EF, U.K.

D. I. Margolin,   Department of Neurology, V.A. Medical Center (116N), 2615 E. Clinton, Fresno, CA 93703, U.S.A.

J. C. Marshall,   Neuropsychology Unit, The Radcliffe Infirmary, Woodstock Road, Oxford OX2 6HE, U.K.

J. Masterson,   Department of Psychology, Birkbeck College, Malet Street, London WC1E 7HX, UK.

R. McCarthy,   Psychology Department, The National Hospital, Queen Square, London WC1N 3BG, U.K.

P. Meara,   Department of Applied Linguistics, Birkbeck College, University of London, Malet Street, London WC1E 7HX, U.K.

J. Morton,   MRC Cognitive Development Unit, 17 Gordon Street, London WC1 0AH, U.K.

F. Newcombe,   Neuropsychology Unit, The Radcliffe Infirmary, Woodstock Road, Oxford OX2 6HE, U.K.

K. E. Patterson,   MRC Applied Psychology Unit, 15 Chaucer Road, Cambridge CB2 2EF, U.K.

E. M. Saffran,   Department of Neurology, Temple University School of Medicine, 3401 North Broad Street, Philadelphia, PA 19140, U.S.A.

S. Sasanuma,   Tokyo Metropolitan Institute of Gerontology, 35–2 Sakaecho, Itabashi-ku, Tokyo–173, Japan.

T. Shallice,   MRC Applied Psychology Unit, 15 Chaucer Road, Cambridge CB2 2EF, U.K.

C. M. Temple,   Neuropsychology Unit, The Radcliffe Infirmary, Woodstock Road, Oxford OX2 6HE, U.K.

M. Vanier,   Montreal Neurological Institute, 3801 University Street, Montreal, Quebec H3A 2B4, Canada.

Phonetic Alphabet

Phonetic symbols (in square brackets) for transcribing vowels and consonants. Column 1 applies to most speakers of American English, Column 2 to most speakers of British English

Vowels			Consonants	
Col. 1	*Col. 2*			
[i]	[i]	head	[p]	pie
[ɪ]	[ɪ]	kid	[t]	tie
[eɪ]	[eɪ]	hay	[k]	key
[ɛ]	[ɛ]	bed	[b]	by
[æ]	[æ]	cat	[d]	dye
[ɑr]	[ɑ]	hard	[g]	guy
[ɑ]	[ɒ]	hot	[m]	me
[ɔ]	[ɔ]	saw	[n]	not
[ʊ]	[ʊ]	could	[ŋ]	rang
[oʊ]	[oʊ]	go	[f]	fox
[u]	[u]	who	[v]	view
[ər]	[ə]	bird	[θ]	thigh
[ʌ]	[ʌ]	hut	[ð]	thee
[aɪ]	[aɪ]	high	[s]	sea
[aʊ]	[aʊ]	how	[z]	jazz
[ɔɪ]	[ɔɪ]	boy	[ʃ]	shy
[ɪr]	[ɪə]	here	[ʒ]	vision
[er]	[ɛə]	care	[l]	lie
[aɪr]	[aɪə]	hire	[w]	we
			[r]	rat
			[j]	you
			[h]	he

Note also:

[ju]	[ju]	new	[tʃ]	chime
			[dʒ]	jive

XIII

ALPHABET PHONETIQUE
(Prononciations des mots, placées entre crochets)

VOYELLES

[i] il, vie, lyre
[e] blé, jouer
[ɛ] lait, jouet, merci
[a] plat, patte
[ɑ] bas, pâte
[ɔ] mort, donner
[o] mot, dôme, eau, gauche
[u] genou, roue
[y] rue, vêtu
[ø] peu, deux
[œ] peur, meuble
[ə] le, premier
[ɛ̃] matin plein
[ɑ̃] sans, vent
[ɔ̃] bon, ombre
[œ̃] lundi, brun

CONSONNES

[p] père, soupe
[t] terre, vite
[k] cou, qui, sac, képi
[b] bon, robe
[d] dans, aide
[g] gare, bague
[f] feu, neuf, photo
[s] sale, celui, ça, dessous, tasse, nation
[ʃ] chat, tache
[v] vous, rêve
[z] zéro, maison, rose
[ʒ] je, gilet, geôle
[l] lent, sol
[ʀ] rue, venir
[m] main, femme
[n] nous, tonne, animal
[ɲ] agneau, vigne

---

[h] hop! (exclamatif)
['] haricot (pas de liaison)

[ŋ] mots empr. anglais, camping
[x] mots empr. espagnol, jota; arabe, khamsin, etc.

SEMI-CONSONNES

[j] yeux, paille, pied
[w] oui, nouer
[ɥ] huile, lui

Source: Dictionnaire Alphabetique et Analogique de la Langue Francaise
(Supplement). 1970, Paris: le Robert.

General Introduction

Consider how reading aloud is normally accomplished. When we read *steam* as "steam," precisely how do we carry out this conversion of print to speech? One can conceive of two different ways in which such conversion might be achieved. On the one hand, reading *steam* aloud could be accomplished by accessing a store of previously learned information about words—a "mental lexicon"—and retrieving from that store the particular phonological form associated with the specific orthographic form *steam*. Here information concerning just the one word *steam* serves as the basis for reading aloud. An alternative possibility is that the reader uses knowledge about correspondences between orthography and phonology at a level smaller than that of the whole word: any such correspondence would apply to many of the words in the reader's vocabulary. Correspondences of this kind could operate on units of various sizes up to, but not including, the whole word. One such unit is the letter or letter combination and its corresponding phoneme. For example, if the word *steam* were broken up into the orthographic units *s, t, ea,* and *m,* and if the phonemic correspondences for these, /s/, /t/, /i/, and /m/, were retrieved and then blended together, the appropriate phonological form /stim/ would result.

Most current models of reading aloud entail some version of this distinction between two procedures for converting print to phonology, although the models differ in the ways in which the two procedures are characterised. In some models (e.g. Coltheart, 1978), the procedure for retrieving whole phonological forms corresponding to specific known words is referred to as the *lexical* procedure (because it depends upon word-specific information) whereas the procedure involving correspondences between orthographic and phonological units at a level smaller than the word is called the *non-lexical* procedure, because it is considered to depend on general rules rather than word-specific information. Although such general rules might be *acquired* via experience with words, the view is that the rules are *used* independently of word-specific knowledge when reading aloud is based on subword units.

Other theorists, however, reject this view, denying that a separate non-lexical system of rules is the basis of reading aloud at the subword level (e.g. Glushko, 1979; Marcel, 1980). Instead, it is argued that subword orthographic units and their phonological correspondences are obtained by reference to knowledge about correspondences at the word level, using procedures for segmenting word representations.

Nevertheless, both "dual-route" theorists and those who reject the idea of a purely non-lexical rule system accept the distinction with which we began this introduction, namely that a word like *steam* can be read aloud either (1) by reference to knowledge specific to that one word or (2) by reference to knowledge about subword-size segments that occur in many words. This distinction is specified here (both in the process model depicted on the book jacket and in the discussion in this introductory section) simply in terms of two *levels* of translation from orthography to phonology—a word level and a subword level. The reason for this choice of terminology is that it is relatively neutral theoretically: it makes no commitment as to the *size* of the units involved in the subword level, nor about their source (lexical or non-lexical). Different theories of reading aloud make different claims about both the size and the source of these subword units.

We have illustrated the distinction between the word-level and the subword-level procedures for reading aloud with reference to the example word *steam*, for which either procedure should yield a correct reading response. A crucial implication of this distinction, an implication around which much work on normal and abnormal reading has been organised, is that the two procedures are not capable of producing correct responses for every type of orthographic input. There are letter strings that cannot be assigned an appropriate phonological code by the word-level procedure; and there are other letter strings that cannot be assigned a correct phonological code by the subword-level procedure, even though for a string like *steam* either procedure yields a correct code.

The word-level procedure allows correct reading aloud only when the orthographic stimulus is a *word*. If instead the input is a non-word like *vib* or *slint*, there will be no means by which the word-level procedure can compute an address for the phonology corresponding to the whole orthographic string. Application of the word-level procedure to a non-word would yield either simply no response, or else a response which is a word orthographically close to the non-word—a "visual error" such as reading *slint* as "sling" or "stint."

In contrast, the subword level procedure guarantees correct reading aloud only when the orthographic stimulus is a regularly spelled word or a non-word. Subword-level translation makes use of correspondences between orthographic and phonological units that are typical of many words, and therefore cannot successfully deal with words like *pint* or *yacht*, which contain atypical spelling–sound correspondences. Application of the sub-word-level procedure to words containing such atypical correspondences ("irregular" or "exception" words) would usually yield a mistranslation of the atypical segment—a "regularisation error" such as reading *pint* to rhyme with *hint*. This is so whether the subword-level procedure works via non-lexical rules or by analogy with lexical entries.

According to this general approach to modelling oral reading, then, correct reading of non-words *requires* a procedure for *subword*-level translation from orthography to phonology, whereas correct reading of words irregular in spelling–sound correspondence *requires* a procedure for *word*-level translation. One way to investigate this approach is to study oral reading by experimental work with skilled adult readers, testing deductions from particular models embodying this distinction between reading procedures. Another way is to study patterns of oral reading in neurological patients who were skilled readers prior to their brain damage. If the distinction between the two procedures is valid, and if in addition the neural mechanisms representing these procedures are so located in the brain that it is possible for brain damage to disrupt one and not the other procedure, then various deductions can be made concerning what patterns of reading impairment should be observed.

If it is the procedure for subword translation from orthography to phonology that is impaired or abolished, the consequence will be that a patient will read *words* aloud correctly (by addressing their whole-word phonology) but will fail when asked to read *non-words*. This pattern, referred to as phonological dyslexia (or phonological alexia), was first described by Beauvois and Derouesné (1979) and by various others since. A particularly clear recent example is the patient W.B. (Funnell, 1983): after his stroke, W.B.'s success in oral reading of real words (even words "difficult" on a variety of dimensions) was around 90%, whereas he was completely unable to read the simplest of non-words.

If, on the other hand, it is the procedure for translating at the word level that is impaired, the consequence will be that a patient will correctly read aloud words with a regular spelling–sound correspondence (e.g. *mint*) and also regularly spelled non-words (e.g. *slint*) but will make errors when asked to read irregular words (like *pint*). This pattern, referred to as surface dyslexia, was first described in any detail by Marshall and Newcombe (1973), and by various others since. It is the primary subject of this book.

If word and subword levels of translation from orthography to phonology are indeed separable procedures in the sense that disruption of one may have no effect on a person's ability to utilise the other, then we would expect to find surface dyslexic patients for whom oral reading of regular words (and non-words) was simply normal. Whatever the size of orthographic segment involved in the subword level, and whether such segments are obtained and translated by non-lexical rule or by analogy with other words possessing the same segments, a functioning system for subword translation should produce correct pronunciations of regular words like *sheet* and non-words like *sheem*. The two surface dyslexic patients originally presented by Marshall and Newcombe (1973), however, made frequent errors when asked to read regular words aloud. If this continued to be true of the further cases described where oral reading apparently relies upon subword translation, then one would begin to have grave doubts about the view that the subword procedure can operate normally when the word-level procedure is impaired. We now know, however, that oral reading of regular words (and non-words) *can* be normal in patients with this general pattern of acquired dyslexia: the case described by Shallice, Warrington, and McCarthy (1983) provides such evidence, and particularly clear support comes from the patient described by Bub, Cancelliere, and Kertesz in Chapter 1 in this book. At least as a working hypothesis, then, the view that the two procedures for oral reading are separable seems tenable. In some patients both procedures are damaged— presumably this was why Marshall and Newcombe's two surface dyslexics were impaired at reading regular words—but this itself does not constitute evidence against the view that the two procedures can be independently damaged.

It should be emphasised that when we speak of the procedure for subword translation, we mean to include not only the appropriate segmentation of the orthographic string and the correct conversion of these segments to their phonological equivalents but also the assembly or blending of the phonological segments into a whole response. Thus all of these components must operate correctly to enable a subword-level system to function normally. In patients with impaired operation of the subword-level procedure, one therefore can seek to specify the precise component of the procedure that is malfunctioning. Attempts to do this may be found in the chapters by Temple, by Newcombe and Marshall, and by Derouesné and Beauvois.

As already indicated, we must be able to demonstrate that each procedure for oral reading can function within the normal range of performance when the other is impaired, if we are to claim that the two procedures are indeed separate. This requirement seems to be satisfied for both the whole-word level (by phonological dyslexic patients whose oral reading of real words is essentially normal) and the subword level (by surface dyslexic patients whose oral reading of words regular in spelling–sound correspondence is essentially normal). What about the other side of the coin: the *degree* of impairment of the impaired procedure when only one of the procedures is disrupted? We noted earlier that at least one patient has been described in whom the subword level was *abolished* with the word-level procedure essentially intact: W.B. correctly read aloud 90% of real words and 0% of non-words (Funnell, 1983). On the other hand, no case has yet been reported with *total* disruption of the word-level procedure and preservation of the subword-level procedure. Total disruption of the word-level procedure should result in essentially *no* correct pronunciations of highly irregular words such as *vase* or *yacht*; but in all cases of surface dyslexia so far described, some such words could still be read. Therefore, one must conclude that, for the cases of surface dyslexia studied to date, the word-level procedure for translating from orthography to phonology either (1) is preserved for some *lexical entries* but not others, or (2) has a fluctuating pattern that enables it to succeed on some *occasions* but not on others. Whatever the nature of the word-level impairment, it is clear that it is sensitive to word frequency (see Chapter 1).

Thus far we have simply referred to the "word-level procedure" for reading aloud. Like the subword procedure, however, this must in fact involve several different components, which appear in the diagram on the book jacket. At a minimum, according to this model, correct word-level assignment of phonology to orthography requires that the printed word be recognised in (i.e. be matched to an entry in) the orthographic lexicon and that this entry then address the corresponding entry in the phonological lexicon. The model also suggests that a semantic interpretation of the word may, but in the normal system need not, mediate between orthographic recognition and phonological output when oral reading occurs. Impairment of one or more of these components then constitutes a disruption of the procedure for word-level oral reading, which may force reliance on the subword procedure. Although *any* pattern of oral reading deriving primarily from a reliance upon the subword procedure tends to be called surface dyslexia, various different impairments in the word-level procedure may be causal factors; therefore we should in fact anticipate a variety of rather different patterns in connection with surface dyslexic performance. For example, a patient with a defect of orthographic recognition, and a patient with a defect of phonological output, might both rely upon the subword level for oral reading; but in other respects the two patients would show very different patterns of impairment. That such different patterns do emerge is one of the main themes of this book. Thus one must not expect the syndrome label "surface dyslexia" to specify precisely how every patient so characterised will perform. What different surface dyslexic patients have in common is that they rely to an abnormal degree upon the subword procedure for translating from orthography to phonology. Both the nature of the word-level impairment responsible for this reliance, and the extent to which the subword procedure is intact, will vary from case to case.

We have already referred several times to the "book-jacket" model of reading, which is reproduced in Fig. 1. It represents a minimal process model to which all (or most) of the contributions to this volume at least roughly conform. The notational conventions that it uses are as follows: A solid box represents a processing mechanism and/or knowledge store; a solid line (with arrows) represents the flow of information between two processing components; dotted lines with arrows that depart from (or terminate in) thin air represent interconnections the exact status of which, vis-à-vis both the information they transmit and their loci of departure and arrival, is disputed. The main source of such uncertainty in this diagram corresponds to the controversy about whether the subword procedure is non-lexical or lexical. If it is non-lexical, then the first stage of the procedure (orthographic segmentation) will follow Preliminary Visual Analysis of the letter string; if lexical, then the orthographic segmentation necessary for subword translation will occur in the orthographic lexicon. Because this issue is unresolved, we locate the initiation of the subword procedure in thin air somewhere between Preliminary Visual Analysis and Orthographic Recognition; for parallel reasons, we locate the termination of this procedure in thin air between Output Phonology and the Response Buffer. The symbol >.....< is intended to acknowledge another controversy, regarding the nature and size of the units involved in translation from orthography to phonology. In some models, such units come in only two sizes—whole words and graphemes (i.e. the individual letters and letter clusters that correspond to single phonemes); in other models, these units can additionally take a range of sizes in between the two extremes. One of the ways in which one can attempt to resolve such controversies is by studying surface dyslexia.

REFERENCES

Beauvois, M. F., & Derouesné, J. (1979). Phonological alexia: Three dissociations. *Journal of Neurology, Neurosurgery, and Psychiatry,* **42,** 1115–1124.

Coltheart, M. (1978). Lexical access in simple reading tasks. In G. Underwood (ed.), *Strategies of Information Processing.* London: Academic Press.

Funnell, E. (1983). Phonological processes in reading: New evidence from acquired dyslexia. *British Journal of Psychology,* **74,** 159–180.

Glushko, R. J. (1979). The organisation and activation of orthographic knowledge in reading aloud. *Journal of Experimental Psychology (Human Perception and Performance),* **5,** 674–691.

Marcel, A. J. (1980). Surface dyslexia and beginning reading. A revised hypothesis of the pronunciation of print and its impairments. In M. Coltheart, K. Patterson, & J. C. Marshall (eds), *Deep Dyslexia.* London: Routledge and Kegan Paul.

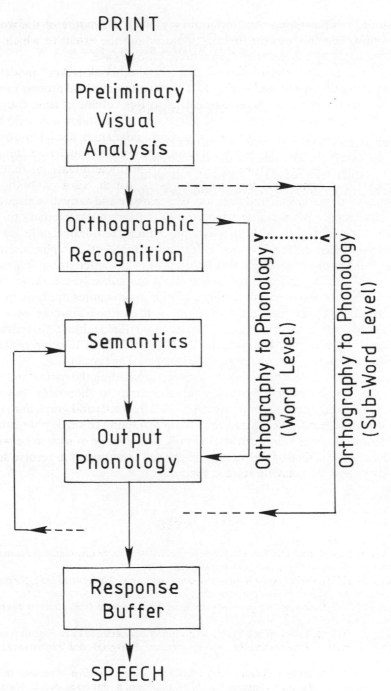

FIG. 1. A minimal model of reading aloud and reading for meaning.

Marshall, J. C., & Newcombe, F. (1973). Patterns of paralexia: A psycholinguistic approach. *Journal of Psycholinguistic Research*, **2**, 175–199.

Shallice, T., Warrington, E. K., & McCarthy, R. (1983). Reading without semantics. *Quarterly Journal of Experimental Psychology*, **35A**, 111–138.

ACKNOWLEDGEMENT

We are grateful to the Medical Research Council, and in particular Dr Joan Box, for making it possible for the contributors to this volume to spend a most productive three days together, discussing surface dyslexia, in the pleasant surroundings of Wolfson College, Oxford.

CASE STUDIES OF ACQUIRED SURFACE DYSLEXIA

Introduction

Nineteenth- and early twentieth-century neurolinguistic inquiry has one striking and peculiar characteristic: either the theory is clear and explicit but the data that fall within the domain of the model are only vaguely sketched, or the data are transparent but the theory is woefully insubstantial. Nowhere is this strange double dissociation more apparent than in studies of acquired disorders of reading.

For example, a complex of symptoms now termed "deep dyslexia" (Marshall & Newcombe, 1973) was described in considerable detail in papers published between 1895 and 1931 (Marshall & Newcombe, 1980; Obler, 1984). The inability to read orthographically legal non-words, the gross impairment of "function word" reading, and the presence of frank semantic paralexias (to single words) were all clearly outlined. Yet theoretical analysis of this constellation of symptoms did not progress beyond the claim that the patient manifested "associative loss" or an inability to analyse a whole into its parts. By contrast, a theoretical analysis of a complex of symptoms now termed "surface dyslexia" (Marshall & Newcombe, 1973) *was* explicitly formulated (see, for example, Lichtheim, 1885; Wernicke, 1885). This analysis involved the notion of "non-lexical" or "pre-lexical" phonological recoding of print (which is referred to with greater generality as "subword-level recoding" in the General Introduction to this book). The data adduced by Wernicke and Lichtheim were, however, so amorphous that it is frequently very difficult to tell exactly what the patient did when attempting to read.

Let us elaborate this seemingly paradoxical claim. In the case reports of nineteenth-century neurologists, the descriptions and diagrams whereby the acquired dyslexias were interpreted clearly stated that *all* reading for meaning was mediated by the centre for auditory *speech* imagery (Lichtheim, 1885; Wernicke, 1885). The sole path from the centre for "visual representations" to the "concept centre" is via the centre for auditory word representations. (Lichtheim's diagrams do, however, allow for correct reading aloud without semantic involvement; but, in this eventuality too, visual representations are converted into articulatory form via the centre for auditory word images.) Stated in this general form, the claim is equivalent to the hypothesis of Rubenstein, Lewis, and Rubenstein (1971) that prelexical phonological recoding is *obligatory* in visual word recognition, a claim echoed by Laberge (1972), who states categorically that "written material *must* (our italics) be coded into phonological form to be comprehended." We now know that this conjecture is false (Coltheart, Patterson, & Marshall, 1980). None the less, the written word *can* be converted to "sound" prior to comprehension, and one question at issue in this book is how this conversion takes place.

In the first modern description of surface dyslexia, Marshall and Newcombe (1973) interpreted their patient's reading as follows: pronunciation of the printed word usually occurred by means of grapheme–phoneme correspondence rules (GPCs) and comprehension of the printed word was mediated by the phonological output of this GPC routine. Historically speaking, it is not clear that this interpretation would apply to many of the nineteenth-century cases of acquired dyslexia who were reported to read by a phonologically mediated procedure. For example, in case 3 of Lichtheim (1885), the patient (J.U.S.) was reported, in the acute phase, to understand nothing of the printed or handwritten word, although he could *name* most letters correctly. Furthermore, "he can make up letters into words, and he can read aloud by spelling; but it is evident that the sense of the word remains closed to him." During the course of recovery, Lichtheim notes that J.U.S. "makes out the meaning better" when he reads aloud, and that later still "he understands short words at once." Even so, "longer ones take him an interval, during which he seems to put them together: he used to repeat them, but this being forbidden he appears to spell them inwardly." Transposed into current terminology, it would seem that J.U.S. was reading via the overt or covert use of letter names, which function as the access code for semantic interpretation. This syndrome—letter-by-letter reading—and its historical background is described by Patterson and Kay (1982). There may well be "mixed" cases, however, in which patients use a combination of letter-naming and letter-sounding in order to cope with the printed word (see, for example, patients T.P. and K.C. in Patterson & Kay, 1982, and the discussion by Shallice & McCarthy, Chapter 15 in this book). Similarly, it would appear that some patients, in the course of the evolution of the deficit, move from (predominantly) using letter names to using letter sounds (see patient M.B. in Newcombe & Marshall, 1973). Nowhere in Lichtheim's paper, however, does he make an explicit distinction between letter names (e.g. $c \rightarrow$/si/) and letter sounds (e.g. $c \rightarrow$/kə/ or /sə/). In part, this odd oversight may be due to the (even odder) persistence throughout Europe of the Graeco-Roman ABC method of teaching reading (see Huey, 1908, Chapter 13).

A similar failure to distinguish between letter-by-letter reading and surface dyslexia can be seen in the English-language literature. For example, Elder (1897) described a case of alexia without agraphia, with minimal aphasic involvement. The patient, M.P., had some difficulty in recalling proper names and a "slight impairment of her memory for events." Information relevant to her dyslexia is reported as follows:

> On testing her eyesight I found that she could see objects quite well, that she saw letters well and could name them slowly, but that she could not put them into words. When, however, I spelled short words aloud for her she could pronounce the word from the sound, but often in a slow and disjointed manner. She herself could read in this way, viz. by reading the letters aloud and pronouncing the word from the sound of the letters, but this could only be done with the smaller words. She could write voluntarily, but she could not read what she had written, although she could make out the letters and figures (p. 159).

Elder's use of the expression "the sound of the letters" does not, in the context of his description, provide an explicit, unambiguous account of the patient's strategy.

As far as we are aware, the first author to make the unequivocal distinction between letter sounds and letter names is Störring (1907). Störring opens his discussion: "We may now proceed to derive from pathological cases an answer to *the question whether reading and writing always takes place literally, i.e. letter by letter*." The first case he cites (a patient of Sommer's) could name most letters correctly; when required to read the word *band*, the patient spelled out the letters without error but "after prolonged attempts" articulated "bank" and then "bar" before giving up "in despair." Sommer then "pronounced (the sounds) to him"; the patient could combine *a, u, s* into "aus" but failed totally with *B,u,c,h*, and *H,a,n,d*. Sommer's explanation was that "mere succession of letters is not sufficient to constitute words" and that "the succession must take place at a definite speed." But Störring notes that "if we are to utilize these data it is important to know whether the constituent sounds or the constituent letters of words were pronounced to the patient." This crucial observation of Störring's seems to have had little or no effect upon subsequent developments in the interpretation of reading and writing disorders, and indeed he failed to apply his own distinction to the interpretation of reading. Part of the problem, of course, is that throughout the nineteenth century, the term *letter* was used for what we would now refer to as a *phoneme*.

Current concepts of phonology (and an appropriate terminology) were first introduced by Baudouin de Courtenay and by the Prague School (Trubetzkoy & Jakobson). It may thus be no accident that the first really convincing outlines of surface dyslexia and surface dysgraphia were provided by Jakobson's friend, the Soviet neuropsychologist Alexander Romanovitch Luria.

Luria (1947, English translation 1970) argues that the fluent, mature reader, especially when reading text, employs a direct visual route: "The experienced reader grabs only the general contour of a word and the characteristic configuration of its major letters which usually constitute its root part. On the basis of this he guesses the meaning of the word as a whole." But if this "sight vocabulary" is unavailable (either because an unfamiliar word is encountered or due to pathology) a rule-governed (grapheme–phoneme) strategy must be employed, based upon the sub-lexical analysis of the written stimulus and its phonological realisation. When, consequent upon brain damage, this extra-lexical route is itself impaired, Luria distinguishes two types of functional disorder. In the first variety, the patient's difficulty arises from "impairment of the ability to remember the phonemes represented by different letters." In the second variety, "the difficulty arises when he is required to read groups of letters forming sequential patterns, for he has lost the schemata whereby letters appearing in sequences unite to form syllables. He is unable to look ahead and by noting the context of a given letter, pronounce it correctly (p. 355)." Problems of this second type can exist at either of two functional loci: at input when a particular letter has more than one phonological realisation, the correct variant depending upon the graphemic context (cf. English rule of *e*, whereby the vowel undergoes a regular alternation in such pairs as *fin* versus *fine*); at output when the precise articulatory realisation of a particular phoneme is dependent upon smooth "blending" (co-articulation constraints) of phonic constituents.

In Luria's analysis, then, the extra-lexical routine for reading must consist of (at least) three subcomponents: (1) correct segmentation of the letter string; (2) retrieval of appropriate grapheme–phoneme correspondences; (3) accurate synthesis of the phoneme string into syllables and words (see Luria, 1970, p. 355). Many current models of extra-lexical reading follow, and elaborate, the structure of Luria's account of extra-lexical reading (Colt-heart, 1978; Newcombe & Marshall, 1981; Temple & Marshall, 1983; and the chapters by Derouesné and Beauvois, and by Temple, in this book).

There are few clinical reports of the characteristic symptomatology of surface dyslexia prior to Marshall and Newcombe (1973). Partial failure of grapheme–phoneme correspondence rules had been observed (although not described in these terms) by Alajouanine, Lhermitte, and Ribaucourt-Ducarne (1960). Presented with *lit*, one of their patients initially read the word correctly—/li/—but then "corrected" his response to /lit/, indicating thereby his unstable control of the conversion rule that, in French, terminal *t* is regularly silent. Earlier, Lyman, Kwan, and Chao (1938) had described a fully bilingual patient (Chinese-English) who had especial difficulties when reading English words containing silent consonants. The patient of Lyman et al. would often attempt to sound out the words segment by segment, a phenomenon also observed by Dubois-Charlier (1971) who reports such *conduits d'approche* as *appauvrissait*→"ap . . . appauv . . . pauvri . . . appauv-riss."

The importance of studying "surface dyslexia" in a variety of languages (and, where possible, in biscriptal patients) had previously been stressed by Luria (1960, 1970). The *overt* manifestations of surface dyslexia and dysgraphia, he points out (Luria, 1970), will depend to a considerable extent upon the precise form of the mapping from orthography to phonology that is represented in the language: "The writing disorder . . . may be especially severe if the patient writes in a relatively nonphonetic language such as French or English, i.e. in a language in which the spelling of words often does not correspond to the pronunciation (p. 333)." Bilingual patients (Luria, 1960) can accordingly provide a subtle assay of the interaction between underlying damage to neuronal structures and the differing phenotypic expressions of that damage in different orthographies (where with respect to lesion localisation the patient is, of course, his own control). Thus Luria (1970, p. 334) reports that his bilingual patient Falk could easily write words correctly to dictation in Russian (where the orthography is highly regular), but he frequently confused homophonic words when writing to dictation in French (which contains both large numbers of silent letters and many differently spelled versions of the same sound sequence). Falk wrote "le maire" as *le mère* (despite the meaning having been glossed when the dictation was given); similarly, he wrote "je le vois" as *je le voix*, and "il le voit" as *il le voix*. The errors are phonologically appropriate but the orthography is incorrect vis-à-vis meaning and grammatical form.

In an attempt to account for surface (as well as other patterns of) dyslexia, Marshall and Newcombe (1973) conjectured that the normal reader could utilise, in parallel, two routes for reading aloud (and comprehension). One route associated the visual addresses of words with their appropriate semantic representations; the other route converted visual addresses into phonological form via the operation of grapheme–phoneme conversion rules. Overt articulation of an input word, they argued, could then be triggered either from the semantic representation of the word or from its phonological representation. If, due to pathology, access to the semantic route (from visual addresses) was impaired, the patient must rely on phonological recoding, this latter representation acting now as the sole input both to semantic information and to the routines required for overt pronunciation.

In a phonetically irregular orthography, like English, reliance on such an extra-lexical route will run foul of numerous words whose pronunciation is not derivable from general rules. Marshall and Newcombe (1973) accordingly noted that their patients J.C. and S.T. (called "surface dyslexics") had

> especial difficulty with the context-sensitive nature of grapheme–phoneme mappings. That is, ambiguous consonants (whose phonetic value depends upon the graphemic context in which they are placed) and markers (such as terminal *e*) which have themselves no phonetic value but rather specify the realization of some other part of the word .... (p. 191)

When these patients overgeneralized a correspondence rule, for example, by overtly pronouncing the silent *t* in *listen*, the word was interpreted semantically as the (erroneous) response (i.e. "liston ... that's the boxer, isn't it?").

Writing to dictation was not studied in J.C. or S.T. because both men were too impaired in this task to produce a meaningful corpus for analysis. De Agostini (1977), however, noted that patients who wrote "phonetically" would appear to be more seriously impaired if they were French (where the orthography is highly irregular) than if they were Italian (where there is a very consistent relationship between phonological and orthographic form). None the less, Italian does have some ambiguous correspondences. The syllable /ku/, for example, can legally be written as either *cu* or *qu* in syllable initial position, or as *ccu* or *cqu* in non-initial position. De Agostini discovered a small group of Italian aphasics who did indeed produce incorrect but phonemically plausible errors on writing to dictation (e.g. "acquaio"→*accuaio*; "acquaio"→*aquaio*).

If reading is extra-lexical in surface dyslexia, it should follow that non-words (whose "correct" pronunciation must, by definition, be regular) should be read no less successfully than (regular) words. Kremin (1980) reported a French-speaking patient (F.R.A.) whose errors on word reading were, for the most part, interpretable in terms of unstable grapheme–phoneme correspondences, and who did indeed have well-preserved non-word reading. The patient also manifested "surface dysgraphia" in that errors on writing to dictation were frequently accurate or plausible as a phonological transcription of the stimulus (e.g. "ciseaux"→*sizo*, "escabeau"→*escabo*, "héros"→*hérot*, "hormis"→*hormi*). This patient is further described and discussed in Chapter 7 in this book.[1]

Further studies of surface dysgraphia in French were reported by Beau-

---

[1] It should be noted that this patient is sometimes referred to as F.R.A. and sometimes as B.F.

vois and Derouesné (1981), although their term for this pattern of spelling impairment was "lexical or orthographic agraphia." Their patient (R.G.) wrote virtually all non-words (even long, complex ones) perfectly to dictation, but made substantial numbers of errors when writing even very common words that were orthographically ambiguous or irregular (e.g. "pigeon"→*pijon*, "église"→*aiglise*, "tank"→*tanq*, "copeau"→*copot*, "photo"→*fauto*). The patient showed an interesting qualitative dissociation between the pattern of his reading and writing disorder. His reading of non-words was severely impaired relative to his fairly well-preserved word reading (phonological dyslexia); he was frequently unable to read back the phonologically correct but neologistic responses that he had himself produced when writing to dictation.

The reading performance of R.O.G., reported by Shallice and Warrington (1980), was quite similar to that displayed by J.C. and S.T. (Marshall & Newcombe, 1973). Words were sounded out very slowly, a strong "regularity effect" was found on the Coltheart word list (Coltheart, Besner, Jonasson, & Davelaar, 1979), and all the errors involved "misapplication of a grapheme/ phoneme conversion rule" (e.g. *broad*→/broɑd/).

It would seem that for J.C., S.T., and R.O.G. the semantic system itself is well preserved but *access* to it from print is impaired. Warrington (1975), however, described three patients (whose *primary* diagnosis was associative agnosia) who had an impairment of the semantic memory system per se. These patients too should, *ex hypothesi*, read aloud by a "phonological route" (either sub-lexical or whole word), as indeed they did. One of these patients (E.M.), who suffered from a progressive dementing illness, initially showed only a small discrepancy between her ability to read regular and irregular words, but the magnitude of the effect increased dramatically as her condition deteriorated (see also Schwartz, Marin, & Saffran, 1979; Schwartz, Saffran, & Marin, 1980). Shallice and Warrington (1980) accordingly propose that the phonological route does not operate solely on graphemes (i.e. letters or letter combinations that map on to one phoneme) but that the route may additionally translate "larger visual units including syllables and short words." They hypothesise that: "The ease of operation of the route would vary with the frequency in the language with which a particular letter combination occurs with a particular sound and inversely with the frequency with which alternative pronunciations of the letter string occur (p. 123)." As they point out, such a mechanism would presuppose that different "parsings" of the letter string be made, with the phonological route accepting "the most word-like as valid" (see also Marcel, 1980). On this account, "regularity" would not be a dichotomous variable, but rather subject to degrees (Shallice & Warrington, 1980): ". . . as the phonological route becomes increasingly impaired so the frequency with which a particular visual-auditory mapping of a letter combination would need to occur in order to be utilized, would increase (p. 123)." This line of argument ("levels of irregularity") is further developed by Shallice, Warrington, and McCarthy (1983), and by Shallice and McCarthy (Chapter 15 in this book).

By contrast, Coltheart (1978, 1982) has argued for a much "purer," more restricted phonological route that only translates the orthographic units ("graphemes") whose phonic representation is a single phoneme; for each grapheme the phonic realisation provided by the translation rules is the most frequent correspondence. Coltheart (1982) demonstrated that the regularity effect shown by six subjects with surface dyslexia (some acquired, some developmental) is consistent with that shown by a computer program (McIlroy, 1977) that "relies almost entirely on a set of letter–sound translation rules." The program's ability to perform homophone matching (a task where the subject must decide whether the two words of a printed pair such as *ferry/fury* and *berry/bury* are identical in pronunciation) also parallels that of the surface dyslexics. One of these (human) cases of acquired surface dyslexia (A.B.) is reported in more detail in Coltheart, Masterson, Byng, Prior, and Riddoch (1983). For this patient, there is little or no reason to suppose that any "units intermediate between the whole word and the grapheme are used when converting print to phonology," a conclusion that would also seem to be true of the French-speaking patient (A.D.) studied by Deloche, Andreewsky, and Desi (1982). Both A.B. and A.D. also manifested phonological spelling (surface dysgraphia). Thus A.B. wrote "genuine" as *jenuwen*; A.D. wrote "cerveau" as *cervot*.

To date, most published cases of surface dyslexia have also shown surface dysgraphia (but cf. Newcombe & Marshall, 1984). One would not, however, expect surface dysgraphia to be the simple inverse of surface dyslexia (in English or French, at least). Grapheme–phoneme correspondence rules cannot just be reversed in order to give phoneme–grapheme correspondences. This issue is further developed by Hatfield and Patterson (1983), who provide an intensive analysis of the writing performance of T.P., a case previously mentioned with regard to her reading by a combination of letter naming and letter sounding (Patterson & Kay, 1982). Hatfield and Patterson (1983) also make the point that surface dyslexia and surface dysgraphia will fail to exhibit a precise parallel due to the differential role of comprehension in reading and writing/spelling. When reading, the surface dyslexic is attempting to gain access to the meaning of the input word; in writing, the meaning is usually known and hence "for a patient like T.P. . . . there will be little or no motivation to generate 'meaningful' spellings." One might therefore expect a higher proportion of neologistic spellings in surface dysgraphia than neologistic readings in surface dyslexia. In the latter case, some patients at least attempt to constrain their output by reference to the *phonological* form of known words.

Thus far, we have tended to describe cases of "surface dyslexia" as if the term referred to a single, constant syndrome. But the patients differ from one another in a variety of ways. They differ in the other disorders of higher cognitive functioning that can be associated with "surface dyslexia." And, more crucially, they differ in the precise form of phonological reading they display. That is, the phonological route can itself be impaired at several different functional loci, and also the failure to use the "semantic" route can result from impairment at a variety of stages. In short, whatever its value as a "shorthand" way of referring to patients, "surface dyslexia" is *not* a single, stable syndrome with a precise list of criteria that can be applied to patients for the purpose of differential diagnosis. Once this fact is realised, there are two methodological-cum-theoretical paths that the investigator can take. One can multiply the number of "subtypes" of surface dyslexia, or one can renounce classification into syndromes. For any complex skill, based upon a number of subprocesses and interconnections between them, the possible ways in which the process as a whole can in principle fractionate becomes astronomically large. Thus Marshall (1984) notes that the (very) simple model of reading proposed in Marshall and Newcombe (1973) predicts the existence of 16,383 varieties of dyslexia ($2^n - 1$, where n is the number of components of the model). To have more *syndromes* of acquired dyslexia than there are patients studied is probably not wise. The alternative, then, is to stop thinking in terms of syndromes (and the generalisability of results from one patient to another). Rather, we should regard the construction of general models as the primary aim of cognitive neuropsychology. The performance of an individual patient may thus constitute a counter-example to a particular theoretical model, even if the patient's pattern of performance is unique. Further remarks on the inadequacies of "syndrome thinking" can be found in Caramazza (1984), Coltheart (1984), Marshall (1982), and Schwartz (1984).

The "minimal model" of reading to which all (or most) of the contributions to this volume conform is shown in diagram form in Fig. 1 of the General Introduction. The chapters in the first section of this book address some of the disputed issues that the "minimal model" raises and they attempt to specify in more detail the structure and operation of the postulated routes and representations.

Bub, Cancelliere, and Kertesz accept that written words can be "translated directly into phonology, without prior access to semantic representation" and ask the question: "Which stimulus items are translated into sound as whole words, and which items are mediated by analytic, subword correspondences?" Newcombe and Marshall draw attention to the necessity for "graphemic parsing" of an input letter string if subword units are to be converted to sound. (This parser does not appear on our "minimal model" but is mentioned in the General Introduction to this book.) They present evidence that pathology can so reduce the "window size" of the graphemic parser that words are transcoded individual letter sound by individual letter sound. Saffran notes that the fully isolated operation of a grapheme–phoneme conversion route would transform most irregular words into neologistic output. Yet some subjects with "surface dyslexia" have a strong tendency to produce real words as output. Does this imply that a strict separation of lexical and non-lexical reading routes cannot be justified? Or can the standard model cope with such findings without extensive modification or *ad hoc* pleading?

REFERENCES

Alajouanine, Th., Lhermitte, F., & de Ribaucourt-Ducarne, B. I. (1960). Les alexies agnosiques et aphasiques. In Th. Alajouanine (ed.), *Les Grandes Activités du Lobe Occipital*. Paris: Masson.

Beauvois, M. F., & Derouesné, J. (1981). Lexical or orthographic agraphia. *Brain*, **104**, 21–49.

Caramazza, A. (1984). The logic of neuropsychological research and the problem of patient classification in aphasia. *Brain and Language*, **21**, 9–20.

Coltheart, M. (1978). Lexical access in simple reading tasks. In G. Underwood (ed.), *Strategies of Information Processing*. London: Academic Press.

Coltheart, M. (1982). The psycholinguistic analysis of acquired dyslexias: Some illustrations. *Philosophical Transactions of the Royal Society*, **B298**, 151–164.

Coltheart, M. (1984). Acquired dyslexias and normal reading. In R. N. Malatesha & H. A. Whitaker (eds.), *Dyslexia: A Global Issue*. The Hague: Martinus Nijhoff.

Coltheart, M., Besner, D., Jonasson, J. T., & Davelaar, E. (1979). Phonological encoding and the lexical decision task. *Quarterly Journal of Experimental Psychology*, **31**, 489–507.

Coltheart, M., Patterson, K., & Marshall, J. C. (eds.). (1980). *Deep Dyslexia*. London: Routledge and Kegan Paul.

Coltheart, M., Masterson, J., Byng, S., Prior, M., & Riddoch, J. (1983). Surface dyslexia. *Quarterly Journal of Experimental Psychology*, **35A**, 469–495.

De Agostini, M. (1977). A propos de l'agraphie des aphasiques sensoriels: Etude comparative italien-francais. *Langage*, **47**, 120–130.

Deloche, G., Andreewsky, E., & Desi, M. (1982). Surface dyslexia: A case report and some theoretical implications for reading models. *Brain and Language*, **15**, 12–31.

Dubois-Charlier, F. (1971). Approche neurolinguistique du problème de l'alexie pure. *Journal de Psychologie*, **68**, 39–67.

Elder, W. (1897). *Aphasia and the Cerebral Speech Mechanisms*. London: H. K. Lewis.

Hatfield, F., & Patterson, K. E. (1983). Phonological spelling. *Quarterly Journal of Experimental Psychology*, **35A**, 451–468.

Huey, E. B. (1908). *The Psychology and Pedagogy of Reading*. Cambridge, Massachusetts: MIT Press.

Kremin, H. (1980). Deux stratégies de lecture dissociables par la pathologie. *Grammatica*, **7**, 131–156.

Laberge, D. (1972). Beyond auditory coding. In J. F. Kavanagh & J. G. Mattingly (eds.), *Language by Eye and by Ear*. Cambridge, Massachusetts: MIT Press.

Lichtheim, L. (1885). On aphasia. *Brain*, 7, 433–484.

Luria, A. R. (1947). *Traumatic Aphasia*. The Hague: Mouton. (Translated 1970)

Luria, A. R. (1960). Differences between disturbances of speech and writing in Russian and in French. *International Journal of Slavic Linguistics and Poetics*, **3**, 13–22.

Lyman, R., Kwan, S., & Chao, W. (1938). Observations on alexia and agraphia in Chinese and in English. *Chinese Medical Journal*, **54**, 491–516.

McIlroy, M. D. (1977). Synthetic English speech by rule. *Computer Science Technical Report No. 14*. New Jersey: Bell Telephone Laboratories.

Marshall, J. C. (1982). What is a symptom-complex? In M. A. Arbib, D. Caplan, & J. C. Marshall (eds.), *Neural Models of Language Processes*. New York: Academic Press.

Marshall, J. C. (1984). Toward a rational taxonomy of acquired dyslexias. In R. N. Malatesha & H. A. Whitaker (eds.), *Dyslexia: A Global Issue*. The Hague: Martinus Nijhoff.

Marshall, J. C., & Newcombe, F. (1973). Patterns of paralexia: A psycholinguistic approach. *Journal of Psycholinguistic Research*, **2**, 175–199.

Marshall, J. C., & Newcombe, F. (1980). The conceptual status of deep dyslexia: An historical perspective. In M. Coltheart, K. Patterson, & J. C. Marshall (eds.), *Deep Dyslexia*. London: Routledge and Kegan Paul.

Newcombe, F. & Marshall, J. C. (1973). Stages in recovery from dyslexia following a left cerebral abscess. *Cortex*, **9**, 329–332.

Newcombe, F., & Marshall, J. C. (1981). On psycholinguistic classifications of the acquired dyslexias. *Bulletin of the Orton Society*, **31**, 29–46.

Newcombe, F., & Marshall, J. C. (1984). Task- and modality-specific aphasias. In F. C. Rose (ed.), *Progress in Apasiology*. New York: Raven Press.

Obler, L. (1984). Dyslexia in bilinguals. In R. N. Malatesha & H. A. Whitaker (eds.), *Dyslexia: A Global Issue*. The Hague: Martinus Nijhoff.

Patterson, K. E., & Kay, J. (1982). Letter-by-letter reading: Psychological descriptions of a neurological syndrome. *Quarterly Journal of Experimental Psychology*, **34A**, 411–442.

Rubenstein, H., Lewis, S. S., & Rubenstein, M. A. (1971). Evidence for phonemic recoding in visual word recognition. *Journal of Verbal Learning and Verbal Behavior*, **10**, 645–657.

Schwartz, M. F. (1984). What the classical aphasia categories can't do for us, and why. *Brain and Language*, **21**, 3–8.

Schwartz, M. F., Marin, O. S. M., & Saffran, E. (1979). Dissociations of language function in dementia: A case study. *Brain and Language*, **7**, 277–306.

Schwartz, M. F., Saffran, E., & Marin, O. S. M. (1980). Fractionating the reading process in dementia: Evidence for word-specific print-to-sound associations. In M. Coltheart, K. Patterson, & J. C. Marshall (eds.) *Deep Dyslexia*. London: Routledge and Kegan Paul.

Shallice, T., & Warrington, E. K. (1980). Single and multiple component central dyslexic syndromes. In M. Coltheart, K. Patterson, & J. C. Marshall (eds.), *Deep Dyslexia*. London: Routledge and Kegan Paul.

Shallice, T., Warrington, E. K., & McCarthy, R. (1983). Reading without semantics. *Quarterly Journal of Experimental Psychology*, **35A**, 111–138.

Störring, G. (1907). *Mental Pathology in its Relation to Normal Psychology*. London: Swan Sonnenschein.

Temple, C. M., & Marshall, J. C. (1983). A case study of developmental phonological dyslexia. *British Journal of Psychology*, **74**, 517–533.

Warrington, E. K. (1975). The selective impairment of semantic memory. *Quarterly Journal of Experimental Psychology*, **27**, 635–657.

Wernicke, C. (1885). Einige neurere Arbeiten über Aphasie. *Fortschritte der Medizin*, **3**, 824–837.

1 Whole-word and Analytic Translation of Spelling to Sound in a Non-semantic Reader

D. Bub, A. Cancelliere, A. Kertesz

Some recent models of written word processing have suggested that whole-word information can be translated directly into phonology, without prior access to semantic representation (e.g. Baron, 1977; Morton & Patterson, 1980). Consistent with this suggestion and with previous reports (Funnell, 1983; Schwartz, Saffran, & Marin, 1980), a patient, M.P., is described who has grossly impaired comprehension but is nevertheless clearly using lexical knowledge to pronounce written words. Evidence will be presented that strongly indicates that oral reading is not mediated by semantic access, so that written word pronunciation is based, at least in part, on direct lexical connections between orthographic and phonological representations.

In addition to providing support for a word-specific route from print to sound, the present chapter explores in detail the *extent* to which lexical knowledge is preserved in the patient. It will be shown that whole-word pronunciation is retrieved for only a certain percentage of items and that, on other occasions, M.P. relies on a more analytic mechanism that incorporates common correspondences between spelling segments and their phonology.

Partial failure of the lexical route is apparent when M.P. is asked to read words with an irregular spelling–sound correspondence. She can read some of these items correctly, indicating that word-specific information is accessed, but remaining responses are produced by using general principles of spelling–sound translation to assemble phonology. As a result, M.P. makes numerous regularisation errors. Her oral reading of regular words and of non-words, however, is extremely accurate relative to exception words over a wide range of different spelling patterns. Thus, M.P. clearly retains a sophisticated grasp of the relationships between orthography and pronunciation, which stands in marked contrast to her loss of whole-word specifications.

We assessed M.P.'s reading performance with a large number of exception and regular words to document the breakdown in her whole-word knowledge and the consequent reliance on a more stereotyped, rule-based approach to written word pronunciation. Her regularisation errors were also examined for clues about the mechanism used to pronounce those written words that are not mapped on to their correct lexical address. Finally, we tried to determine what aspect of whole-word specification has been lost for these items; some evidence suggests that M.P.'s functional impairment is localised at the level of phonological retrieval rather than at the level of orthographic representation for words. This possibility will be discussed after presenting a detailed account of M.P.'s ability to process written words along semantic, lexical, and phonological dimensions.

CLINICAL HISTORY

M.P., a 62-year-old right-handed female, was struck by a motor vehicle on 11 April 1979. Following emergency hospitalisation, she was found to have lost a large quantity of blood and to have sustained obvious trauma to the skull and scalp.

Two weeks after an operative procedure to relieve left temporal lobe herniation, M.P. underwent preliminary speech and language assessment. She remained drowsy and lethargic during testing. There was no answer to any form of questioning other than to echo the question or to respond, "This I ask, hurry up and let me low." Naming consisted of neologisms and perseveration. Speech was a mixture of semantic jargon, neologisms, and literal paraphasias. The examiner noted, however, that despite profound comprehension loss, oral reading of both words and sentences was executed rapidly and accurately.

COMPREHENSION

A series of comprehension tests was conducted approximately 3 years after M.P.'s accident. The results point to a major and persistent loss of comprehension for language, together with anomia, paraphasia, and jargon. Oral reading of words, nonsense words, and sentences, however, was remarkably intact, with rapid, fluent, and prosodically appropriate performance occurring in the absence of any understanding.

Peabody Picture Vocabulary Test (PPVT)

The written equivalent of the PPVT (Dunn, 1965) was administered to M.P. Testing was discontinued when M.P. made six errors over eight consecutive trials. The raw score obtained was 31, which is equivalent to an age level of 2.8 years. On the auditory version of the PPVT, the raw score was 21, equivalent to an age level of 2.0 years.

1. Word–Word Semantic Categorisation

Twenty-six trials were administered, each consisting of four words printed in uppercase letters. An additional word, semantically related to one of the four items, was presented alongside the array and was underlined (e.g. chair, apple, boy, hat, table). M.P. was asked to select one word from the four choices that was semantically similar to the test stimulus. The position of the critical word was randomised across trials.

In order to ensure that M.P. understood the nature of the task, 12 preliminary trials were constructed using pictures instead of words. She was requested to choose the item that was most similar to the test picture. Eleven out of twelve responses were correct for this task.[1] Immediately afterwards, the procedure was repeated, but with words instead of pictures. It was carefully reiterated that the word that was conceptually similar to the underlined word was the target item. M.P. scored 9 out of 26 correct responses, a level of accuracy expected by chance.

An analogous task was administered orally to M.P., involving 20 word-pairs, half of which were semantic associates (e.g. hand, foot). She was asked to judge whether items in each pair were semantically related or unrelated. Trials were presented in random order. Eleven out of 20 responses were correct, indicating chance performance.

2. Picture–Word Semantic Categorisation

M.P. was shown a black-and-white line drawing which was accompanied by four written words (e.g. tree (picture), *shoe, flower, pen, hand*). She was required to choose the word that was most similar conceptually to the picture, using the same instructional technique as before. Seven out of 20 responses were correct, a score expected on the basis of chance alone.

3. Card Sorting

Twenty-one semantic categories were selected and five exemplars from each were individually typed in uppercase lettering on white cards. M.P. was presented with 15 randomised stimuli on a given trial, chosen from three categories (e.g. food, vehicles, furniture) and was asked to place each card

---

[1] We do not feel that M.P.'s performance on this test constitutes good evidence that semantic access is possible for pictures but not words, because many of the pictures could have been matched on the basis of physical attributes alone. We used pictures primarily as an instructional device, to maximise the possibility that M.P. understood the basic requirements of the categorisation task, and we therefore took no measures to preclude the use of physical characteristics as a way of achieving a correct response.

under the appropriate heading. Category headings were printed in capital letters on white cards.

Forty-nine out of 105 items (49/105) were correctly classified, which is slightly greater than would be expected by chance alone ($\chi^2 = 7.8$, $P < 0.01$). The nature of the responses, however, suggested only a very minimal grasp of semantic relationships for a few written words. On no occasion were all the words correctly assigned to a particular category and misclassification of items was frequently noted under the same heading that produced three or four correct responses. Thus, M.P. correctly placed the words *August, March, June,* and *May* under the category heading *months,* but she also included the words *coffee, juice,* and *foot.* Similarly, *minute, hour, year,* and *month* were assigned to the heading *time,* but so were *pilot* and *nurse.*

It is conceivable that some misclassifications were due to failure to comprehend the meaning of the category heading rather than the inability to categorise the stimuli themselves. For example, M.P. may have incorrectly placed *square, triangle,* and *circle* under the category *furniture,* even if these words were perceived as being shapes, simply because the heading itself was not understood. In order to correct for this possible artefact, the *maximum* number of words from the same semantic class assigned to a given heading was counted correct, regardless of whether this was appropriate to the meaning of the actual category. Thus, if *pliers, drill,* and *hammer,* for example, were assigned to *body parts,* along with *neck,* then the number of correct responses was designated three instead of one. Using this procedure, a score of 56/105 was obtained, a level of accuracy which did not differ significantly from that occurring with the more rigorous scoring procedure ($\chi^2 = 1.6$, $P > 0.1$).

4. Reading Latency for Semantically Primed Words

The results of the previous tests indicate that semantic access is severely limited for both spoken and written words; before concluding that reading is not mediated via semantic access, however, we felt that one final search should be conducted for any possible contribution of meaning to M.P.'s reading, using a task that does not require *explicit* recognition of the relationship between words along a semantic dimension.

This additional evidence is necessary because forced choice tests may not always provide a complete measure of language competence in patients with impaired comprehension. For example, lack of attention, failure to understand the task or to perceive the relevant dimension connecting the test and related target item could all contribute to depressed performance which does not accurately reflect the extent of single-word comprehension. Furthermore, it may be the case that automatic components of semantic activation are still intact in certain aphasics (cf. Milberg & Blumstein, 1981) even though additional processing, which allows overt judgement of semantic category, is not available.

For these reasons, M.P. was administered a reading task that is highly sensitive to any influence of semantic association between words and that does not require overt judgement of meaning. This involved reading words which were preceded by semantically related items or by words that were not associated with the target stimuli. For normal subjects, naming is significantly faster by approximately 50 msec when words are preceded by a semantic associate compared to RT for target words preceded by semantically unrelated stimuli (Meyer, Schvaneveldt, & Ruddy, 1975). Moreover, this result is also obtained when patients with comprehension difficulty are required to perform lexical decisions (Milberg & Blumstein, 1981) in spite of the fact that these same patients show impairment in categorising words in a forced choice paradigm. If M.P. were to show similar effects of semantic priming, then the argument that oral reading occurs without access to semantic representation would clearly be invalid.

Thirty word-pairs were selected consisting of a stimulus and its primary associate, from standardised norms of word association. All words were concrete, high-imagery items. Stimuli were presented foveally for 500 msec, with a 1-second interval between trials. M.P. was required to read each word aloud when it appeared, as quickly and as accurately as possible. Thirty practice trials were administered, using words that did not appear in the experiment. Naming latency correct to the nearest millisecond was measured with a timer and voice-activated relay.

Two blocks of 60 trials were presented, consisting of 15 words followed by a semantically associated target item and 30 filler trials, comprising the remainder of the experimental stimuli in random order. Prime-associate pairs used in block 1 served as random filler trials in block 2, while the 30 filler trials in block 1 were regrouped for block 2 and comprised the prime-associate stimuli. In this way, it was possible to compare naming latency for primed target words with naming latency for the same items preceded by semantically unrelated stimuli. Mean naming latency is illustrated in Table 1.1. All of M.P.'s responses were correct.

It can be seen that no facilitation occurred for semantically primed words,[2] in spite of the fact that performance was well within the normal range

TABLE 1.1
Mean Naming Latencies and Standard Deviations for
Semantically Primed and Unprimed Words

Primed		Unprimed	
Mean (msec)	SD (msec)	Mean (msec)	SD (msec)
588	71	594	79

[2] The experiment was repeated using a slightly different technique—naming latency for primed items was compared with latency for a control list matched in terms of frequency and length. The results confirmed the absence of any priming effect.

SD-B*

of speed and accuracy. Difficulties in interpreting excessively slow or inaccurate responses, often encountered when speeded tasks are administered to brain-damaged patients, consequently do not apply in this instance. Taken together, the results of the semantic priming and forced choice tests of comprehension are clearcut—M.P. retrieves phonology for the majority of written words without accessing semantic representation.

LEXICAL PROCESSING

Having established that M.P.'s reading is not based on semantic processing, the status of her whole-word knowledge is now examined. Does M.P. retrieve word-specific information when she reads or does she mainly rely on general correspondences between spelling and sound?

In order to test for the presence of word-specific connections underlying her performance, two aspects of oral reading were considered. First, some evidence for lexically mediated pronunciation would be obtained if it were shown that M.P. retained an ability to read exception words, as it is generally assumed that phonology for these items cannot be correctly produced by translating spelling segments into sound.

We also used a second measure to determine whether M.P. had access to lexical representation, which involved naming latency for words that varied in frequency.

Studies with normal subjects indicate that high-frequency words are read faster than low-frequency words (Forster & Chambers, 1973; Frederiksen & Kroll, 1976). One interpretation of this is that word pronunciation is usually based on a search through lexical addresses with faster access to more common items. If M.P.'s oral reading is mediated by a similar process, then in addition to the evidence obtained from preserved accuracy for orthographically irregular words, reading latency for high-frequency (HF) words should be faster than reading latency for low-frequency (LF) words, confirming the presence of whole-word mapping from print to sound.

This possibility was tested by presenting M.P. with 160 single-syllable five-letter words, half of which were greater than 55 per million (HF words) in frequency (Kucera & Frances, 1967) and half of which (LF words) were less than 15 per million. In addition, 40 words in each frequency group were regular, while 40 were irregular, in their spelling–sound correspondence.

Stimuli were presented individually to M.P. for oral reading in two blocks of trials consisting of regular and exception words respectively, which were administered separately over a 48-hour period. We hoped in this way to avoid any potential encoding bias that may occur when two words with the same spelling pattern and different pronunciations (e.g. *home, come*) are presented in the same list (see Seidenberg, Waters, Barnes, & Tanenhaus, 1984). Each stimulus was displayed for 500 msec at fixation by means of a slide projector and electronically controlled shutter. An interval of approximately 2 sec occurred between items. Reading latency was measured for each response by means of a millisecond timer and voice-activated relay. Pronunciations were also tape-recorded and later transcribed for analysis. Prior to the experimental series, 20 practice trials were administered, during which M.P. was encouraged to respond as quickly and as accurately as possible. Mean latencies for *correct* responses and error scores are displayed below in Table 1.2.

TABLE 1.2
Naming Latency and Number of Errors for High-frequency (HF) and
Low-frequency (LF) Regular and Exception Words

		Latency		
		Mean *(msec)*	*SD* *(msec)*	*No. of* *errors*
Regular	HF	619	96	2
	LF	671	119	1
Exception	HF	627	99	3
	LF	651	183	11

M.P. is clearly able to pronounce a large number of exception words correctly, although her performance for regular words is considerably more accurate. Nevertheless, as reading of exception words is quite possible, it is apparent that M.P.'s pronunciation cannot be based on spelling–sound translation alone.

This conclusion is further supported by the marked influence of word frequency on naming latency; HF items were pronounced, on average, 52 msec more rapidly than LF items for regular words and 24 msec more rapidly for irregular words.[3] The results, therefore, strongly indicate that M.P. is able to pronounce written words by accessing lexical information, in spite of the fact that further processing at a semantic level does not occur.

ORTHOGRAPHIC AND LEXICAL PROCESSES IN READING

There is some evidence from the previous experiment to suggest that whole-word retrieval of phonology does not extend to all words. Whereas regular words were almost always correctly read, a substantial number of exception words were mispronounced as regularisations (see Table 1.3), particularly

---

[3] Word frequency had a smaller effect in naming latency for exception words because many of M.P.'s slower responses were also incorrect and were therefore not included in the analysis. If these latencies are averaged as well, the means for HF and LF words are 627 msec (SD = 99) and 690 msec (SD = 183) respectively.

TABLE 1.3
Incorrect Pronunciations for HF and LF Words.
Responses for Exception Words Are
Regularisation Errors

Stimulus	Type	Response
drink	HFR	/brɪŋk/
plane	HFR	/plæŋk/
crank	LFR	/kreɪn/
phase	HFE	/feɪzi/
laugh	HFE	/lɔg/
touch	HFE	/taʊtʃ/
steak	HFE	/stik/
vogue	LFE	/vɒgju/
ghoul	LFE	/gaʊl/
queue	LFE	/kjui/
gauge	LFE	/gɔdʒ/
suede	LFE	/su'wid/
suite	LFE	/sʊ'waɪt/
guile	LFE	/gʊ'waɪl/
cough	LFE	/kaʊg/
yacht	LFE	/jætʃt/
flood	LFE	/flud/

when LF items were presented. It should be emphasised that these LF words would be perfectly familiar to normal readers, as Table 1.3 illustrates.

This increase in errors for less common exception words points to a loss of lexical specification that is most severe at the lower end of the frequency spectrum, forcing M.P. to use an alternative procedure for oral reading. Given that her performance for regular words is near perfect, we infer that she relies on an intact grasp of the most typical correspondences between spelling and sound to assemble a response for items that cannot be pronounced via word-specific associations.

In the present section, we explore more fully the different processes responsible for M.P.'s oral reading. We have thus far described performance for short, single-syllable words that are orthographically fairly simple; does her understanding of general spelling–sound relationships hold true for more complicated orthographic patterns as well? We also wished to obtain a better description of the deterioration in M.P.'s word-specific reading for less familiar items; does the tendency to produce regularisations occur abruptly at a certain frequency level or is there a gradual failure in the extent of her whole-word knowledge as items become less familiar? We therefore administered a relatively large sample of exception words to her, which varied progressively across a range of frequency values. Finally, we were interested in examining the regularisation errors M.P. produces for different exception words in order to obtain some idea of the spelling units she identifies when converting letter sequences into sound. Do mispronunciations reflect the analysis of individual graphemes (Coltheart, 1978), for example, or are larger orthographic segments, such as word endings (Shallice, Warrington, & McCarthy, 1983), incorporated in M.P.'s responses?

Reading of Exception and Regular Words—A Closer Look

An extensive list of regular and exception words, which contained examples of many different spelling patterns, was compiled and administered to M.P. for oral reading. As a preliminary framework within which to classify stimuli and assess M.P.'s pronunciation, items were defined as regular or exceptional on the basis of Venezky's (1970) description of spelling–sound correlations, which categorises regularities at the level of individual graphemes. Stimuli included examples of: (1) letters (or letter clusters) with invariant assignment of phonemes, regardless of position or orthographic context (e.g. *tch* is always pronounced /tʃ/); (2) letters that require consideration of contextual information for correct pronunciation (e.g. *c* before *a, o, u* is pronounced /k/, otherwise /s/; and (3) pronunciations that are not predicted by (1) and (2). On average, 15 stimuli were selected from each of 60 predictable and unpredictable correspondences, resulting in approximately 900 words. These were presented individually and in random order to M.P. for oral reading over a period of 5 days. All responses were tape-recorded and later transcribed. An additional list of nonsense words, taken from Glushko (1979), was also administered to M.P. for oral reading; these consisted of 43 items generated by changing the initial consonant of a regular word and 43 items generated from an exception word by a similar procedure.

Pronunciation Accuracy

1. *Nonsense Words.* M.P. read correctly all 43 nonsense items obtained from regular words. She assigned an irregular pronunciation to 4 out of 43 of the stimuli derived from exception words (/wɒʃ/ for *wush*, /blɛd/ for *blead*, /wɒl/ for *wull*, and /grɒk/ for *grook*) and used regular spelling–sound correspondences for remaining responses.

2. *Words.* The percentage scores for individual orthographic patterns within regular and exception word categories are shown in Table 1.4. It can be seen that performance is markedly influenced by regularity, so that very accurate pronunciation occurred when words were presented that are definable by rules of print-to-sound translation. Because this was the case even for regularities that depend on contextual information, such as position (e.g. the influence of *ll* on the vowel varies for medial and terminal locations, cf. *fallacy* versus *fall*) and letter cues (*c* before *e, i,* and *y* is rendered as /s/,

TABLE 1.4
Percentage Accuracy Scores for Consonants and Vowels in Regular and
Exception Words

		Regular Words	
Letter	Examples	No. of words	% Correct
B as /b/	brake, ebb, ball	24	100
C as /k/	porcupine, talc, zinc	14	100
C as /s/	circuit, tacit, fallacy	14	93
CH as /tʃ/	chance, orchard, lunch	11	100
D as /d/	defect, respond, dagger	28	100
F as /f/	free, raft, flood	25	100
G as /g/	gold, dagger, magnificent	21	100
G as /dʒ/	region, virgin, vegetable	7	100
G silent	sign, gnome, benign	22	41
H as /h/	hard, exhale, harvest	14	100
J as /dʒ/	jest, junk, jar	8	100
K as /k/	king, kind, speak	9	100
K silent	knife, knee, knight	5	100
L as /l/	lump, wolf, bulk	16	100
L silent	chalk, calm, half	6	83
M as /m/	mark, mendicant, mandate	24	100
N as /n/	band, hand, churn	26	100
N silent	hymn, damn, solemn	3	67
P as /p/	plan, harp, lump	27	100
Ph as /f/	sphere, phone, phenomenon	10	100
R as /r/	rasp, term, train	23	100
S as /s/	mistake, scare, aspire	22	100
S as /z/	design, resign, resound	10	100
T as /t/	tow, table, tomato	25	100
T as /ʃ/	initial, patient, reaction	9	67
Th as /ө/	cloth, thumb, breath	10	100
V as /v/	cave, vigour, solve	14	100
W as /w/	swan, award, aware	21	100
X as /ks/	exactly, mixture, maximum	10	100
Y as /j/	voyage, year, canyon	9	100
Vwl + CV	pope, rude, induce	20	95
Vwl + Cns + L/R + Vwl	zebra, ladle, microbe	16	94
Vwl + funct. compound + Vwl	luxury, axe, chicken	15	100
Vwl + cluster of Cns's	annal, cabbage, gossip	11	100
Vwl + word final Cns or Cns unit	hard, cloth, run	17	100
Final E or Cns + E(LE, RE, STE)	paste, haste, mistake	27	100
Vwl + R + Vwl + Vwl or R + Vwl + junct.	cure, glory, wire	20	100
Vwl + R + Vwl + Cns or RR	borrow, arid, miracle	14	100
Vwl + R + Cns or juncture	carve, formula, spur	15	100
Vwl + final L, LL or medial L + Cns	call, bill, troll	10	90

Vwl + medial LL	fallacy, trolley, bullet	9	100
Vwl + final L + Cns	chalk, belt, yolk	11	100
Secondary vwl patterns (major)	bait, reign, teach	55	90
Total		707	$\bar{x} = 96\%$

Exception Words

Letter	Examples	No. of words	% Correct
B silent	debt, subtle, doubt	3	67
Ch as /k/	ache, school, character	8	44
Ch as /ʃ/	machine, chef, moustache	8	20
Ch silent	yacht	1	0
G as /ʒ/	garage, mirage, massage	7	14
H silent	honest, hour, vehicle	6	67
P silent	coup, receipt, corps	4	0
S silent	aisle, debris, island	4	0
S as /ʃ/	sugar, sure	3	100
T silent	buffet, debut, mortgage	4	25
Vwl + Cns + E	have, police, prestige	26	27
Vwl + R + Vwl	are, safari, very	5	100
Vwl + RR or R + CV	siren, urine, worry	6	50
Vwl + R + Cns	scarce, sergeant, attorney	3	33
Vwl + Cns cluster	kind, bold, child,	27	46
Vwl + cluster + GH	weigh, tough, cough	30	50
Secondary Vwl pattern (minor)	said, siege, head	79	60
Total		224	$\bar{x} = 41\%$

Correspondences are considered regular if they are invariant or if their alternate forms are predictable on the basis of contextual features (e.g. *k* before *n* is silent, word final *gn* becomes /n/, etc.). Vwl = vowel; Cns = consonant; CV = consonant–vowel cluster.

otherwise as /k/), M.P. clearly has the ability to use sophisticated generalities in retrieving phonology—pronunciation is not merely based on the mapping of individual letters to sound.

In contrast to the accurate performance obtained for regular words, M.P.'s reading of exception words is frequently incorrect, with the overwhelming majority of errors dictated by inappropriate but valid application of spelling–sound principles. Thus, minor correspondences are pronounced as major correspondences, unpredictable final *e* patterns are pronounced according to the rule of vowel lengthening, etc. Significantly, however, oral reading for exception words is only partially impaired, consistent with previous evidence indicating that specification is retained for a substantial proportion of items within the lexicon. In order to verify that whole-word identification deteriorates for *less common* words, we assessed the effect of word frequency on reading accuracy within the present corpus by dividing items into groups that varied incrementally from 25 or less per million to words greater than 400 per million. Results for both regular and exception stimuli are depicted in Fig. 1.1. Reading accuracy for exception words falls systematically as word frequency diminishes (although even at very low frequencies some capacity for correct pronunciation is retained), whereas scores remain consistently high for regular patterns. M.P. therefore experiences progressive difficulty in accessing word-specific phonology as items become less familiar, and depends more often on general correspondences between spelling and sound to assemble pronunciation.

Units of Spelling–Sound Translation

What is the nature of the orthographic information M.P. uses to read words that do not achieve lexical specification? Inspection of regularisation errors suggests that her analysis of letter clusters is not restricted to one type of spelling unit, but that different segments, varying in size and specificity, can mediate retrieval of phonology. Thus, certain errors provide strong

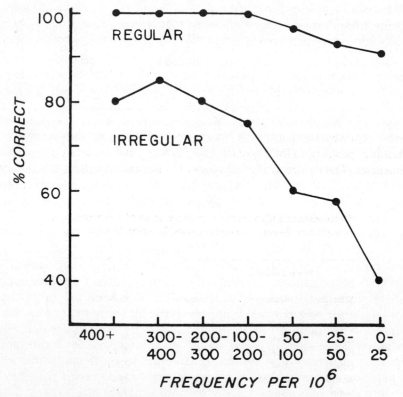

FIG. 1.1   Pronunciation accuracy for regular and exception words as a function of frequency. Spelling patterns tested are described in Table 1.4.

evidence that entire word endings are used to assemble a response; for example, the words *womb* and *tomb* are rendered as "wome" /woɷm/ and "tome" /toɷm/ (see Table 1.5), which can only be explained by assuming that M.P. has accessed the pronunciation incorporated in the word *comb* to synthesise a response.

Other regularisations, however, suggest an additional approach to oral reading that involves more analytic processing of relational units. Consider, for example, the response "milled" /mɪld/, which M.P. produces for the word *mild*. The stimulus itself is not irregular if the correspondence for the whole *ild* ending is taken into account, because the medial vowel for all words terminating with this segment is consistently rendered as /aɪld/ (i.e. *child, mild, wild*). At a more general level, however, the *ild* category can be considered exceptional, because other words ending in *l* plus a final consonant are usually assigned a short pronunciation (e.g. *hilt, milk, film*). M.P.'s regularisation of *child* in accordance with these quite general instances therefore implies the ability to assign phonemic values independently of a given lexical analogue, so that performance is mediated, at least on some occasions, by relatively abstract relationships between spelling and sound. (Patterson and Morton, in Chapter 14 of this book, put forward similar evidence from normal readers indicating that phonological assembly incorporates correspondences that are not determined by whole-word analogy.)

LEXICAL IMPAIRMENT—RECOGNITION OR RETRIEVAL?

Lexical representation is partially impaired in M.P., as indicated by the increasing proportion of regularisation errors that occur at lower word frequencies. The nature of the impairment is not entirely clear, but the most

TABLE 1.5

Regularisations Incorporating Pronunciation of Word Endings and More General Correspondence Between Spelling and Sound

Word Endings		General	
Stimulus	*Response*	*Stimulus*	*Response*
dough	/dʌf/	mind	/mɪnd/
cough	/kʌf/	blind	/blɪnd/
bomb	/boɷm/	kind	/kɪnd/
bough	/bɒf/	leather	/liðər/
womb	/woɷm/	fought	/faɒt/
tomb	/toɷm/	mild	/mɪld/
bead	/bɛd/	wild	/wɪld/

reasonable assumption is that for words pronounced via principles of spelling–sound correspondence, the lexical entries are completely lost. An alternative possibility must also be considered, however. Conceivably, M.P. encounters difficulties during *retrieval* of phonology when mispronunciations occur, so that even though lexical information is accessed, her responses incorporate processing segments that are smaller than those existing for whole words.

One way of checking on this account is to examine M.P.'s ability to make lexical decisions: if irregular words that are habitually mispronounced are still discriminated from non-words at better than chance accuracy, then clearly some form of lexical information is available to M.P. that is distinct from phonological specification. Preliminary testing, however, showed no ability to perform lexical decisions, even when the possibility of recognition was maximised by using high-frequency regular words. M.P.'s responses were invariably positive (i.e. "Yes, that's a word") for both words and nonsense items, despite repeated reminders from the examiner that half the stimuli were nonsense words.

M.P.'s failure on this task was initially surprising, given the evidence that lexical information was available to her in other tests. We noted, however, that judgements for words were executed rather rapidly, whereas she often puzzled over non-words and repeated them several times before responding. Perhaps, then, words were indeed recognised as lexical items, whereas responses for non-words were incorrect because M.P. failed to adopt an appropriate criterion for distinguishing positive from negative items. One possibility, given the nature of the error pattern, is that *orthographic* and *whole-word* familiarity were confused, leading to positive responding for all items with legal spelling patterns, regardless of their status as real words. A further test of M.P.'s ability was therefore devised, using a lexical discrimination task rather than a lexical decision paradigm. Four groups of 36 trials were generated, each trial consisting of a word and a nonsense word displayed horizontally in random order on a white card; such an arrangement, it was thought, might encourage M.P. to focus more selectively on lexical cues by providing an explicit contrast between this source of information and orthography.

Trials were formed in the following manner: 68 words were selected so that half were irregular items that M.P. consistently mispronounced on previous testing. The remaining 34 were regular words, closely balanced with the irregular words for frequency and length. Nonsense words were generated by changing the *first* letter of each word only, so that the orthographic pattern was preserved. This resulted in nonsense words with regular spelling patterns (e.g. *plock* formed from *block*) and nonsense words with irregular patterns (e.g. *macht* formed from *yacht*). Trials comprised regular words paired with regular nonsense words (e.g. RR—*brain, plock*), regular words and irregular nonsense words (RI—*king, macht*), irregular words and regular nonsense words (IR—*yacht, krade*), and irregular words and irregular nonsense words (II—*leopard, rubtle*). Stimuli were presented twice over a 3-week period, using different word–non-word pairings for each test session. M.P. was required to select the stimulus on every card that represented a real English word. On RR and II trials, orthographic cues are balanced between words and nonsense words as both are either regular or irregular, and M.P. may thus be forced to attend to lexical aspects of the stimuli rather than spelling structure. Assuming that internal representation of irregular words is more intact than would be expected on the basis of oral reading, performance on II (and RR) trials should be well above chance accuracy. On IR trials, however, a non-word with a very frequent configuration is opposed to a word with a highly infrequent pattern. If M.P. inappropriately attends to orthographic familiarity, as we assume, then the incorrect response for IR word–non-word combinations should often be selected and performance on these trials will consequently be very poor.

Results, displayed in Table 1.6, strongly support the assumption that M.P. retains some ability to discriminate lexical exemplars from non-words, even for irregular words that are mispronounced; performance was significantly better than chance for both RR ($\chi^2 = 9.6$, $P < 0.01$) and II ($\chi^2 = 15.6$, $P < 0.01$) items. In contrast, M.P. failed to choose correctly on the majority of IR trials (14/34 correct), consistent with the hypothesis that whole-word knowledge tends to be ignored when orthographically familiar non-words are juxtaposed with irregular words. Such an outcome, incidentally, rules out the possibility that M.P. accurately chooses words on II and RR trials simply because she recognises them as items encountered during previous testing. If non-words (which had never been presented to M.P. before) are frequently selected as positive items on IR trials, whereas words are most often selected in other conditions, processing is clearly sensitive to more abstract properties of the stimuli than short-term familiarity.

The evidence therefore suggests that at least some of M.P.'s regularisations involve defective retrieval of phonology, while the ability to recognise the target lexically remains intact. Her performance also implies, incidentally, that word–non-word discriminations need not require semantic access, because this kind of processing is severely limited for M.P., nor even the retrieval of lexical phonology, which she fails to obtain for exception words

TABLE 1.6
Percentage Correct for Lexical Discriminations

Condition	% Correct
RR (Regular word, Regular non-word)	76
RI (Regular word, Irregular non-word)	85
II (Irregular word, Irregular non-word)	82
IR (Irregular word, Regular non-word)	41

that are correctly identified in the discrimination task. M.P. is apparently able to base her decisions solely on *orthographic* descriptions of lexical items, even though information from other levels of representation (i.e. semantic and phonological) is unavailable.

We should emphasise, however, that M.P.'s accuracy, though better than chance, was far from perfect. Thus, it is not the case that she recognises all the items that she fails to pronounce as whole words. A reasonable conclusion, in view of the overall pattern of results, is that certain regularisations (perhaps those associated with low-frequency words) might well reflect global impairment to whole-word orthographic addresses, whereas other errors (conceivably produced by words of intermediate frequency) could take place subsequent to lexical access, at the level of whole-word pronunciation.

DISCUSSION

The severe comprehension deficit observed in M.P., as well as the absence of any priming effect for naming latency, indicate that reading is not based on semantic encoding. Nevertheless, it is clear that whole-word information still mediates oral reading: naming latency was strongly influenced by word frequency, suggesting that a lexically mediated process underlies performance. This supports the interpretation that M.P. processes many written words via direct visual access to a phonological lexicon independently of semantic representation, which is consistent with evidence put forward from a previous case report of lexical-non-semantic reading (Schwartz et al., 1980).

It is clear, however, that M.P. is not always able to retrieve lexical phonology from print; on some occasions pronunciation can only be assembled via general correspondences between spelling and sound. Results indicate, furthermore, that her capacity for whole-word reading strongly depends on familiarity—she is less likely to obtain word-specific phonology for lower-frequency items and the number of regularisation errors increases accordingly.

Some recent findings suggest that M.P.'s reliance on principles of spelling–sound translation to pronounce low-frequency words may in fact also be characteristic of normal performance under certain circumstances. Seidenberg, Waters, Barnes, and Tanenhaus (1984) have reported that subjects' oral reading of low-frequency exception words is slower relative to matched regular words, whereas latency for high-frequency words does not differ as a function of regularity. These authors conclude that very familiar written words are rapidly pronounced by direct lexical look-up, which results in equivalent reading latencies for both regular and exception items. Whole-word reading becomes inherently more difficult as word frequency decreases, however, and spelling–sound correspondences are used instead to generate candidate pronunciations. Latencies for exception words are consequently slower because their phonology cannot be specified on the basis of common spelling–sound relationships, and further processing is needed for a correct response.

In terms of this analysis, M.P.'s performance can be seen as an outcome of the way written word pronunciation occurs in the normal system. Her relatively preserved ability to read high-frequency exception words is consistent with a closer association between orthography and lexical phonology for these items, whereas regularisations point to the existence of an additional mechanism which can assemble pronunciation when word-specific mapping from print is unavailable.

We cannot determine, given the available evidence, whether such a mechanism utilises information stored independently of the lexicon or whether whole-word representation is always used to assemble pronunciation. The fact that M.P. does retain a partially intact lexicon certainly allows for the possibility that her grasp of print-to-sound translation relies entirely on correspondences retrieved from known words. Analysis of regularisation errors indicates, however, that spelling–sound conversion is not limited to segments obtained from words that share the same orthographic pattern as the target item. Some of M.P.'s mispronunciations could have been produced in this way but other errors occurred because smaller, more analytic units mediated oral reading. Although lexical entries may perhaps form the basis for responding, M.P.'s performance captures spelling–sound relationships that are not directly linked to specific whole-word exemplars.

ACKNOWLEDGEMENTS

We wish to thank Patrick Brown for assistance during initial stages of the research. The chapter was written while the first author held a Postdoctoral Fellowship from the Medical Research Council of Canada.

REFERENCES

Baron, J. (1977). Mechanisms for pronouncing printed words: Use and acquisition. In D. LaBerge and S. J. Samuels (eds.), *Basic Processes in Reading: Perception and Comprehension*. Hillsdale, NJ: Lawrence Erlbaum Associates Inc.

Coltheart, M. (1978). Lexical access in simple reading tasks. In G. Underwood (ed.), *Strategies of Information Processing*. New York: Academic Press.

Dunn, L. M. (1965). *Manual for the Peabody Picture Vocabulary Test*. Minnesota: American Guidance Service Inc.

Forster, K. I., & Chambers, S. M. (1973). Lexical access and naming time. *Journal of Verbal Learning and Verbal Behavior*, **12**, 627–635.

Frederiksen, J. R., & Kroll, J. F. (1976). Spelling and sound: Approaches to the internal lexicon. *Journal of Experimental Psychology: Human Perception and Performance*, **2**, 361–379.

Funnell, E. (1983). Phonological processes in reading: New evidence from acquired dyslexia. *British Journal of Psychology*, **74**, 159–180.

Glushko, R. J. (1979). The organization and activation of orthographic knowledge in reading aloud. *Journal of Experimental Psychology: Human Perception and Performance*, **5**, 674–691.

Kucera, H. & Francis, W. N. (1967). *Computational Analysis of Present-day American English*. Providence, RI: Brown University Press.

Meyer, D. E., Shvaneveldt, R. W., & Ruddy, M. G. (1975). Loci of contextual effects on visual word recognition. In P. M. A. Rabbitt & S. Dornic (eds.), *Attention and Performance 5*. New York: Academic Press.

Milberg, W. & Blumstein, S. E. (1981). Lexical decision and aphasia: Evidence for semantic processing. *Brain and Language*, **14**, 371–385.

Morton, J. & Patterson, K. (1980). A new attempt at an interpretation, or, an attempt at a new interpretation. In M. Coltheart, K. Patterson, & J. C. Marshall (eds.), *Deep Dyslexia*. London: Routledge & Kegan Paul.

Schwartz, M. F., Saffran, E. M., & Marin, O. S. M. (1980). Fractionating the reading process in dementia: Evidence for word-specific print-to-sound associations. In M. Coltheart, K. Patterson, & J. C. Marshall (eds.), *Deep Dyslexia*. London: Routledge & Kegan Paul.

Seidenberg, M. S., Waters, G. S., Barnes, M. A., & Tanenhaus, M. K. (1984). When does irregular spelling or pronunciation influence word recognition? *Journal of Verbal Learning and Verbal Behavior*, **23**, 383–404.

Shallice, T., Warrington, E. K., & McCarthy, R. (1983). Reading without semantics. *Quarterly Journal of Experimental Psychology*, **35**, 219–234.

Venezky, R. L. (1970). *The Structure of English Orthography*. The Hague: Mouton.

APPENDIX

Reading Errors

ache	/ætʃ, eɪtʃ/	brooch	/brutʃ/
acre	/'ækrə/	bruise	/bru'waɪz/
aisle	/'eɪzəl/	buffet	/'bʌfɪt/
align	/ə'lɪgən/	calm	/kæ'ləm/
allege	/æ'lidʒ/	camouflage	/kæmoʊ'fleɪg/
architect	/ɑr'tʃɪtɛkt/	champagne	/tʃæm'pægən/
assign	/ə'sɪgən/	chaos	/'tʃeɪɒs/
attorney	/ɑ'tɔrni/	character	/'tʃæræktə/
aye	/'eɪjə/	chauffeur	/tʃaʊ'fjur/
barrage	/'bærɪdʒ, bɑ'reɪdʒ/	chef	/tʃɛf/
bead	/bɛd/	chorus	/'tʃɔrəs/
bear	/bɪər/	circuit	/sər'kjuɪt/
benign	/bə'nɪgən/	clientele	/'klaɪəntil/
biscuit	/bɪs'kjuɪt/	collie	/kɒ'laɪ/
blind	/blɪnd/	corps	/kɔrps/
blood	/blud/	corsage	/'kɔrsɪdʒ/
bomb	/boʊm/	cougar	/koʊgər/
bough	/bɑf/	cough	/kʌf/
bought	/baʊt/	coup	/kaʊp/
bowl	/baʊl/	coyote	/'kɔɪoʊt/
broad	/broʊd/	debris	/'dɛbrəs/

debut	/di'bʌt/	parachute	/pærə'tjut/
design	/də'zɪgən/	paradigm	/pærə'dɪgəm/
dough	/dʌf/	pear	/pɪər/
drought	/draʰt/	pilot	/'pɪlət/
facade	/fæ'keɪd/	police	/poʊ'laɪs/
find	/fɪnd/	poll	/pɒl/
flood	/flud/	porpoise	/pɔr'pɔɪz/
foot	/fut/	pour	/paʊr/
fought	/faʊt/	prestige	/prɛs'tɪdʒ/
garage	/ga'reɪdʒ/	pursuit	/pər'sjuət/
gauge	/gɔdʒ, gə'judʒ/	ratio	/'rætɪoʊ/
ghoul	/gʰaʊl/	ravine	/ræ'vaɪn/
giraffe	/gə'ræf/	receipt	/rə'sipt/
gnaw	/'gənɔ/	regime	/rə'dʒaɪm/
gnome	/gə'noʊm/	resign	/rə'zɪgən/
grind	/grɪnd/	rhinoceros	/raɪnoʊkərɒs/
harem	/'heɪrəm/	rouge	/raʊdʒ/
have	/heɪv/	route	/'roʊtɪ/
heir	/hɛər/	routine	/ru'taɪn/
hicrarchy	/haɪr'ɑrtʃɪ/	sardine	/sɑr'daɪn/
hymn	/'hɪmən/	scheme	/stʃim/
initiate	/ɪ'nɪtɪeɪt/	sergeant	/sər'dʒɪnt/
island	/'ɪzlænd/	sieve	/siv/
isle	/'aɪzəl/	siren	/'sɪrən/
key	/keɪ/	sleight	/sleɪt/
kind	/kɪnd/	soot	/sut/
leather	/liðər/	spatial	/'spætɪəl/
leisure	/'liʒər/	steak	/stik/
lose	/loʊz/	subtle	/'sʌbtɪl/
malign	/mə'lɪgən/	suit	/suət/
marine	/mə'raɪn/	suitor	/'suətər/
massage	/'mæsɪdʒ/	taught	/tæft/
mechanic	/mə'tʃænɪk/	thought	/θaʊt/
mild	/mɪld/	tomb	/toʊm/
mind	/mɪnd/	tortoise	/tɔr'tɔɪz/
mirage	/'mərɪdʒ/	touch	/taʊtʃ/
morale	/mɒ'reɪl/	tow	/taʊ/
mortgage	/mɔrt'geɪdʒ/	treachery	/'tritʃərɪ/
moustache	/'mʌstæk/	urine	/ju'raɪn/
move	/moʊv/	vehicle	/vɛ'hɪkəl/
nought	/naʊt/	were	/wʰɛr/
nuisance	/'njuəsæns/	whose	/hoʊs/
orchestra	/ɔr'tʃɛstrə/	wild	/wɪld/
orchid	/ɔr'tʃɪd/	womb	/woʊm/
ought	/aʊt/	wrought	/raʊt/
own	/aʊn/	yacht	/'jætʃɪt/

Nonsense Word Reading

Regular Pseudowords		Exception Pseudowords	
beed	/bid/	bild	/bɪld/
beld	/bɛld/	bint	/bɪnt/
bink	/bɪŋk/	blead	/blɛd/
bleam	/blim/	bood	/bud/
bort	/bɔrt/	bost	/bɒst/
brobe	/broʊb/	brove	/broʊv/
cath	/kæθ/	cose	/koʊz/
cobe	/koʊb/	coth	/kɒθ/
dold	/doʊld/	dere	/dɪər/
doon	/dun/	domb	/dɒm/
dore	/dɔr/	doot	/dut/
dreed	/drid/	drood	/drud/
feal	/fil/	fead	/fid/
gode	/goʊd/	gome	/goʊm/
grool	/grul/	grook	/grʊk/
hean	/hin/	haid	/heɪd/
heef	/hif/	heaf	/hif/
hode	/hoʊd/	heen	/hin/
hoil	/hɔɪl/	hove	/hoʊv/
lail	/leɪl/	lome	/loʊm/
lole	/loʊl/	lool	/lul/
meak	/mik/	mear	/mɪər/
moop	/mup/	mone	/moʊn/
mune	/mjun/	moof	/muf/
nust	/nʌst/	nush	/nʌʃ/
peet	/pit/	pild	/pɪld/
pilt	/pɪlt/	plove	/ploʊv/
plore	/plɔr/	pomb	/pɒmb/
pode	/poʊd/	poot	/put/
pold	/poʊld/	pove	/poʊv/
prain	/preɪn/	praid	/preɪd/
sheed	/ʃid/	shead	/ʃɪd/
soad	/soʊd/	sood	/sud/
speet	/spit/	sost	/sɒst/
steet	/stit/	speat	/spit/
suff	/sʌf/	steat	/stit/
sust	/sʌst/	sull	/sʌl/
sweal	/swil/	sweak	/swik/
taze	/teɪz/	tave	/teɪv/
weat	/wit/	wead	/wid/
wosh	/wɒʃ/	wone	/woʊn/
wote	/woʊt/	wull	/wʊl/
wuff	/wʌf/	wush	/wʊʃ/

2 Reading and Writing by Letter Sounds

F. Newcombe and J. C. Marshall

INTRODUCTION

In *any* model that countenances the existence of a non-lexical route underlying reading aloud, that route must consist of (at least) four distinct components: In the first place, the representations derived by visual analysis must be assigned "abstract letter identities"; second, the string of individual letters so constructed must be explicitly parsed into graphemic constituents; third, sight–sound correspondence rules must assign a phonological representation to each element of the parsed letter string; finally, the sequence of phonological elements so assigned must be "blended" (by phonetic rules) into fully specified phonetic segments (in syllables) that can trigger motor commands to the speech musculature.

Current arguments about the nature of the non-lexical route are concerned with the precise form of functioning involved, with particular regard to stages two and three; the overall functional architecture of the indirect route is not in question, except, of course, by those scholars who deny that there is such a route (Glushko, 1979, 1981; Henderson, 1982; Marcel, 1980). For the present discussion of non-lexical reading we shall adopt the following terminology: A letter is a single orthographic unit, irrespective of case, typeface, or individual variation in handwriting; the Greek alphabet thus comprises 24 letters, the English alphabet 26. By contrast, a grapheme consists of *one or more* letters such that the sequence (letter string ⩾ 1 letter) is normally pronounced as *one* phoneme. Thus, in *break*, the final *k* is a single grapheme, and the medial digraph *ea* is also a single grapheme (Coltheart, 1978). This use of the term "grapheme" corresponds with Venezky's (1970) term "functional spelling unit." It is an empirical issue whether the sight–sound correspondences involved in non-lexical reading are represented as grapheme–phoneme correspondences (under the foregoing definition). Coltheart, Masterson, Byng, Prior, and Riddoch (1983) have argued, with supporting evidence from acquired and developmental surface dyslexia, that it is psychologically correct to characterise the indirect route in this fashion. Their position implies that, *prior* to the assignment of correspondences, the input letter string must be parsed into the appropriate graphemes or functional spelling units (Coltheart, 1978). Thus the five letters of *sheep* should be parsed into the three graphemes (sh) + (ee) + (p) that constitute the correct input to the system of correspondence rules. And the five letters of *yacht* should be parsed as (y) + (a) + (ch) + (t). Thus the non-lexical route would yield the pronunciation /jætʃt/. The *correct* pronunciation, of course, contains only three phonemes, and this discrepancy between the number of graphemes in *yacht* and the number of phonemes illustrates the irregularity of the word's spelling–sound correspondence.

In contrast, Shallice, Warrington, and McCarthy (1983) have proposed a "multi-level system in which word-form units of a number of different sizes can be translated into a phonological form." It follows on their account that the non-lexical route must parse input strings into chunks of variable length, with all the attendant problems of control that such systems bring with them. (See Shallice and McCarthy, Chapter 15 in this book, for proposed solutions to some of these problems.) These "graphemic chunks" will often be larger than a grapheme; thus *ain* (as in *plain* or *rain*) could, on this account, be associated with a stored pronunciation. The final segmentation of *plain* that is input to the correspondence rules may, according to the model of Shallice et al., contain no explicit representations of graphemes; in other words, the parse could produce the bracketing (*pl*) + (*ain*). The problem, however, with multi-unit mechanisms is to specify how the system "knows" which units are appropriate to the word at hand. If *a* and *i* are translated as letters the system will generate /æ/ + /ɪ/; if additionally the digraph *ai* is translated, the system will also have available the (regular) pronunciation /eɪ/ . . . to say nothing of the divergent pronunciations /aɪ/, /æ/, /ɛ/, and /i/. How could such a system "choose" a "best bet" translation?

One solution to the control problem would be to segment input strings on an initially left-to-right basis but allow successive letters to over-rule earlier parses (and hence change the sight–sound correspondences that earlier parses regularly imply). As a (very) simple example, consider how the correct vowel pronunciation in *book* might be achieved by such a system:

1. $b \rightarrow [/b/]$.
2. $bo \rightarrow [/b/ + (o) \rightarrow /ɒ/]$.
3. $boo \rightarrow [/b/ + (oo) \rightarrow /u/]$.
4. $book \rightarrow [/b/ + (ook) \rightarrow /ʊk/]$.

A similar mechanism was proposed by Marcel (1980), although in the context of a model in which successive segmentations were derived lexically, that is, from look-up of words that contained the letter strings in question. It is not, however, essential to the proposal that the device should run lexically; if the mechanism works at all it should work equally well as an expanded set of grapheme–phoneme correspondence rules. A related notion was first put forward by Holmes (1973), who argued that failure to apply such context-sensitive grapheme–phoneme correspondences was a characteristic feature of reading performance in some cases of acquired and developmental dyslexia. Whatever the eventual outcome of such arguments, it is clear that graphemic parsing must play a critical role in any analysis of the non-lexical route (Coltheart, 1978).

We might expect, then, that different kinds of parsing deficit will underlie many of the superficially distinct forms of dyslexia. In particular, one might conjecture that brain damage could reduce the "window" of the scanning mechanism to one character. And indeed the first patients to be studied under the rubric "surface dyslexia" (J.C. and S.T.) were interpreted as frequently translating from orthography to sound on a letter-to-letter basis (Holmes, 1973, 1978; Marshall & Newcombe, 1973, 1977) in the sense that subsequent context did not override, say, the assignment of short i ($/\iota/$) to words that, consequent upon a following consonant $+ e$, required long i ($/a\iota/$), as in *fine*. Although the response patterns of J.C. and S.T. were somewhat too complex to be described *solely* in these terms, the generalisation does capture one important aspect of their performance. More germane to the present study is the paper by Derouesné and Beauvois (1979). They discussed four patients with a severe defect of the non-lexical route (phonological dyslexia) and conclude that some of these cases were worse at reading non-words that contained 2:1 correspondences of letters to phonemes (e.g. *au* in *cau*) than non-words with solely 1:1 correspondences (e.g. *iko*). Further details of the parsing problem in phonological dyslexia can be found in Chapter 16 in this book. One should be able to throw more light upon the graphemic parser and its possible malfunctions by documenting cases in which the *majority* of errors can be explained by postulating that window size has very often been reduced to one (letter) character. It is to this end that we present the following case. Since proliferation of terminology has apparently become the *sine qua non* of studies of the acquired dyslexias, we shall call the pattern of performance "letter-sound reading"; it could equally well be termed "letter-by-letter reading", except that the latter term has been preempted for those patients who read solely by the assignment of letter names (Patterson & Kay, 1982). Letter names, in English, often consist of two phonemes; our case assigns *one* phoneme to each letter of the input word, and hence the condition could also be called "phoneme-by-phoneme" reading.

CASE REPORT

M.S. was born on 12 March 1960. His medical history was uneventful until he sustained a severe closed head injury in a road traffic accident on 21 October 1978. On admission to hospital he was deeply unconscious with a very slugglish response to painful stimuli. Four days after the injury he was fully conscious but confused and talking irrelevantly. A month after the accident, his behaviour was so violent as to require intramuscular sedation; the consultant psychiatrist who saw him gave as his opinion that M.S. had organic brain damage with "catastrophic reaction" and poor memory. On 22 November, M.S. was transferred to a psychiatric hospital where he was noted to be disorientated in time and place. He was finally discharged from hospital on 12 January 1979, and spent several months in a day centre where he was reported to have had "special tuition in reading." A year later, the consultant psychiatrist reported that M.S. had very poor memory and considerable difficulty with writing and spelling, although he performed simple arithmetic tasks reasonably well. The first psychological examination was carried out by a senior clinical psychologist on 1 June 1979. Intellectual functions were judged to be "close to normal limits"; the principal difficulty was with reading, although some word-finding deficits and generalised memory impairment were also found. M.S. was "usually able to identify individual letters, but was able only to read words after he had identified each constituent letter in turn."

M.S. was first examined by one of us (F.N.) in May 1981, and subsequently in June and November 1981, for the purpose of a medico-legal assessment. Further studies were then carried out in 1982 and 1983 to describe more precisely the nature of his reading and writing problems.

NEUROPSYCHOLOGICAL PROFILE

Throughout these and subsequent psychological examinations, M.S. was fully cooperative. The salient feature was a striking discrepancy between severely impaired performance on long-term memory and some language tasks, and normal scores on other tests of skill and ability that do not rely heavily on these functions. For example, he obtained an IQ in the normal range on the performance scale of a well-standardised test of general ability (Wechsler Adult Intelligence Scale) and on another reliable test of non-verbal general intelligence (Progressive Matrices). His understanding of spoken language was unimpaired: on the Token Test, M.S. performed quickly and accurately, making only two errors on the final section. He was given a test for grammatical comprehension (TROG), devised by Dr Dorothy Bishop, in which each of 80 spoken sentences was to be matched to one of four pictures

(Bishop, 1982). The elements tested include active/passive, affirmative/
negative, singular/plural, comprehension of embedded relative clauses, prep-
ositions, and comparatives. M.S. made no errors. Against that pattern of
performance, the evidence of gross deficits on reading, writing, and memory
tasks is the more striking.

He showed a severe impairment of long-term memory, for both verbal and
non-verbal material. His recall of short paragraphs, read to him by the
examiner, was meagre; and he was unable to reproduce any of the content of
these paragraphs 1 hour later, without forewarning. Similarly, his performance on a task requiring him to recognise unfamiliar faces (presented once
and then included in a collection of new faces) was well below the normal
range for men of his age. There was further evidence of impaired non-verbal
memory on a task using a different material: very poor delayed recall of a
geometrical figure that he had had ample time to copy three-quarters of an
hour before the delayed memory test.

The significantly low verbal IQ (79), compared with a performance IQ (90)
within the normal range, reflected memory deficits that resulted in low scores
on tests of span (ability to repeat a list of numbers), vocabulary, and general
knowledge (or "factual memory").

There was additional evidence of gross memory impairment from his
difficulty with a face–name learning task that has proved particularly
sensitive to the learning difficulties shown by young subjects with closed head
injury (Oddy, 1979). Even more striking was his inability to recognize any of
27 photographs of famous personalities. His errors included Prince Philip
identified as Presidents Carter or Reagan, James Hunt as Barry Sheen, and
Princess Margaret as the Queen. It is interesting that the faces were identified
as personalities within the same professional sphere: a finding reminiscent of
the semantic errors of aphasic patients (especially in spontaneous speech and
object naming) and also of the "category effect" found in normal face
recognition (Bruce, 1979).

Although the reading and writing of four-digit numerals were performed
without error, word reading and spelling were grossly impaired and there is
no reason to assume that this severe deficit preceded the accident. In fact, the
few documents available—including a school book—show that his pre-
traumatic performance was well within normal limits.

His attempts to read and spell were not haphazard and, accordingly, did
not suggest lack of cooperation or attention. On the contrary, they were
patently rule-bound to the extent that it was possible to predict the errors
that he made. He was able to follow only very simple rules for converting
print to sound (reading) or sound to print (writing to dictation). Using this
strategy, he was able to read and write to dictation some simple, orthographically regular words (e.g. *pig, hat, wed*). Irregular words presented an almost
insuperable problem (*whom* pronounced as /wə/-/hɒm/; *shoe* pronounced as

/sə/-/hɒ/-/i/; *fight* pronounced as /fɪg/-/hʌt/). In addition, he very frequently confused *b* and *d* (*did* pronounced as "bib"; *dug* pronounced as "bug"), and often gave both readings in successive attempts (*broad*→/broɷ-æd ... droɷ-æd/).

M.S. has a permanent reduction of vision. Careful testing, by Dr Graham Ratcliff, using a Harms perimeter, showed "a dense right homonymous hemianopia with macular sparing." Colour vision, as measured by the Farnsworth–Munsell 100-Hue Test, was unimpaired. He made only four minor errors, reversing the order of two of the pairs, in the total sample of 48 stimuli.

A summary of the psychological tests results is given in Table 2.1.

NEUROLOGICAL STATUS

A neurological examination, conducted by a consultant neurosurgeon in February 1981, found no abnormality in the cranial nerves with the exception of a visual field defect. Nevertheless, visual acuity, as measured by naming letters in fine print, was unimpaired (J1) in both the left and right eye; fundi were normal. There was no unsteadiness of gaze; pupils were large but reacted equally to light. He could hear a whisper in either ear at a distance of 1 metre. Examination of the limbs showed normal power in the upper limbs, but some spasticity in the lower limbs. The plantar responses were flexor. Coordination was virtually normal in the upper limbs, except for a tremor on drawing, and was poor in the right lower limb, being a little better in the left.

A CT scan, carried out on 6 January 1981, showed "slight but generalized dilation of the left lateral ventricle affecting in particular the left trigonal region and the left temporal horn. In addition, the right temporal horn is slightly dilated. The sulci are slightly more prominent on the left than on the right in particular in the posterior part of the Sylvian fissure." It was concluded that there was "slight generalized atrophy of the whole left hemisphere, in particular the left temporo-parietal region, and of the right temporal region."

CHARACTERISTICS OF READING AND WRITING

M.S. was asked to read, write to dictation, and spell orally 100 words from the Stanovich and Bauer (1978) list. This contains two sets of 50 words, distinguished in terms of their "regularity," in relation to the most common grapheme–phoneme correspondences in the language. (Thus *dint, hint, lint, mint,* and *tint* are regular, *pint* irregular.) The two sets are matched for letter length and word frequency. As a check on the reliability of the findings, the

TABLE 2.1
Psychological Test Results

Standard Cognitive Tests

Progressive matrices: Score 52/60 IQ equiv > 117
WAIS: Verbal IQ = 79, Performance IQ = 90

	Raw Score	Scaled Score
Information	4	4
Arithmetic	7	7
Similarities	13	10
Digit span	5 + 3	6
Vocabulary	17	3
Digit symbol	39	7
Picture completion	12	9
Block design	37	11
Picture arrangement	20	9
Object assembly	22	7

Language Tasks

Token comprehension test	64/66 correct
Bishop's comprehension test (TROG)	80/80 correct
Reading	Schonell's RA = 5.5 yrs
Spelling	Schonell's SA = 6.5 yrs
Oldfield–Wingfield Object Naming	22/36 correct
Picture description	Normal

Memory Tasks

Story recall	Immediate 7:8 7:8
(Wechsler Memory Scale I)	Delayed (1 hour) 0:0
Rey Osterrieth	Copy = 34/36 (normal)
	"Strategy" score = 13/36 (impaired)
	Delayed recall score = 12.5/36 (impaired)
Memory for faces	35/60
(unfamiliar faces, recurring	(> 2 SD below mean)
format)	
Face naming	0/27
(photographs of famous	
personalities)	
Face–name learning task	8/40
	(> 2 SD below mean)

---

same tests were carried out after a 5-month interval. M.S. performed very poorly. On first presentation he read correctly twelve of the regular and only three of the irregular words; on re-testing 5 months later, he read six regular words and one irregular. The words read correctly on testing sessions 1 and 2 are shown in Table 2.2. It will be seen that the words read correctly on second presentation are a proper subset of those read correctly on first presentation.

TABLE 2.2
Reading Aloud

Regular	(1)	(2)	Irregular	(1)	(2)
snob	√	√	police	√	√
alarm	√	√	doll	√	×
open	√	√	dollar	√	×
soft	√	√			
hand	√	√			
blast	√	√			
motor	√	×			
honey	√	×			
fancy	√	×			
grow	√	×			
hunter	√	×			
fuse	√	×			

The same set of words was presented for writing to dictation. On first testing, M.S. wrote seven regular and one irregular word correctly; on second testing, 5 months later, he correctly wrote six regular and two irregular words. The specific words written correctly are shown in Table 2.3. (Although one may dispute the "regularity" of a few of the words so classified by Stanovich and Bauer, the overall pattern is clear.)

Oral reading errors show a strong tendency to assign a phonetic value to each letter of the stimulus item. (Some examples are given in Table 2.4.) Thus *ph* is not assigned the value /f/; rather each letter of the digraph is given a separate phonological representation (*ph*→/pə/ . . . /hə/).

Errors in writing to dictation tended to preserve, in simplified orthography, the phonetic shape of the stimulus; letter names are sometimes used, as in *kos*. Examples are shown in Table 2.5. To the extent that M.S. consistently simplifies the orthography when writing to dictation, it should follow that he

TABLE 2.3
Writing to Dictation

Regular	(1)	(2)	Irregular	(1)	(2)
snob	√	√	pint	√	√
soft	√	√	police	×	√
hand	√	√			
host	√	√			
blast	√	√			
along	√	×			
alarm	√	×			
charm	×	√			

TABLE 2.4
Errors in Oral Reading

phrase→/pə'hə'ræsi/	*treat*→/tə'ri'æt/
touch→/tɒ'kə'hə/	*suit*→/su'ɪt/
whom→/wə'hɒm/	*cheap* /kə'hə'æp/
aisle→/æ'ɪ'sli/	*fight*→/fɪg'hʌt/
guess→/gə'ɛs/	*thumb*→/tə'hʌm'bə/
match→/mæt'kə'hə/	*chasm*→/sə'hæs'ɛm/
float→/flɒ'æt/	*advice*→/æd'vɪκi/

will be more successful at reading his own writing errors correctly than he is at reading their conventional forms (where "correctly" means that M.S. recovers the original word). It should furthermore follow that the original regularity effect should disappear. M.S. was accordingly asked to read back his own written responses (right and wrong) to the two previous presentations of the dictation task (Stanovich & Bauer, 1978). Both predictions were confirmed. On first testing, M.S. read correctly 25/50 originally regular words (including 7 that he spelled correctly), and 22/50 originally irregular words (including one that he spelled correctly); on second testing, he read correctly 23/50 originally regular words (including 5 that he spelled correctly), and 20/50 originally irregular words (including 1 that he spelled correctly). The correctly read words are given in Tables 2.6 and 2.7.

Tables 2.8–2.11 compare his ability to read the target words written in conventional orthography (regular and irregular) and his own orthography (where on writing to dictation his orthography differs from the norm). That the numbers in each table do not add up to 50 reflects the fact that M.S. occasionally produced the correct spelling of the words dictated to him (see Tables 2.6 and 2.7).

It will be seen that, overall, when a word is conventionally regular, M.S. is still four times as likely to read correctly his own misspelling; when a word is conventionally irregular, M.S. is thirteen times more likely to read correctly his own misspelling. For a letter sound-by-letter sound reader, regular vowel digraphs, regular consonant clusters, and "rule of *e*" are irregular. In other words, regularity is in the route of the reader.

TABLE 2.5
Errors in Writing to Dictation

"whom"→*hum*	"wheel"→*wel*
"guess"→*ges*	"chaos"→*kos*
"shoe"→*shu*	"thumb"→*fum*
"hour"→*owa*	"cliché"→*klesha*

TABLE 2.6
Reading Own Spellings (1)

Regular	Irregular
along→along	pint→pint
snob→snob	POLECE→police
alarm→alarm	FRAZ→phrase
soft→soft	KAFA→cafe
hand→hand	ONIST→honest
host→host	BER→bear
blast→blast	WUMUN→woman
KLIK→click	GES→guess
WIP→whip	BIZE→busy
OPUN→open	LIKA→liquor
PLAT→plate	DOL→doll
FLOT→float	IUN→iron
FANSE→fancy	DOLA→dollar
HOLDA→holder	GON→gone
TRET→treat	WURD→word
TON→tone	WONT→want
WEL→wheel	NOB→knob
MOTA→motor	FUM→thumb
HUNE→honey	BLUD→blood
ALIK→alike	FLUD→flood
KLASIS→classes	METUL→metal
SUK→suck	SO→sow
GRO→grow	
HUNTA→hunter	
ALON→alone	

LEXICAL DECISION

By the same token, it can safely be predicted that M.S. will make many errors in lexical decision tasks. Ignorance of the "rule of *e*," for example, will result in a large number of false negatives; in fact, the expectation must be that M.S.'s bias will be to reject words rather than accept non-words. That was precisely the pattern of his response on two lexical decision tasks. First, M.S. was asked to sort a randomised deck of 43 regular words and 43 regular pseudowords taken from Glushko (1979, Table A1). Each stimulus word was typed on a separate card and no time pressure was exerted. As can be seen from Table 2.12, the salient feature was his rejection of words. The second set of material (Masterson, 1983) comprised 160 stimuli. The core stimuli were 20 three-letter words and 20 three-letter non-words. Additional sets were generated by adding terminal *e* and/or *s*. Thus the stimuli included:

TABLE 2.7
Reading Own Spellings (2)

Regular	Irregular
snob→snob	police→police
soft→soft	KAFE→cafe
hand→hand	ONIST→honest
host→host	BER→bear
blast→blast	WUMUN→woman
ULONG→along	GES→guess
KLIK→click	BIZE→busy
WIP→whip	KARM→calm
ULARM→alarm	DOL→doll
OPUN→open	IUN→iron
FING→thing	DOLU→dollar
KAP→cape	GON→gone
FLOWT→float	NOR→gnaw
FANSE→fancy	WURD→word
GOZ→goes	WONT→want
HOLDU→holder	NOB→knob
MOTU→motor	ONU→honour
HUNE→honey	BLUD→blood
LIKWID→liquid	FLUD→flood
SUK→suck	METUL→metal
GRO→grow	
HUNTU→hunter	
SUMIT→summit	

TABLE 2.8

Regular (1)	Own (1)	No. of Responses
√	√	6
√	×	1
×	×	24
×	√	12

TABLE 2.9

Irregular (1)	Own (1)	No. of Responses
√	√	3
√	×	0
×	×	28
×	√	18

TABLE 2.10

Regular (2)	Own (2)	No. of Responses
√	√	2
√	×	0
×	×	27
×	√	16

TABLE 2.11

Irregular (2)	Own (2)	No. of Responses
√	√	0
√	×	0
×	×	30
×	√	19

TABLE 2.12
Correct Lexical Decision

Lists	Words	Non-words
Glushko (1979)	23.3%	88.4%
Masterson (1983)	31.3%	90.9%

wag	wags	wage	wages
nag	nags	nage	nages
pag	pags	page	pages
vag	vags	vage	vages

Again M.S. rejected a substantial proportion of real words (including *way, ton, huge, tar, sons, car,* and *tins*). In contrast, few non-words were wrongly classified (see Table 2.12).

COMPREHENSION OF THE WRITTEN WORD

M.S. does not comprehend the written word directly, with the exception of a small sight vocabulary of high-frequency and salient (for him) words; these include *police, pint, beer,* and a number of terms associated with rock music (e.g. *metal, fuse,* and *purple*). M.S. was given 60 written words from

Coltheart's homophone matching task, and asked to define them without previously letter naming or reading them aloud (see Coltheart et al., 1983). He succeeded with only seven. For 47 of the stimuli he was unable to suggest a definition. On one occasion only did he define a homophone as its mate (*nun*→"I ain't got none"); and once he gave both interpretations (*sum*→"that's sum ... maths ... or when you goes to shop and says 'I want some fags' ... two things for the one thing, we're doing pretty well"). The other four responses were *ale*→"kind of a path"; *paste*→he mimed kneading dough; *bare*→"it's an island ... Barry Island"; *sale*→"name of a woman, I used to fancy her, Sally." M.S. was also shown 26 homophone pairs from this list (e.g. *piece–peace; nose–knows*) and asked to point to the stimulus that matched our verbal definition (e.g. "the opposite of war," "the part of your face you smell with"). His performance was at chance (26/52 correct). Coltheart's synonym judgement task (high-imageability pairs) was given in shortened form. On this task, he was asked to judge whether pairs of words (e.g. *ocean–sea; joy–bag*) were or were not closely related in meaning. M.S. performed very poorly to written presentation (3/12 correct) though he was usually able to respond to oral presentation (11/12 correct).

As a final example of surface interpretation of the written word, we may consider the following description of how M.S. says he would use, in a sentence, a word he was attempting to read: "If you came up to me and said 'I'm going to get your head kicked in,' then I'd say '*Oh, ah* ... and who's going to do it?'" The written stimulus was, of course, *oar*.

CONCLUSIONS

M.S. manifests a particularly pure form of extra-lexical reading. Despite an adequate aural vocabulary his sight vocabulary is extremely limited. To all intents and purposes (save recognition of some titles on record sleeves) he is unable either to read aloud or to comprehend either by direct association between visual and oral word forms or by semantic mediation between visual and oral word forms.

His sole access to the pronunciation and meaning of the printed word is accordingly via a grapheme–phoneme translation route. This route, how-ever, is also impaired. It is not possible to derive an accurate (extra-lexical) phonic translation of English (or French) without the ability to segment the input letter strings into graphemes (which may consist of more than one letter). M.S. can only segment such input into *single* letters (which are then transcoded into phonological form). Consistent with his use of the phonic route, M.S. does show a "regularity" effect, but fails to read correctly even those *regular* words that demand parsing into multi-letter graphemes. The disorder of the phonic route is "pure" in that all of his errors can be attributed to an impaired mechanism of orthographic parsing. The phonic translations that he produces are all "valid" (see Chapter 11 in this book) in that they occur in substantial numbers of English words. Similarly, "blending" is basically intact; M.S. produces a smooth output rendition of many English words that do not require parsing into multi-letter units; when parsing is required (but unavailable to M.S.) he either inserts "schwas" to preserve continuity or selects the phonic value of the letter name. With the exception of a very small sight vocabulary, M.S.'s comprehension of the written word depends entirely upon the output of his *one letter–one phoneme* mapping rules.

As in previous cases of "surface dyslexia" the qualitative form of M.S.'s writing deficit matches the form of his reading deficit. When writing to dictation, M.S. is essentially encoding the continuous, enciphered input into a discrete sequence of phonemes that he then transcribes into print on the basis of *one phoneme = one letter*. This system is supplemented by the use of letter names when the phonemes of the input stimulus have no direct association with simple letter sounds; thus "you" is written as *U*. Once again, M.S.'s errors are all valid (with the exception of *b/d* confusions) and he in fact produces a remarkably accurate transcription, given that the code available to him is the English alphabet rather than the International Phonetic Alphabet. That M.S. uses an anglicised International Phonetic Alphabet as his internal code for reading and writing is confirmed by the dramatic superiority with which he can read his own spellings as compared with even "regular" English orthography.

The extreme purity of M.S.'s deficit is consistent with the claim that the extra-lexical reading route is both functionally and anatomically distinct from reading routes based upon *word forms*. It is unclear how *single-route* theories could cope with the extreme dissociation we have described.

REFERENCES

Bishop, D. V. M. (1982). *Test for Reception of Grammar*. Abingdon, Oxford: Thomas Leach Ltd (printed for the MRC).

Bruce, V. (1979). Searching for politicians: An information-processing approach to face recognition. *Quarterly Journal of Experimental Psychology, 31*, 373–395.

Coltheart, M. (1978). Lexical access in simple reading tasks. In G. Underwood (ed.), *Strategies of Information Processing*. London: Academic Press.

Coltheart, M., Masterson, J., Byng, S., Prior, M., & Riddoch, J. (1983). Surface dyslexia. *Quarterly Journal of Experimental Psychology, 35A*, 469–495.

Derouesné, J., & Beauvois, M.-F. (1979). Phonological processing in reading: Data from alexia. *Journal of Neurology, Neurosurgery, and Psychiatry, 42*, 1125–1132.

Glushko, R. J. (1979). The organization and activation of orthographic knowledge in reading aloud. *Journal of Experimental Psychology: Human Perception and Performance, 5*, 674–691.

Glushko, R. J. (1981). Principles for pronouncing print: The psychology of phonography. In A. M. Lesgold, & C. A. Perfetti (eds.), *Interactive Processes in Reading*. Hillsdale, NJ: Lawrence Erlbaum Associates Inc.

Henderson, L. (1982). *Orthography and Word Recognition in Reading*. London: Academic Press.

Holmes, J. M. (1973). Dyslexia: A neurolinguistic study of traumatic and developmental disorders of reading. Unpublished PhD. thesis, University of Edinburgh.

Holmes, J. M. (1978). "Regression" and reading breakdown. In A. Caramazza, & E. B. Zurif (eds.), *Language Acquisition and Language Breakdown: Parallels and Divergences*. Baltimore, Md: Johns Hopkins Press.

Marcel, A. J. (1980). Surface dyslexia and beginning reading. In M. Coltheart, K. E. Patterson, & J. C. Marshall (eds.), *Deep Dyslexia*. London: Routledge & Kegan Paul.

Marshall, J. C., & Newcombe, F. (1973). Patterns of paralexia: A psycholinguistic approach. *Journal of Psycholinguistic Research*, **2**, 175–199.

Marshall, J. C., & Newcombe, F. (1977). Variability and constraint in acquired dyslexia. In H. Whitaker, & H. A. Whitaker (eds.), *Studies in Neurolinguistics*, Vol. 3. New York: Academic Press.

Masterson, J. (1983). Surface dyslexia and the operation of the phonological route in reading. Unpublished PhD thesis, Birkbeck College, University of London.

Oddy, M. (1979). Follow-up study of cognitive performance in young head-injured males. Talk given at 4th Workshop of Trauma International, Groningen, May 1979.

Patterson, K. E., & Kay, J. (1982). Letter-by-letter reading: Psychological descriptions of a neurological syndrome. *Quarterly Journal of Experimental Psychology*, **34A**, 411–441.

Shallice, T., Warrington, E. K., & McCarthy, R. (1983). Reading without semantics. *Quarterly Journal of Experimental Psychology*, **35A**, 111–138.

Stanovich, K. E., & Bauer, D. W. (1978). Experiments on the spelling-to-sound regularity effect in word recognition. *Memory and Cognition*, **6**, 410–415.

Venezky, R. L. (1970). *The Structure of English Orthography*. The Hague: Mouton.

APPENDIX

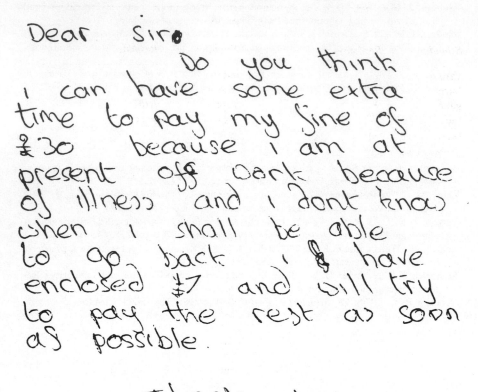

Dear Sir,

Do you think
i can have some extra
time to pay my fine of
£30 because i am at
present off work because
of illness and i dont know
when i shall be able
to go back i have
enclosed £7 and will try
to pay the rest as soon
as possible.

Thank you

Fig. 2.1   A letter written by M.S. prior to his accident.

DER SUR

DU YU FINK ^i_I KAN AV SUM EKSTRA TIM TU PA MI FIN UV £30

BEKOZ ^i_I AM AT PREZ^U_ENT OF WURK BEKOZ UV ^iLNES ^AN_{AND I} ^i DONT

NO WEN ^i_I SHAL BE ABUL TU GO BAK ^i_I AV ENKLOZD £7 AN WIL TRI

TU PA THE REST AZ SUN AZ PASUBUL

FANK YU

Fig. 2.2   A prediction (by Professor Victoria Fromkin) of how M.S. would write the same letter after his accident. (M.S. now writes in uppercase letters, with the exception of an occasional lowercase *i*.)

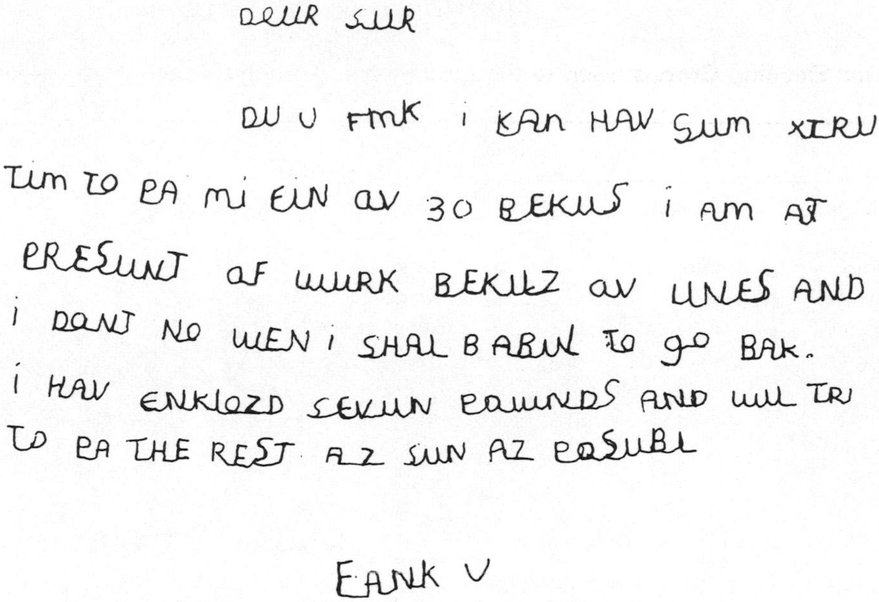

DEUR SUR

DU U FINK i KAN HAV SUM XTRU
TIM TO PA mi EIN AV 30 BEKUS i AM AT
PRESUNT AF WURK BEKUZ AV UNES AND
i DONT NO WEN i SHAL B ABUL TO go BAK.
i HAV ENKLOZD SEVUN POWNDS AND WIL TRI
TO PA THE REST AZ SUN AZ POSUBL

EANK U

Fig. 2.3 The letter as written to dictation by M.S. after his accident.

It should be noted that the orthographic representation provides an excellent transcription of M.S.'s normal dialect (e.g. "think" is "fink" in his accent).

3 Lexicalisation and Reading Performance in Surface Dyslexia

E. M. Saffran

The errors that surface dyslexics make in reading aloud are commonly taken to reflect the use of a non-lexical procedure for mapping orthography onto phonology. The reliance on non-lexical procedures in surface dyslexia is, in turn, cited as support for the view that there are separable lexical and non-lexical routes in oral reading.

Marcel (1980) has challenged this line of argument, on the grounds that the oral reading errors of surface dyslexics are subject to lexical influences. In support of this view, he offers observations on two patients studied by Marshall and Newcombe (1973). Contrary to the expectation that errors generated by non-lexical mapping procedures should consist largely of non-words, the majority of their errors were word substitutions; *incense* was read as "increase", *gauge* as "jug", and so on. There were also indications that reading accuracy was affected by lexical variables such as word frequency and part-of-speech (Marshall & Newcombe, 1973). These effects led Marcel to question the standard interpretation of reading performance in surface dyslexia, as well as the dual route view of reading which it supported (see also Kay & Marcel, 1981).

Lexical influences in surface dyslexic reading clearly need to be assessed, though their implications for the dual route model may not be as dire as Marcel has suggested. Since it appears that lexically-based reading is to some extent preserved in surface dyslexia, variables like frequency and part-of-speech could well determine whether a word can be read via the lexical procedure: indeed, as shown in Chapter 1, the ability of a surface dyslexic to read a word lexically *can* depend on word frequency. Furthermore, utilisation of a non-lexical phonological translation procedure does not preclude lexical involvement at a point *subsequent* to phonological encoding of the letter string; for example, lexical units could be activated on the basis of partial phonological information.

53

Attempts to explain these effects are, however, premature in view of the paucity of relevant data. As yet, there have been no investigations specifically designed to study lexical influences on reading performance in surface dyslexia. This study seeks to provide such evidence by examining whether the lexical status of alternate pronunciations of a vowel grapheme influences the oral reading response to that grapheme. More specifically, is a surface dyslexic more likely to produce an incorrect pronunciation for a vowel grapheme if that incorrect pronunciation yields a word, as opposed to a non-word? And is a surface dyslexic more likely to produce a correct pronunciation for a vowel grapheme if the incorrect pronunciation yields a non-word, as opposed to a word? The results demonstrate that lexicalisation can be a potent factor in the reading performance of a surface dyslexic.

CASE REPORT

This study is based on a corpus of reading responses from L.L., a 15-year-old female who suffered a closed head injury as a result of a traffic accident in September 1981. At the time of injury, she was in her second year of high school, where she had been receiving good grades. L.L. was comatose for approximately 1 month following the accident. A CT scan performed during this period indicated diffuse white matter injury and a punctured left basal ganglion haematoma. Residual neurological deficits at the time the present data were gathered (February–May 1982) included hyperactive reflexes in both lower extremities, ataxic gait, and peripheral constriction of both visual fields.

L.L.'s performance on psychological tests was indicative of generalised intellectual impairment. On a WISC-R administered in June 1982, L.L. obtained a verbal IQ of 80 and a performance IQ of 67, scores that represent a considerable decline from estimated pre-morbid levels. Her Wechsler Memory Quotient at this time was 76. L.L.'s speech was mildly dysarthric and somewhat anomic. She demonstrated moderate impairments in auditory comprehension and word retrieval on a Boston Diagnostic Aphasia Examination (BDAE) administered in January 1982; by the time a second BDAE was given in June 1982, these deficits had largely cleared. Deficits in reading and writing are described in the following section.

READING AND WRITING

L.L.'s reading was markedly impaired. Her z scores on the oral reading and reading comprehension subtests of the BDAE administered in January 1982 ranged from -1 to -2.2. To specify the nature of the impairment, she was given a battery of tasks that are sensitive to features of the various forms of acquired dyslexia as described, for example, by Shallice and Warrington (1980) and by Patterson (1981).

1. Letter Identification

L.L. named uppercase letters without error, and made 2/24 errors in upper-/ lowercase matching (*Qq* and *Ff*). Her ability to identify letters was not affected by the size of the array in which the target letter was embedded. Attentional dyslexia (Shallice & Warrington, 1977) was therefore ruled out.

2. Effect of Word Length

Given a set of words between three and seven letters long that were matched for frequency across word length, L.L. read correctly 10/10 three-letter words, 8/10 four-letter words, 4/10 five-letter words, 7/10 six-letter words, and 4/10 seven-letter words. Errors on this task were not systematically distributed across letter positions; 4/17 errors involved initial letters and three involved final letters. Though L.L.'s reading speed increased monotonically with word length, response latency varied considerably within sets of words of a given length and appeared closely related to accuracy. Only in one instance did L.L. name letters aloud when reading. Thus, though L.L.'s performance was affected by word length, she did not appear to be reading letter by letter (cf. Patterson, 1981).

3. Effect of Spelling-to-Sound Regularity

The Coltheart list of 39 regular and exception words (Coltheart, Besner, Jonasson, & Davelaar, 1979) was administered twice, first on 8 February 1982 and again on 27 April 1982 (see Appendix I for a complete list of L.L.'s responses). On both occasions, L.L. read correctly 29/39 regular and 18/39 irregular words (scoring first attempts only). Of the 62 words that were misread, 36 were misread on both occasions. A discrepancy between regular and irregular words is, of course, the cardinal feature of surface dyslexia. L.L.'s errors were similar to those reported in other surface dyslexics: regularisations (e.g. *sword*→/swɔrd/; *gone*→/goɔn/); insensitivity to contextual constraints (e.g. *spade*→/spæd/); misplaced stress (e.g. *distress*→ /'dɪstrɛs/); letter additions (e.g. *spade*→spred/), etc.

4. Reading of Non-words

Non-word reading was investigated using a set of 10 four-letter pseudowords derived from real words by changing one letter. Performance was 70% correct, as compared with 80% correct on real words of equal length and similar composition. The ability to read non-words can be relatively well preserved in surface dyslexia (Shallice, Warrington, & McCarthy, 1983; see also Chapter 1 in this book).

TABLE 3.1
Examples of L.L.'s Spelling Errors

Written to Dictation		Spelled Aloud	
"calf"	cafe	"spade"	SPAD
"coal"	kool	"flood"	FLOUD
"frame"	fraim	"stupid"	STOUPID
"steak"	steek	"gone"	GAWN[a]
"twin"	twine	"spend"	SPEAND
"flood"	flod	"castle"	CHASTLE

[a] A permissible phonetic spelling for this word in L.L.'s dialect.

Spelling was not investigated systematically. Examples of L.L.'s spelling errors may be found in Table 3.1. She appears to be using a phonological strategy, as has been noted in other surface dyslexics whose spelling has also been studied (e.g. Coltheart, Masterson, Byng, Prior, & Riddoch, 1983). However, her ability to spell phonologically does not appear to be entirely adequate (note, in particular, the errors on vowels).

Further study of L.L.'s reading performance was undertaken, initially with the aim of investigating her ability to utilise spelling–sound rules as a function of rule frequency and complexity. Lists of words and non-words exemplifying various rules were generated for this purpose. This project was not completed, due to L.L.'s unavailability. However, the corpus of reading responses that was obtained from L.L. proved suitable for the analysis of lexicalisation effects that is now described.

THE LEXICALISATION ANALYSIS

The analysis examines lexical influences on the pronunciation of vowel letters that have alternative phonological realisations. Thus, for example, the letter i may be pronounced as the short vowel /ɪ/ or as the long vowel /aɪ/. The long-vowel pronunciation occurs in the context iCe (where C = consonant). This is, of course, an instance of the "silent e" rule, which applies to other vowels as well ($aCe \rightarrow$ /eɪ/, $oCe \rightarrow$ /oʊ/, etc.).

Suppose that an acquired dyslexic patient lacks perfect control over these rules of vowel pronunciation, and that the realisation of the vowel grapheme is affected by the lexical status of alternative pronunciations, in that there is a tendency to choose responses that are themselves words. If so, the patient should make fewer errors on words like $line$, where the alternative short-vowel pronunciation would yield a non-word (/lɪn/), than on words like $pine$, where the short-vowel pronunciation would result in another word (pin). A

TABLE 3.2
The Conditions Used in the Lexicalisation Analysis

Condition	Stimulus	Example	Response	Example
W–*W	VCe	ripe	VC	rip
	VC	tap	VCe	tape
W–*NW	VCe	trade	VC	/træd/
	VC	slip	VCe	/slaɪp/
NW–*W	VCe	slame	VC	slam
	VC	lin	VCe	line
NW–*NW	VCe	yate	VC	/yæt/
	VC	kip	VCe	/kaɪp/

* = Lexical status of error response produced by incorrect lengthening or shortening of the vowel.

similar prediction applies to the reading of non-words: more errors should occur on non-words like *grine*, where the short-vowel pronunciation yields a word (*grin*), than on non-words like *crine*, where the short-vowel pronunciation does not yield a word.

The full set of stimulus types used in this analysis is illustrated in Table 3.2. If lexicalisation affects L.L.'s reading performance, her error rate should be greater on the W–*W and NW–*W conditions, where the incorrect pronunciation would yield a word, than on W–*NW and NW–*NW, where the incorrect pronunciation would not yield a real word.

A test of this prediction was carried out on an appropriate subset of the oral reading responses obtained from L.L.

Method

The data used in this study were selected from the corpus of 1018 oral reading responses that had been obtained from L.L. The materials used to elicit these responses consisted of lists of words and non-words, which were selected to exemplify a number of spelling–sound rules; these included correspondences based on single letters (e.g. most consonants and certain pronunciations of vowels) as well as correspondences based on letter combinations (e.g. *ph, ch, oa, oo,* and the rule of silent *e*). Each list consisted of about 200 stimuli, half of them words and half pronounceable non-words, exemplifying several different rules and arranged in random order. The lists were administered in five sessions between February and May 1982.

The stimuli were typed on 8 × 13-cm cards that were presented one at a time for oral reading. The task was self-paced. L.L.'s responses were recorded on tape and subsequently transcribed phonetically.

Data Analysis

For the purposes of the present study, all responses to monosyllabic stimuli containing *aCe, iCe, aC(k)*, or *iC(k)* were selected for analysis. Several letter strings appeared more than once in the stimulus lists; in such cases, only the first presentation of the string was analysed. On some trials, L.L. gave more than one response to a stimulus (e.g. *blame*→/blæm/, "blame"); in these instances, only the first response was scored. Letter strings were assigned to conditions (W–*W, W–*NW, etc.) *on the basis of pronunciation*; thus, for example, a pseudohomophone like *phan* would be classified as a W–*W.

Results

Table 3.3 contains a summary of L.L.'s performance across the conditions outlined in Table 3.2. Inspection of the bottom row of the table, which lists the overall percentage of correct responses for each condition, indicates that there was an effect of lexicalisation. Performance is clearly best in the W–*NW condition, where the incorrect pronunciation of the vowel would result in a non-word, and worst in the NW–*W condition, where the incorrect pronunciation results in a word.

Statistical tests (Fisher Exact Probability Test) of the lexicalisation effect were carried out by comparing performance on W–*W vs. W–*NW, and on NW–*W vs. NW–*NW, for each of the vowel types separately. As can be seen from Table 3.3, five of the eight comparisons were statistically significant. Of the three cases in which lexicalisation effects were not obtained, two involved *iCe* stimuli. Of the four vowel graphemes tested, overall performance was, in fact, best for *iCe* stimuli (75% correct, as opposed to 54–56% correct for the other stimulus types). This might reflect more adequate control over a mapping "rule" for *iCe*, as compared with the other string types tested; or, conceivably, /aɪ/ might be, for L.L., a preferred, or default, pronunciation for *i* ("when in doubt pronounce *i* as /aɪ/").

The possibility that preferences of this sort were affecting L.L.'s reading performance was investigated by examining her pronunciation of *o* in different graphemic contexts: in *oCe* and *oa*, where the correct realisation is /oω/; in *oo*, which should be realised as /u/; and in *oC*, where the correct pronunciation is /ɒ/. These data are summarised in Table 3.4. L.L. makes relatively few errors on strings for which /oω/ is the correct realisation; her error rate is higher for /u/ and /ɒ/, and where she makes an error, she most frequently substitutes the /oω/ pronunciation. These results suggest that L.L. has a bias towards pronouncing *o* as /oω/.

We are cautioned, however, by the results of the lexicalisation analysis to consider the possible role of lexicalisation in this effect: that is, was the composition of the stimulus set such that there were more opportunities to

TABLE 3.3
Results of the Lexicalisation Analysis

String Type	W–*W	W–*NW	Significance	NW–*W	NW–*NW	Significance	Percentage Correct
(C)CaCe							56
No. of tokens	19	26		15	24		
No. read correctly	9	20	$P < 0.05^a$	3	16	$P < 0.05$	
No. read as /æ/	10	5		10	5		
No. other errors	0	1		2	3		
(C)CaC(k)							54
No. of tokens	18	16		11	12		
No. read correctly	15	14	N.S.	2	10	$P < 0.01$	
No. read as /eɪ/	2	2		7	1		
No. other errors	1	0		2	1		
(C)CiCe							75
No. of tokens	18	16		9	14		
No. read correctly	13	13	N.S.	7	10	N.S.	
No. read as /ɪ/	5	2		2	2		
No. other errors	0	1		0	2		
(C)CiC(k)							55
No. of tokens	13	11		7	14		
No. read correctly	5	8	$P = 0.05$	2	10	$P = 0.05$	
No. read as /aɪ/	7	1		5	2		
No. other errors	1	2		0	2		
$\bar{x}$ percentage correct	62	80		33	72		

[a] Fisher Exact Probability Test, One-tailed.

TABLE 3.4
Evidence of a Preferred Pronunciation for the Letter o

String Type	No. of Tokens	Correct Vowel Pronunciation	Actual Vowel Pronunciation (Percentage Occurrences) /oʊ/	/u/	/ɒ/	Other
oCe, oaC	36	/oʊ/	89	0	11	0
ooC	20	/u/	30	55	10	5
oC, ock	21	/ɒ/	33	0	67	0

lexicalise the letter strings as /oω/ words, as compared with other pronunciations of *o*? To exclude lexicalisation as a factor, the analysis must be restricted to NW–*NW strings. In the case of *oCe* and *oaC*, there were eleven such items, all of which were read correctly; in the case of *oC* and *ooC* there were nine, five of which were realised as /oω/. This effect is statistically significant (Fisher Exact Probability Test, $P = 0.01$). Thus there is evidence that L.L.'s oral reading performance is affected by certain letter pronunciation preferences, as well as by lexicalisation.

Given that lexicalisation does affect reading in L.L., one might ask, further, whether her performance is influenced by the relative frequency of alternative lexical choices. To examine this question, Kucera–Francis (Kucera & Francis, 1967) frequencies were obtained for both the W and *W words in the W–*W condition (Table 3.3). If frequency is a determining factor, L.L.'s responses should be biased towards the more frequent of the alternative lexicalisations. This effect was not obtained. Of the 64 W–*W pairs for which relative frequencies could be determined (in cases where only one item was listed in the Kucera–Francis table, the unlisted item was assumed to be lower in frequency), L.L. produced the more frequent word in 34 cases and the less frequent in 30. However, in many of the pairs, the two words were relatively close in frequency. A further investigation of frequency effects was therefore performed by analysing W–*W pairs in which the frequencies of the two words differed by at least an order of magnitude; of the 21 such cases, the more frequent word was produced in 13. This effect was not significant (Binomial Test, $P = 0.2$).

DISCUSSION

These results, together with the evidence cited by Marcel (1980), argue convincingly that, for at least some patients with a surface dyslexic pattern of reading performance, there is a significant lexical influence on the assignment of pronunciation. This influence is not characteristic of all "surface dyslexic" patients (see, for example, cases H.T.R. of Shallice, Warrington, & McCarthy, 1983; and M.P. of Bub, Cancelliere, & Kertesz, Chapter 1 of this book), nor would one expect it to be (Hatfield & Patterson, 1983). As lexicalisation *can*, however, be a major feature, it is necessary to consider at what point in the reading process, and in what manner, lexical effects are exerted.

According to the standard view of reading in surface dyslexia, phonological transcription of the letter string generally occurs prior to, and is then in fact the precondition for, lexical access (e.g. Marshall & Newcombe, 1973; Patterson, 1981). The lexicalisation effect would seem to suggest that lexical information impinges on the putatively pre-lexical translation process. How might this occur?

Impaired ability to access the lexicon by means of orthographic input is generally thought to be at the root of the surface dyslexic's reading problem. If orthographic access is completely blocked, the surface dyslexic would have to rely entirely on grapheme–phoneme translation. This would produce a total inability to read irregular words, and this has not yet been observed in any patient. Instead, it would seem that the ability to access the lexicon orthographically is partially preserved in all cases of surface dyslexia so far reported. If so, access via a *malfunctioning* orthographic route might conceivably account for the effects observed in L.L. Her errors might be interpreted, for example, as involving letter additions (e.g. *brid*–bride, *grim*–grime) or deletions (e.g. *jare*–jar, *dime*–dim). The problem for this, or any other orthographic account for that matter, is that the errors involve vowel graphemes almost exclusively. It is difficult to understand why vowels should be any more vulnerable than consonants to the vagaries of an orthographic process. It is, rather, at the level of grapheme–phoneme translation, where mapping rules for consonants tend to be simpler and more consistent than those that encode vowels, that one would expect such differences to occur.

The nature of the errors suggests, then, that the mode of lexical entry is phonological, as has generally been assumed to be the case in surface dyslexia (but see Marcel, 1980). The most obvious interpretation of the lexicalisation effect is that a patient like L.L. generates alternative mappings for a letter string, that these alternate mappings are referred to the lexicon, and that selection from among these alternatives is lexically determined. The data also indicate that the mappings for a given vowel grapheme $V(X)(Y)$ are constrained to the set of plausible mappings for V (an *a*, for example, rarely elicits an *o* pronunciation) and that the alternative mappings for V may be differentially weighted (viz. Table 3.4).

How are these alternative mappings generated? In the case of complex vowel graphemes, like *VCe*, multiple mappings could result from operation of a letter-string segmentation process, or parser, of the type proposed by Shallice and his co-workers (Shallice & Warrington, 1980; Shallice, Warrington, & McCarthy, 1983; Shallice & McCarthy, Chapter 15 in this book; see also Kay & Marcel, 1981; Marcel, 1980). A feature of the proposed parsing process is that it is exhaustive, in other words, it segments the letter string in all possible ways. A word like *lake*, for example, might be segmented as [l][ake], [la][k][e], [l][a][k][e], etc. The multiple outputs of the parser could conceivably serve as the basis for alternative realisations of the vowel.

There are serious problems with this account, however. First, multiple bracketings cannot explain L.L.'s frequent production of long-vowel pro- nunciations for graphemes that encode short vowels (Table 3.3); there is no way that [VCe] segments can be generated from *VC* strings. Furthermore, if short-vowel pronunciations of *VCe* stimuli reflect the encoding of [VC][e] bracketings of the strings, one might expect the implementation of such a bracketing to result in pronunciation of the stranded final *e*—that *lake*, for example, would be read not as "lack" but as "lackey." No examples of such an effect are to be found in L.L.'s corpus. This is not a reflection, however, of a general reluctance on L.L.'s part to voice final *e*. In fact, she had a preference for articulating final *e* in other contexts: of 44 *VCCe* strings, she pronounced 24 with a terminal /i/ (e.g. *hedge*→/hɛdʒi/, *punge*→/pʌndʒi/, *tible*→/tɪbli/).

These observations suggest, moreover, that it may be incorrect to characterise a surface dyslexic patient's deficit in terms of the size of the orthographic units that are mapped onto phonology. An account along these lines has been proposed by Shallice and his co-workers (Shallice, Warrington, & McCarthy, 1983; Shallice & McCarthy, Chapter 15 in this book). These authors suggest that surface dyslexia lies on a continuum bounded on one end by "letter sound by letter sound" reading, in which the mapping units are limited to single letters (see Newcombe & Marshall, Chapter 2 in this book, for a case that fits this description), and by semantic dyslexia, in which the mapping units encompass several letters but are still submorphemic, on the other end (Shallice, Warrington, & McCarthy, 1983). If the graphemic units that are mapped onto phonology are small, as they are assumed to be in surface dyslexia, pronunciation rules that span several letters (the rule of silent *e*, for example) will not be respected. The data for terminal *e* suggest, however, that L.L.'s mispronunciation of vowel graphemes did not reflect the size or composition of the mapping units she was using, but rather ambivalence with respect to their phonological realisation. L.L. appeared to be utilising *VCe* (or possibly *CVCe*) segments in mapping from print to phonology; the problem was that she was unsure what the phonological realisation of these segments should be.

The data from L.L. suggest the following account of her reading. Phonological translation of the letter string is performed by means of a grapheme–phoneme translation process that permits alternative mappings for certain graphemes (for *VCe* and *VC*, for example). Hence, a single letter string may generate conflicting phonological representations. Whether this is a normal property of the grapheme–phoneme translation process is an unresolved issue, discussed further in Chapters 11 and 14 in this book. The output of the translation process is referred to the phonological lexicon. If a lexical entry is accessed, a pronunciation will be generated lexically (i.e. lexicalisation will occur); if not, articulatory encoding will be based directly on the output of the phonological translation process. To account for errors like *incense*→"increase," where the discrepancies between stimulus and response are not easily explained by the limitations of the grapheme–phoneme translation process, requires the further assumption that lexical access may occur on the basis of partial phonological information.[1] A problem with this assumption is that it allows almost any response to be explained on the basis of lexicalisation. It is clearly necessary to set criteria for the degree of disparity between stimulus and response that can be tolerated under a lexicalisation model. Alternatively, an error like *incense*→"increase" may be a result of approximate visual access, involving the orthographic lexical route.

The necessity to consider possible lexicalisation effects greatly complicates the interpretation of surface dyslexic performance in a case like L.L. To what extent, for example, do a surface dyslexic's correct responses to orthographically regular words reflect lexicalisation on the basis of partial phonological information, as opposed to the adequacy of grapheme–phoneme translation? Could some of the phenomena described by Coltheart et al. (1983), which suggest that comprehension of printed words may be based on correct phonological translation even with homophonic exception words (giving the definition of *bold* when presented with *bowled*, for example), be explained in the same manner? Errors that might be interpreted as "visual," implying that they originate at an orthographic level of processing, could also, in many cases, be explained as phonologically based lexicalisations (e.g. *lose*→"loss," *check*→"cheek," from Appendix I).

To assess phonological translation abilities independently of lexicalisation effects, it is necessary to use either a restricted set of stimuli—NW–*NW non-words, as in the present study—or, as Jackie Masterson shows in the note appended to this chapter, to present non-words under blocked rather than mixed-list conditions.

ACKNOWLEDGEMENTS

The author would like to thank Dr David Caplan for assistance with the preparation of stimulus materials and transcription of the responses. Preparation of the manuscript was supported by grant NS 17326-01S1 from the National Institute of Health.

---

[1] One can surmise, furthermore, that it is where lexical access is based on partial specification of the lexical entry that factors like word frequency are most likely to enter. This may explain why frequency effects were not obtained in the present study, though Marcel (1980) found them in the Marshall and Newcombe (1973) corpus. There were seldom large discrepancies between stimulus and response in L.L.'s corpus, perhaps because the letter strings that were used were relatively simple. From the examples given, it appears that there may have been greater discrepancies in the data used by Marcel.

REFERENCES

Coltheart, M., Besner, D., Jonasson, J.-T., & Davelaar, E. (1979). Phonological encoding and the lexical decision task. *Quarterly Journal of Experimental Psychology,* **31,** 489–507.

Coltheart, M., Masterson, J., Byng, S., Prior, M., & Riddoch, J. (1983). Surface dyslexia. *Quarterly Journal of Experimental Psychology,* **35A,** 469–496.

Hatfield, F. M., & Patterson, K. E. (1983). Phonological spelling. *Quarterly Journal of Experimental Psychology,* **35A,** 451–468.

Kay, J., & Marcel, A. (1981). One process, not two, in reading aloud: Lexical analogies do the work of non-lexical rules. *Quarterly Journal of Experimental Psychology,* **33A,** 397–414.

Kucera, H., & Francis, W. N. (1967). *Computational Analysis of Present-day American English.* Providence, RI: Brown University Press.

Marcel, A. J. (1980). Surface dyslexia and beginning reading: A revised hypothesis of the pronunciation of print and its impairments. In M. Coltheart, K. E. Patterson, & J. C. Marshall (eds.), *Deep Dyslexia.* London: Routledge & Kegan Paul.

Marshall, J. C., & Newcombe, F. (1973). Patterns of paralexia: A psycholinguistic approach. *Journal of Psycholinguistic Research,* **2,** 175–199.

Patterson, K. E. (1981). Neuropsychological approaches to the study of reading. *British Journal of Psychology,* **72,** 151–174.

Shallice, T., & Warrington, E. K. (1977). The possible role of selective attention in acquired dyslexia. *Neuropsychologia,* **15,** 31–41.

Shallice, T., & Warrington, E. K. (1980). Single and multiple component central dyslexic syndromes. In M. Coltheart, K. E. Patterson, & J. C. Marshall (eds.), *Deep Dyslexia.* London: Routledge & Kegan Paul.

Shallice, T., Warrington, E. K., & McCarthy, R. (1983). Reading without semantics. *Quarterly Journal of Experimental Psychology,* **35A,** 111–138.

APPENDIX I

Coltheart Words

	Irregular Words			Regular Words	
Stimulus	*Response*		*Stimulus*	*Response*	
	(2/82)	*(4/82)*		*(2/82)*	*(4/82)*
gauge	/geɪg/	/geɪg/	grill	+	+
aunt	+	+	gang	+	+
laugh	+	+	treat	+	+
break	+	/brik/	dance	+	+
steak	+	+	slate	/slæt/	+
debt	/dɛbt/	/dɛpt/		/sæt/	
pint	/pɪnt/	/pɪnt/	cult	+	+
sign	+	+	pine	+	+
mortgage	/mɔrtgeɪ/	/mɔrtgeɪ/	base	+	+
castle	/keɪstli/	/keɪstli/	distress	/dɪskres/	/dɪstrəs/
come	+	+	sherry	+	+

APPENDIX I—*continued*

Irregular Words			Regular Words		
Stimulus	Response (2/82)	(4/82)	Stimulus	Response (2/82)	(4/82)
glove	+	/gloɷv/	take	+	/tæk/
love	+	+	spade	/sprɛd/	/spæd/
shove	/ʃoɷv/	/ʃoɷv/	turn	+	+
lose	/lɔs/	/loɷs/	shrug	+	+
move	+	+	save	/soɷ/	+
prove	+	/proɷv/		+	
gone	+	/goɷn/	sort	+	+
gross	/græs/	+	spend	+	+
bury	+	+	kept	+	+
borough	/bɔrʌg/	/bɑroɷ/	quick	+	/kwɛk/
through	/ɵroɷ/	+	duel	+	+
	/ɵroɷrʌg/		capsule	+	+
scarce	/ʃɛɑki/	+	splendid	/splɛnd/	+
	/ʃækəri/		strewn	+	+
answer	+	+	county	/kɒnti/	+
sword	/swɔrd/	/swɔrd/	spear	+	+
yacht	/jɒtʃt/	/jækt/	trout	+	+
sure	+	+	free	/frɛʃ/	+
blood	+	+	horse	+	+
flood	+	floɷd	tooth	+	/taɷɵ/
cough	/kɒŋ/	/kɔd/	barge	+	+
	/tʃʌndʒ/		throng	+	/ɵraɷŋ/
through	/trɒŋk/	/traɷg/	plug	+	+
bowl	+	+	mile	+	+
soul	+	+	check	/tʃik/	+
build	/boɷld/	+	shampoo	+	+
biscuit	/bɪskjut/	+	protein	/broɷtin/	+
circuit	/sər/	/sərkjut/		/proɷtaɪn/	
	/sərkʌt/		stupid	/stʌpt/	+
subtle	/sʌbtəl/	/sʌbtəl/	run	+	+
sew	/su/	/su/	fresh	+	/freɪz/
broad	/broɷd/	+			

APPENDIX II

Oral Reading Corpus Used in the Lexicalisation Analysis

		String Type: aCe	
Stimulus	*Response*	*Stimulus*	*Response*
stape	stap	tape	+
slame	+	wage	wag
frame	+	mage	/mæg/
stare	star, stray	vage	/veɪgd/
blame	blam, /bleɪn/	prake	/præk/
snape	snap	cane	can
shake	+	babe	/bæb/
flape	/freɪp/	cake	+
wate	what	case	+
stake	stack	dame	+
trade	+	game	+
rate	rat	gave	+
take	+	lake	+
stame	+	made	+
snake	snack	bake	back
glape	+	cage	/kæj/, /kæg/
chale	/tʃɔl/	came	+
date	+	cape	cap, cape
yate	/yæt/	cave	+
rage	+	dare	+
rake	+	gate	+
hane	+	gaze	+
mate	+	lane	+
vake	+	make	make, /mæk/
nabe	made	lape	lap
mafe	+	dafe	+
yake	yak	lare	+
fane	fan	sade	sad
mase	/meɪoɷs/, +	dake	+
jame	jam	tave	take
vame	+	wase	+
bave	+	chase	+
hake	+	pake	pack
gade	+	tase	+
yame	yam	snase	+
fape	/fæp/	trake	track
mave	+	base	+
jare	jar	brake	/bræk̩/

APPENDIX II—*continued*

String Type: aCe

Stimulus	Response	Stimulus	Response
vate	+	safe	+
baze	+	tale	+
gake	+	rare	/rɒr/
race	+	sake	sack
rape	rap	wace	+

String Type: aC, aCk

Stimulus	Response	Stimulus	Response
hack	+	back	+
blam	blame	phat	pal, fat
brack	branch	phan	/feɪn/
fram	frame	gram	+
rat	+	frab	+
cack	cake	plan	+
brak	+	chat	+
stack	+	shat	+
star	+	than	+
bak	+	trag	+
tak	+	that	+
flap	+	drab	+
slam	+	trab	+
cak	+	twam	/tweɪm/
shack	shake	drag	+
tack	take	grab	+
trad	trade	mag	+
snack	+	han	+
wat	wait	yat	+
snap	+	prack	+
mack	match	ran	+
snak	+	can	+
mak	make	rack	+
frack	+	mat	+
tap	+	chap	+
rag	+	phap	fake
vack	+	sack	+
vag	+	swam	+
wag	/weɪg/		

APPENDIX II—*continued*

String Type: iCe

Stimulus	Response	Stimulus	Response
blide	bind, blind	kile	+
gise	+	fice	+
yite	/yuti/	fite	fit
slide	+	kine	+
chipe	chip	fise	+
pride	+	fipe	+
site	sit	twine	twin
skide	skid	spine	+
kipe	+	dime	dim
vite	+	slime	+
life	+	rite	+
hire	+	wine	+
like	+	pine	+
rife	+	gripe	+
rike	+	stripe	strip
mile	+	bride	/brɪd/
nice	+	line	+
rice	+	swine	+
ride	+	tribe	+
mine	+	white	+
rise	+	fine	+
ripe	+	bime	/bɪm/
size	+	brine	/brin/
hine	+	gride	+
pline	+	slipe	+
prime	/frɛn/	chine	+
bine	+	crime	+
grine	+	swime	+
trine	+		

APPENDIX II—*continued*

String Type: iC, iCk

Stimulus	Response	Stimulus	Response
skid	+	slit	+
sit	+	swim	/swaɪm/
blid	blind	thip	+
slid	slide	glit	+
yit	+	clip	+
prid	pride	drip	+
drim	+	win	+
drin	+	grip	+
crim	crime	strip	stripe
chin	+	pin	pine
slim	+	grid	/graɪb/
slip	+	bim	+
grim	grime	twin	twine
crig	/grɪg/	spin	/spʌn/
plip	+	dim	dime
plim	/plaɪm/	kit	kite
kip	+	brid	bride
bin	+	lin	+
vit	+	swin	+
chip	+	trib	tribe
prid	pride	whit	+
phip	/faɪp/	ship	sheep
frim	+		

APPENDIX III

Data exactly comparable to those collected from L.L. and presented in Table 3.3 of Chapter 3 were collected from the developmental surface dyslexic C.D., who is fully described in Coltheart et al. (1983). A mixed list of words and non-words was presented to C.D. for oral reading. From this list, items ending in the structures vowel + consonant + final *e* or vowel + consonant + *e* + *s* (where the vowel should be long) and items ending in the structures vowel + consonant or vowel + consonant + *s* (where the vowel should be short) were extracted for analysis. The results of this analysis are given in Table 1. Incorrect responses to these items were mostly errors in which the wrong vowel length was used (25/34). As was observed with L.L., C.D.'s reading responses, whether the stimulus was a word or a non-word, were more likely to be correct when a response using the alternative vowel length is not a word than when it is a word. In other words, reading accuracy is affected by the lexical status of potential alternative responses.

This lexicalisation tendency might be regarded as a relatively fixed property of the putatively "non-lexical" reading system. Alternatively it might be a strategy voluntarily adopted by L.L. and C.D. as a response to the fact that the item list presented to them consisted of a mixture of words and non-words. Evidence that might help to distinguish between these possibili-

APPENDIX III: TABLE 1
Mixed-list Presentation

	W–*W	W–*NW	NW–*W	NW–*NW	Total
Vowel, consonant, e					
No. correct	6 (86%)	7 (100%)	1 (17%)	2 (40%)	16 (64%)
No. incorrect	1	0	4	3	8
Other incorrect	0	0	1	0	1
Vowel, consonant					
No. correct	5 (71%)	7 (100%)	3 (43%)	4 (100%)	19 (76%)
No. incorrect	0	0	3	0	3
Other incorrect	0	0	1	0	3
Vowel, consonant, e, s					
No. correct	2 (40%)	4 (80%)	0 (0%)	2 (40%)	8 (42%)
No. incorrect	3	0	2	3	8
Other incorrect	0	1	2	0	3
Vowel, consonant, s					
No. correct	3 (60%)	4 (100%)	1 (25%)	2 (40%)	10 (56%)
No. incorrect	2	0	3	1	6
Other incorrect	0	0	0	2	2
Total correct	16 (67%)	22 (96%)	5 (24%)	10 (53%)	53 (61%)

APPENDIX III: TABLE 2
Single (Non-word) List Presentation

	*NW–*W*	*NW–*NW*
Vowel, consonant, e		
No. correct	4 (36%)	4 (31%)
No. incorrect	2	5
Other incorrect	5	4
Vowel, consonant, (k)		
No. correct	0 (0%)	2 (29%)
No. incorrect	1	0
Other incorrect	1	5
Total correct	4 (31%)	6 (30%)

ties is provided by further data from C.D., collected on an occasion when all the items she was given to read were non-words (and she was informed of this). The set of 120 non-words given included 33 with the terminal structure vowel + consonant + final *e* or vowel + terminal consonant(s). The results are given in Table 2. The numbers of stimuli involved here are very small, but the data do suggest that no lexicalisation tendency was operating here. Hence the results provided by C.D. might be taken as indicating that the principle of choosing among alternative phonological translations of a letter string by favouring those phonological representations that are themselves words is a strategy adopted in conditions where the dyslexic reader knows that many of the items presented for reading will in fact be words. In other words, lexicalisation may not be a fixed property of the procedures used for reading non-words, but a strategy used to make selections from alternative outputs generated by these procedures.

J. Masterson

II

COMPREHENSION IN SURFACE DYSLEXIA

▌▌ Introduction

Conceptions about surface dyslexia, in fact about reading disorders generally, indeed about neuropsychological deficits even more generally, are changing rapidly. One significant aspect of change is the growing realisation of or emphasis on the fact that symptoms (or even symptom complexes) rarely imply unique causes. One symptom of surface dyslexia is that, in a phonologically non-transparent orthography like English or French, a patient pronounces a common printed word in a way that is phonologically plausible but lexically incorrect (e.g. *pint*→/pɪnt/, rhyming with "mint"). The functional accounts of this symptom given initially (e.g. Marshall & Newcombe, 1973) or even more recently (e.g. Coltheart, 1981; Patterson, 1981) suggested, either explicitly or implicitly, that this behaviour might have a unique cause. In terms of a model like that on the jacket of this book, whenever a word fails to achieve access to the component labelled "Orthographic Recognition," this would force oral reading to rely on the use of subword-level correspondences between orthography and phonology, yielding regularisation errors like *pint*→/pɪnt/. Shallice and Warrington (1980) were the first authors to caution against the single-cause error with respect to surface dyslexia, noting that reliance on the assignment of phonology to subword orthographic units might be provoked by any one of several different impairments in the procedures for addressing the output phonology for a whole familiar written word. This point had been previously neglected despite the fact that the early models (from Marshall & Newcombe, 1973, onwards) permitted this variety of deficits affirmed by Shallice and Warrington.

It is a clear prediction from the book-jacket model that, if a patient *did* have a deficit in orthographic word recognition, it is not only his lexically correct oral reading (of irregular words) that should suffer, *but also his comprehension of these words*. Conclusions about the functional locus of the deficit for a surface dyslexic patient thus require data on the patient's comprehension of written words. And indeed either anecdotal (Marshall & Newcombe, 1973) or experimental (Coltheart, Masterson, Byng, Prior, & Riddoch, 1983) comprehension data for some patients did yield an answer compatible with the idea of an "early" lexical deficit, that is an impairment either of orthographic word recognition or of access from orthographic recognition to semantics. Thus such patients, if pronouncing *pint*→/pɪnt/, would fail to obtain any meaning for the word, and if pronouncing *bear*→"beer" would understand the word as referring to an alcoholic drink rather than a large animal.

The chapters in this section, on the other hand, describe four patients who might regularise *bear* as "beer" in oral reading but nevertheless correctly understand the target word as referring to an animal. With the exception of a few examples of this phenomenon in a case previously reported by Deloche, Andreewsky, and Desi (1982), the patients presented here are the first to reveal this pattern. There are interesting and theoretically important differences among these patients, but these are not detailed here, as an introduction should not divulge the whole story. The reasons why these four chapters form a coherent section, however, is that they share a concern with the following three issues.

1. As already indicated, these chapters illustrate how an assessment of reading comprehension as well as of oral reading is absolutely vital to a functional, theoretical account of any patient's pattern of reading performance. Indeed, a satisfactory account of a patient's reading will require investigation of more than the various aspects of reading skill. Some components of the cognitive system for reading, such as orthographic recognition, contribute *only* to reading; but other subsystems involved in oral reading, such as output phonology, are in many models also crucial components of non-reading tasks like object naming and spontaneous speech. All four chapters (perhaps especially Chapter 6 by Margolin, Marcel, & Carlson) stress the fact that in some patients, a reading and a naming deficit may in fact reflect one and the same impairment.

2. Again as already indicated, the chapters in this section reflect the concern not to equate symptoms with deficits. In fact, this concern amounts to a shift in the conception of neuropsychological syndromes. All the patients described in this section are accorded the syndrome label "surface dyslexia"—which is appropriate as a quick and useful way to communicate, but only as that. These patients are alike in that they sometimes or usually derive

oral reading responses for words by assigning phonology to subword-sized orthographic segments. In other respects, however, the patients differ from each other and even more from other patients called surface dyslexics. The implication of this variability is not that we must abandon the useful shorthand of syndrome *labels*, but rather that, if we use syndromes in this way, we must not expect to be able to offer a single theoretical account of a syndrome. Each patient's specific pattern of performance requires its own interpretation; generalisation must be from each patient to a functional model and not from one patient to another. Further arguments along these lines can be found in Marshall (1982, 1984) and Coltheart (1984), as well as in various places throughout this book.

3. Finally, the chapters in this section (perhaps especially Chapter 7 by Goldblum) are germane to another important issue. Many cognitive tasks such as oral reading can no doubt be accomplished by more than one routine or strategy. To what extent does a patient's performance reflect a genuine impairment to one routine as opposed to the choice (deliberate or unconscious) of some other strategic option for accomplishing the task? Neuropsychologists often simply adopt the former interpretation without considering the latter. Either explicit instructions to the patient to try to use the putatively unavailable routine or the employment of task variants which should specifically mobilise that routine are, as Beauvois and Derouesné (1982) have emphasised, essential dimensions of neuropsychological research. If the range of possible strategies is, as it should be, specified by the model, then the functional description of how a patient accomplishes a task may not depend on whether an alternative routine is actually unavailable to him or only eschewed by him. None the less, a more complete account of the patient's pattern of abilities and deficits does demand this distinction. Furthermore, the notion that a strategy that is both available to the person and adequate to the task might yet be ignored raises intriguing questions regarding compatibilities between tasks and strategies.

REFERENCES

Beauvois, M. F., & Derouesné, J. (1982). Recherche en psychologie cognitive et rééducation: Quels rapports? In X. Seron (ed.), *Rééduquer le Cerveau*. Brussels: Pierre Mardaga.

Coltheart, M. (1981). Disorders of reading and their implications for models of normal reading. *Visible Language*, XV(2), 245–286.

Coltheart, M. (1984). Acquired dyslexias and normal reading. In R. N. Malatesha & H. A. Whitaker (eds.), *Dyslexia: A Global Issue*. The Hague: Martinus Nijhoff.

Coltheart, M., Masterson, J., Byng, S., Prior, M., & Riddoch, J. (1983). Surface dyslexia. *Quarterly Journal of Experimental Psychology*, 35A, 469–495.

Deloche, G., Andreewsky, E., & Desi, M. (1982) Surface dyslexia: A case report, and some theoretical implications for reading models. *Brain and Language*, 15, 12–31.

Marshall, J. C. (1982). What is a symptom-complex? In M. A. Arbib, D. Caplan, & J. C. Marshall (eds.), *Neural Models of Language Processes*. New York: Academic Press.

Marshall, J. C. (1984). Toward a rational taxonomy of the acquired dyslexias. In R. N. Malatesha & H. A. Whitaker (eds.), *Dyslexia: A Global Issue*. The Hague: Martinus Nijhoff.

Marshall, J. C., & Newcombe, F. (1973). Patterns of paralexia: A psycholinguistic approach. *Journal of Psycholinguistic Research*, **2**, 175–199.

Patterson, K. E. (1981). Neuropsychological approaches to the study of reading. *British Journal of Psychology*, **72**, 151–174.

Shallice, T., & Warrington, E. K. (1980). Single and multiple component central dyslexic syndromes. In M. Coltheart, K. Patterson, & J. C. Marshall (eds.), *Deep Dyslexia*. London: Routledge and Kegan Paul.

4 Routes to Meaning in Surface Dyslexia

J. Kay and K. E. Patterson

INTRODUCTION

"Liston ... that's the boxer" is an oft-quoted response to the target word *listen* made by a patient J.C., described by Marshall and Newcombe (1973) in a seminal psycholinguistic study of acquired reading disorders. It quite clearly illustrates two characteristics of the symptom complex *surface dyslexia*; first, that the pronunciation of a written target word frequently happens to be an incorrect though phonologically appropriate rendering, and second, that if comprehension is demonstrated, it is of the given response, rather than of the target word (Coltheart, Masterson, Byng, Prior, & Riddoch, 1983).

It has been widely assumed that, in the course of reading a word like *listen* aloud, we first gain access to an abstract orthographic representation of its visual form in some sort of internal word store, or lexicon. From this point, the phonological representation /lɪsn/ can be addressed in one of two ways: either by a direct connection between lexical orthography and phonology, or via a mediating semantic representation which allows the word to be correctly understood (Morton, 1979; Morton & Patterson, 1980). This approach also necessitates the existence of a second system for assembling pronunciations from print, as we can pronounce unfamiliar written letter strings that have no stored lexical representations. A popular candidate has been a system comprising a set of context-sensitive rules for the translation of individual graphemes of a string into corresponding phonemic values (Coltheart, 1978). Such grapheme–phoneme correspondence (GPC) rules are held to be independent of stored lexical knowledge, although derived from such knowledge in the first instance, and are believed to be equivalent to standard linguistic rules of English pronunciation (e.g. Venezky, 1970; Wijk, 1966). In psychological descriptions of these linguistic rules, each grapheme is invariably assigned its most frequent phonemic value (that is, the value that occurs in the largest number of words containing that unit in context). One consequence of this "all-or-none" GPC assignment is that irregular or GPC rule-breaking words like *great* or *head* (which contain a less common pronunciation of the vowel digraph *ea*) will be given incorrect or "regularised" pronunciations (e.g. /grit/ and /hid/), which could only be corrected by the products of lexical processing.

On those occasions in surface dyslexic reading in which written words are mispronounced, access to lexical phonology (by either process) has plainly been denied. Because these words are also misunderstood (even if preserved comprehension in other modalities can be demonstrated), it is assumed that the impairment arises at a stage prior to that at which meaning is determined. This might be at the level of (1) access to orthographic lexical representations; (2) orthographic lexical representations themselves; or (3) transmission of information from these representations to both semantic and lexical phonological systems. Laying these three alternatives aside for the present, impairment at the level of lexical input orthography has the consequence within this framework of forcing reliance on non-lexical GPC processes. As a result, GPC rule-governed pronunciations will be produced, which for the majority of English words (those that obey linguistic rules of spelling–sound regularity) will be correct. However, a proportion of words like *listen*, which contain less common or exceptional GPCs, will be pronounced as if they were regular, with a "regularised" pronunciation (i.e. /lɪstən/). Phonological specifications constructed with the aid of GPC rules are used to gain access to semantic information. Coltheart et al. (1983) assume that this is achieved via a connection between the non-lexical GPC system and an input system that deals with the recognition of spoken words; that is, words are comprehended as if they had been spoken rather than written. In consequence, when an incorrect response to a target word corresponds to the spoken form of another word, the target word will be understood, as we have seen, in terms of that response.

In all published cases of surface dyslexia, irregular words are sometimes read aloud correctly. On the account of surface dyslexia we have just described, pronunciations of irregular words may only be produced by access to their specific lexical representations; hence it would appear that lexical phonology is on occasion tapped successfully in all cases so far described. As Coltheart et al. (1983) have demonstrated, however, successful retrieval of lexical phonology does not always result in correct comprehension because of the presence of homophones in the language. Thus, in a task that required the subject first to define and then to pronounce the target word, they discovered that the meaning of an irregularly pronounced word such as *bury* was often confused with that of its homophone ("fruit on a tree"), *even though it was read aloud successfully*. They suggest that, in such instances, the direct lexical connection between orthography and phonology was operational, although the communication from orthography to meaning (a critical step in disambiguating homophonic words) is nonetheless prevented.

Thus, Coltheart et al. (1983) distinguish two distinct methods of "phonological reading" in surface dyslexia. In the first, successful lexical orthographic access is not achieved, resulting in GPC rule-generated responses (which in the case of irregular words are incorrect). In the second, successful access to lexical orthography and retrieval of lexical phonology is achieved (so that even irregular words are correctly pronounced). In both cases, however, communication between lexical orthography and semantic descriptions is lacking, so that phonological influences upon reading comprehension can be discerned (homophone confusions, for example).

In this chapter, we present oral reading data from a patient with severe nominal dysphasia. The patient, E.S.T., may also be described as a surface dyslexic reader on the basis of features distinguished by Coltheart et al. (1983). Thus, he finds it more difficult to read irregular than regular words correctly, and produces regularisations of irregular words. He sometimes misunderstands the target word, his definition agreeing with his mispronunciation. In addition, though, our patient on occasion demonstrates correct understanding of an irregular word for which he none the less produces a regularised pronunciation (e.g. *foot*→"body and its my shoe, my /fut/"). We investigated the nature of his reading disability and its connection with his acute disturbance of naming.

CASE REPORT

E.S.T. (born in 1923), strongly right-handed, is highly educated, with an honours degree in mechanical engineering, and has a small engineering business. He is a man, to quote his consultant neurologist, of "robust Lancastrian personality," providing him with the optimism and determination to struggle through a long history of neurological illness.

In 1968, when E.S.T. was 45 years old, he was admitted to the Regional Neurological Centre in Newcastle. He complained of a number of episodes during the previous 9 months of confusion and dizziness, several of which involved loss of consciousness. In the later attacks, he also reported that he was aware of voice-like noises in his head, that his speech was disturbed, and that he had lost the ability to name familiar people and things. A preliminary diagnosis of symptomatic temporal lobe epilepsy was made, and E.S.T. was treated with anticonvulsants. At the same time, electroencephalography, carotid angiography, and gamma encephalography were carried out, the sum of which suggested a left temporal, or temporo-parietal, space-occupying lesion extending almost to the midline and of uncertain depth. Test findings strongly indicated an infiltrating gliomatous tumour. There was a marked absence, however, of raised intracranial pressure or focal neurological abnormalities. In consequence, and because it was felt that a biopsy or exploratory surgery would result in rapid mental and physical deterioration, his condition was simply monitored.

In 1970, EEG, isotope-scan, and left-carotid angiography showed no expansion of the tumour, and a benign meningioma was therefore suspected. There were still few significant neurological signs, apart from fleeting attacks of nominal dysphasia.

By 1976, however, his speech was getting worse, his word-finding difficulties were becoming more severe, and it was becoming difficult for him to continue with his work. This time, a carotid angiogram indicated a considerable increase in the mass of the slow-growing tumour. An EMI scan revealed an area of increased density in the left temporo-parietal region, which extended posteriorly to the occipital region and approached the midline. There was also a marked shift of the lateral ventricles and a pineal shadow to the right side. Perimetry of his visual fields indicated a right homonymous hemianopia with sparing of the macula.

Surgery was finally carried out in 1977. A pre-operative EMI scan showed that the overall size and appearance of the mass had not significantly changed since the scan of a year earlier. A large left temporal meningioma (11.0 × 6.5 × 6.0 cm) was removed from the lateral ventricle where it was arising from the choroid plexus. No difference in visual fields and visual acuity was found from the pre-operative testing.

Prior to his operation in 1977, it was noted that, apart from "a mild expressive dysphasia," E.S.T. also had a "severe degree of dyslexia." No elaboration of this statement is supplied. However, post-operative assessment in the Speech Therapy Department of Newcastle General Hospital indicated that his word-finding and reading difficulties were greater than they had been before surgery. With regard to his reading, it was observed that he read aloud letter-by-letter, "associating individual letters with a word (e.g. s = star; w = Warrington) then building up the whole word."

We began to see E.S.T. approximately 4 years after surgery, and studied his language abilities in a number of sessions that took place over a 12-month period. He no longer uses this overt letter-naming strategy, but frequently correctly spells out the letters of a word in the course of producing a pronunciation.

CLINICAL ASSESSMENT OF LANGUAGE ABILITIES

Spontaneous Speech

E.S.T. has obvious word-finding difficulties in his spontaneous speech, which are well masked by his use of substitute words and circumlocutions. His speech is restricted in content, although it is fluent and in general grammatical and functional communication is achieved. His speech is also marked by literal or phonemic paraphasias, and occasional jargon (see Table 4.1).

Repetition

Repetition of single words is generally good, with only 4/78 errors on the Coltheart, Besner, Jonasson, and Davelaar (1979) list of regular and irregular words. He made 4/24 errors in repeating non-words. Errors on both words and non-words were phonemic paraphasias (e.g. *distress*→/dɪstrɛf/), although there was one instance in word repetition where he made a phonemic followed by a semantic paraphasia (e.g. *sword*→"/sɔld/ ... fighting"). His ability to repeat phrases from the Boston Diagnostic Aphasia Examination (Goodglass & Kaplan, 1972) was somewhat impaired (5/8 correct on high-probability phrases, only 2/8 correct on low-probability phrases), with frequent intrusions of semantic paraphasias (e.g. *The phantom soared across the foggy heath*→"The phantom flew over the garden").

Elicited Naming

E.S.T. was asked to name 150 black-and-white photographs of common domestic objects grouped into 12 categories (e.g. kitchen equipment, tools). He instructed us that "these are the things that I have problems with, so it's

TABLE 4.1
A Sample of E.S.T.'s Spontaneous Speech

E.S.T. was asked to describe his working career at British Oxygen. He speaks with a definite Lancashire accent.

J.K.: "So when did you come back to Newcastle?"

E.S.T.: "I've been there twice actually ... hmm ... I went, aye I went, from there I went for British Oxygen, and British Oxygen offered me a job up here ... Of course British Oxygen's closed down over 'ruddy place ...'s a tragedy really ... well, they offered me a job there ... /kʌnfəs si wɛrə wɛrə jə/ like, I forget what, what me name was ... I could never remember /wɛrə/ name, it 'ud a lot of words on it, lotta words on it, that was it ... assistant so and so, so and so, so and so ... (laughs) ... I've often thought many times after, what the hell I was ... the manager ... what they were trying, what they were finding out was that ... if I was okay, 'n the man, the manager was going ... going to, going t'another ... to London, you see ..."

---

worth listening to!" The photographs were presented in random order, and he was given unlimited time. Although he generally indicated that he knew what each object was (either by gesture or by explication; for a bottle of shampoo, for example, he said "rub it on your head if you're washing"), he only successfully named 46% of the items. As his difficulty is in naming rather than in recognising these items, we conclude that E.S.T.'s is not an agnosic but an anomic disorder.

On many of the occasions in which he initially failed to retrieve an object's name, he correctly supplied the initial sound and number of letters of the word (e.g. *plate*→"five in it, begins with /p/"; *biscuits*→"about eight in it, its /b/"). In other instances, he repeatedly used linguistic context to try and evoke the name (e.g. *slippers*→"shoes, socks . . . have you got . . . shoes, pair of shoes . . . not a hard pair of shoes . . . take these off and put on my . . ."). Pease and Goodglass (1978) report that these were the most effective cues in attenuating word-finding difficulties (providing comprehension was intact); E.S.T. spontaneously supplied such cues and although we did not formally investigate their effectiveness, it is our impression that he was often helped in retrieving the correct word in this way.

On the Coughlan and Warrington (1978) naming tests, he named without hesitation 6/15 objects presented visually, 6/15 objects presented tactually, and 5/15 objects from oral description. As in other reported cases of "classical" anomia, therefore, our patient's word-finding difficulties would appear to be independent of the modality in which stimuli are presented (Geschwind, 1967).

Auditory Comprehension

E.S.T.'s auditory comprehension (at least of the single words corresponding to presented objects) is considerably superior to his ability to name these objects. None the less, he shows some impairment in his ability to understand abstract and low-frequency items. On the four-choice picture–word matching test of Shallice and McGill (unpublished), for example, he was 97% correct in selecting the picture to match concrete words (his single error was on the low-frequency item, rosary), compared with 60% correct on abstract words (e.g. boredom), and only 33% correct on abstract emotional words (e.g. agony) (chance = 25%). On the Coltheart synonym matching test (unpublished) he was 100% correct in judging synonymity of concrete word-pairs (e.g. magazine–journal), but 83% correct in matching abstract pairs (e.g. origin–source) (chance = 50%).

From the 150 black-and-white photographs of common domestic objects that he had previously been required to name, we selected 25 groups of four pictures that were closely related in meaning (but were neither visually nor phonologically confusable), e.g. pineapple, grapes, lemon, pear. E.S.T. was asked to point to the target picture immediately after the experimenter had named the object. He made no errors on this task, although he was considerably slower than a number of control subjects who were also tested.

Oral Reading of Single Words

On clinical tests of reading, E.S.T. managed to pronounce only 44.6% of the words of the Schonell (1942) graded word reading test successfully; on the more difficult New Adult Reading Test (Nelson & O'Connell, 1978), which is composed of uncommon irregular words, this dropped to 8% (4/50) (his four correct pronunciations were of the words *subtle, equivocal, drachm, abstemious*). Generally, his reading is very slow and laboured and is characterised by multiple attempts to pronounce the stimulus word (e.g.*appeared*→"/æpəːd/ ... /æpəːd/ ... /æpɛəd/ ... /æpɛəd/ ... it's /æpɛə/"). Except for *b/d* confusions, letter-naming is unaffected.

We next examined E.S.T.'s performance on the Coltheart et al. (1979) list of matched regular and irregular words. As E.S.T. typically produced a string of utterances for each target word, only the first response was initially counted. He was more successful in reading the regular than irregular words of the Coltheart et al. (1979) list (27/39 compared with 22/39 respectively), although the difference between the two word-types does not reach significance (McNemar's test: $N = 21$; $B = 6$). He made an average of 2.3 attempts to pronounce each irregular word and eventually gave up on 11 of them. He needed fewer attempts at regular words (an average of 1.5 attempts per word) and failed to obtain the correct pronunciation of only two. The final difference between the two word groups is significant (McNemar's test: $N = 13$; $B = 2$; $P < .05$).

The largest single category of error responses to irregular words (8/17) consisted of "regularisations" (e.g. *break*→/brik/). In addition, a number of errors on both word sets were classified as non-phonological, "orthographic" errors (3/17 on irregular words; 5/12 on regular words). All of these error responses corresponded to existing words, and involved either letter changes (e.g. *rob*→/rʌb/, *tooth*→/tiə/) or letter additions or deletions (e.g. *circuit* →səkl/, *scarce*→/skɛə/). There was a single stress error (*distress*→/'dɪstrɪs/), although this type of error was commoner when there was more opportunity for it in the polysyllabic words of the Schonell and NART lists. The remainder, which could not be unambiguously classified in one of these three categories, was assigned to a fourth, "other" category.

On occasions in which E.S.T. mispronounced the word in front of him, but spontaneously told us what he thought it meant, he was sometimes incorrect in a style that has been described for other surface dyslexic patients (e.g. *heir*→"/hɛə/ ... not horses ... there's four feet on them (*hare?*)"). There were several instances, however, in which he apparently understood at least something of the veridical meaning (e.g. *choir*→"this is easy ... /tʃ/ ... /tʃ/ ... singing ... now I'm lost with the /tʃɔ/ ... /kɔ/"). In addition, there were two examples in which the target word was both irregular and a homophone, and where it was correctly pronounced, but assigned the meaning of the other word (e.g. *soul*→"on my shoes ... /soʊl/").

Oral Reading of Non-words

E.S.T. was faster and more accurate in reading non-words than words aloud (the corpus of non-word pronunciations is shown in Appendix I). For example, he took around 14 minutes to read 80 non-words (whereas reading of 80 words from which such non-words were derived might take him well over 1 hour). He produced a total of 67/80 "appropriate" responses, in which non-words were pronounced like visually similar rhyming words (e.g. *tave* like *save* or *have*). Cases in which any constituent grapheme of the string was assigned a phonemic value which it does not receive in the same context in a real word, were regarded as "inappropriate" error responses. Half of the non-words were derived from a visually similar word set that contained both regular and irregular rhyming words (e.g. *jear* may rhyme with either *fear* or *bear*). Following Glushko (1979), these were termed "inconsistent" non-words, and were contrasted with the remainder of non-words that were derived from visually similar word sets which are consistently pronounced in a regular fashion (e.g. *jeap* rhymes with *leap, heap, reap*, etc.). Consistent and inconsistent non-words were presented in random order. Of the 33 inconsistent non-words given appropriate responses, 13/33 were pronounced like visually similar irregular words (e.g. *jear*→/dʒɛə/).[1]

Lexical Decision

The task of deciding whether a presented letter string is a real word can be achieved by accessing (in the case of a word) its lexical orthographic entry. If surface dyslexics rely on phonological recoding in lexical decision, in the same way as they are assumed to do in reading aloud, then their performance on lists of regular words/non-words should be substantially better than on lists of irregular words/pseudohomophones. On the latter lists, non-words which sound like real words should be falsely accepted as words; irregular

---

[1] According to the notion of "all-or-none" GPC assignment outlined in the introduction to this chapter, non-words should invariably be assigned pronunciations that correspond to the commonest phonemic values of their constituent graphemes. Glushko (1979) has reported that this is certainly not always the case for normal subjects: "inconsistent" non-words were sometimes pronounced like visually similar irregular words. It is also not the case for our patient: 39% of his non-word pronunciations comprised the less frequent pronunciation of the vowel grapheme or digraph.

TABLE 4.2
Lexical Decision Performance

	Regular Words Non-homophonic Non-words	Irregular Words Pseudohomophonic Non-words
Coltheart words		
False-positive rate	0.00	0.21
Hit rate	1.00	0.87
d'	4.64	1.94
Concrete nouns		
False-positive rate	0.07	0.23
Hit rate	0.93	0.93
d'	2.94	2.21

words that become non-words when pronounced regularly should be falsely rejected.

E.S.T.'s lexical decision performance on the Coltheart regular and irregular word list is shown in Table 4.2. In addition his performance on 30 regular and 30 irregular nouns, matched for frequency, length, and number of syllables, is also shown. In both cases, "pseudohomophonic" non-words that sound the same as real words (e.g. *brane*) were used as distractors with irregular words. Non-homophonic non-words acted as distractors with regular words.

For E.S.T., the two comparisons demonstrate a regularity effect in lexical decision. Only on the Coltheart words, however, does this difference attain the expected sort of magnitude. Moreover, it is clear from examination of Table 4.3 that E.S.T. is considerably better in making correct lexical decision judgements to the Coltheart words (and more especially, the irregular word set), than in determining their pronunciations.

TABLE 4.3
Comparison of Oral Reading and Lexical Decision Performances on the Coltheart et al. (1979) Words

Proportion Correct	Regular Words	Irregular Words
Oral reading	0.69	0.56
Lexical decision	1.00	0.87

Homophone Matching

E.S.T. was given the homophone matching task devised by Coltheart et al. (1983). Without sounding them aloud, he was required to judge whether word pairs and non-word pairs would sound identical if pronounced. In half of the word pairs, both words were regular, but in the remaining half, only one of the words was regular, the other was irregular. The task cannot be successfully carried out on the basis of visual similarity judgements since non-homophonic distractor pairs were matched to the homophonic pairs on this dimension (e.g. *loan–lone* vs. *loan–long*; *sew–so* vs. *new–no*; *phex–feks* vs. *brex–feks*). E.S.T.'s performance is illustrated in Table 4.4. Coltheart et al. (1983) suggest that a regularity effect should again be present on this task, because the use of phonological recoding (when and if lexical orthographic access fails) should result in the production of incorrect phonological specifications for irregular members of homophone pairs (e.g. *sew*→/su/ would be judged not to rhyme with *so*→/soɷ/). Regular word matching should succeed both when lexical orthographic access is achieved and when a rule-governed phonological code is generated by the GPC system. Regular word-matching may also be superior to non-word matching that can only successfully utilise the GPC system. The results shown in Table 4.4 indicate that E.S.T.'s regular word matching is indeed better than irregular word matching, but interestingly it is a little worse than non-word matching ($\chi^2 = 7.589$; df = 2; $P < .025$).

Tests of Written Comprehension

We have seen that there were a few examples in E.S.T.'s reading of the Schonell, NART, and Coltheart et al. words, which suggest that he understood at least something of the meaning of the target word while producing an incorrect response. Unfortunately, however, he did not usually comment on a target word's meaning, and when he did he was often not precise enough for us to be sure what he meant: e.g. *siege*→"a /sig/ ... a /sig/ ... a /sig/ ... everybody ... /sig/ ... you're all there ... everybody there ... a /sig/ and you don't want anybody else to come in."

TABLE 4.4
Homophone Matching Performance

	Regular Words	Irregular Words	Non-words
False-positive rate	0.12	0.22	0.04
Hit rate	0.98	0.78	0.96
d′	3.22	2.17	3.50

Sometimes approximate knowledge of the target word's meaning was demonstrated, but no actual reading response was produced: e.g. *thyme*→"I think I know what this is ... something to do with a bird, not a bird .. it grows ... something that grows ... it doesn't fly, it grows and smells nicely." In the initial sets of reading responses, we found in fact only two convincing examples of preserved comprehension of the target word with incorrect pronunciation (the first two examples shown in Appendix II, which gives examples of this type of response).

To investigate further E.S.T.'s reading comprehension abilities, we asked him first to define and then to pronounce the target word (following the procedure of Coltheart et al., 1983). For stimulus materials, we again used the Coltheart et al. (1979) words. As E.S.T. has a demonstrable impairment in auditory comprehension of abstract and low-frequency words, we also used our own list of 30 regular and 30 irregular concrete nouns, matched for frequency, length, and number of syllables. In addition, we took the 30 regular and 30 highly irregular ("OPD") words from Parkin's (1982, Appendix A) lists. E.S.T. was shown each word for a maximum of 2 seconds (in an attempt to combat his tendency to produce multiple responses to the target), and then asked first, to say what the word meant, and second, to pronounce it. We took only his first responses and assigned them to one of eight categories:

1. Where his comprehension and pronunciation response were both correct.
2. Where his definition fitted the target word, but the word itself was mispronounced. Mispronunciations in this category could be of any kind, either phonologically related to the target word (e.g. *gauge*→ "something about a railway ... /gɔdʒ/"), or an error in stress assignment (e.g. *canoe*→"boat, small boat that you get in (mimicks side-to-side paddling) ... no, I'll have to spell it ... /'kænu/"), or orthographically related to the target word (there were no instances of this kind).
3. Where his definition fitted the target word, but where he did not attempt a pronunciation (e.g. *snail*→"it's something with ... going into the grass ... and this damn little thing is going into there ... it's a ... little ... up and down, goes under the grass, and when the birds come and pick it off ...").
4. Where his comprehension response was incorrect, although his pronunciation was correct (e.g. *raid*→"water ... r,a,i,d ... raid ... I was thinking of rain").
5. Where his comprehension response agreed with his pronunciation, both responses being wrong. Within this category are responses that are classically associated with surface dyslexia, where the response is either phonologically related (e.g. *meringue*→"/mɛrɪŋgju/ ... sounds

like, I'll see you next week . . . /miriŋgju/ (me ring you)"), or orthographically related (e.g. *prank*→"wood . . . /plæŋk/").

6. Where his comprehension response was incorrect and where he did not attempt a pronunciation (e.g. *flock*→"a guess . . . women's clothes").
7. Where he indicated that he did not know what the word meant and he subsequently did not attempt a pronunciation, or the pronunciation supplied was incorrect, usually corresponding to a non-word (e.g. *device*→"no, I'm lost altogether . . . /dɛskraib/").
8. The final category was made up of "other" responses, which included cases where his definition may have fitted the target word, but was too vague for us to classify with reasonable confidence (e.g. *empire*→"I think it's the Queen's . . . the Queen . . . something regarding the Queen").

The proportion of responses in each category is shown in Table 4.5. Forty-seven percent of regular and 42% of irregular words were both defined correctly (to our satisfaction) and pronounced correctly. Examining the "errors" that he made on this task (where either comprehension or pronunciation or both were incorrect), we find examples in which he clearly understood something of the correct meaning of the target word while failing to produce a correct pronunciation. This phenomenon made up 11% of his total responses and 19% of his errors for the regular word set, and 11% of

TABLE 4.5
Comprehension and Pronunciation of Regular and Irregular Words

Category of Response	Proportion of Regular Words	Proportion of Irregular Words
1. "Appropriate" definition, correct pronunciation	0.47	0.42
2. "Appropriate" definition, incorrect pronunciation	0.05	0.08
3. "Appropriate" definition, no pronunciation attempted	0.06	0.03
4. "Inappropriate" definition, correct pronunciation	0.04	0.00
5. "Inappropriate" definition, incorrect pronunciation	0.06	0.07
6. "Inappropriate" definition, no pronunciation attempted	0.13	0.11
7. "No definition attempted, incorrect pronunciation	0.11	0.14
8. Other	0.07	0.14

total responses and 20% of errors for the irregular word set. The majority of mispronunciations of irregular target words were regularisations (e.g. *pier*→/paiə/). There was also one error in stress assignment, and one phonetic error. Errors on regular target words consisted mainly of phonemic paraphasias (e.g. *stupid*→/stubl/).

The "classic" surface dyslexic miscomprehension error (in category 5) occurred less often than responses which indicated some understanding of the target word (in categories 2 and 3). E.S.T.'s errors in this category mainly consisted of visual errors on regular words, with slightly more phonological than visual errors on irregular words. His visual errors always corresponded to existing words.

We next tested E.S.T.'s comprehension of written words by taking 15 of the words that he had apparently understood but had either mispronounced, or given no oral reading response, and we devised three definitions. One was correct, the second corresponded to that of a phonologically related word (his error pronunciation in most cases), and the third corresponded to that of a visually similar word: e.g. target word = *gauge*; definition = (1) distance between rails of a railway track; (2) deep valley with steep sides (*gorge*); (3) dig something out with your hands (*gouge*).

The definitions were matched as far as possible for length and semantic and syntactic complexity. Each target word was presented visually for 2 seconds; the three definitions were then read aloud to E.S.T. and he was asked to indicate the one which matched by saying either "one", "two", or "three". (The order of presentation of each type of definition was randomised across the 15 target words.) After each trial he was asked to name the target word for us. As one can see from Table 4.6, he correctly chose 12/15 definitions, but produced the right pronunciation on only half of these 12 occasions. This result would appear to suggest that E.S.T. can indeed often understand something of a visually presented target word that he cannot successfully pronounce. (Of the remaining six responses, he made no attempt at pronunciation in three instances, he produced one phonologically plausible rendering [e.g. *route*→/root/] and two orthographically related words [*tsar*→/stɑ/; *quay*→/kju/].) In the 3/15 cases where he picked the wrong definition, his phonological response was related to his incorrect choice, rather than to the correct definition. Immediately after this test, E.S.T. was again shown the 15 target words and required simply to read them aloud. There was no time limit. His performance is also shown in Table 4.6. He managed to pronounce seven of the words correctly. They had all previously been identified by definition, although only three of them had been successfully pronounced immediately post-trial.

Coltheart et al. (1983) discovered the existence of "homophone confusion" errors in surface dyslexic reading in which homophones with an irregular spelling–sound correspondence were successfully pronounced, but

TABLE 4.6
Matching Written Words with Their Correct Definitions, Followed by
Immediate and Post-trial Pronunciations

Target Word	Selected Definition	Immediate Pronunciation	Post-trial Pronunciation
thumb	√	√	√
route	√	/roɑt/	√
foot	√	√	/fut/
scene	√	√	√
tongue	√	—	/tɒŋg/
beret	berry	/bɛri/	/dɛrət/, /bɛrət/
honour	√	√	√
gauge	√	—	/gɔdʒ/
tsar	√	/stɑ/	√
cough	√	√	/koɑtʃ/
orchestra	orchard	/ɒrɪndʒ/, no	/ɔtʃɛstrə/
choir	chore	/tʃɑ/	/tʃɔ/
psalm	√	—	√
quay	√	/kju/	√
dough	√	√	/boɑ/, /bu/

nevertheless incorrectly defined (e.g. *bury*→"fruit on a tree"). They suggest that in these cases, the correct lexical orthographic specification has provided access to a lexical phonological representation (otherwise non-lexical GPC rules would have yielded incorrect phonological specifications) but has been unable to provide access to meaning. The assessment of E.S.T.'s reading comprehension abilities was extended to include the definition followed by pronunciation of 15 homophone pairs, utilising the procedure described above. One member of each pair was an irregular word (e.g. *break*); the other was regular (e.g. *brake*). The two words from a given pair were presented on separate occasions. He saw half of the regular words and half of the irregular words in one test session, and then the remainder of each word set 1 week later. There were only four instances of apparent homophone confusions; only one occurred when the target word was irregular (e.g. *mown*→"when you /moɑn/ that your breakfast is late, think of the poor fellows in Chittagong"). In the remaining cases the word targets were all regular, and we therefore cannot judge whether the phonology used to gain access to semantic descriptions was obtained via lexical or non-lexical systems.

DISCUSSION

The investigation of surface dyslexic reading has typically focused on the patient's frequent inability to read aloud single words. It is a common observation that words that do not obey standard linguistic rules of English pronunciation (so-called irregular words) are often mispronounced with a regularised, rule-governed pronunciation. It has been assumed that on such occasions, access to abstract orthographic representations in a visual input lexicon cannot be achieved and oral reading is therefore driven by a system of non-lexical GPC rules (Coltheart, 1978). Phonological specifications produced non-lexically will therefore be used to gain entry to word meanings, because access to this domain of word knowledge is unavailable via an orthographic code. Regular words, which will be correctly pronounced by non-lexical phonological assignment, will in consequence be correctly understood (providing comprehension systems are intact). On the other hand, incorrect phonologically recoded pronunciations of irregular words will not only fail to access correct semantic descriptions of target words, but will also access inappropriate descriptions in cases in which these pronunciations correspond to the spoken form of other words (e.g. *gauge*→"a big dip, /gɔdʒ/"). Thus, the formal study of surface dyslexic comprehension of single written words by Coltheart, Masterson, Byng, Prior, and Riddoch (1983), in which patients were asked to define the meaning of a target word before pronouncing it, led these authors to claim that in this acquired reading disorder "silent reading comprehension is often mediated by prior phonological recoding; *this is always the case when the phonological recoding is incorrect*" (p. 485, emphasis added).

Access to Appropriate Meaning in Surface Dyslexic Reading

The case of the patient E.S.T. (and also the patients discussed by Deloche, Andreewsky, & Desi, 1982; Goldblum; Chapter 7 in this book; Kremin, Chapter 5; Margolin, Marcel, & Carlson, Chapter 6) indicate that the strong claim made by Coltheart et al. is clearly false. We have documented examples in which E.S.T. gives an appropriate definition followed by an incorrect, apparently phonologically recoded, reading response (e.g. *gauge*→"something about a railway, /gɔdʒ/"). We would claim that on such occasions, a correct lexical orthographic code has been used to access the correct semantic description in a cognitive system, but that retrieval of corresponding lexical phonology, either via semantics or by a direct lexical orthography–phonology connection, is impaired. Hence, for pronunciation, the patient is forced to rely on phonological recoding, despite the fact that comprehension has been adequately achieved.

As we have seen, E.S.T.'s recorded difficulty in retrieving lexical-phonological forms is not confined to oral naming of written words. As one would expect, this difficulty also manifests itself in elicited naming with visual and tactual presentation, in naming from description, and in spontaneous speech. Rather than concentrating on the single dimension of oral reading performance, therefore, we might do well to look at the whole pattern of naming impairments and consider whether there is a common deficit which underlies these disorders, as indeed is suggested by Margolin, Marcel, and Carlson (Chapter 6 in this book). In the investigation of modality-independent naming disorders, impairment or impairments at a number of different levels of word retrieval have been considered. In the main, work has focused on three likely candidates (e.g. Berndt, Caramazza, & Zurif, 1983): (1) a central level of semantic integration of language; (2) transmission from information at this level to an abstract phonological level; (3) a level of abstract phonological representations. With reference to the pattern of impairments exhibited by our patient, let us consider these three loci in turn. First, let us examine the possibility of a deficit at a central semantic level.

A weight of evidence has accumulated to suggest that severe naming disorders can be associated in some patients with structural impairments of semantic descriptions, which result in the deterioration of all but broad semantic categories or "spheres" of meaning (e.g. Caramazza & Berndt, 1978; Goodglass, 1980). Thus, Zurif, Caramazza, Myerson, and Galvin (1974) demonstrated that aphasic patients with poor written and auditory comprehension and acute naming difficulties were unable to make semantically principled groupings from among triads of written words (e.g. *ferocious, trout, tiger*). Grober, Perecman, Kellar, and Brown (1980) showed that the disruption of lexical semantic knowledge in such aphasic patients is not random, however, and is far from total. Their patients could rapidly and accurately decide that *chair* belongs to the category of *furniture*, but were slower and less accurate to decide that *rug* also belongs. These aphasics also showed a tendency to accept examples that are not members of a category, but share some semantic overlap (e.g. *window* and *furniture*). Grober et al. claim that this finding reflects an almost idiosyncratic organisation of semantic knowledge, with the determinants of boundaries of category membership "ill-defined or fuzzy."

In addition, there appears to be a strong reciprocal relationship between a breakdown at a semantic level and the production of semantic paraphasias in elicited naming (Buckingham & Rekart, 1979; Gainotti, 1976). An implication of this finding is that the patient in some sense does not know that his oral response, derived from an ill-defined semantic description, is incorrect. This is most definitely not the case with E.S.T.; in confrontation naming and in spontaneous speech, he tends to produce circumlocutions rather than semantic paraphasias. That is, he not only knows what he wants to say, but, to quote William James, "the wraith of the name is in it."

In tests of auditory comprehension that did not require the production of a verbal response, E.S.T. performed at a relatively unimpaired level, at least with concrete nouns. He was, for example, able to select the correct photograph to match a spoken word from among semantically related foils.

He was able to identify pairs of concrete nouns as synonyms. On an English version of a written word sorting task, on which Lhermitte, Derouesné, and Lecours (1971) showed that patients with posterior lesions violated semantic descriptions either by grouping words that were semantically unrelated, or failing to group semantically related words, E.S.T. performed within the normal range. In the light of these admittedly few test findings, we suggest that E.S.T. does not appear to have a central lexical comprehension deficit in understanding concrete concepts, which is therefore not the primary cause for his word-finding difficulties with such items.[2] This does not of course mean that we are denying *any* influence of selective comprehension difficulties (even at the single-word level in the case of abstract words) in his oral naming deficit.

We are left then with two other candidates: impairment of access to lexical phonological representations, or impairment to the representations themselves.

There are three sources of evidence that appear to be inconsistent with (but do not rule out) the hypothesis of a deficit in output phonology. First, E.S.T. is generally able to repeat single words; he repeated the majority of the Coltheart et al. words successfully, for example, although he had great difficulty in reading them aloud. Success in single-word repetition may require relatively preserved lexical phonology, though it is also possible, as Morton and Patterson (1980) have observed, that such success can be attributed to some form of non-lexical "acoustic-phonological process," necessary for the repetition of spoken non-words. E.S.T. was indeed able to repeat non-words, though he was a little worse in doing so than in repeating words. Second, we have seen that when E.S.T. spontaneously supplies the initial sound of the word he is seeking, or is given the initial sound as a phonemic cue in tasks of confrontation naming, he can often rapidly retrieve the correct name. This would suggest, as Luria (1970) has observed, that it is in access to lexical phonology, rather than in the representations themselves, where the primary disturbance lies. Third, we should note that E.S.T. is sometimes able to read aloud irregular words that on another reading test he had been unable to pronounce. If damage has occurred at this level, therefore, it would appear to be of a transitory rather than a permanent nature. As Warrington and Shallice (1979) have argued, this pattern of unpredictable success or failure suggests an access impairment, whereas consistent failure implies structural deficits to the representations themselves. Thus, the pattern that we have observed would at least appear to reflect, to use the distinction made by Weigl and Bierwisch (1970), an impairment of performance rather than underlying phonological competence.

---

[2] We are well aware that our claim is subject to at least two important criticisms. First, that the tests of comprehension that we employed are perhaps not all that precise. Second, that the deficit in comprehension for abstract words is certainly a complication for our interpretation.

The remaining alternative states that E.S.T.'s major difficulty lies in the transmission of information from the semantic to the lexical phonological level. Although this proposal can account for the modality-independent difficulties in confrontation naming that have been observed, it *cannot* also account for the severe disturbance of irregular word reading, for the following reason. According to the model of word recognition and production that we have considered, written words can be successfully pronounced either by accessing their meanings in a semantic system, which mediates between abstract orthographic and phonological representations, or by a direct connection between lexical orthography and phonology. If the major impairment is in the transmission of information between meaning and phonology, it should therefore still be possible for oral reading to be achieved by the direct lexical route. In consequence, not only should confrontation naming be considerably worse than oral reading of irregular words, but there should also *be* no observable deficit in oral reading of irregular words, neither of which was the case for our patient. To account for the pattern of impairments exhibited by E.S.T. in terms of an access difficulty, one therefore has to postulate that his naming difficulties result from a failure to access lexical phonology from semantics, but that his dyslexic difficulties result from an additional failure to access lexical phonology from lexical orthography.

Clearly, it is more parsimonious to attribute E.S.T.'s anomic and dyslexic difficulties to a single cause. One way that allows us to do this, and yet still maintain our view that actual lexical phonological forms are relatively preserved, is by postulating that threshold levels, which must be reached for the representations to become available, are abnormally raised in our patient (see Morton & Patterson, 1980, for a similar proposal that is used to account for semantic paralexias in deep dyslexic reading). Except for their augmented thresholds, there is little wrong with the representations themselves. This kind of access difficulty would apply equally to two sources of incoming information: from semantics and from lexical orthography. It might also accord well with our observations on cueing: the heightened threshold of a particular representation will only be breached with extra information such as that conveyed by a phonemic cue. With the additional assumption that threshold levels are fluctuating rather than stable, one can also explain why E.S.T. is sometimes able to successfully pronounce an irregular word, but is unable to do so on another occasion.

Miscomprehension in Surface Dyslexic Reading

Examples in which the target word was clearly misunderstood in terms of the spoken response were present in E.S.T.'s reading. As we have seen, this type of miscomprehension has been accounted for with the assumption of difficulties in access to an orthographic input lexicon. How does this interpretation square, however, with our earlier claim that lexical ortho-graphic entries are generally spared in E.S.T.? We wish to claim that in his case, lexical orthography *is* generally accessible, both when the target word is understood and when its appropriate meaning is unavailable. In both types of response there is a failure to retrieve correct lexical phonology, and if pronunciation is required, it is usually mediated by non-lexical phonology. In examples in which the target word is misunderstood in terms of the phonologically recoded response, access to the appropriate meaning speci-fied by an orthographic code has been denied.

If the appropriate meaning specified by an orthographic code is unavail-able, it would appear that E.S.T. makes use of a number of sources of information, both orthographic and phonological, in an attempt to under-stand the target word. Thus, the majority of pronunciation errors to irregular words that were misunderstood, were phonological regularisations of the written letter string, and his definitions were tailored accordingly (e.g. *chute*→"telling you how to write ... a /tʃutə/"; *plait*→"for your teeth, /pleit/"). On the other hand, the remainder of his error responses, particularly on regular words, were visually similar to the target word, with a correspond-ing definition (e.g. *chime*→"that's the ... I know what it is ... in the ... top of a building, when you have coal ... that is ... old house with coal ... building ... that bit is the /tʃɪmni/"; *spend*→"go quickly ... /spid/").

Note that the mispronunciations in single-word reading which we classi-fied as visual errors (letter changes, additions, or deletions, in the main) always corresponded to existing words. In considering the production of visual errors in surface dyslexic reading, Coltheart et al. (1983) argued that they do not reveal the use of an "approximate visual access" strategy, discussed in relation to a similar phenomenon in "deep" dyslexia (Coltheart, 1980; Patterson, 1978). According to the approximate visual access account, visually similar lexical representations and their meanings are accessed along with those corresponding to the target. If either the actual representation or its specified semantic description is blocked in some way, then the patient's only alternative (apart from making no response at all) is to rely on visually similar counterparts. The primary argument against this provenance of visual errors in surface dyslexic reading put forward by Coltheart et al. is that visual errors can be non-word responses (even when the stimulus is a word). Non-words by definition do not have lexical entries, and therefore cannot be produced as a result of a strategy of approximate visual access.

As we have already observed, E.S.T. did not produce visual errors that could be judged to be non-words, and we speculate that for him, such errors did arise as products of a lexically determined strategy. Of course, in seeking the referent specified by the wrong semantic description, E.S.T. would still be subject to the same difficulties in arriving at its name. Interestingly, E.S.T. sometimes appeared to have accessed not only the correct meaning of the stimulus, but also the meaning of a visually similar word. In reading the word *pine*, for example, he said, "I think it's something which grows high and tall ... possibly twenty yards high ... pretty close to the next one ... a /pain/," but he seemed puzzled and rather unsure. He then wrote down the letter string *pian* and said he was also thinking about a /tʌŋki tʌŋk/, wriggling his fingers at the same time as if he were playing a piano!

Homophone Confusions with Irregularly Spelled Homophones

As already mentioned, Coltheart et al. (1983) discovered that an irregularly spelled homophone could be correctly pronounced in surface dyslexic reading, but confused with the meaning of its phonological twin (e.g. *mown*→"to be unhappy, sad"). This finding suggests that correct lexical phonology has been accessed, in this case by a direct orthography–phonology link (because phonological recoding would supply an incorrect response), although an appropriate semantic description has not been reached by its lexical orthographic entry.[3] This represents, according to Coltheart et al., a second form of "phonological reading"; that is via the output logogen system rather than via the non-lexical grapheme–phoneme system. In the course of our examination of E.S.T.'s reading abilities, we observed only three instances of homophone confusions with irregularly spelled homophones. In searching for cases in a formal test, we found a number of exemplars of homophone confusions; but these occurred, with one exception, only to words with a regular spelling–sound correspondence (e.g. *stake* →"you could have to eat ... I think it's a /steik/ of meat"). On these occasions, pronunciation could equally have been gained by non-lexical phonological recoding. Perhaps we should not be too surprised at the low incidence of this type of error, however. It is assumed that the patients

---

[3]In the light of recent findings and theories (e.g. Glushko, 1979; Marcel, 1980; Shallice, Warrington, & McCarthy, 1983), an alternative account of this phenomenon is worth considering. According to the model of the non-lexical process that we have so far considered, an irregular word like *mown* (which contains a less common pronunciation of the vowel digraph -*ow*-) will be assigned the most frequent, GPC pronunciation (e.g. /maʊn/). The correct pronunciation of such words can only be obtained by accessing word-specific phonological entries. If one assumes that the non-lexical process assigns GPCs on a probabilistic rather than all-or-none basis, however (so that less common correspondences are sometimes assigned), or if it can also operate on orthographic–phonological units larger than the grapheme and phoneme, such as the subsyllable or vowel–consonant segment (e.g. -*own*→/oʊn/ or /aʊn/), then one might expect such a non-lexical routine to sometimes supply responses of the *mown*→/moʊn/ kind. The pronunciations of irregular homophones would therefore have the same provenance (i.e. non-lexical) as the mispronunciation (and miscomprehension) errors typically described in surface dyslexia, and would not reflect an alternative form of phonological reading (i.e. via lexical phonology).

described by Coltheart et al. experience great difficulty in accessing the cognitive system via lexical orthography. If a word is *recognised* by the latter system, it can be successfully read aloud, even when it is an irregular homophone, but it may be misunderstood. E.S.T.'s major difficulty, however, lies in retrieving lexical phonology, rather than in lexical orthographic access, or even access to systems of meaning. An irregularly spelled homophone is therefore more likely to be understood than pronounced correctly.

SUMMARY

As Coltheart, Masterson, Byng, Prior, and Riddoch (1983) have observed, reading comprehension had not until recently been systematically investigated in surface dyslexia. None the less, it has been widely assumed that a semantic description is rarely attained directly from lexical orthography. Rather, as Marshall and Newcombe (1973) reported, comprehension appeared to be based solely on the phonologically recoded form of the printed word. As Shallice and Warrington (1980) have pointed out, however, phonological reading can in principle occur from impairment at one of several different stages of lexical processing: at the stage of gaining access to lexical orthography, for example, or at the stage of retrieving lexical phonology. (Note that according to the model of oral reading espoused in this chapter, impairment to the semantic system alone will not precipitate phonological reading, because a direct lexical orthography–phonology connection would still be available.)

We have described a patient, E.S.T., who appears to rely on phonological recoding in reading aloud, but who nevertheless sometimes demonstrates correct understanding of the presented word, even if it is mispronounced. This phenomenon is reported by other authors in this book, and has also been investigated by Deloche, Andreewsky, and Desi (1982). We have argued that the primary impairment in E.S.T.'s case is in gaining access to lexical phonology rather than to lexical orthography. As one might expect from this hypothesis, the difficulties that he faces are not confined to oral reading, but are also manifested in other domains of language use that require access to lexical phonology, such as elicited naming and spontaneous speech. Like Margolin, Marcel, and Carlson (Chapter 6 in this book), we would emphasise the connection between the nature of this type of oral reading disorder and acute disturbances of naming.

The common thread that links all of the patients who have so far been described in the work on surface dyslexia is the presence of phonological reading. We have argued, however, that there will always be a number of ways of producing a particular symptom. Thus, although these patients show this phenomenon, with the pattern of oral reading that it characteristically produces, an obvious distinction can be made between the patients in their ability to access the semantic system in the normal fashion in oral reading. We therefore wish to conclude with the caveat that to draw these apparently dissociable disorders together under the umbrella of the term "surface dyslexia" (albeit as "input" or "output" forms of the same syndrome) may prove, in the light of future theoretical and empirical research, to be of questionable validity.

ACKNOWLEDGEMENTS

The authors wish to express their gratitude to E.S.T. for his time and patience in the course of this study. They also wish to thank Mrs. Susan Clark (Department of Speech Therapy, General Hospital, Newcastle-upon-Tyne) for her considerable assistance in testing E.S.T., and Professor John Hankinson (Regional Neurological Centre, Newcastle-upon-Tyne) for his permission to cite neurological details of the case. Finally they wish to thank Dr. Ruth Lesser for her comments on the manuscript. This research was supported by a Project Grant to the first author from the Medical Research Council.

REFERENCES

Berndt, R. S., Caramazza, A., & Zurif, E. (1983). Language functions: Syntax and semantics. In S. J. Segalowitz (ed.), *Language Functions and Brain Organization*. New York: Academic Press.

Buckingham, H. W., & Rekart, D. M. (1979). Semantic paraphasia. *Journal of Communication Disorders*, **12**, 197–209.

Caramazza, A., & Berndt, R. S. (1978). Semantic and syntactic processes in aphasia: A review of the literature. *Psychological Bulletin*, **85**, 898–918.

Coltheart, M. (1978). Lexical access in simple reading tasks. In G. Underwood (ed.), *Strategies of Information Processing*. London and New York: Plenum Press.

Coltheart, M. (1980). Reading, phonological encoding and deep dyslexia. In M. Coltheart, K. E. Patterson, & J. C. Marshall (eds.), *Deep Dyslexia*. London: Routledge & Kegan Paul.

Coltheart, M., Besner, D., Jonasson, J.-T., & Davelaar, E. (1979). Phonological encoding and the lexical decision task. *Quarterly Journal of Experimental Psychology*, **31**, 489–507.

Coltheart, M., Masterson, J., Byng, S., Prior, M., & Riddoch, J. (1983). Surface dyslexia. *Quarterly Journal of Experimental Psychology*, **35A**, 469–495.

Coughlan, A. D., & Warrington, E. K. (1978). Word comprehension and word retrieval in patients with localised cerebral lesions. *Brain*, **101**, 163–185.

Deloche, G., Andreewsky, E., & Desi, M. (1982). Surface dyslexia: A case report and some theoretical implications to reading models. *Brain and Language*, **15**, 12–31.

Gainotti, G. (1976). The relationship between semantic impairment in comprehension and naming in aphasic patients. *British Journal of Disorders of Communication*, **11**, 57–61.

Geschwind, N. (1967). The varieties of naming errors. *Cortex*, **3**, 97–112.

Glushko, R. J. (1979). The organization and activation of orthographic knowledge in reading aloud. *Journal of Experimental Psychology: Human Perception and Performance*, **5**, 674–691.

Goodglass, H. (1980). Disorders of naming following brain injury. *American Scientist,* **68,** 647–655.

Goodglass, H., & Kaplan, E. (1972). *The Assessment of Aphasia and Related Disorders.* Philadelphia: Lea & Febiger.

Grober, E., Perecman, E., Kellar, L., & Brown, J. (1980). Lexical knowledge in anterior and posterior aphasics. *Brain and Language,* **10,** 318–330.

Lhermitte, F., Derouesné, J., & Lecours, A. R. (1971). Contribution à l'étude des troubles semantiques dans l'aphasie. *Revue Neurologique,* **125,** 81–101.

Luria, A. R. (1970). *Traumatic Aphasia.* The Hague: Mouton.

Marcel, A. J. (1980). Surface dyslexia and beginning reading: A revised hypothesis of the pronunciation of print and its impairments. In M. Coltheart, K. E. Patterson, & J. C. Marshall (eds.), *Deep Dyslexia.* London: Routledge & Kegan Paul.

Marshall, J. C., & Newcombe, F. (1973). Patterns of paralexia. *Journal of Psycholinguistic Research,* **2,** 175–199.

Morton, J. (1979). Word recognition. In J. Morton, & J. C. Marshall (eds.), *Psycholinguistics Series 2.* London: Elek.

Morton, J., & Patterson, K. E. (1980). A new attempt at an interpretation, or an attempt at a new interpretation. In M. Coltheart, K. E. Patterson, & J. C. Marshall (eds.), *Deep Dyslexia.* London: Routledge & Kegan Paul.

Nelson, H. E., & O'Connell, A. (1978). Dementia: The estimation of premorbid intelligence levels using the new adult reading test. *Cortex,* **14,** 234–244.

Parkin, A. J. (1982). Phonological recoding in lexical decision: Effects of spelling–sound regularity depend on how regularity is defined. *Memory and Cognition,* **10,** 43–53.

Patterson, K. E. (1978). Phonemic dyslexia: Errors of meaning and meaning of errors. *Quarterly Journal of Experimental Psychology,* **30,** 587–601.

Pease, D. E., & Goodglass, H. (1978). The effects of cuing on picture naming in aphasia. *Cortex,* **14,** 178–189.

Schonell, F. J. (1942). *Backwardness in Basic Subjects.* Edinburgh: Oliver & Boyd.

Shallice, T., & Warrington, E. K. (1980). Single and multiple component central dyslexic syndromes. In M. Coltheart, K. E. Patterson, & J. C. Marshall (eds.), *Deep Dyslexia.* London: Routledge & Kegan Paul.

Shallice, T., Warrington, E. K., & McCarthy, R. (1983). Reading without semantics. *Quarterly Journal of Experimental Psychology,* **35A,** 111–138.

Venezky, R. L. (1970). *The Structure of English Orthography.* The Hague: Mouton.

Warrington, E. K., & Shallice, T. (1979). Semantic access dyslexia. *Brain,* **102,** 43–63.

Weigl, E., & Bierwisch, M. (1970). Neuropsychology and linguistics: Topics of common research. *Foundations of Language,* **6,** 1–18.

Wijk, A. (1966). *Rules of Pronunciation for the English Language.* Oxford: Oxford University Press.

Zurif, E. B., Caramazza, A., Myerson, R., & Galvin, J. (1974). Semantic feature representations for normal and aphasic language. *Brain and Language,* **1,** 167–187.

APPENDIX I

Oral Reading of 40 "Consistent" and 40 "Inconsistent"
Non-words

Consistent Non-words		Inconsistent Non-words	
heef	/hif/	toof	/tuf/
rane	/reɪn/	rone	/roʊn/
munt	/mʌnt/	rint	/rɛnt/
sede	/sid/	lere	/lɛə/
sond	/sin/	nind	/naɪnd/
fent	/fɛnt/	pimb	/pɪm/
pench	/pɛntʃ/	gouch	/gaʊtʃ/
prain	/preɪn/	preak	/preɪk/
joon	/dʒun/	bour	/bɔ/
sade	/seɪd/	sead	/sid/
grolm	/groʊl/	groll	/grɒl/
wosh	/wɒʃ/	nush	/nʌʃ/
bret	/brɛt/	brut	/brʌt/
moop	/mup/	mook	/muk/
gorp	/gɔp/	gowl	/gaʊl/
prold	/prɒld/	gront	/graʊnt/
forch	/fɔtʃ/	fouth	/faʊʃ/
doon	/dun/	snood	/snud/
taze	/teɪz/	tave	/teɪv/
cath	/kæə/	coth	/kɒə/
yean	/jun/	yead	/jəːd/
sheef	/ʃif/	shome	/ʃ . . ʃoʊm/
stode	/stoʊd/	stose	/stoʊt stoʊs/
pold	/pɒld/	polf	/pɒlf/
jamb	/dʒæm/	jomb	/dʒɒm/
hest	/hɛst/	nost	/nɒst/
beed	/bid/	gaid	/geɪd/
pode	/poʊd/	pove	/poʊv/
spon	/spɒn/	spow	/spaʊ/
coom	/kum/	stoll	/stoʊl/
trewn	/trun/	trown	/troʊn/
grell	/grɛl/	stoul	/stoʊl/
bire	/baɪə/	bive	/baɪv/
joot	/dʒut/	soad	/soʊd/
suff	/suf sʌf/	wull	/wɒl/
feech	/fitʃ/	fough	/faʊʃ/
chail	/tʃeɪl/	pould	/poʊld/
sneal	/sneɪl/	dreat	/drɛt/
pealth	/pil . . pɛlə/	peath	/pɛə piə/
jeap	/dʒip/	jear	/dʒɛə/

APPENDIX II

Examples in Which E.S.T. "Appropriately" Defined,
But Mispronounced the Target Word

soloist	/soɑlɪst/ ... singing /soɑlɪst/ /soɑlɪst/ ... he's a /soɑlɪst/.
steak	I'm going to eat something ... it's beef ... you can have a /sə/ ... different ... costs more ... a different da di da ... used to know ... in Yankee land ... great big ... it's ridiculous ... far better with a small size ... with potatoes ... things which cost more are often more tasty ... /skɪp/ /skeɪp/.
shampoo	Don't need much, haven't got much on my head ... if I wanted to wash ... /'ʃægən/.
spear	It's a black man ... and they have a /spi/ ... /speɪd/ fighting, it's a ... /spɛə/.
trout	That I'd eat it ... it's a fish ... and just after the war in London ... I thought I'd get one ... didn't have things like that ... /traɪət/ ... /trit/ ... /treət/ ... /troɑt/ ... /troɑt/ ... /troɑət/ ... /troɑt/ ... /trɒt/ ... /troɑt/ ... /troɑt/ ... fish.
stupid	/stju/ ... /stjʌbl/ ... /stjubl/ ... six in it ... if it's something, a fellow is a bit thick ... he doesn't understand things ... /stʌbl/.
thumb	Something to eat, no, on your hands ... /ɵʌmp/, /ɵrə/ not /ɵʌmp/.
canoe	Boat, small boat that you get in (mimicks side-to-side paddling) ... no I'll have to spell it ... /'kaenu/.
foot	Body, and it's my shoe ... f, o, o ... or is it /fə/ ... /ud/, eating? ... /fut/.
route	Driving in your car, and you've come to ... on the ground ... r, o, u ... /raɑt/ ... no, putting everybody in a /raɑt/.
pier	In the sea, we haven't got one here, but we have one in ... falling down now ... begins with p ... /paɪə/ ... (drew a picture of a pier) ... /paɪ/.
tongue	Mouth ... something ... have to spell it to myself ... t, o something with teeth ... /tʌnɪkəl/ ... where I'm supposed to be at the moment (showed dental appointment card).
grill	Eating, cooking, /graef/ ... /grɪf/ ... can't even spell it now, but that's what I was thinking, but it could be another.
gauge	That is something about a railway ... that's as much as I've got, train /gɔdʒ/.
tsar	That's a damn good 'un ... many years ago, before you and I were born, in Russia ... one of the Billy Bloggs was whatever he was ... he's the, what they used to call the Queen, or the

King ... they used to kill each other off ... busy place ... I can't spell it ... it begins with t ... the Queen ... the King of Russia ... /ti/ ... /stɑ/ /tɑ/.

wharf   Yes, that's er ... something with river ... and it's ... in a river ... boat ... something about boats ... /wɔd/, /hɔd/.

beret   That I don't know ... it's either something to eat, stuff that grows half way up a tree, not an apple, like an apple (*berry?*) ... I'm only guessing ... or a jacket, on your head ... /dɛrək/ ... /bɛrək/.

mauve   /mɑv/, a /mɑv/, a /mɑv/ jacket, it's the colour of a ... a /mɑv/ lady ... I don't suppose a fellow would have a /mɑv/ on ... if I mixed blue and red I'd probably have /mɑv/.

5 Routes and Strategies in Surface Dyslexia and Dysgraphia

H. Kremin

Surface dyslexia was first described by Marshall and Newcombe in 1973. Carrying out a taxonomic analysis of patients' reading errors, the authors distinguished two subjects whose paralexias resulted from a "partial failure" in the application of grapheme–phoneme correspondence rules (GPCs). Later, Marshall (1976) defined four features of surface dyslexia:

1. "Can read (some) nonsense syllables."
2. "Errors are typically phonologically similar to the stimulus."
3. "Errors are frequently phonologically possible but non-existent lexical forms."
4. "Semantic reading of the visual stimulus is determined by the (frequently erroneous) phonology of the response." (p. 114)

Subsequent research on reading disorders became more and more a matter of theoretical concern. Surface dyslexia and deep dyslexia—both originally described as patterns of reading errors—were used as prototypes for the description of processes of reading. Indeed, most of the authors concerned with reading assumed that there are two routes for reading a given word: a "direct" route from print to meaning and a "phonological" route by grapheme-to-phoneme conversion. In the framework of the information-processing approach the direct route is lexical, namely bypassing pre-lexical phonology and retrieving the phonology of words from the lexicon as a whole. In contrast, the phonological route is considered to be a non-lexical and rule-governed process: the letter string is pronounced by the application of grapheme-to-phoneme translation, and so words and nonsense syllables are treated alike. This second reading route allows access to semantics only *after* the application of GPCs (probably) by auditory checking procedures.

Both routes yield correct pronunciations for regular words, but only the direct lexical route would guarantee the correct pronunciation of irregular words. Indeed, Shallice and Warrington (1980) presented a case of surface dyslexia whose deficit was limited to the reading of irregular words. This patient, R.O.G., thus seems to represent a purer syndrome than J.C. and S.T., the two principal cases of Marshall and Newcombe (1973).

In more recent studies on new cases (Deloche, Andreewsky, & Desi, 1982; Kremin, 1980) data tend to accumulate that cannot easily be dealt with in the framework of a purely non-lexical treatment of information: although these patients used grapheme-to-phoneme translation for oral reading, their reading errors showed an influence of the part of speech dimension and erroneous responses were often self-corrected. Furthermore, in one patient the error pattern for words and non-words was not the same, and many words that could not be read aloud were none the less understood (Kremin, 1980). These results suggest—because of the involvement of lexical dimensions—that language disturbances other than the total unavailability of the direct lexical route might play a role in grapheme-to-phoneme reading. I therefore claimed that the typical error pattern of surface dyslexics' oral reading does not result from a single component syndrome (Kremin, 1982). I tentatively proposed instead that surface dyslexic reading may result from two different underlying causes: a disruption at the level of visual word recognition (which was the standard interpretation of the syndrome) *or* a disruption at the level of post-lexical phonological output (which seemed to apply more typically to our patients' reading behaviour—Kremin, 1980, 1982).

The purpose of this chapter is to furnish more data for such a view. I describe a patient whose reading errors were mainly phonological in nature and argue that, in this case, the oral reading pattern is due to a functional lesion occurring at a later stage than the level of visual word recognition; in the terminology of Morton and Patterson (1980), which I follow, this stage is referred to as the "visual input logogen system."

CASE REPORT

H.A.M., a 35-year-old, right-handed woman with high-school education, had a cerebral accident on 25 March 1980, while giving birth.[1] The

---

[1]H.A.M. was seen in April 1980. At that time I just started to speculate about a possible relationship between surface dyslexia and surface dysgraphia (see Kremin, 1980). I therefore administered *separate* lists for the dictation of words and for the dictation of nonsense syllables. This was done in order to "prevent" the patient from using a non-lexical transcoding strategy in writing words. (Such peripheral writing strategy may be reinforced by the presentation of mixed stimuli.) H.A.M.'s surface dysgraphic writing performances were discussed at the meeting of "Arbeitsgemeinschaft für Aphasieforschung und -behandlung," Maastricht, 1980.

neuropsychological standard examination (see Boller & Hécaen, 1979) was conducted in the second half of April and revealed the following characteristics: The patient had no problems with orientation in time and space. Auditory comprehension of isolated words (to match with pictures) was well preserved. Verbal comprehension in terms of execution of commands was perfect for oral and written material. The patient showed good remote episodic memory. Her short-term memory as assessed by digit span was very poor in the beginning but improved to four digits 1 month after her accident. Her oral naming was poor in all modalities (visual, auditory, tactile, varying between 20% and 25% correct responses). On the Verbal Fluency Test, she produced 18 words (normal). There were no signs of apraxia, agnosia, or acalculia. No disturbance of sensitivity was noted but the motricity of the face was weak on the right side. Examination of the visual fields showed a right homonymous hemianopia. In the middle of April the patient's spontaneous language showed phonemic paraphasias, (rare) verbal substitutions, and word-finding difficulties, but her language seemed rather normal when recorded on 5 May 1980. A CT scan showed a spontaneous hyperdensity in the parieto-temporal region (middle and posterior territory of the left Sylvian artery).

Special testing of H.A.M.'s reading, writing, naming, and repetition performances started on 25 April—1 month after her accident—and was conducted for 10 days.

READING

When administered the "Standard Reading Test" of our laboratory (see Hécaen & Kremin, 1976) H.A.M. produced only 10% errors for letters, 8% for words, and 30% for nonsense syllables. Moreover, all her initial reading errors were successfully self-corrected. As we could not detect any problems concerning her comprehension of written material, H.A.M. would hardly have become a "case" if we had not been intrigued by the fact that, during "screening," she seemed to write dictated nonsense syllables more easily than dictated words. When finally given a list of irregular words (see Goldblum, Chapter 7 in this book, for descriptive details of the list), the patient's reading errors turned out to be similar to those produced by F.R.A. (B.F.), our first patient with surface dyslexia (see Kremin, 1980, and Goldblum, Chapter 7. Please note that F.R.A. and B.F. are one and the same patient). Indeed, H.A.M. read these words more successfully than B.F., committing only 21 errors on 60 words. As for B.F., however, the majority of H.A.M.'s oral reading errors were "phonological" in nature, that is, they can be accounted for by the application of GPCs (irrespective of the conventional pronunciation of the letter string) and/or by a partial failure in the application of these rules. The patient's reading errors on this list are reproduced in Table 5.1.

TABLE 5.1
H.A.M.'s Reading Errors on Irregular Words

Stimulus	French Pronunciation	English Translation	H.A.M.'s Oral Reading Response
phénix	/feniks/	phoenix	→/feni/ /fenir/ /fenir/ je ne comprends pas ce que cela veut dire.
album	/albɔm/	album	→/alb/ /albym/.
stagner	/stagne/	to stagnate	→/sta/ /sta/ olala! ... un stagiaire ... ça pourrait être un stagiaire oui.
ration	/rasjɔ̃/	ration	→/ra/ /ratj/ /ratjɔ̃/ /ra ... **ra-sjɔ̃** une **ration**
anguille	/agij/	eel	→une aiguille.
rhum	/rɔm/	rum	→du /rym/ (rhume).
bénitier	/benitje/	holy water basin	→/beni/ **bénitier**.
dompteur	/dɔ̃tœr/	tamer	→/dɔ̃ptœr./
condamné	/kɔ̃dane/	condemned	→kɔ̃damme/**condamné**.
initier	/inisje/	to initiate	→/ini/ /iniks/ **initier**.
cation	/katjɔ̃/	cation	→/ka/ **cation** qu'est-ce que c'est ce mot? ... /kasjɔ̃/ ...
quotient	/kɔsjã/	quotient	→continent non ça va pas ... conscient ... conscient oui.
tas	/ta/	pile	→/tak/ /tas/ /**ta**/ un **tas**.
chrétien	/kretjɛ̃/	christian	→/ʃe/ /ʃe/ **chrétien**.
lien	/ljɛ̃/	link	→/li/ /li-ã/ le **lien**.
moelle	/mwal/	marrow	→/moɛl/ **moelle**.
cholestérol	/kolɛsterol/		→/ʃolɛste/ **cholestérol**.
élection	/elɛksjɔ̃/	election	→/elɛktjɔ̃/ /elɛktjɔ̃/ /elɛks/ ah! c'est pas pareil! les **élections**.
régner	/renje/	to rule	→/reg/ régler non! **régner!**
fuel	/fjul/	fuel	→/fyɛl/ /fyl/ comment on appelle ça ... du /fwal/ non pas du /fwal/ (do you know what it means?) pour chauffer ... du /fyl/ du /fwal/ du /pwal/ (poêle?) non on ne l'appelle pas comme ça ... (examiner: du /fjul/) oui du **fuel**.
toast	/tost/	toast	→/toa/ /twal/ non! ... /twal/ (toile?) ... qu'est-ce que ça veut dire ça un **toast** on le mange ... un /tɔks/ non pas un /tɔks/ un /taks/ non plus ... /toask/ ça ne se prononce pas comme ça /to/ ... un /toast/.

H.A.M.'s oral reading responses are printed in **bold** type if they correctly reproduce the target word.

Our working hypothesis was that H.A.M.—as well as B.F.—may belong to the second type of surface dyslexic reader who is characterised by "normal" semantic access via the visual input logogens but in whom (for reasons to be described) oral output is often achieved by assembling phonology on the basis of left-to-right reading of the letter string.

H.A.M.'s oral reading was thus analysed with regard to linguistic components of the written stimuli. We furthermore tested the patient's comprehension of written words and compared oral output from reading with the oral output from other tasks such as repetition and naming. The patient's performances in writing are also discussed in more detail.

The Influence of Linguistic Variables

It is now a generally accepted view that the regularity of word spellings exhibits a crucial influence on the reading performances that result from a non-lexical reading routine, that is from left-to-right assignment of a sound-form to a given written letter string (by correspondences between single graphemes and phonemes and/or between clusters more complex than the single unit). Accordingly nonsense syllables would be read as well as words with regular spelling-to-sound associations. Moreover, such a reading routine should not depend on lexical parameters for the reading of words. We therefore checked for the influence of lexical dimensions on our patient's oral reading of regular words.

It can be seen from Table 5.2 that H.A.M.'s oral reading was not influenced by either the part-of-speech or the concrete/abstract dimension or the frequency of the presented regular words. If we compare the patient's oral reading of regular and irregular words, the latter seem to be more error prone: 19/160 = 12% errors on regular words (Table 5.2); 21/60 = 35% errors on irregular words (see p. 107).

The Influence of Meaningfulness on Oral Reading

We checked for the influence of stimulus length of the visual input in terms of number of letters. According to the standard interpretation of surface dyslexia words are (often or mainly) read as if they were nonsense syllables, that is, without semantic access via orthography. Thus the meaningfulness of the presented letter string should not play a crucial role for the reading of items of same length. H.A.M. was thus administered another 220 words,

TABLE 5.2
H.A.M.'s Errors in Reading of Regular Words (List I)

High-frequency words (N = 40)	7 (17.5%)
Low-frequency words (N = 40)	3 (7.5%)
Concrete nouns (N = 20)[a]	4 (20%)
Abstract nouns (N = 20)[a]	2 (10%)
Function words (N = 40)[a]	3 (7.5%)

[a]Lists contain stimuli of various frequencies that are balanced across the three lists.

TABLE 5.3
Oral Reading of Words and Non-words (List II): Influence of Number of Letters

% Error	I (2–4)	II (5–8)	III (9 and More)
Total number of items (N = 220)	(N = 32)	(N = 119)	(N = 69)
Words: 24%	9%	28%	23%
Total number of items (N = 100)	(N = 21)	(N = 64)	(N = 15)
Non-words: 38%	14%	41%	60%

including many long words, and 100 nonsense syllables that were derived from words by substitution of one or two phonemes. It can be seen from Table 5.3 that the length of the letter string was a crucial variable for dissociating the reading of words from the reading of nonsense syllables: H.A.M.'s reading of isolated words seemed little influenced by the number of constituent letters whereas her oral reading of nonsense syllables seemed to be systematically influenced by the length in letters of the stimuli. Because the number of items in each category is not balanced—this is a *post-hoc* analysis—we did a statistical analysis of the data (standard Bayesian inference methods). The comparison of the patient's oral reading of short items (group I, with 2–4 letters) did not yield statistical significance with regard to meaningfulness ($P = .30$). The reading of longer letter strings, however, differed significantly in this respect with words being read more successfully than nonsense syllables ($P = .05$ for group II; $P = .003$ for group III).

We also analysed the influence of stimulus length in terms of number of syllables of the oral output. The descriptive data (which are represented in Table 5.4) resemble those with regard to length in terms of constituent letters.

TABLE 5.4
Oral Reading of Words and Non-words (List II): Influence of Number of Syllables

% Error	1	2	3	4 and More
Total number of items (N = 220)	(N = 46)	(N = 86)	(N = 64)	(N = 24)
Words	11%	24%	33%	17%
Total number of items (N = 100)	(N = 28)	(N = 39)	(N = 33)	—
Non-words	18%	44%	52%	—

From the foregoing data it is thus not possible to conclude whether the found effect of length is due to a problem of visual input or of oral output. A further comparison of oral output in reading and in repetition should answer this question (see later).

In fact, the meaningfulness of the letter string did not only play a role when first erroneous responses were considered but also with regard to the patient's subsequent reading behaviour. Indeed, 70% of the initial reading errors on words were successfully self-corrected as opposed to only 25% successful self-corrections on nonsense syllables. (Note that all but one attempt at self-correction on words resulted in a correct final response.) This difference is not an important detail per se (because successful self-corrections on words may also occur, we think by chance, through the use of "auditory checking procedures"; I discuss this particular point later in more detail). But H.A.M.'s reading of nonsense syllables resulted, with only one exception, in the production of nonsense syllables. Because the non-word stimuli differed from real words in only one or two phonemes, one would, however, expect many more nonsense syllables to be (mis-)corrected into words if the patient's strategy for self-correction depended only on the (secondary) analysis of the auditory input from the oral reading response.

(Remember also that most of the non-words were visually rather close to real words. Nevertheless the patient did not misperceive them as words. Consider, for example, the non-word *esquiman*, which differs only slightly from the word *esquimau*. H.A.M.'s reading of this nonsense syllable, however, resulted in another non-word (→/ɛskimãs/).

Finally, it should be underlined that on 12 occasions H.A.M. spontaneously read a target word with the corresponding (indefinite) article in French: *langouste*→"une langouste", *écrevisse*→"une écrevisse." Note that producing the article indicates that the patient knows that the target is a noun. This knowledge, however, is not supposed to be forthcoming from the non-lexical route of phonological reading.

Analysis of Reading Errors

We analysed the "nature" of the patient's oral reading errors (list II). We considered whether her errors were visual or phonological, a combination of both, or purely "syllabic" (that is, part of the stimulus was produced and then "aborted" for fluent reproduction). The results that are represented in Table 5.5 indicate that H.A.M. produced more phonological than visual errors on both words and nonsense syllables. The "nature" of the reading errors thus does not seem to reveal a different reading behaviour with regard to the meaningfulness of the letter string.

Independently of the nature of the reading errors (visual, phonological, etc.), H.A.M. almost exclusively produced neologisms. We therefore checked

TABLE 5.5
Oral Reading of Words and Non-words: Error Analysis (% Error of Total Errors)

	Self-correction	Visual	Phonological	Visual/ Phonological	Syllabic	Omission	Other
Words	70%	30%	51%	2%	13%	0	4%
Non-words	25%	31%	50%	17%	3%	0	0

for a possible relationship between error source and successful self-correction on words. It turns out that H.A.M. successfully self-corrected all her syllabic readings but none of the (few) mixed (visual/phonological) errors. Moreover, she successfully self-corrected 73% of her "visual" errors and 71% of her phonological errors. This pattern, together with the high overall percentage of self-correction, suggests that H.A.M.'s "visual" errors do not occur at the level of the visual input logogens. As pointed out and discussed in more detail in several other chapters in this book (e.g. Temple, Chapter 11; Derouesné & Beauvois, Chapter 16; and Saffran, Chapter 3), "visual" errors may also occur either at a later stage within the direct route or within the phonological route itself. Because of the almost parallel error pattern for words *and* non-words we would locate both the patient's visual and phonological errors within the non-lexical reading routine. Note, however, that the patient attempted to self-correct words more often and more successfully than non-words. (I come back to this point later.) A rather typical error in reading words (but not non-words) was "syllabic" reading, that is, she would start to pronounce the first syllable(s) of a letter string, "abort" her production and then self-correct herself with reference to the lexicon, e.g. *Birmanie* /birmani/ →/birmã/ "Birmanie"; *cholestérol* /kɔlesterɔl/→ʃolɛs/ "cholestérol". H.A.M. rarely produced multiple answers (and if so, only on irregular words). Generally she produced the target correctly, produced one error, or produced one error with a successful self-correction following immediately. Her oral reading errors on real words resulted (with only four exceptions) in nonwords; her oral reading of non-words, with one exception, resulted in the production of non-words. Her numerous phonological errors seem to depend on two different factors:

1. In reading words and non-words the patient had severe problems with the application of the correct GPC rule. In fact, she seemed to apply these rules rather randomly and without context sensitivity, e.g. *ovac* /ovak/→"ovas"; *docile* /dɔsil/ (submissive)→/doki/ "docile"; *algérien* /alʒerjẽ/ (algerian)→ /alge/ "algérien"; *gorison* /gorisɔ̃/→ /ʒorisɔ̃/; etc.
2. In reading words the patient often applied a spelling-out strategy from

left to right, thus misregarding the conventional pronunciation of words, e.g. *moelle* /mwal/ (marrow)→/mɔɛl/ *moelle*. Left-to-right reading seems to be indeed the main source of errors on words even when they are comprehended as shown by the patient's comment, e.g. *fuel*→ /fuɛl/ ... /fyl/ "comment on appelle ça ... du /fwal/ non pas du /fwal/" (do you know what it means?) "pour chauffer ... du /fyl/ du /fwal/ du /pwal/" (poêle?) "non on ne l'appelle pas comme ça" (examiner: du /fjul/) "oui du *fuel*."

This left-to-right reading would "explain" why H.A.M.'s oral reading does not depend solely on the regularity (vs. irregularity) of the presented words, but also on the "degree of orthographic ambiguity" of the presented stimulus. This notion was introduced by Beauvois and Derouesné (1981) for their analysis of surface dysgraphia. Ambiguous letter strings (words *and* non-words) would be those where the choice between possible grapheme–phoneme transcodings is determined by sequential conversion rules (they thus contrast with irregular words that require lexical knowledge for correct pronunciation). It seems plausible that the notion of orthographic ambiguity also plays a role for oral reading by a non-lexical routine. If so, it may explain the similarity of H.A.M.'s error pattern on words and non-words: the subject who proceeds—for oral production—by a strict left-to-right analysis of the letter string will know the adequate phoneme for the letter *g*, for example, only *after* having considered the following context ($g + a$→/ga/ but $g + e$→ /ʒe/). Perhaps the patient has "treated" (at least sometimes) only those letters that are pronounced right away without sequential context sensitivity. H.A.M.'s syllabic reading, together with her numerous self-corrections, seems to substantiate such a view; for example:

Birmanie (birmani)→/birmã/ "birmanie"
garde-manger (gardmãʒe)→/ʃa/ ʒar /ʒardmãʒe/ "garde-manger"
docile (dosil)→/doki/ "docile"
douane (duan)→/duã/ "douane"
algérien (alʒerjẽ)→/alge/ "algérien".

H.A.M.'s oral reading performance on *irregular* words fits into the general pattern described above: she committed 24% visual, 52% phonological, and 19% mixed visual/phonological errors. However, the percentage of successful self-correction (52%) was lower than on the regular words (or list II: 70%). One possible explanation is that the left-to-right reading strategy is less likely to be a successful *self-prompt* to attain the correct output logogen for irregular words. (It seems to be indeed the degree of orthographic ambiguity that may account for H.A.M.'s even better performance on list I—92% final correct readings.) The words of this list are in fact "extremely" regular, that is, there are hardly any letter clusters of orthographic ambiguity. This composition, however, is fortuitous because Beauvois and Derouesné's (1981) variable of orthographic ambiguity was not taken into account. The patient's rare misreadings on this list may indeed be best explained by this variable, e.g. *divin*→"divine", *haut*→"haute", *cambrioleur*→/kam/ /kãbri/ "cambrioleur", *genre*→/gãrə/ "genre."

It should be noted that the patient spontaneously commented on the (two) occasions on which she could not recognise the printed word: *phénix* (phoenix)→/feni/ fenir/ fenir/ . . . "je ne comprends pas ce que cela veut dire" (I do not understand what it means); *cation* (cation)→/ka/ "*cation* . . . qu'est ce que c'est ce mot? . . . /kasjõ/ . . ."

On some other rare occasions the patient tried to "guess" a word, e.g. *stagner*→/sta/ /sta/ "olala! . . . un stagiaire . . . ça pourrait être un stagiaire" (person under instruction); *quotient*→"continent non ça va pas . . . conscient . . . conscient oui." We think that this guessing happened when, exceptionally, the *correct* visual input logogen could not be activated. Knowing, however, that the stimulus was a word, the patient would try to assign some meaning to it on the basis of *visual* resemblance with the written word. What seems to be important, however, with regard to this (rather exceptional) reading behaviour is the fact that H.A.M. did not resort to the grapheme–phoneme conversion that was at her disposal. It thus seems that on the rare occasions where the visual input logogen could not be correctly accessed, H.A.M. behaved like a "non-surface dyslexic" patient and produced a visual whole word error.

Oral Reading of Sentences

H.A.M.'s reading of sentences was worse than and different from her reading of isolated words. She produced a considerable number of whole-word substitutions, some of them having a visual/semantic relation to the target word; for example, *débordent* (overflow)→"débouchent" (to open a bottle, to discharge); *vache* (cow)→"vanne" (water gate); *ferme* (farm)→"fermier" (farmer). Moreover, her phonemic difficulties in word production became more pronounced as documented by numerous entanglements of the "conduction type" (e.g. *locomotive*→"colomotive"; *caravanes*→"a . . . cara-na non! caravanes"). The patient tried to overcome these difficulties by a syllabic reading strategy; for example, *le sacristain fait sonner le bourdon*→"le sa . . . la sa-crista . . . sacristain fait sonner le bourdon . . . bour-don . . . le sacristain . . . sas-cristain fait sorner . . . so- oh! je vais y arriver! . . . le sacristain fait so-nner le bour-don."

COMPREHENSION OF WRITTEN MATERIAL

Lexical Decisions

H.A.M. missed only one word in a lexical decision task in which she had to discriminate words (concrete and abstract nouns of low frequency) from visually similar non-words (N = 90).

Written Comprehension of Single Words

The patient did perfectly on the concrete and on the abstract words of a written word-association test (N = 100).

Written Comprehension of Sentences

H.A.M. was completely successful in judging whether complex sentences were possible or impossible (N = 30). As mentioned earlier, she executed simple and complex written commands without any difficulty. Finally, she had no problems in a written sentence arrangement test: she could rearrange randomly given words into grammatical sentences, and she would put lexemes into the right order to constitute "telegrams." (The sentence arrangement test can detect discrete syntactic disturbances even in patients with apparently normal spontaneous speech—see Kremin & Goldblum, 1975.)

Matching and Comprehension of Written Homophones

H.A.M. was administered our test of recognition of homophonic words. She was presented with 20 different arrays of four written words, in which: (1) the words are all homophones (e.g. *saint* (saint) / *sain* (sane) / *seins* (breasts) / *ceint* (third person, singular, of the verb "ceindre"—to gird) (N = 2); (2) only three of them are homophones (N = 8); (3) only two of them are homophones (N = 8); (4) there is no homophone at all (N = 2). The homophonic words of each array had to be pointed out. H.A.M. omitted only one homophone in a series of three: that is, on one trial of the type (2), she pointed out only two of the three homophonic words.

We also tested the patient's comprehension of half of these homophonic words. She had to identify which of the homophones was related to a given word, for example *bateau* (ship) for the array consisting of the two homophones *porc* (pork) and *port* (harbour) plus the visually similar words *porte* (door) and *parc* (park). H.A.M. executed this test of written homophone comprehension flawlessly. Her performance thus contrasts with J.C.'s impaired comprehension of homophonic words (Newcombe & Marshall,

1981). H.A.M.'s flawless performance suggests that her semantic comprehension of words depends on the visual orthographic input, even in the case of homophonic words.

REPETITION

Repetition of Isolated Items

Repetition of isolated items was reported to be "impossible" on 16 April 1980. Five days later, however, H.A.M. correctly repeated 92% of words (N = 200) and 89% of nonsense syllables (N = 175). The few repetition errors were exclusively of the phonemic type and did not seem to depend on the length of the stimulus for either words or non-words.

H.A.M.'s even better repetition performance (25 April) on subsequent lists presented for direct comparison of oral reading and repetition of same items (see Tables 5.6 and 5.7) is probably due to further recovery.

Repetition of Sentences

As there is no way of testing "irregular" words for repetition, we tried to reinforce a possible semantic/lexical treatment by testing the repetition of sentences. Our hypothesis was that sentence repetition (with the exception of cases with echolalia and/or transcortical aphasia) possibly implies the participation of the cognitive system.

Indeed, H.A.M.'s performance in sentence repetition contrasted with her performance in word repetition: she produced numerous phonemic paraphasias and approximations on the lexical items, e.g. *Les caravanes de dromadaires traversent le Sahara*→"les caravanes de do-dra-daires ... des do ... ah! il y a deux ... traversent le sara- ... le cha ... ch ... cha sara-ra non ... sa- ..." (*you know what it means?*) "oui c'est le ... euh ... il y a du ... comment on appelle ça ... toujours ..." (*du sable*) "oui du sable ... sa ... sara ..." (*sahara*) "... sahara."

Moreover, while repeating sentences, H.A.M. produced semantic and

TABLE 5.6
Comparison of Repetition and Reading of Same Words (N=100):
Influence of Number of Syllables

	Total % Error	1 (N=4)	2 (N=36)	3 (N=45)	4 (N=15)
Repetition	1	0	0	2	0
Reading	30	0	25	38	27

TABLE 5.7
Comparison of Repetition and Reading of Same Non-words (N=90):
Influence of Number of Syllables

	Total % Error	1 (N=26)	2 (N=37)	3 (N=27)
Repetition	1	4	0	0
Reading	40	19	43	56

verbal paraphasias (which never occurred during her repetition of isolated words), e.g. *pelouse* (lawn)→"herbe" (grass); *parc* (park)→"jardin" (garden); *trois grands cèdres* (three huge cedar trees)→"avec un C . . . trois arbres . . . cèdres" (starts with C . . . three trees ... cedar trees); *fusil* (gun)→"avec F . . . fusée . . . fusil" (starts with F . . . rocket . . . gun).

Finally, H.A.M. repeated syntactically "rich" sentences (e.g. *Il s'en est alors remis quoique très tardivement*) more easily than semantically "rich" sentences (e.g. *Le pianiste joue une valse rêveuse de son répertoire*). The patient had the impression that the sentences of the first list were shorter. (In fact, they were not.) With reference to the "semantic" sentences she commented: "C'est là où ça accroche . . . je cherche à donner le sens de la phrase . . . j'arrive pas à répéter" (that's where I have trouble . . . I try to give the sense of the sentence . . . I don't succeed in repeating). The patient thus describes in her own words that, with the participation of the cognitive system, repetition performance worsens, resulting in phonemic paraphasias and in verbal or semantic substitutions.

Comparison of Oral Output in Repetition and in Reading

The same two lists of items (100 words and 90 nonsense syllables) were given for oral reading and for repetition. The results, shown in Tables 5.6 and 5.7, confirm the overall findings mentioned earlier: stimulus length (in terms of number of syllables) does not play a role in repetition (either of words or non-words). In contrast, stimulus length (in terms of number of syllables) is a variable in oral reading, although it seems to exhibit a systematic influence only during H.A.M.'s reading of nonsense syllables.

ORAL NAMING

We already mentioned that H.A.M.'s oral naming performance was poor in all modalities. But she was able to match objects (N = 20) correctly with the corresponding written word in a multiple choice paradigm. (For *glass*, for example, the following written words were presented; the target word (*verre*), one semantic distractor (*bouteille*/bottle), one phonological distractor (*serre*/ greenhouse), and one word without any relation (*micro*/microphone).

Her oral naming performance was characterised by phonemic paraphasias, approximations, and (rare) substitutions. On some occasions the patient spontaneously produced the article that corresponded to the target without being able to name the presented object. We therefore decided to investigate more systematically H.A.M.'s deficit in word retrieval by testing oral naming *plus* gender assignment. Our approach was facilitated by the structure of the French language: in French, every noun has a gender, either masculine or feminine. Gender is sometimes the only key to the semantic representation of spoken words as in, for example, /mɜr/: la *mère* (the mother) and le *maire* (the mayor). This feature of the language, tested in a naming task, should allow us to gather information about the stages of treatment of the presented stimulus. In fact, patients might achieve the concept of an item without being able to access the phonological code of its name. In order to study H.A.M.'s naming problems, 20 items were chosen from the Boston Naming Test, half of them requiring the masculine article in French and half of them of the feminine form. The patient was asked to name the stimulus items *and* their genders. In this task H.A.M. produced 4/20 (25%) correct responses (name and gender). In two more instances the misnamings were close semantic substitutions where the gender corresponded to the erroneous response, e.g. *un loquet* (latch)→"une serrure" (lock). Of the remaining 14 incorrectly named objects, 12 were "identified" as shown by correct gender assignment.

For illustration we reproduce two of H.A.M.'s responses:

spirale (spiral): *une* (feminine)
→"mais c'est une . . . ah! c'est . . . une . . . /bou/ . . . avec un R non plus . . . il y a les escaliers qui sont comme ça mais je me rappelle plus . . . c'est une . . . non (*which letter in the beginning? which sound?*) je ne suis pas sûre . . . une . . . une (*sp-*) spirale."
accordéon (accordion): *un* (masculine)
→"ça c'est un . . . un . . . un instrument de musique . . . c'est un . . . un . . . c'est un . . . un . . . c'est un . . . un . . . il ne marche plus . . . un . . . ah! . . . un . . . un . . . c'est pas le . . . un . . . un . . . (*you know the first letter?*) peut être . . . /prese/ . . . président (patient laughs) . . . un . . . peut être un F . . . non! A! un A! un /mar/ . . . /moricã/ ça va pas . . . un . . . un amour . . . un /maksinõ/ . . . un amour ah je sais! . . . un . . . ça finit par O.N. . . . /ame/ (*it begins with A and ends with ON?*) oui . . . un million non pas un million . . . un . . . un /amaksimom/ non c'est pas ça . . . un a . . . /aks/ . . . non . . . (*accordéon*) oui un accordéon.

H.A.M. thus produced phonemic paraphasias, and verbal and semantic substitutions in oral naming. (It should be explained that the response

TABLE 5.8
Oral Naming: Influence of Number of Syllables of the Target
Word

	Number of Syllables		
	1	*2*	*3*
Number of items	15	16	9
% Error	67%	69%	56%

"président" in connection with the stimulus *accordéon* is not a totally deviant production but, rather, "in the sphere": in fact, the aristocratic president (Giscard d'Estaing) was known to play a very popular instrument, the accordion.) But special testing of naming plus gender assignment seems to lead to the conclusion that in H.A.M. (who proved to be dramatically disturbed in evoking object names) the breakdown of word retrieval occurred *after* the arousal of its semantic representation, the semantic representation being achieved as shown by correct gender assignment. The results suggest that H.A.M.'s naming disturbance is (in spite of her verbal, semantic, and phonemic paraphasias) mainly a problem of retrieval of the adequate phonological form.

Anomia as an output problem is not surprising indeed, but naming performances have not yet been systematically studied in patients with surface dyslexic reading (see, however, Margolin, Marcel, & Carlson, Chapter 6, who report similar findings).

In order to distinguish problems at the level of the output logogens from a possible problem at the level of oral output, that is, response buffer (Morton & Patterson, 1980), we analysed the influence of the length of the stimuli (in terms of number of syllables) on the patient's oral naming performance. It can be seen from Table 5.8 that the number of syllables of the target word to be produced had no influence on H.A.M.'s oral naming.

WRITING

H.A.M.'s copy of a longer text resulted in only one minor error (*siamoise*→ *siamoine*). Her spontaneous writing, in contrast, was poor and full of errors. She correctly gave her name and address; but the description of her daily occupations was limited to *perde de memoige* (probably: perte de mémoire); and *depuis que la santein de ma petite fife va mieux* . . . (probably: depuis que la santé de ma petite fille va mieux . . .).

Although the patient commented: "je ne peux pas vraiment écrire" (I cannot really write), we decided to further investigate her writing impairment

TABLE 5.9
Dictation of Words: Error Analysis (% Error of Total Errors)

Orthographic	Phonological	Other	Omission	Self-correction
88.3	6.3	5.4	0	0

(see p. 106, footnote 1). In total 201 single words and 65 nonsense syllables were given for writing from dictation (mainly items that were also given for oral reading.) The patient was able to write isolated items from dictation. She wrote nonsense syllables much better (19% errors) than words (55% errors).[2] All errors on words written from dictation consisted in non-word productions. Moreover, the majority of these non-words sounded exactly like the target word but did not respect the orthographic conventions of French (see Table 5.9).

Some writing errors occurred because of the omission of a mute letter (e.g. "aéroport"→*aéropor*) or its addition (e.g. "motif"→*motife*). But most of H.A.M.'s writing errors occurred because of grapheme substitutions that, nevertheless, preserved the sound of the target:

"chacun"→*chaquin*; "ration"→*racion*; "printemps"→*au printen*; "chocolat"→*le chocolac*; "lien"→*le lient*; "tas"→*tap*; "noeud"→*neup*; "baptême→*un batteme*; "moelle"→*moile*; "orient"→*l'orian*; "ici"→*issi*; "jabot"→*un jabeau*; "oasis"→*une oasice*; "oeillet"→*un oeuillait*; "ancêtre"→*les encetres*; "haitien"→*haisien*; "photo"→*fautop*; "aiguille"→*aiguye*; "fuel"→*le fioul*; "dinosaure"→*dynosor*; etc.

It is noteworthy that on different occasions H.A.M. would reproduce the same word with different spellings, e.g. "fleau"→*fléod* and *fléot*; "steak"→ *steick* and *steech*. It should be stressed that H.A.M. never wrote down a word without having repeated its sound-form, that she never omitted reproducing a stimulus, and that she hardly made any attempt to correct her erroneous word spellings. These characteristics also apply to other reported patients with phonological spelling, for example by Beauvois and Derouesné (1981) and by Hatfield and Patterson (1983). Another point deserves special attention: from the patient's corpus of word writing from dictation it can be seen that H.A.M. very often assigned the corresponding article to a noun, which, of course, was dictated in isolation. The patient's spontaneous (and correct) gender assignment thus indicates that the word was recognised in the auditory input logogen system.

---

[2] Note that the "better" performance on non-words is due to scoring: in contrast to words, there are no orthographic conventions for the spelling of nonsense syllables; thus any letter string reproducing the sound form of the target is legal.

Of the 150 nouns included in the list the patient spontaneously reproduced 99 with an article (and, with one exception, the article corresponded to the correct grammatical gender of the noun). We thus checked for the possibility that success/failure to retrieve the correct orthographic representation of nouns may be influenced by the patient's spontaneous lexicalisation. H.A.M. showed a certain tendency to write more nouns correctly when the corresponding article was spontaneously produced (51/99 correct) as compared to nouns without gender assignment (12/51 correct). However, because gender assignment was not a task requirement no firm conclusion should be drawn from the data. More important seems to be the fact that, in spite of auditory lexical access, H.A.M.'s writing of many words from dictation turned out to be of the surface dysgraphic type. This seems to suggest that, in terms of the logogen model (Morton, 1980), the connections between auditory input logogen and graphemic output logogen were disrupted and/or that the graphemic output logogen system ("which contains spelling patterns for words," Morton, 1980, p. 132) was not operational. However, as the patient was capable of acoustic-graphemic conversion (as shown by the successful writing of nonsense syllables), presumably H.A.M. used the same conversion mechanism for the production of isolated words from dictation.

In contrast to isolated words, dictated sentences did not result in pure phonological writing but showed agraphic features close to those of her spontaneous writing: "La matinée était fraîche"→*la matinans étant franche*; "Je fis quelques pas dans la cour"→*je fis quelles pas dans la cours*; "Une brume légère se levait de la rivière et masquait la vue de la route derrière les peupliers"→*une bruille laiger se sépevel de la rivielle et masquer la vus de la rout dérient les brebi.*

WRITTEN NAMING

We furthermore tested the patient's written naming of objects (N = 20). Again the same phonological writing occurred as with dictation of isolated words, e.g. scie→*sie*, verre→*vert*, clef→*clai*, etc. It should be stressed, however, that H.A.M. *never* attempted to write the name of an object without having first sounded out the word's phonological form. Indeed, her performance in written naming crucially depended on this sounding-out of the target word (and was a time-consuming task in the light of her problems in oral naming). Note that written naming can be functionally independent of previous or correct oral output (see the cases described by Bub & Kertesz, 1982; Ellis, Miller, & Sin, 1983; Hier & Mohr, 1977; Lhermitte & Derouesné, 1974; Michel, 1979). For the purpose of written naming, however, our patient created a situation similar to the one in writing from dictation: she proceeded by converting a sound-form into a letter string without accessing the orthographic representations of the target word. As a consequence the error patterns of written naming and of writing words from dictation are similar.

RECOGNITION OF ORTHOGRAPHY

Finally, we asked H.A.M. to make lexical decisions on the orthography of words. Ninety items had to be judged: words (*stylo, étain*, etc.), pseudohomophones of words (*stilault, éthin*), and legal nonsense syllables (*stilotte, éthine*). The patient's performance on this lexical decision task (see Table 5.10) indicates that although she reproduced words (when dictated and to written naming) almost exclusively in a phonological form disregarding orthographic conventions, she nevertheless showed reasonable knowledge of orthography when this variable was tested in a recognition task. This pattern of performance favours the view that recognition and production of orthography depend on two separate knowledge stores as suggested by Morton (1980) and, more recently, by Ellis (1982).

In fact, the written productions of both surface and deep dysgraphic writers result in misspellings in spite of the different pathways that are used for written production. For both types of disturbed writing, however, relatively good orthographic *recognition* has been reported. Thus V.S., who suffered from deep dysgraphia, made only 7/75 errors when she had to judge words and nonsense syllables—including her own spelling errors from writing—in a lexical decision task (Nolan & Caramazza, 1983). Moreover, when asked to correct these misspelled items, V.S. was able to correct 76% of her initial writing errors. And R.G., a patient with surface dysgraphia, when confronted with his own misspellings in a reading task often (i.e. in 62% of the cases) did not read anything and made remarks such as "it's not a word," "it's badly written," "oh what a mistake" (Beauvois and Derouesné, 1981, p. 32).

In contrast to H.A.M., two other patients with surface dysgraphia (and surface dyslexia) did have problems with the recognition of orthography (Deloche et al., 1982; Kremin, 1980). The same seems to be true for J.C. and M.S., as their semantic comprehension of homophonic words ("be" vs.

TABLE 5.10
Lexical Decisions on Orthography (N=90)

	% Errors
Real words	4%
Pseudohomophones of words	13%
Non-words	7%

"bee") was impaired (Newcombe & Marshall, 1981, and Chapter 2 in this book). This discrepancy in the performances of various surface dysgraphic patients indicates that a general loss of orthographic representations *can*, but *need* not, occur in surface dysgraphia.

COMMENTS

Our patient's performance in reading isolated items corresponds to three of the four features that Marshall (1976) described as characterising surface dyslexia: (1) H.A.M. can read nonsense syllables; (2) the majority of her reading errors are phonologically similar to the stimulus; (3) she frequently produces non-lexical forms while reading isolated words. But H.A.M. does not show the fourth characteristic, namely that semantic reading comprehension depends on the erroneous reading response. This feature, however, has played the most important role for the formulation of theoretical models about reading processes. Whether authors distinguish two main routes (Coltheart, 1980; Marshall & Newcombe, 1973) or three possible ways to read a word aloud (Morton & Patterson, 1980), their views coincide in the definition of a "phonological" route where a phonological representation is achieved without intermediary semantic access. Indeed, all cases of surface dyslexic patients reported to date (J.C. and S.T. by Marshall & Newcombe, 1973; and Holmes, 1973, 1978; R.O.G. reported by Shallice & Warrington, 1980; F.R.A. reported by Kremin, 1980; A.D. reported by Deloche, Andreewsky, & Desi, 1982; A.B. reported by Coltheart, Masterson, Byng, Prior, & Riddoch, 1983; H.T.R. reported by Shallice, Warrington, & McCarthy, 1983) produced reading errors that can mainly be accounted for by left-to-right mapping of a phonetic value on to a graphemic item.

However, Marshall and Newcombe (1973) also mention that (only) approximately 25% of the reading errors of J.C. and S.T. were neologisms, which (as noted by Marcel, 1980) seems a strong lexical tendency. Holmes (1973) explicitly distinguished a "type of semantically and/or syntactically related error" (p. 122), for example *judgement*→"justice", *govern*→"governor", *enlighten*→"enlightening."

How do we deal with Japanese surface dyslexics who commit semantic errors in reading kanji words (Sasanuma, 1980; Chapter 9 in this book; Sasanuma, Itoh, & Murakami, 1982)? How do we deal with H.A.M.'s "naming" of many written words by spontaneous gender assignment and with F.R.A.'s, A.D.'s and H.A.M.'s preserved written comprehension in multiple-choice paradigms and lexical decision tasks? I propose that these apparent contradictions can be resolved by admitting that some patients, in spite of their surface dyslexic *oral* reading performance, have spared (visual) access to the lexicon and/or semantics. H.A.M., who is obviously surface dyslexic *and* surface dysgraphic, nevertheless showed a fair knowledge of orthography when this variable was tested in a lexical decision task; this finding is at variance with the view that surface dyslexics have lost the orthographic specifications for (some) words in the input lexicon (Marcel, 1980). Finally, could one really explain the numerous reading self-corrections of H.A.M., A.D., and F.R.A. in terms of auditory access to the lexicon "by way of the intact auditory channel" (Holmes, 1973, p. 111)? This seems especially unlikely in the case of F.R.A., whose auditory channel has been described as an "auditory analogue to deep dyslexia" (Goldblum, 1979— B.F. and F.R.A. being the same patient).

I think that many of these apparent contradictions can be enlightened by reconsidering the existing data (see, for example, Shallice & McCarthy's discussion, Chapter 15 of this book, of J.C., S.T., and A.D.). I also think that by now it is experimentally established that two types of surface dyslexic reader ought to be distinguished: one type is characterised by non-semantic reading with pre-lexical phonological output and the other by a post-lexical disturbance of accessing phonology (see Goldblum, Chapter 7; Margolin, Marcel, & Carlson, Chapter 6; Kay & Patterson, Chapter 4—all in this book).

Returning to H.A.M., her reading performance did not show the influence of many of the variables that are difficult to account for from the perspective of a non-semantic reading route. In fact, H.A.M.'s oral reading of isolated words did not show the influence of lexical dimensions such as part of speech and the concrete/abstract dimension. But her reading performance showed a monotonic influence of stimulus length (graphemic and/or syllabic) only for nonsense syllables, not for words. Moreover, she immediately produced words correctly more often than non-words: 21% of overall errors on words vs. 38% of errors on nonsense syllables. According to Shallice, Warrington, and McCarthy (1983), nonsense syllables should be read as easily as (regular) words by a non-semantic reading routine. It is rather H.A.M.'s reading of *irregular* words (pairs of words that contrast on the pronunciability of same sequences of graphemes) that did not differ from her reading of non-words (35% vs. 38%).

The different influence of stimulus length for reading words and non-words seems to indicate that the two types of linguistic material do not have the same status for H.A.M.'s treatment of the letter strings. We thus have to consider whether this difference is due to a problem with the visual input or with the verbal output. Let us start with the verbal output: H.A.M.'s repetition of isolated items (words *and* non-words) is almost perfect and shows no influence of stimulus length (in terms of number of syllables). If we accept the view that there is only one response buffer for verbal output (see Morton & Patterson, 1980), then the effect of the length of the stimuli while *reading* non-words should not be attributed to a general problem at the level of the response buffer, but would rather be due to a disruption at an earlier stage.

H.A.M. typically "recognises" and understands written words immediately, as is shown by her preserved comprehension of written words and by the numerous instances of (correct) gender assignment to the written word. Words must therefore be correctly categorised by the visual input logogen system and processed by the semantic system, both of which can activate the corresponding output logogen. Non-words, too, are immediately "recognised" as such (as demonstrated by H.A.M.'s reasonably good performance in lexical decision tasks and her non-lexical reading of nonsense syllables); but with non-words there is no "target" other than the visual array of the letter string to refer to for oral production (in contrast to words where there are more "targets": the visual array of the letter string, the visual input logogens, and, eventually, the "sense" of the item to be produced). Therefore non-words might be more vulnerable and so become a source of more errors (depending on the length of the letter string).

The length effect for non-words may thus be related to a problem at the level of non-lexical translation from graphemes to phonemes (the more elements there are to translate, the more difficult it is to keep track of them all, in the correct order, etc.). We therefore propose that the observed double effect of (graphemic and/or syllabic) length of the non-word stimuli reflects just one problem, complexity of the *non-meaningful* stimulus to be read. (In fact, this influence of graphemic length on non-word reading seems to be a problem specific to our patient: a 12-year-old control subject read the same list of nonsense syllables and committed only 12% of initial errors and only 3% after self-correction.)

We are confronted with another problem as well: why are the error patterns on words and nonsense syllables so similar (in terms of visual vs. phonological errors)? I mentioned before and stress again here: words are not "seen" and treated in the same way as nonsense syllables, but there is still the possibility that they could be *orally* produced in the same way as non-words, that is by left-to-right grapheme-to-phoneme mapping. H.A.M. may opt for such a "phonological" reading strategy for oral production because of a more general impairment of accessing lexical phonology.

Oral Surface Dyslexic Reading Due to a Post-lexical Disturbance of Accessing Phonology

Let us start our argument with reading and go back to one of the errors we already mentioned: *rhum* /rɔm/ (rum)→"du rhume" /rym/ (a cold). This latter reading error is extremely interesting because of its linguistic characteristics. In fact, both French words, *rhum* (rum) as well as *rhume* (cold), have masculine gender assignment. But the French language permits the generic article only in the case of *rhum* (rum) in expressions such as "Du rhum c'est bien!" (Rum? that's great!), the construction "Du rhume? c'est mauvais!" being illegal. The correct construction in French would be "Un rhume? c'est mauvais!" (a cold? that's bad!). As H.A.M. never showed any difficulties with grammar in any of the numerous tasks that are part of our "standard examination", I propose the following explanation for this reading error: she correctly accessed the input logogen from *rhum* (rum) and treated the stimulus in her semantic system where the adequate generic article to the target was generated (in analogy to "du lait" (milk) or "de la bière" (beer) for example, and, of course, in analogy to H.A.M.'s own production on *onyx*→"de l'onyx"). The actual reading error "du rhume" /rym/ might then have occurred for the following reason: the adequate lexical phonological form (output logogen) is not forthcoming; in order to pronounce the word, which has already been treated and understood, the patient utilises the strategy of grapheme–phoneme conversion that is at her disposal. Thus for *rhum* (rum)→"rhume" (cold), grapheme–phoneme reading (combined with a partial failure in the application of GPCs typical for H.A.M.) results—by chance—in the production of another word that actually exists in the phonological lexicon. This explanation seems to be reinforced by the fact that she read *rhume* /rym/ (cold)→"un rhume" /rym/ (a cold), thus correctly "naming" the stimulus by assignment of the correct *indefinite* article.

Unfortunately we did not ask the patient for her reading comprehension of these particular items. But there are other instances where we did so, and which clearly show that the target word was immediately correctly understood *in spite of* an erroneous oral reading. The example of *fuel* was given earlier; another is:

> *toast*→"/toa/ /twal/ non ... qu'est ce que ça veut dire ça, un *toast* on le mange (patient looks at the written word and tries again) un /tɔks/ non pas un /tɔks/ un /taks/ non plus /toask/ ça se prononce pas comme ça /to/ ... un /toast/."

(In fact, H.A.M. produced only one reading error in which her semantic reading of the stimulus seemed to take place after the production of the oral response: *élection* /elɛksiɔ̃/→"/elɔktjɔ̃/ ... /elɛks/ ... ah! les élections! c'est pas pareil!".)

Let us now turn to H.A.M.'s oral naming. Like Morton and Patterson (1980), I assume that the processes involved in categorising a picture would be located in the cognitive system, which sends a semantic code to the output logogen system where the appropriate phonological code should be produced. H.A.M.'s errors in naming, combined with the preserved ability of correct gender assignment, demonstrate that for her "the appropriate phonological code" is not forthcoming.

Spontaneous language, too, relies on the participation of the cognitive system. It has often been suggested that spontaneous language might be facilitated by being spontaneous, that is only producing (but not re-producing) an utterance. Still, H.A.M.'s spontaneous language was (at least initially) characterised by phonemic paraphasias and approximations as well as by verbal substitutions.

When (supposedly) the cognitive system was engaged during the repetition and reading of sentences, H.A.M. produced phonemic paraphasias and approximations as well as verbal and semantic substitutions. This tendency, though, was less pronounced when reading than when repeating sentences. This difference might be accounted for by the fact that, in *reading* sentences, the target is permanently available and thus offers the possibility of phonological recoding that might block the overt expression of semantic errors in reading aloud. Indeed, when reading sentences, H.A.M. often had recourse to syllabic sounding-out of the items to overcome the initial entanglements on lexemes only.

Finally, what happens when H.A.M. repeats isolated items? She repeated words as perfectly as non-words during the period of "special testing," starting on 25 April 1980. But in the medical record it is stated on 16 April that word repetition was "impossible" (no data are available for this early period). It is, of course, tempting to imagine that H.A.M. quickly developed the strategy of repeating words as if they were nonsense syllables. As the "regularity" of words is not a relevant dimension for word repetition I maintain my hypothesis: remember that there were qualitative differences in H.A.M.'s repetition of isolated words as opposed to words in the frame of a sentence. (I demonstrated elsewhere, in more detail, that the reproduction of (written as well as spoken) words can depend on the use of different pathways according to stimulus presentation—whether in isolation or in the frame of a sentence—see Kremin, 1984.)

An example to illustrate the possibility that "peripheral" strategies (for repetition and/or reading) can indeed be an ingenious discovery of the patient (to compensate for a disturbance) might be taken from our patient F.R.A. (Kremin, 1980). When I saw this patient for a preliminary screening in March 1978, I recorded (while testing her reading comprehension) her oral reading of 10 nouns and 10 pseudoword homophones of nouns (e.g. *cendrier* (ashtray) vs. *sandrié*). The patient read only two real words without error, whereas 9/10 pseudowords were correctly produced. This seems to indicate that F.R.A. read words and non-words differently at this initial period: words by a "direct" pathway (resulting in phonemic paraphasias) and non-words by grapheme–phoneme conversion (resulting in adequate realisations). When extensive testing began 6 weeks later, F.R.A.'s reading of isolated words had improved and showed the characteristic left-to-right mapping strategy of surface dyslexia (see Kremin, 1980). I think it is worthwhile mentioning another feature of F.R.A.'s impairment in this early period: in spite of the bad oral reading performance on real words, the recognition of these items (in a multiple-choice situation with four pictures) was perfect. In contrast, in spite of the almost perfect reading performance on homophonic pseudowords, F.R.A. matched only 4/10 of these items in the same multiple-choice situation. These results seem to suggest that F.R.A.'s comprehension of isolated words did not rely on her phonological output but rather on the orthographic visual input.

H.A.M.'s knowledge of orthography was tested in more detail. The patient's good performances in this regard—both on lexical decisions for words vs. homophonic pseudowords and on the comprehension of homophonic words—thus contrasts with those of some other patients with surface dyslexia. It supports the notion that H.A.M.'s deficit is an output one, while J.C. (Newcombe & Marshall, 1981) and M.S. (Newcombe & Marshall, Chapter 2 in this book) seem to have lost the orthographic input representations for words as their comprehension of written homophonic words was erroneous. That such patients rely on auditory analysis for word comprehension is a consequence of their visual/orthographic impairment.

The presence of semantic comprehension (in spite of erroneous output of the surface dyslexic type) distinguishes our patient's reading behaviour from that of young readers. A 12-year-old child who was given the same list of irregular words to read committed 13/60 reading errors, exclusively of the surface dyslexic type. From Table 5.11 it can be seen, however, that the young reader's oral reading errors were due to non-comprehension of the written stimulus, which was not (yet) part of his sight vocabulary. Consequently the child never made any attempt after meaning and/or self-correction even though some of these words were part of his phonological lexicon. When questioned he indeed knew the meaning of the sound-form /fjul/ and was astonished that the corresponding written word was spelled *fuel*. He knew the sound-form /ljẽ/ and /su/ but did not seem to know the written analogues *lien* and *saoul*.

On the one hand the foregoing observations confirm that the beginning reader's *oral reading pattern* resembles those of subjects with acquired surface dyslexia. On the other hand, they also document that beginning readers and patients like H.A.M. (with a post-lexical disturbance of accessing phonology) differ in their written understanding of the stimuli as well as in their attempts at self-correction of the reading errors. Both points, however, are at variance with some previous accounts (e.g. Marcel, 1980), which viewed the reading errors of both surface dyslexics and beginning readers as resulting from the same underlying cause: the lack of orthographic lexical specifications for words.

I agree with Coltheart (1982) "that, in the limit, every normal reader (...) is surface dyslexic" (p. 157); that is, once in a while every one is confronted with a rare irregular word whose pronunciation is not "automatic" through lexical access. There is, however, evidence that many irregular words can be

TABLE 5.11
Oral Reading of Irregular Words by a Child (Mispronunciations)

Irregular Stimulus Word	Correct Pronunciation	English Translation	Response
chorus	/kɔrys/		→/ʃorys/
paon	/pɑ̃/	peacock	→/paɔ̃/ (you know what it is?) ... un **paon?**
Caen	/kɑ̃/	name of a city	→/kaɑ̃/ (you know what it is?) je connais pas (I don't know).
lien	/ljɛ̃/	link	→/liɑ/ (you know what it means?) je connais pas (you know what it means: un lien/ljɛ̃/?) ah oui.
rhum	/rɔm/	rum	→/rym/ (rhume) (you know what it means?) **rhum?**
dompteur	/dɔ̃toer/	tamer	→/dɔ̃p-toer/ (is that correct?) **dompteur.**
fosse	/fos/	grave	→/fɔs/ (you know what it means?) non.
saoul	/su/	tipsy	→/saul/ (you know what it means?) je connais pas ... (you know what it means: être saoul /su/?) ah oui.
maintien	/mɛ̃tjɛ̃/	maintenance	→mention (is that correct?) non ... /mɛ̃tiɑ̃/ (you know what it means?) non.
faon	/fɑ̃/	fawn	→/faɔ̃/ (you know what it means?) non ... (you know the word faon /fɑ̃/?) non.
poêle	/pwal/	frying pan	→/pwɛl/ (you know what it means?) non.
moelle	/mwal/	marrow	→/moɛl/ (you know what it means?) non.
fuel	/fjul/	fuel	→/fy-ɛl/ (you know what it means?) connais pas ... (you know the word fuel /fjul/?) ah bon!

Correct pronunciations are in **bold** type.

read by the direct lexical non-semantic route to phonology (see Funnell, 1983; Heilman & Rothi, 1982; Schwartz, Saffran, & Marin, 1980), especially when the irregular words are of high frequency (see Bub, Cancelliere, & Kertesz, Chapter 1 of this book). The point I wish to make, with reference to H.A.M. in particular and with regard to the second type of surface dyslexia in general, is that the regularity of words (although it can have an effect on pronunciation) is not the only or even main source for oral misreadings. Kay and Patterson (see Chapter 4 in this book) did not find a statistically significant difference between E.S.T.'s oral reading of the two types of words, and R.F. (Margolin et al., Chapter 6) also had problems reading both regular and irregular words.

In the second type of surface dyslexic reading described here, the "normal" route for word reading (that is, the direct lexical non-semantic route, which, in principle, is error-free; see Morton & Patterson, 1980) is malfunctioning (as it is in deep dyslexia): the patient cannot access the lexical phonology of a written word although it is recognised and comprehended. For the patient with this impairment who has available a routine for non-lexical assignment of phonology, oral reading will not become deep dyslexic but, rather, the surface type.

We therefore reiterate our initial proposal that two different causes of surface dyslexic reading ought to be distinguished, one at the level of the visual input logogens or semantics and another at the level of the phonological output logogens. As both types of patients have available a routine for non-lexical translation of orthography to phonology, their responses in oral reading should yield rather similar patterns. The two types, however, can be distinguished by their different reading comprehension. The first type (with a disturbance at the level of the visual input logogens) shows the characteristic attempt after meaning based on phonological reading responses (or may show no comprehension at all because of a general breakdown of semantic knowledge). In contrast, the second type of surface dyslexic reading (with a disturbance at the level of the output logogens and/or response blocking) exhibits semantic comprehension that correctly refers to the written stimulus.

One can only speculate about whether this problem of accessing post-lexical phonology can be specific to the direct lexical route *for reading*, or whether it necessarily depends on a general breakdown of post-lexical phonology. Cases reported to date seem to suggest that anomia is often a concomitant syndrome of surface dyslexic reading. This seems to be true not only for cases with spared orthographic/semantic access of the written stimuli but also for patients who read without semantics (see Shallice, Warrington, & McCarthy, 1983; Bub, Cancelliere, & Kertesz, Chapter 1 in this book). In this context it should be mentioned that H.A.M. was "clinically" classified as suffering from "pure" anomia. Note, however, that even patients without semantic understanding and a severe naming deficit read many irregular words, probably by direct print-to-sound associations via the lexical non-semantic pathway for reading (Schwartz, Saffran, & Marin, 1980).

Surface Dysgraphic Writing: a Compensatory Strategy?

In the context of possible "compensatory" strategies H.A.M.'s realisations in writing are discussed briefly. The patient's writing from dictation resembles those of other cases with surface dysgraphia (Beauvois & Derouesné, 1981; Hatfield, 1982). For the writing of isolated items to dictation, phoneme–grapheme conversion was virtually unaffected. But in contrast to R.G. (Beauvois & Derouesné, 1981), H.A.M. did not employ this writing strategy either in spontaneous writing or during the dictation of sentences, in other words when the cognitive system is (supposedly) engaged. Furthermore, her productions of the phonological form in written naming depended crucially on having first sounded out the target word. She thus recreated, for her written naming, a situation analogous to the repetition of isolated words. She then proceeded, I believe, by acoustic-graphemic conversions. It appears that H.A.M. had not yet acquired a compensatory strategy for all her writing productions, her spontaneous writing still being "spontaneous," that is, without preceding verbalisation to create the condition (*sine qua non?*) for phoneme–grapheme conversion. The same argument might account for her writing to dictation of sentences: she understands them and wants to write them. But without employing the strategy of (overt or implicit) sounding out, her writing productions are not "phonological," but, rather, predominantly agraphic. This interpretation, of course, remains open to question, especially because I did not have the *présence d'esprit* to voluntarily induce such a compensatory strategy for spontaneous writing by requesting overt verbalisation explicitly; I simply accepted the patient's statement "Je ne peux pas vraiment écrire" (I cannot really write). It is possible, indeed, that there is more than one syndrome of surface dysgraphia (as there is more than one type of surface dyslexia). Still, the factor "onset of testing period after accident" fits the tentatively proposed hypothesis about surface dysgraphia as a possible compensatory strategy (for patients with spared phoneme–grapheme conversion): H.A.M.'s writing was studied only 1 month after her cerebral accident whereas R.G.'s writing performances date from 1–2 (and 5) years after surgical intervention. The same argument may also account for M.S.'s spontaneous writing: his ingeniously surface dyslexic writing of a letter was recorded 3 years after his accident (see Newcombe & Marshall, Chapter 2 in this book).

Digression About Phonological Reading and Comprehension Based upon Auditory Analysis

Instead of a conclusion, I would like to mention some results which have only a loose connection with the case study presented here. Indeed, the literature focusing on acquired reading disturbances often overlaps Broca's aphasia and the syndrome of deep dyslexia and/or impairment of the phonological reading route. Caramazza, Berndt, and Hart (1981), however, mention a patient with Broca's aphasia (B.D.) who not only had no difficulties in reading function words aloud but could, moreover, read 57% of the presented non-words correctly. Goldberg and Benjamins' (1982) case study also points to the possible existence of phonemic coding in Broca's aphasia (their patient was capable of matching orally presented nonsense syllables to their written analogues). Finally, the study by Ross (1983) of a series of aphasic patients suggests that aphasics with both anterior and posterior lesions are capable of phonological processing (during silent reading). So the empirical evidence concerning the relation between phonological reading and concomitant aphasia and/or involved lesion site remains contradictory, and the question is far from being systematically explored.

To present additional information about the complex of problems that remains open to question in this regard, I report some results concerning a large series of subjects with brain damage. The aim was: (1) to furnish data with reference to the hypothesis of semantic comprehension via the auditory channel by testing the subjects' "comprehension" of pseudowords; (2) to see whether aphasics suffering from different cerebral lesion sites behave differently with regard to the oral reading of non-words. In fact, I have administered the little "homophone reading and comprehension test" (mentioned earlier with reference to F.R.A.) to 40 patients suffering from aphasia and to 15 brain-damaged subjects without language and/or reading disturbances. (None of the tested patients had problems in the auditory matching of an orally given word in a multiple-choice situation of four pictures.) All patients were asked

1. To read 10 real words (object names).
2. To read 10 pseudowords, homophones of real words.
3. To point to the corresponding (of four) picture(s) with reference to the (same) written word.
4. To point to the corresponding (of four) picture(s) with reference to the (same) written pseudohomophone.

The following words and pseudowords were to be read and matched:
   Words: lit, chaussure, panier, lunettes, tambour, barque, chaise, vis, robinet, téléphone.
   Pseudowords: trin (train), stileau (stylo), monet (monnaie), oto (auto), sandrié (cendrier), bato (bateau), guent (gant), couto (couteau), phleurre (fleur).

As none of the control subjects made errors on this test they were excluded from the statistical analysis. The descriptive data of the aphasics' performances are represented in Table 5.12.

An analysis of variance (two-factorial ANOVA with two repeated measurement factors) was conducted. Significant ($\alpha = 5\%$) interaction tests for main effects (Kirk, 1968) yielded a significant difference only for comprehension, real words inducing more correct solutions than pseudohomophones in the multiple-choice situation. These results seem to indicate that aphasics (as a group) rely more successfully on orthographic cues for the understanding

TABLE 5.12
Word/Pseudohomophone Reading and Comprehension: Descriptive
Statistics (% Correct)

Subjects (N = 40)	Reading		Comprehension	
	Words	Homophones	Words	Homophones
x̄	84.85	80.57	93.71	79.71
s	33.02	32.35	15.73	27.59
Range	0–100	0–100	20–100	0–100

of a written item than on the auditory analysis of their own oral production on homophonic pseudowords. But they furthermore show that the patients are capable of doing both analyses with a high degree of reliability.

Furthermore a statistical analysis of the data was conducted on the basis of lesion site of the subjects. The aphasics were divided into two subgroups: patients suffering from anterior lesions and patients suffering from posterior lesions of the left hemisphere. An analysis of variance was conducted with subjects nested into two groups and crossed with the crossing of the two factors: type of stimuli (words/pseudowords) and task (oral reading/comprehension). Statistical analysis did not show any significant difference for the performances of the two experimental groups: either for the main effect ($F = .63$) or for the partial effects of type of stimulus and task (all Fs < 1.33).

The patients' individual performances will be discussed only with reference to phonological reading. (The individual performances are reproduced in the Appendix.) It should thus be pointed out that some patients match pseudowords better than they read them (see cases 2, 18, 19). Their performances thus seem to confirm Goldberg and Benjamins' (1982) finding that some anterior aphasics can process pseudowords even in the absence of overt oral reading. Perhaps more intriguingly, there are other cases who read the pseudowords better than they comprehend them (see cases 1, 16, 17, 25, 33, 35). Remember that none of the patients had any difficulty in auditory comprehension (matching of a spoken word with the corresponding picture). This dissociation between relatively good oral reading of pseudowords but poorer understanding of these words seems to indicate that auditory checking procedures (and/or post-phonological semantic access) are not automatically used by all subjects, in spite of an unimpaired auditory channel.

It is possible, however, that surface dyslexic patients have discovered (or that testing methods made them discover) the strategy of subsequent auditory comprehension. I therefore tried to think of an experimental situation that would imitate even more closely that of a surface dyslexic (type I) during his "attempts after meaning." Fifty reading errors were collected from H.A.M. and from F.R.A. All these errors were initially neologisms but were successfully self-corrected by the patients. These non-words were pronounced and two control subjects were asked to listen and to report the words that resemble those neologisms. The hypothesis was, of course, that this situation should parallel that of a surface dyslexic patient in the case of non-semantic reading relying exclusively on auditory checking mechanisms by an intact auditory channel. The two controls correctly identified 22 and 24 (44% and 48%) of the targets respectively; they both interpreted 4 (8%) neologisms as real words—but these words did not correspond to the targets and self-corrections of the patients; finally, the two control subjects produced 24 and 22 (48% and 44%) "omissions," that is, no existing word that resembled the neologism they just heard came to their minds. This experiment shows that the control subjects were not very successful in their "attempts after meaning" with regard to auditorily given neologisms. They "recognised" only about half of the target words; however, *all* these neologisms were "understood," that is, successfully self-corrected by the patients. I therefore think that F.R.A. and H.A.M. did not use auditory checking procedures. Rather, they relied on visual/orthographic analysis for the comprehension of written words.

ACKNOWLEDGEMENTS

Part of this work was supported by an individual fellowship from the Fondation Fyssen, Paris. I am endebted to Klaus Willmes for statistical advice and grateful to the editors for their helpful comments. Particularly I would like to thank Karalyn Patterson and Tim Shallice.

REFERENCES

Beauvois, M. F., & Derouesné, J. (1981). Lexical or orthographic agraphia. *Brain*, **104**, 21–49.
Boller, F., & Hécaen, H. (1979). L'évaluation des fonctions neuropsychologiques. Examen standard de l'Unité de Recherches Neuropsychologiques et Neurolinguistiques (U.111) de l'INSERM. *Revue Psychologie Appliquée*, **29**, 247–266.
Bub, D., & Kertesz, A. (1982). Evidence for lexicographic processing in a patient with preserved written over oral simple word naming. *Brain*, **105**, 697–717.
Caramazza, A., Berndt, R. S., & Hart, J. (1981). Agrammatic reading. In F. J. Pirozzolo, & M. C. Wittrock (eds.), *Neuropsychological and Cognitive Processes in Reading*. New York: Academic Press.
Coltheart, M. (1980). Reading, phonological recoding and deep dyslexia. In M. Coltheart, K. Patterson, & J. C. Marshall (eds.), *Deep Dyslexia*. London: Routledge & Kegan Paul.
Coltheart, M. (1982). The psycholinguistic analysis of acquired dyslexias: Some illustrations. *Philosophical Transactions of the Royal Society of London*, **B298**, 151–164.
Coltheart, M., Masterson, J., Byng, S., Prior, M., & Riddoch, J. (1983). Surface dyslexia. *Quarterly Journal of Experimental Psychology*, **35A**, 469–495.

Deloche, G., Andreewsky, E., & Desi, M. (1982). Surface dyslexia: A case report and some theoretical implications to reading models. *Brain and Language*, **15**, 11–32.

Ellis, A. W. (1982). Spelling and writing and reading and speaking. In A. W. Ellis (ed.), *Normality and Pathology in Cognitive Functions*. New York: Academic Press.

Ellis, A. W., Miller, D., & Sin, G. (1983). Wernicke's aphasia and normal language processing: A case study in cognitive neuropsychology. *Cognition*, **15**, 111–144.

Funnell, E. (1983). Phonological processes in reading: New evidence from acquired dyslexia. *British Journal of Psychology*, **74**, 159–180.

Goldberg, T., & Benjamins, D. (1982). The possible existence of phonemic reading in the presence of Broca's aphasia: A case report. *Neuropsychologia*, **20**, 547–558.

Goldblum, M. C. (1979). Auditory analogue of deep dyslexia. *Experimental Brain Research*, Supplementum II, 397–405.

Hatfield, F. M. (1982). Diverses formes de désintégration du langage écrit et implications pour la rééducation. In X. Séron, & C. Laterre (eds.), *Rééduquer le Cerveau? Logopédie, Psychologie, Neurologie*. Brussels: Pierre Mardaga.

Hatfield, F. M., & Patterson, K. E. (1983). Phonological spelling. *Quarterly Journal of Experimental Psychology*, **35A**, 451–468.

Hécaen, H., & Kremin, H. (1976). Neurolinguistic research on reading disorders resulting from left hemisphere lesions. Aphasic and "pure" alexias. In H. Whitaker, & H. A. Whitaker (eds.), *Studies in Neurolinguistics* (Vol. 2). New York: Academic Press.

Heilman, K. M., & Rothi, J. (1982). Acquired reading disorders: A diagrammatic model. In R. N. Malatesha, & P. G. Aaron (eds.), *Reading Disorders: Varieties and treatments*. New York: Academic Press.

Hier, D. B., & Mohr, J. P. (1977). Incongruous oral and written naming. *Brain and Language*, **4**, 115–126.

Holmes, J. M. (1973). Dyslexia: A neurolinguistic study of traumatic and developmental disorders of reading. Unpublished PhD. dissertation, University of Edinburgh.

Holmes, J. M. (1978). Regression and reading breakdown. In M. Caramazza, & E. Zurif (eds.), *The Acquisition and Breakdown of Language: Parallels and divergencies*. Baltimore: Johns Hopkins University Press.

Kirk, R. E. (1968). *Experimental Design: Procedures for the Behavioral Sciences*. Belmont, Calif.: Brooks/Cole.

Kremin, H. (1980). Deux stratégies de lecture dissociables par la pathologie: Description d'un cas de dyslexie profonde et d'un cas de dyslexie de surface. In *Etudes Neurolinguistiques*. Université de Toulouse, Le Mirail, *Grammatica*, **7**, 131–156.

Kremin, H. (1982). Alexia: Theory and Research. In R. N. Malatesha, & P. G. Aaron (eds.), *Reading Disorders: Varieties and treatments*. New York: Academic Press.

Kremin, H. (1984). Comments on pathological reading behavior due to lesions of the left hemisphere. In R. N. Malatesha, & H. A. Whitaker (eds.), *Dyslexia: A global issue*. NATO ASI Series D: Behavioural and Social Sciences. No. 18. The Hague: Martinus Nijhoff.

Kremin, H., & Goldblum, M. C. (1975). Etude de la compréhension syntaxique chez les aphasiques. *Linguistics*, **154/155**, 31–46.

Lhermitte, F., & Derouesné, J. (1974). Paraphasies et jargonaphasie dans le langage oral avec conservation du langage écrit. *Revue Neurologique*, **130**, 21–38.

Marcel, T. (1980). Surface dyslexia and beginning reading: A revised hypothesis of the pronunciation of print and its impairments. In M. Coltheart, K. Patterson, & J. C. Marshall (eds.), *Deep Dyslexia*. London: Routledge & Kegan Paul.

Marshall, J. C. (1976). Neuropsychological aspects of orthographic representation. In R. J. Wales, & E. Walker (eds.), *New Approaches to Language Mechanisms*. Amsterdam: North Holland.

Marshall, J. C., & Newcombe, F. (1973). Patterns of paralexia: A psycholinguistic approach. *Journal of Psycholinguistic Research*, **2**, 175–199.

Michel, F. (1979). Préservation du langage écrit malgré un déficit majeur du langage oral. *Lyon Médical,* **241** (3), 141–149.

Morton, J. (1980). The logogen model and orthographic structure. In U. Frith (ed.), *Cognitive Processes in Spelling.* London: Academic Press.

Morton, J., & Patterson, K. (1980). A new attempt at an interpretation or, an attempt at a new interpretation. In M. Coltheart, K. Patterson, & J. C. Marshall (eds.), *Deep Dyslexia.* London: Routledge & Kegan Paul.

Newcombe, F., & Marshall, J. C. (1980). Transcoding and lexical stabilization in deep dyslexia. In M. Coltheart, K. Patterson, & J. C. Marshall (eds.), *Deep Dyslexia.* London: Routledge & Kegan Paul.

Newcombe, F., & Marshall, J. C. (1981). On psycholinguistic classifications of the acquired dyslexias. *Bulletin of the Orton Society,* **31,** 29–46.

Nolan, K. A., & Caramazza, A. (1983). An analysis of writing in a case of deep dyslexia. *Brain and Language,* **20,** 305–328.

Ross, P. (1983). Phonological processing during silent reading in aphasic patients. *Brain and Language,* **19,** 191–203.

Sasanuma, S. (1980). Acquired dyslexia in Japanese: Clinical features and underlying mechanisms. In M. Coltheart, K. Patterson, & J. C. Marshall (eds.), *Deep Dyslexia.* London: Routledge & Kegan Paul.

Sasanuma, S., Itoh, M., & Murakami, S. (1982). Acquired dyslexia in Japanese: A case of "surface dyslexia." *Ann. Bull. RILP,* **16,** 195–204.

Schwartz, M. F., Saffran, E. M., Marin, O. S. M. (1980). Fractionating the reading process in dementia: Evidence for word-specific print-to-sound associations. In M. Coltheart, K. Patterson, & J. C. Marshall (eds.), *Deep Dyslexia.* London: Routledge & Kegan Paul.

Shallice, T., & Warrington, E. K. (1980). Single and multiple component central dyslexia syndromes. In M. Coltheart, K. Patterson, & J. C. Marshall (eds.), *Deep Dyslexia.* London: Routledge & Kegan Paul.

Shallice, T., Warrington, E. K., & McCarthy, R. (1983). Reading without semantics. *Quarterly Journal of Experimental Psychology,* **35A,** 111–138.

APPENDIX

Reading and Comprehension of Words and of Homophonic Pseudowords
by Aphasic Subjects

Subjects (N=40)	Oral Reading of Words (N=10)	Oral Reading of Pseudowords (N=10)	Matching of Words (N=10)	Matching of Pseudowords (N=10)
"Anterior" Aphasics				
1	9	10	10	6
2	0	0	10	5
3	10	9	9	9
4	10	10	10	10
5	10	10	10	10
6	10	10	10	10
7	10	10	10	10
8	10	9	10	9
9	10	6	10	6
10	10	10	7	8
11	10	10	10	10
12	10	6	10	6
13	10	9	10	9
14	10	10	10	10
15	10	10	10	10
16	10	10	7	6
17	10	8	9	5
18	0	0	9	5
19	0	0	10	9
20	0	0	8	0
"Posterior" Aphasics				
21	10	10	10	10
22	10	10	10	8
23	10	8	10	10
24	4	1	7	3
25	2	9	9	4
26	10	10	10	10
27	10	10	10	10
28	3	4	2	1
29	10	10	10	10
30	10	9	10	9
31	10	10	10	10
32	10	10	10	10
33	9	10	9	7
34	10	10	10	10
35	9	9	9	5
36	10	9	10	10
37	10	8	10	6
38	10	10	10	10
39	10	10	10	9
40	10	9	10	9

6

Common Mechanisms in Dysnomia and Post-semantic Surface Dyslexia: Processing Deficits and Selective Attention

D. I. Margolin, A. J. Marcel, N. R. Carlson

INTRODUCTION

This chapter addresses itself to several issues. First, it reports a variety of reading impairment not previously described. In doing so, it emphasises a relationship between dysnomia and dyslexia, which have so far usually been discussed separately. The apparent interaction and commonality of resources used in visual object naming and oral reading of printed words are relevant to whether the semantic representations of objects and words are common or separate. Second, an additional area of interest concerns the different types of responses made by the patient in question to a printed word she could not read, which often differed qualitatively to the same word on different occasions. This raises several issues related to the currently predominant information-processing approach to acquired dyslexias. At the moment, symptom patterns are understood in terms of loss of one or another type of information or process. Response variability as reported here may be better understood in terms of factors concerning the *use* of information and processes such as strategies, selective attention, coordination of information, and pragmatics.

The criteria for the designation of surface dyslexia have, until now, remained as specified by the investigators who coined this term—Marshall and Newcombe (1973). Prototypically, one of their patients, J.C., appeared to be reading non-lexically, and his reading comprehension was determined by the pronunciation which he assigned to the written word (e.g. *begin*→ /bɛgɪn/ and defined as "that's collecting money").

In the terminology of the recent information-processing literature, surface dyslexia is most commonly viewed as due to a deficit in the orthographic input lexicon (Marcel, 1980; Patterson, 1981, p. 166), its closest equivalent in Shallice's (1981) model, the visual word-form system, or its equivalent in Morton and Patterson's (1980) model, the visual input logogen system. In other words, the tendencies to regularise spelling-to-sound correspondences in oral reading and to understand one's spoken response rather than the printed stimulus are seen as due to loss or inaccessibility of entries in a system that lexically categorises complete printed words and gives access to their meanings and their complete phonology. Consequently, the reader is forced to use the correspondences of sub-lexical segments of orthography and phonology. However, it must be noted that Shallice and Warrington (1980, p. 120) suggested that surface dyslexia could arise from deficits at a number of points in lexical processing.

These same information-processing models of reading, however, predict the existence of another type of surface dyslexia. Consider the flow diagram presented in Fig. 6.1, which differs in terminology but not in substance from the aforementioned models. In this model there are three pathways or routes that can be utilised in oral reading. One pathway utilises direct transfer of information from the orthographic input lexicon to the phonological output lexicon. A second pathway includes both of these lexicons but utilises the semantics of printed words for retrieval of their phonology. The third pathway differs from the other two in that it is non-lexical. In this route, phonology is assigned to letter strings in terms of sub-lexical segments. Although this pathway is depicted here as utilising grapheme-to-phoneme correspondences (GPCs), the size of the orthographic unit may be variable (Shallice, Warrington, & McCarthy, 1983). Furthermore, in normal readers this pathway may not be entirely non-lexical (Glushko, 1979; Kay & Marcel, 1981; Marcel, 1980). Based upon evidence from patients with acquired dyslexia, however, it has been suggested that the non-lexical pathway can function independently from lexical processes (Shallice et al., 1983).

The phonological output lexicon depicted in Fig. 6.1 is utilised in spontaneous speech, object naming, and oral reading. Thus, a disturbance at this critical stage of processing would affect all of these skills. With regard to speech and naming, a deficit of output phonology is usually regarded as the underlying cause of anomic aphasia (Caramazza & Berndt, 1978; Goodglass, 1980). Such patients have word-finding difficulties that can be manifested in several ways; empty circumlocutory responses (e.g. "its one of those things, you know, what do you call them?"), descriptive circumlocutions, commonly of a functional nature (e.g. "you pound in nails with it"), or creative word

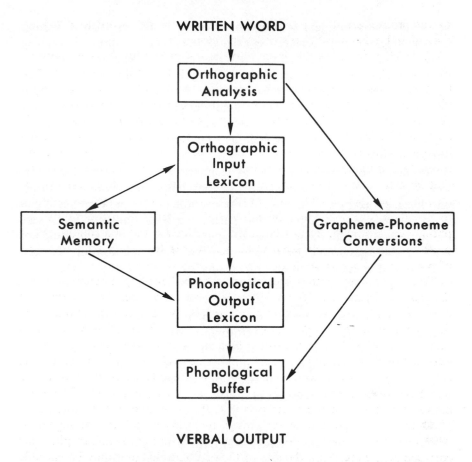

FIG. 6.1   Putative information-processing stages underlying reading.

substitutions (e.g. "time telling blades" for the hands of a watch, or "temperature clock" for a thermometer).

Reading aloud would also be affected by a disturbance of the phonological output lexicon. The effect on reading comprehension is more difficult to predict because the orthographic input lexicon has direct access to semantic memory. Data from deep dyslexic patients (Coltheart, Patterson, & Marshall, 1980) indicate that considerable reading comprehension, particularly for highly imageable and/or concrete words, can be accomplished via this direct access to semantics.

Patients with disturbance of the phonological output lexicon, who have difficulty in retrieving lexical phonology from semantics, could make several types of response when required to read aloud a written word. For example, they could use a non-lexical procedure, which would result in a reading pattern associated with surface dyslexia, such as regularisation of irregular words and the improper assignment of stress and syllabification. However, if the process of sub-lexical conversion of orthography to phonology utilises or converges on the output lexicon (see Marcel, 1980), then problems in output phonology would compromise even a sub-lexical strategy of pronouncing printed words. Alternatively they could generate a response based on the available semantic information, such as a circumlocution or a semantically related substitution.

The details of this latter type of response would be very interesting because they might tell us something of the quality of the semantic information generated by a written word. For example, it would be interesting to see if the response to a word that such a patient could not read were qualitatively similar to the responses to a picture or object that s/he could not name. These data would bear upon theories of the relationship between semantic codes involved in the processing of words versus objects (e.g. Beauvois, 1982; Carr, McCauley, Sperber, & Parmalee, 1982; Paivio, 1971; Warrington, 1975).

The behaviour of the patient reported here was consistent with a post-semantic deficit. Her linguistic performance was probed with particular attention to studies that would relate to the issue of the convergence and divergence of cognitive processes underlying reading and naming. In addition her behaviour raises questions about several aspects of the currently predominant approach to acquired dyslexias.

CASE REPORT

R.F., a 39-year-old strictly right-handed woman, suffered a major head trauma on 7 November 1981, in a motor vehicle accident. Until then, she had been working as a secretary, was educated through 1 year of college, and had no history of learning disability. As a result of the head trauma she suffered a left temporo-parietal intracerebral haemorrhage that required surgical removal. A CT scan performed 9 months later (see Chapter 18) demonstrated a loss of tissue in the left temporal lobe (including Wernicke's area) and the left inferior parietal lobe (including parts of the supramarginal and angular gyri). Following the accident she was globally aphasic, had right-sided weakness and a right superior quandrantanopsia. She improved steadily so that when we first saw her, $2\frac{1}{2}$ months after the trauma, she had a typical anomic aphasia, fluent, but with a marked paucity of content words (her language profile taken at the end of February 1982 is charted in Fig. 6.2).

She rarely made phonological paraphasias and she could repeat words (10/10 on the Boston Diagnostic Aphasia Exam, Goodglass & Kaplan,

RATING SCALE PROFILE OF SPEECH CHARACTERISTICS

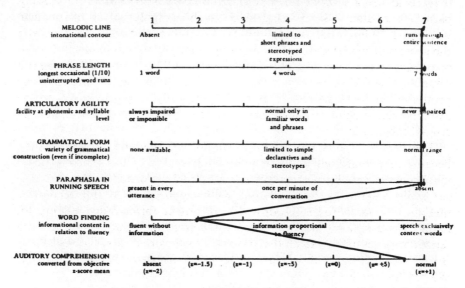

FIG. 6.2   R.F.'s language performance profile on the Boston Diagnostic Aphasia Examination (Goodglass & Kaplan, 1972) at the end of February 1982.

1972), and pseudowords (50/55 correct on the Goldman–Fristoe–Woodcock (GFW) sound–symbol test, Woodcock, 1976) quite well. She repeated eight out of eight high-probability sentences from the Boston Diagnostic Aphasia Exam without error (e.g. "I stopped at his front door and rang the bell"), but failed to repeat four out of eight low-probability sentences (e.g. "The Chinese fan had a rare emerald"). Auditory comprehension on this aphasia test was near normal.

Despite her good performance on repetition tasks, she did have problems with phonological analysis. On the GFW test of sound analysis (Woodcock, 1976) she was required to pronounce the first phoneme of aurally presented non-word speech sounds (e.g. to the sound /tʃɪd/ she was to say /tʃ/). She scored correctly on 19/28 trials. This is the seventh percentile for her age group. On the GFW test of sound blending she had to pronounce a word based upon its component phonemes, which were sequentially presented aurally (e.g. /k/ + /æ/ + /t/ → /kæt/). She scored correctly on 7/33 trials (seventh percentile for age group).

Spelling was problematic. Eighteen words from the Larsen–Hamill test of spelling (Larscn & Hamill, 1976) were dictated to her to be spelled orally. She spelled seven of these correctly. Ten of the eleven errors were visually similar (i.e. 50% of the letters the same) to the target (all spelling responses are listed in Appendix I). Three of these ten errors were simply due to the insertion of an extraneous terminal *e* (e.g. "had" → h,a,d,e). Seventeen different words from this list were dictated for written spelling. She wrote seven correctly. All of the ten written errors were visually similar to the target, three of them resulting from the extraneous terminal *e*. Two oral spelling errors ("section", "s,e,x,s,h,o,n"; "political", "p,o,l,i,t,e,c,a,l") and one written spelling error ("legal"→*leagle*) were non-words, which were homophonic with the target, and one written spelling error was nearly homophonic ("district"→*districk*).

In another spelling task, her responses were qualitatively quite different. When asked to write the names of 20 pictures from the Peabody Picture Vocabulary Test (Dunn, 1959) she was only able to write two of them correctly. Twelve of the errors were semantically related (e.g. truck→*car*). Her other errors consisted of two unrelated real words, three omissions, and one incomplete response (all responses are listed in Appendix I).

On the GFW test of non-word spelling (aural presentation of target, written spelling) she scored correctly on 3 out of 50 trials (below 1st percentile for age; all responses are listed in Appendix I).

Non-linguistic functions were relatively intact. The Wechsler Adult Intelligence Scale (Wechsler, 1958) verbal IQ was 79, the performance IQ was 88, and the full scale was 83. Her memory for autobiographical events occurring before and after the accident was excellent.

READING AND NAMING PERFORMANCE

We studied R.F. over a period of 8 months. Testing was carried out in two blocks; January–February 1982 and August–September 1982. Where appropriate, longitudinal changes in performance are described.

R.F.'s naming strategy was typical of many anomic patients and has remained relatively constant. She would usually indicate immediately that she recognised the object and then describe or mime its use. For example, when trying to name a picture of logs she said, "you can use them for . . . fire . . . put them in your stove . . . you cut them off . . . your tree." In January she could name only 14/50 objects from the first part of the Peabody Picture Vocabulary Test (Dunn, 1959). She rarely made paraphasic errors in naming. In contrast to her naming there has been a qualitative change in her reading. Therefore, the reading data will be presented in two sections according to the date of the testing.

January–February 1982

R.F. had great difficulty reading aloud individually presented words. Often her errors were non-words that were not phonologically or visually close to the target word or only partly so (e.g. *history*→/ˈhæstɪn/, *piano*→/bɪlən/). When she mispronounced a word she usually recognised her error and made several attempts to self-correct (e.g. *theory* →/ɵiraɪz/→/ɵi ə raɪz/). When trying to read words with more than one syllable she would often experiment with different syllabifications and/or stress patterns (e.g. *belief*→/ˈbɛl ɪk/→/bɛˈlɪk/). She was more successful in decoding the first part of words and often seemed to guess at a phonological completion for the word (*flower*→"flown"). This strategy is somewhat similar to that employed by beginning readers (Marcel, 1980), the difference being that in R.F.'s case it operated without a consistently effective lexical constraint, because some of her responses were non-words (e.g. *instance*→"instrake").

Occasionally, words were more effectively transcoded, producing surface dyslexic types of errors (e.g. *castle*→/ˈkæstəl/, *fact*→/feɪkt/, *cellar*→/sɛlˈlar/). Often she would spell out a word letter by letter before or after an attempt to read it. This letter-by-letter approach was rarely successful. Frequently, she would misname letters, which would then influence her reading (e.g. she spelled *key* as "r,e,y," and said /rɛdəl/). About 70% of the time even when she correctly spelled a word she still could not articulate it. At this time she had a digit span of five forward and three backward and a letter span of four to five forward and three backward, but she could not articulate even some three-letter words that were spelled to her orally. This indicates that her inability to pronounce words after her own oral spelling was due to problems in performing letter-to-phoneme transformations, and/or in synthesising these phonemes into a phonological whole, and not to a verbal short-term memory deficit. This analysis is consistent with the documented phonological deficits discussed earlier.

Sometimes she would spontaneously demonstrate that she knew the meaning of a word that she could not read. For example, when asked to read the word *machine* she said, "that's in your car, /ˈmaɪkənəl/". In addition, about 1–2% of her reading errors were semantically related to the target (e.g. *baby*→"child," *wife*→"woman").

Despite evidence for some word comprehension her functional reading was severely limited. For example, she could not follow simple written commands such as *wave goodbye* or *touch your nose*. Her ability to follow the same commands presented orally was normal. In an attempt to define more specifically the deficit(s) underlying this severe dyslexia, the following special tests were presented.

Evaluation of Cognitive Processes Underlying Reading

1. Visual Perception.   Her visual acuity was 20/40 in the right eye and 20/20 in the left eye with corrective lenses. She scored in the 50–75th percentile on the Raven's Progressive Matrices Standard Form (Raven, 1960). She could match an orally presented word with its written counterpart. There were three distractors; a visually and phonologically similar word, a semantically related word, and an unrelated word (e.g. target = brush, distractors

= bush, comb, doll). She performed this test rapidly and scored 29/30 correct. All of these data indicate that her difficulties cannot be attributed to visual perceptual problems.

2. Orthographic Knowledge.   Her knowledge of English orthography was tested in a variety of ways. In a forced-choice paper-and-pencil test she had to decide which of two letter strings was a properly spelled word. The distractor differed from the target by only one letter. The position of the altered letter was varied across the words. The two letter strings were presented one above the other. The target words were selected from both the regular and irregular word lists of Baron and Strawson (1976), for a total of 80 pairs of letter strings. Twenty-five of the non-words (32%) included consonant digrams that do not occur in English (e.g. *sgeat, tolr*). The remainder of the non-words contained only orthographically permissible digrams. She was correct on 76/80 trials although she could read only five of the words.

In a computerised lexical decision task, uppercase letter strings (four to six letters in length) were presented singly on a CRT screen. The test was administered in two parts on the same day. In the first part, there were 50 high-frequency (> 50/million) words; in the second part there were 50 low-frequency (< 2/million, Thorndike & Lorge, 1944) words. In each part 25 orthographically legal non-words were produced by altering one or two letters of 25 list words (e.g. *mother→mopher, person→peston*), and 25 orthographically illegal non-words were produced by rearranging the letters of the remaining 25 list words (e.g. *window→owwdnt, forest→ftsreo*). As seen in Table 6.1, she was quite good at distinguishing between high-frequency words and orthographically illegal non-words, and less good at distinguishing between lower-frequency words and orthographically illegal non-words. When the decision was between words and orthographically legal non-words, her performance deteriorated, and the frequency effect was seen again.

TABLE 6.1
Discriminability of Visually Presented Words and Non-words
(January/February)

Words	Non-words	Hit Rate %	False-positive Rate %	d'
High frequency	Orthographically illegal	94	4	3.29
Low frequency	Orthographically illegal	68	9	1.83
High frequency	Orthographically legal	94	24	2.24
Low frequency	Orthographically legal	68	42	0.68

Despite these problems with orthography she was able to score correctly on 27/30 trials in which she had to match a picture of an object with its written name. There were three distractor words, one visually related, one semantically related, one unrelated (e.g. for the target picture of a leaf the list of written words consisted of *leaf, leap, branch,* and *shoe*). She could only read five of the target words aloud, all of which she correctly matched. Chance score for the 25 words that she could not read would have been 6.25 correct. She scored 22 correct ($\chi^2 = 20.18$, $P < .005$). She also scored correctly in 33/50 trials in which she had to match one of several pictures with its written label. In this task, she was shown one page of the Peabody Picture Vocabulary Test (four pictures) and the target word. Although there is no consistent phonological or semantic relationship between the pictures on a given page, they are sometimes semantically related (e.g. skirt, jacket, mitten, belt). She was able to read 15 of the written labels, all of which she matched correctly. Chance score for the remaining 35 trials would have been 8.75; she scored 18 ($\chi^2 = 5.18$, $P < .025$).

Although these studies demonstrate some ability to match words and pictures, the interpretation of the results is problematic because the matching could be performed on the basis of orthographic, phonological, or semantic codes. In an attempt to disambiguate the results, three sections of the La Pointe and Horner (1979) Comprehension Battery for Aphasia were administered. In the first section, the task is to match a picture (e.g. bus) with its written label in the presence of two visually similar word distractors (*sub* and *bun*). In the second section the distractors are phonologically related (e.g. target = *pie*, distractors = *sky* and *buy*). In the third section the distractors are semantically related (e.g. target = *cigar*, distractors = *pipe, smoke*). Unfortunately, the results were not differential since the scores were, respectively, 8, 9, and 8 out of 10 correct. Results of other tests, however, suggest that her ability to match stimuli on the basis of phonological coding was severely limited.

3. From Orthography to Phonology. In an assessment of *orthographic variables*, R.F. had to indicate whether a pair of visually presented words rhymed or not. Eighty pairs of words were prepared according to a 2×2 design using visual similarity and rhyming as variables. Thus there were 20 pairs of words in each of four conditions; visually similar rhymes (e.g. plain–train), visually similar non-rhymes (e.g. stir–star), visually dissimilar rhymes (e.g. fly–tie), and visually dissimilar non-rhymes (e.g. sing–black). As seen in Table 6.2, her ability to make rhyme judgements was very poor. Furthermore, the pattern of hits and false-positives indicated that her rhyme judgements were heavily influenced by visual similarity. It is interesting to note that in the case of the visually similar non-rhymes, only the vowels differed in each pair. Given the fact that R.F. was heavily influenced by visual

TABLE 6.2
Discriminability of Rhymes and Non-rhymes Based on Visual Similarity
(January/February)

	Hit Rate	False-positive Rate	d'
Visually similar	(16/20) 80%	(13/20) 65%	0.445
Visually dissimilar	(11/20) 55%	(4/20) 20%	0.97

similarity, the fact that vowels differed appears not to have mattered; in other words it really is *visual* similarity to which she was subject. Incidentally, this of course does not necessarily mean that R.F. was deficient in deriving lexical phonology and segmenting it, but may mean that she relied on visual cues when available.

The effects of *lexical variables* such as word frequency or imageability on reading performance have provided useful information in the study of acquired disorders of reading (e.g. Patterson, 1981). In order to assess the effect of these variables on R.F.'s reading, the following stimuli were prepared. One hundred words were chosen from the Paivio, Yuille, & Madigan (1968) corpus of words. There were 25 words in each of four cells, which were created by independently varying imageability and frequency.

Only 18 words were read correctly, and only 20/82 errors (24%) were real words (Appendix II). The visual and phonological relationship between the target and real word error was variable (e.g. *thought*→"telegraph," *soul*→ "salt").

As seen in Table 6.3, there was a highly significant main effect of frequency but no significant main effect of imageability, nor was there any significant interaction (Empirical Logistic Transform Method, Cox, 1970). The lack of an imageability effect distinguished R.F. from patients who appear to be relying predominantly on a semantic route in oral reading (deep dyslexics). The significance of the frequency effect is less clear but it may reflect the use

TABLE 6.3
Effects of Frequency and Imageability on Reading Aloud
(January/February)

	Frequency[a]			Imageability[b]	
	High	Low		High	Low
Reading			Reading		
+	17	1	+	12	6
−	33	49	−	38	44

[a]$\chi^2 = 17.34$ $(P < .005)$. [b]$\chi^2 = 2.44$ $(P > .05)$.

of the direct pathway between the orthographic input and phonological output lexicons (Schwartz, Saffran, & Marin, 1980), preservation of whose entries or connections may well be affected by frequency (Bub, Cancelliere, & Kertesz, Chapter 1 in this book).

In an assessment of R.F.'s ability to derive or assemble phonology from print she was given a standardised test of *non-word reading* (GFW test of reading of symbols, Woodcock, 1976). Stimuli were three- to six-letter pronounceable non-words presented with five words per page, displayed horizontally. She produced acceptable pronunciations for only eight of the stimuli, all of which were one syllable long (complete data in Appendix III).

R.F. displayed very poor non-word reading and made reading errors (to both words and non-words) that differed phonologically from the target letter string, so her pattern of oral reading performance cannot plausibly be described as the output from an intact routine for converting orthographic segments to phonology. To the extent that it did contribute substantively to her oral reading, this routine must have been significantly impaired at some point. Alternatively or additionally, one could interpret some of her word-reading errors as the output of representations in the phonological lexicon, which were not only of reduced accessibility but actually disrupted. There are two ways in which the phonological output lexicon could influence reading of non-words. In the first case consider the suggestion made by Marcel (1980) that the phonological output lexicon consists of phonological segments organised and bound together by structural rules of combination, and that the "non-lexical" process of orthographic-to-phonological translation converges in retrieval of phonological segments on the ouput lexicon. If this lexicon is compromised, then non-lexical reading that utilises it will also be compromised. Suggestive evidence of such organisation comes from phonological dyslexics whose non-word reading is better for pseudohomophones (AKE) than for non-homophonic non-words (AVE) (see Derouesné & Beauvois, Chapter 16 in this book; Patterson, 1982). The alternative account is that R.F. did not use one routine alone, but tried to use both lexical and non-lexical procedures to derive a phonological response. The former (impaired) would distort the latter.

4. Semantic Processing.   As mentioned earlier, R.F. occasionally demonstrated that she had at least partial semantic information about words that she could not read. The following tests were administered to explore further her reading comprehension.

On the Reading Comprehension Battery for Aphasia (La Pointe & Horner, 1979), she scored 9/10 correct in a task of sentence to picture matching (one sentence and three pictures). In this test, however, most of the sentence to picture matchings can be performed based upon comprehension of the verb or the direct object only (e.g. "He stood before the judge" or "He wrote for an hour"). On the same battery she could only match 2/10 written paragraphs to a referentially appropriate picture. However, this might well be due not to a deficit in lexical semantics but to a problem in a post-lexical buffer, because, as noted earlier, she had problems repeating some sentences. In an odd-word-out test (Albert, Yamadori, Gardner, & Howes, 1973) she had to choose the semantically unrelated word from a list of either four or five words (e.g. *glove, hat, shoe, pail, shirt*). She performed well above chance, scoring 9/14 correct (chance = 3). Thus it appears that R.F. gained adequate semantic information from single printed words on a majority of occasions.

Two experiments suggested that her problems in reading and naming were not due mainly to a deficit in semantics per se, but due either (1) to a problem with accessing or use of semantics from written stimuli; or (2) to a deficit in adequately accessing entries in the phonological output lexicon from either pictures or printed words *alone*; or (3) to a combination of these two deficits.

In the first experiment, R.F. attempted to read 50 words (names of objects) and name 50 pictures (depicting the words). The 50 words and pictures were each presented twice. On one presentation if she failed to read the word or name the picture she was orally given a semantic cue (e.g. "you drive it" for *car*), on the other if she failed she was given a phonological cue (the sound of the first phoneme). The order of cues was counterbalanced for each potential word and picture failure. The results are shown in Table 6.4. There was a significantly greater effect of semantic than phonological cues for oral reading of words ($\chi^2 = 9.58$, $P < .005$), and the reverse pattern for naming pictures of objects ($\chi^2 = 4.62$, $P < .05$).

The results of this double-cueing experiment can be interpreted preliminarily as follows. The semantic cues do not greatly help R.F. to name pictured objects because they provide her with no additional information to that which she has already derived. In fact, she often spontaneously provided a very similar semantic circumlocution (as a self-cue) when she first saw the stimulus picture. The phonological cue, however, is effective since it serves to "prime" her compromised output lexicon. In the case of oral reading, the converse is the case. The phonological cue was less effective because R.F.

TABLE 6.4
Effects of Semantic and Phonological Cues on Words and Pictures (January/February)

	Words[a]			*Pictures*[b]	
	Semantic Cue	Phonological Cue		Semantic Cue	Phonological Cue
+	17	4	+	5	13
−	20	29	−	25	26

[a]$\chi^2 = 9.58$, $P < .005$. [b]$\chi^2 = 4.62$, $P < .05$.

could often spontaneously generate the first phoneme from the written word. The relative success of the semantic cues was most probably due to helping semantic access to the output lexicon. In any case pictures and words probably supplied qualitatively different, and potentially complementary, information to R.F. To explore the possibility that these two types of stimuli are complementary the second experiment was carried out.

In this task R.F. had either to read a word, name a picture with the same label as the word, or produce the label when both the name and picture were shown (same stimuli as in aforementioned experiment). These three trials were presented in counterbalanced fashion. She read 31/50 words and named 22/50 pictures. All but three of the 22 picture names were included in the successfully read words. Therefore, a total of 34 different lexical tags were produced when the stimuli were presented individually. (Incidentally her unaided performance on this task was considerably better than in the previous experiment with the same words and pictures. This may be due in part to practice and in part to recovery during the intervening 6 weeks.)

When the stimuli were presented simultaneously, however, she provided the correct lexical tag on 44/50 trials (32 of the previous 34, + 12 of the 16 previously missed tags) (see Table 6.5). The difference between the performance on the individual and the simultaneous presentation was significant ($\chi^2 = 5.83$, $P < .025$).

At this point we will suggest one type of account of R.F.'s performance with pictures and words. It is reasonable to suppose that normally (in the unimpaired person) entries in the phonological lexicon are accessible and able to be activated from each of (1) entries in the orthographic input lexicon; (2) semantics; and (3) segmented or partial phonological information. We suppose that entries in R.F.'s phonological lexicon are of reduced accessibility. Whereas specifications from one route may be insufficient, additional specifications from another route and of another kind will often provide the extra information to retrieve adequately the complete and appropriate phonological lexical entry. A slightly different account of these effects is

TABLE 6.5

Effects of Individual Versus Simultaneous Presentation of Pictures and Words on Ability to Generate Phonological Tags (March)

	Individual	Simultaneous
Tagged		
+	34	44
−	16	6

$\chi^2 = 5.83$, $P < .025$.

proposed in the discussion of the role of attention at the end of this Chapter. But for the moment we can say that the facilitation effects represent a convergence of information between the two classes of stimuli.

To summarise all of the preceding data, in the early part of 1982 R.F. had impairment in the following: orthographic input lexicon, orthographic access to semantics, accessing the phonological output lexicon, non-lexical conversion of orthographic to phonological segments.

August–September 1982

R.F.'s change in performance over the 7 months is summarised in Table 6.6. There was some improvement in her naming ability but this was not statistically significant. She had named 14/50 pictures of objects in January and she named 23 of these in August ($\chi^2 = 3.48$, $P > .05$). The only qualitative change in her naming performance was that, in addition to descriptive circumlocutions and miming, she now used familiar phrases (syntagmatic cues) to prime her response. For example, when trying to name the picture of a brush she said, "to do your hair, you brush your hair, it's a brush." The change in her reading performance was more impressive. She had successfully read 18/100 words in January and she read 44 of these in September ($\chi^2 = 15.9$, $P < .005$). Whereas only 24% of her reading errors had resulted in real words in January, 37% (21/56) were real word errors in September ($\chi^2 = 7.51$, $P < .01$). All of these changes in her reading performance pointed towards an improved access to lexical output phonology. In addition there was now a highly significant effect of both imageability and frequency (Table 6.7). Incidentally, although it is coincidental that R.F. showed exactly the same pattern of performance in relation to manipulation of imageability and frequency, it should be noted that there was by no means a complete overlap of the words producing the two scores. The increased influence of imageability may suggest that at this date R.F. either had better access to semantics from orthography or was making more use of it in oral reading.

She was also given a list of words to read taken from Coltheart et al. (1979). This list consists of 39 orthographically regular (e.g. *grill*) and 39 irregular (e.g. *gauge*) words, presented in randomised order (in fact she was

TABLE 6.6
Comparison of R.F.'s Language Performance in Early and Late 1982

Test	Jan./Feb.	Aug./Sept.
Naming	14/50	23/50
Reading	18/100	44/100
Matching word to pictures	33/50	44/50
Matching picture to words	17/20	28/30

TABLE 6.7
Effects of Frequency and Imageability on Reading Aloud (Aug./Sept.)

	Frequency[a]			Imageability[b]	
	High	Low		High	Low
+	33	11	+	33	11
−	17	39	−	17	39

[a]$\chi^2 = 19.64$, $P < .005$. [b]$\chi^2 = 19.64$, $P < .005$.

tested on only 38 words of each type since one word in each set was inadvertently left out). She correctly read 19 of the regular words, plus an additional 7 self-corrections. She correctly read 13 of the irregular words plus an additional 7 self-corrections. This trend in favour of regular words was not significant ($\chi^2 = 2.73$, $P > .05$). Forty-eight per cent of her errors on the list were real words. Her non-word errors were now much closer to the targets. Thirty-eight per cent of new total errors were categorised as "surface" dyslexic errors based upon the following criteria: (1) no violations of spelling-to-sound rules except at the level of individual lexical conventions. This category includes regularisations in the sense of assignment of the most frequent phonological equivalences of sub-lexical orthographic segments and the concomitant syllabifications and vocalisation of "silent" letters (e.g. *pint*→/pɪnt/; *subtle*→/sʌbtəl/); (2) no violation of grapheme-to-phoneme rules, but violation of contextual rules at the letter-string level (e.g. *city*→/kɪti/; *late*→/læt/); (3) violations of individual grapheme–phoneme correspondences, including addition or deletion of phonemes (e.g. *pine*→ /pæn/; *gang*→/grɛŋ/). Her surface dyslexic errors are listed in Appendix IV.

R.F.'s failure to show a significant regularity effect is actually due to the large number of errors she made on both regular and irregular words, some of which were lexical substitutions, some surface dyslexic errors. Indeed these data are entirely consistent with our earlier explanation (p. 149) for R.F.'s distortions in reading non-words; namely, that either or both (1) the non-lexical procedure converges on the (compromised) phonological output lexicon, or (2) she is attempting to use both the non-lexical and lexical procedures.

The most striking change in R.F.'s reading involved the emergence of a new behaviour. She now made descriptive circumlocutory responses when reading that were very similar to the circumlocutions made when trying to name objects. In fact some were virtually identical although given on different sessions; for example,

reading the word *caboose*→"that's the back of the train, that's the very last one on the train . . ."

naming picture of caboose→"that's the back of the train, the very last one on the train . . ."

reading the word *key*→"how drive your car and get in your home when you lock the door."

naming pictures of keys→"these are what you open your car door with."

She also utilised other strategies in reading that had previously been observed in her naming, including miming the use of the referent (e.g. playing a piano) and using syntagmatic aids (e.g. saying "you are a (pause) gentleman," when trying to read the word *gentleman*).

In order to obtain more data regarding the degree of overlap between the reading and naming responses, the following two tasks were constructed. A corpus of 20 written words (concrete nouns), which had previously engendered descriptive circumlocutory responses, was selected. R.F. was shown the corresponding pictures to name. Three were named correctly. The remaining 17 responses were all descriptive circumlocutions. All but two of these were similar in content to the circumlocution generated in response to the corresponding word. For example, for the written word *diamond* she said "they're very expensive, money," and for the picture of a diamond she said, "jewellery, it can be very expensive."

In the complementary task she was given 47 written concrete nouns to read, each of which corresponded to a picture to which she had previously generated a descriptive circumlocutory response. She was able to read 15 of these words. Of the 32 errors, 22 were descriptive circumlocutory responses, 9 of which resembled the circumlocution that she had made in response to the picture of the same name. For example, for the picture of a waffle she said, "breakfast, you make them for breakfast," and for the word *waffle* she said, "oh, I make these for the kids for breakfast." Ten other representative examples of convergent circumlocutory responses are shown in Appendix V.

In both naming and reading R.F. is demonstrating that she has access to semantic information but not to the specific phonological lexical entry. There was a marked parallelism, if not identicality, between R.F.'s circumlocutions to the equivalent items in the two tasks. Note that this parallelism is in both the form of words used and in the semantic features marked. This suggests that what is common in these two tasks is not only accessing lexical phonology (i.e. the output lexicon), but the semantic representations of objects and words themselves. It is noteworthy that the similarity in circumlocutions occurred at a time when the increased imageability effect suggests a greater use of semantics in oral reading. Whereas other authors have emphasised the differences in the semantic representations of pictures and words based upon normal (Paivio, 1971) or clinical neuropsychological (Warrington & Shallice, 1979) studies, our data indicate that under certain circumstances pictures and words can produce a very similar activation pattern in semantic memory. This is consistent with recent evidence from normal subjects that picture and word interaction can occur at a semantic level (Carr et al., 1982). A model featuring convergence of information processing at the semantic level for pictures and words is presented in Fig. 6.3.

Although certain words that were shown to R.F. activated semantic information, it is evident from a number of the preceding tasks that semantic access was far better overall for pictures than for words. In early 1982 this discrepancy was more marked than it was later in the year. A similar pattern of deficits was observed in the patient A.R., reported by Warrington and

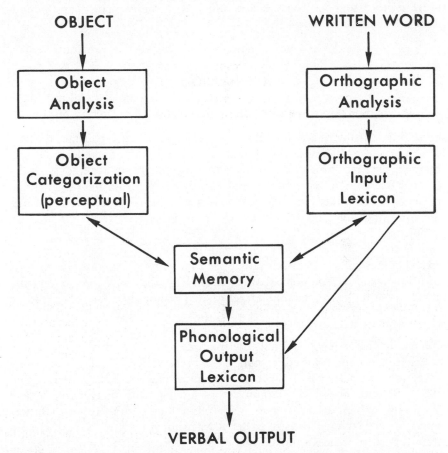

FIG. 6.3 Putative information-processing stages underlying reading and naming. The non-lexical process is omitted for simplicity. (Note: This figure begs the question of the existence of a direct connection between Object Categorization and the Phonological Output Lexicon, analogous to that from the Orthographic Input Lexicon. To our knowledge no data exist to support such a connection.)

Shallice (1979). The greater problem with orthographic than pictorial access to semantics seen in these patients may not be due entirely to the specific effects of their acquired lesions. This pattern may be due, in part, to differences in the way these stimuli are normally processed. It is well documented, for example, that whereas words can be read faster than pictures can be named, pictures can be categorised by superordinate category more rapidly than words (Potter & Faulconer, 1975). Similarly, Carr et al. (1982) have found that semantic activation in normals accrues more rapidly for pictures than for words. The greater loss of semantic access for words as compared to pictures following an acquired lesion might thus reflect a pre-morbid processing bias towards semantic activation by pictures and phonological activation by words.

DISCUSSION

R.F. in Relationship to Other Surface Dyslexics

Should R.F. really be considered with other cases showing a surface dyslexic reading pattern? She does not show a significant effect of regularity in oral reading, she cannot read non-words with a high degree of accuracy, and her errors often contain segments phonologically distant from the target. What evidence is there, then, that she reads via a non-lexical procedure? Consider the following suggestion made by an anonymous reviewer: "R.F. has an impairment in accessing the output lexicon, and is partly anomic and partly a neologistic jargon aphasic. In object naming she cannot access appropriate lexical entries sufficiently from semantics to attempt a response. In reading, additional partial phonological information from the direct connection from input to output lexicon enables target-related neologisms. All of her reading is in fact lexical." This cannot be a complete explanation of R.F.'s performance for several reasons. There are two points as regards the role of jargon aphasia in R.F.'s reading. First, the main evidence that neologistic jargon arises from a compromised lexicon is the preservation of the phonological "skeleton," namely syllable structure and stress pattern (Ellis, Miller, & Sin, 1983). Second, neologistic jargon errors arising from unavailable lexical phonology exhibit a consistency in the phonological substitutions (Butterworth, 1979). Neither of these patterns was shown by R.F. Next, there are certain positive indices that she was on many occasions using a sub-lexical procedure. First, she sometimes used a letter-by-letter strategy. Second, when reading larger orthographic segments she would still attend to one (non-morphemic) part of the word at a time, sometimes actually covering the rest of the word. Third, the errors in Appendices III, IV, and VI are too similar to the "surface" errors of Marshall and Newcombe's patients to be discounted, and they fall within the criteria listed on p. 153.

As we have suggested earlier, R.F.'s failure to show a significant regularity effect, poor non-word reading, and phonological distortions are not necessarily evidence against her using a non-lexical procedure, but may arise from her additional attempts to use a compromised lexical procedure. Thus, while she fails to satisfy the superficial criteria of surface dyslexia, the evidence from reading strategies and error analysis qualifies her to be included on the grounds of reliance on sub-lexical procedures.

As described in the first report of surface dyslexia (Marshall & Newcombe, 1973), J.C.'s reading comprehension for a word appeared to be mediated by his oral response. R.F. also occasionally displayed this type of error. For example, she read *bury* as /bjurɪ/ and said "where you buy beer" (brewery), or read *fact* as "fast" and said "you fast in the Catholic church." However, the majority of the time an incorrect articulatory response by R.F. did not seem to interfere with her comprehension. A corpus of samples where she demonstrated at least partial comprehension with incorrect phonology is presented in Appendix VI. This was true even when the incorrect reading would have led to an alternative definition (e.g. *pen*→"pine"). It is clear that incorrect oral reading did not necessarily signify improper comprehension of a word, nor did the articulatory response necessarily dominate the ultimate interpretation of the written word.

Another of R.F.'s reading errors is particularly interesting. When given the word *apple* to read she said "I just froze these . . . I cut them off the tree . . . to make pie", and then read the word as /eɪpəl/. The inability to retrieve the proper phonological tag for the word apple, despite apparently adequate semantic activation, is indicative of a problem at the level of lexical output phonology. At the same time she offers a reading response that is suggestive, at least on this occasion, of a moderately functioning non-lexical process of orthographic-to-phonological transformation. Like previous patients with surface dyslexia or "semantic dyslexia" (Shallice et al., 1983), R.F. demonstrates a problem in accessing lexical output phonology while retaining at least partial use of non-lexical phonology. R.F.'s pattern, however, is unlike that in previously described cases in that she sometimes simultaneously demonstrates access to semantics, failure to access (correct) lexical output phonology, and use of (partially functioning) non-lexical phonology. In this she is like some other patients reported in this book by Kay and Patterson (Chapter 4), by Kremin (Chapter 5), and by Goldblum (Chapter 7).

The patients reported in this book by Kay and Patterson (E.S.T.), Goldblum (B.F.) and Kremin (H.A.M.) follow the pattern of post-semantic dyslexia for some words. However, none of these three patients nor R.F. represents a pure form of post-semantic surface dyslexia. According to models of language functioning like the one presented in Fig. 6.3, a pure post-semantic surface dyslexic would be anomic in spontaneous speech and in confrontation naming. Comprehension of written words would be normal but the task of translating print into phonology would be restricted to the non-lexical route. This formulation produces the testable prediction that there is a group of anomic patients who have more trouble reading aloud irregular than regular words, but can comprehend both types of words. Despite the ability to comprehend single words it is likely that functional reading would be limited, as there is evidence that reading text for comprehension depends on accessing the phonology of words and holding them in short-term memory (Baddeley, 1979; Kleiman, 1975; Vallar & Baddeley, 1984).

Selective Attention and Coordination of Codes

From the beginning, one of the most striking aspects of R.F.'s behaviour has been the variety of responses that she makes when trying to read a written word. For any given word, she may provide a descriptive circumlocution, or attempt to sound it out, or spell it aloud, or mime the use of an object to which the word refers, or provide a syntagmatic clue. Even for the same word, the type of approach is quite variable from one session to another. We wish to suggest that overselective attention or limited capacity can account for both this and another aspect of R.F.'s performance.

Several models of reading, both interactive (Becker, 1976; Keele & Neill, 1978; McClelland & Rumelhart, 1981) and non-interactive (Marcel, 1983) hold that when normal people read a word there is automatic parallel activation of several different cognitive codes. These could include visual, orthographic, semantic, phonological, and motor codes. The term "automatic" is used here to refer to a process that does not require intention or conscious awareness, nor interferes with other ongoing mental activity (Posner, 1978, p. 91). In interactive models, the diverse codes activated by the orthographic stimulus interact to facilitate and verify one another. For example, facilitation of orthographic processing by a semantic code is documented in the semantic priming effect in the lexical decision task (e.g. Meyer & Schvaneveldt, 1971). Although the initial activation of codes is automatic, conscious attention can direct the process of integration of codes and modulate the degree of activation for any particular code.

In R.F.'s case there was clearly a problem with the activation and coordination of cognitive codes. Whereas she could sequentially provide orthographic, semantic, phonological, or praxic/gestural (miming) information about a word or picture, these bits of information usually did not summate to produce a correct response. In fact some of her responses indicated that phonological and semantic codes were functioning independently. For example, when asked to read the word *camel* she said, "that's what you take a picture with, camel, no!, this is an animal, a camel." Apparently, the orthographic stimulus had activated semantic and phonological codes that were discordant. Her auditory comprehension was good enough, however, to verify the correct response in the final analysis. The activation of information (particularly for phonological coding) was no longer automatic and had indeed become very effortful.

This shift from an automatic process to a process that requires attention has important implications. Even a normal person has limited information-processing capacity for intentional tasks, and the allocation of processing to one task often occurs at the expense of other tasks. This general principle has been instantiated in a number of experimental studies that pit attention to semantic and phonological processing against one another. For example, Henik, Friedrich, and Kellogg (1983) have shown that the semantic priming effect on a lexical decision task in normals is influenced by the nature of the task performed on the prime word. When instructed to name the primes the expected semantic priming effect was observed. When subjects had to perform a letter search task on the prime, however, there was no semantic priming effect. Similarly when a person monitors an aurally presented sentence for phonemic or specific-word targets, the amount of semantic content understood is significantly reduced (Johnson, 1980). When children sound out new words (by non-lexical rules) they often fail on already familiar words in the same phrase (MacKinnon, 1959). Likewise, when people read a list of non-words, an unexpected final exception word tends to be regularised, *wolf* being pronounced /wɒlf/ (Midgley-West, 1977), which seems to show the non-lexical process operating without the normal domination of the lexical process. Conversely, attention to semantic content reduces both proof-reading efficiency (Smith & Groat, 1979) and the speed with which phonemic and other analytic targets are detected (Green, 1977).

Thus, attention can certainly be biased to one type or another of processing of words, or to one level or another of linguistic analysis. This principle is of even more importance in evaluating the behaviour of brain-damaged patients. Any given response (e.g. a semantic paralexia, a visual error, a misapplication of GPCs, or letter-by-letter reading) cannot be taken as the only possible response. In order to investigate the full range of responses it is necessary to provide specific instructions in order to direct the patient's attention and consequently their strategy. Beauvois (1982) has shown this principle operating in a case of optic aphasia. We suggest that this biasing may account for the variability in the type of response R.F. gave when reading. When attending to semantics she would give a circumlocution, when attending to phonology she would give a surface dyslexic or letter-by-letter response. The crucial deficit according to this account is that usually she did not spontaneously combine information derived from the different types of processing.

There is likely to be a great deal of variability between patients in the extent to which they spontaneously utilise all available reading or naming strategies. Patients like R.F. are quite willing to try multiple strategies, which accounts, at least in part, for the marked variability in their performance. Presumably, other patients might not spontaneously demonstrate the full range of their residual information-processing capacity.

Such attentional and strategic factors can also account for the facilitation effects in R.F.'s object naming and reading. Consider the two experiments with pictures and words, one using complementary semantic and phonological cues and the other using single versus dual presentation of pictures and words. We still assume, as in the account proposed earlier (p. 151), that entries in R.F.'s phonological lexicon are of reduced accessibility, but make the following additional suggestion. It is plausible that a patient with a neurological deficit may rely more on one than another means to the same end (a point that is also indicated by the data of Beauvois, 1982). We would like to speculate that presentation of a picture induces predominantly semantic processing, whereas presentation of an orthographic stimulus induces predominantly phonological processing (given, of course, that such processes are extant). In terms of this account, in both the cueing and the dual-presentation experiment R.F. was induced to utilise additional information to that biased by the stimulus, where relying on a single type of information was inadequate to access her relevant phonology. Thus in reading aloud words, she would have relied on accessing phonology via the direct lexical route or via segmental correspondences. Simultaneous pictures or semantic information either helped activate phonological lexical entries via the semantic route to speech or aided her to use the semantics of the written word (either by priming semantic entries for orthographic access or by drawing attention to that route). The effect of printed words on pictures may have helped R.F. to do more than circumlocute, by drawing attention to the phonological "name" or by providing at least partial phonology. At any rate, the very effectiveness of providing complementary types of information and cues, supports the suggestion that R.F. was spontaneously attending to only one of the two types of information potentially available to her.

Finally, shifting of attention from one level or type of analysis to another provides one explanation for the coexistence of surface dyslexia and letter-by-letter reading observed in R.F. and other patients (e.g. Marshall & Newcombe, 1973, patient S.T.). Considerations of attentional mechanisms may also affect our interpretation of semantic paralexias and the deep dyslexia syndrome.

Semantic Paralexias, Circumlocutions, and Fluency

Semantic paralexias (e.g. *boy*→"girl") can be considered the *sine qua non* of deep dyslexia (Coltheart, 1980a). R.F.'s descriptive circumlocutions (e.g. *table*→"that's what we eat on at home, in the kitchen ...") and her syntagmatic responses (e.g. *brush*→"you brush your hair") are similar to semantic paralexias in that they convey at least partial knowledge of word meaning and usage. The length of these responses may be determined by factors not directly related to the reading process (e.g. bias to the lexicon versus semantics; situational pragmatics). In addition, patients who are fluent in their spontaneous speech, like R.F., would be more likely to make circumlocutory errors than patients who are agrammatic and non-fluent, like most deep dyslexics. This interpretation is supported by the fact that some deep dyslexics make descriptive circumlocutory errors as well as semantic paralexias (e.g. *legality*→"solicitors or uh, jury, no, parliament," Coltheart et al., 1980, p. 422).

In order to explore this idea the following task was administered. R.F. was given the same list of 20 words (concrete nouns) to read on two separate occasions (1 week apart). On the first occasion she was instructed not to respond aloud to the stimulus until she had read the word to herself and could give the correct response. On the second occasion she was told to read aloud without further instruction. The responses under both conditions are listed in Appendix VII. As can be seen, eight of the responses in the unconstrained condition were good examples of descriptive circumlocutions (the first eight responses listed) while on three occasions (the first three listed) the constrained response was similar to semantic paralexias seen in deep dyslexic patients. The nature of her response was thus, to some extent, under strategic control.

Further support for this argument is provided from examination of her written versus oral naming. Although it was common for her to provide long-winded circumlocutory responses in oral naming this was not the case for written naming. As discussed earlier, about two-thirds of her writing errors were single-word semantic paralexias (e.g. "truck"→*car*, Appendix I). Apparently the writing task itself served to constrain her responses.

Viewing circumlocutions and semantic paralexias as fundamentally the same type of response has several implications. First, this interpretation offers some insight into the deficits underlying the semantic paralexia, which is still an unresolved issue. Theoretically, semantic paralexias could be due to a problem of orthographic access to semantics, a problem within the semantic system, a problem with access from semantics to phonology, or a problem within the phonological output lexicon itself. It has also been suggested that some semantic paralexias reflect inherent limitations of the semantic route for reading operating without benefit of other procedures for obtaining the phonology for a written word (Newcombe & Marshall, 1980). We have already discussed the fact that R.F.'s descriptive circumlocutions when trying to name objects and read words were sometimes very similar. All available evidence indicates that her naming difficulties were due to a problem in accessing the phonological output lexicon. Presumably then, her circumlocutions when reading were also due to such a post-semantic deficit.

The hypothesis that circumlocutions are due to a post-semantic deficit and that semantic paralexias are abbreviated circumlocutions accounts for the finding that deep dyslexic patients are often aware that their semantic paralexic responses are incorrect (Kapur & Perl, 1978; Patterson, 1978), and that some of these patients make such paralexic responses despite apparently normal comprehension of the target word (Patterson, 1979). According to the abbreviated circumlocution hypothesis these patients' reading performance is limited by their verbal fluency and not by their comprehension. In other words, they are reporting what they can say about the word rather than what they know about the word.

To the extent that at least some semantic paralexias are indeed abbreviated responses, this also has two important implications for Coltheart's (1980b) view of semantic errors. He distinguished between two types: (1) the shared-feature semantic error (*table*→"chair"), where target and response are of the same syntactic category and share all but the more specific semantic features; and (2) the associative semantic error (*merry*→"Christmas"), where target and response are often from different syntactic categories and have different semantic features. Let us first focus on associative semantic paralexias, which Coltheart proposes are due to a failure to restrict verbal output to the appropriate element in a field of activation occasioned by associative spread of excitation in the lexicon. Consider R.F.'s syntagmatic response "you brush your hair" to the word *brush*. This could be condensed into the associative paralexia, *brush*→"hair." Now consider her descriptive circumlocution to the word *table*, "that's what we eat on at home, in the kitchen ..." There are three different abbreviated versions of this response (i.e. *table*→"eat",→"home",→"kitchen"). Each of these would be classified as an associative semantic paralexia. Yet the full response is an explication of some of the functional and locative semantic features of the type supposedly underlying the shared-feature semantic error. Indeed, in the case of "you brush your hair," it is not clear whether the phrase was intended to help the utterance of the target word or as a definition, bearing in mind that quite normal people often find it difficult to define a word without using it in a phrase ("you brush your hair with it"). Thus the potentially abbreviated nature of the semantic paralexia might mask important differences in the type of putative extended response underlying the shortened overt response. In other words, there might be more than one type of associative semantic paralexia. Some may be shortened forms of phrases intended to help utterance of the target, others may be shortened descriptions or definitions.

Although only a few of R.F.'s circumlocutions could be comfortably abbreviated into shared-feature semantic errors, one might extend the previous argument to suggest that the shared-feature semantic error is also an abbreviated circumlocution. If this were the case it would provide an alternative explanation to that suggested by Coltheart (1980b). He proposed that some of the more specific semantic features of the target word are lost or inaccessible. The alternative is that the block can occur in accessing output phonology rather than within semantic memory. Existing data on reading comprehension in deep dyslexic patients is not sufficiently analytic to differentiate between these two hypotheses. Such data as we have suggest that the deep dyslexic symptoms of *some* patients are due to one deficit and those of *other* patients may be due to the other deficit (Morton & Patterson, 1980).

Semantic paralexias have provided the single most important piece of neuropsychological evidence for direct orthographic access to semantics. As discussed in the previous section, however, the activation of information within semantic memory by written words is an automatic process in normal readers. R.F.'s reading and naming responses, however, were often quite effortful. If, as we have proposed, the semantic paralexias produced by deep dyslexics are equivalent to R.F.'s responses, then we should be cautious in extrapolating about normal reading processes based upon these errors.

Syndromes, Deficits, and Strategies

The information-processing approach to acquired reading disorders that has proliferated during the past decade holds great promise for providing substantive and durable contributions to our understanding of higher cortical functions. Although this approach has been much more quantitative than the more classical neuroanatomical approach, it shares with it a fondness for syndrome making. Syndrome labels are a useful shorthand, but they do provide the temptation to force patients into one category or another. In reality, the great majority of patients display a combination of deficits that is not easily labelled. There are two aspects to the (even tacit) use of the concept of syndrome.

First, at present there is an emphasis on defining syndromes in terms of observed patterns of behaviour (i.e. a symptom complex). Further, a syndrome is seen as a definition of a patient. Thus surface dyslexia, deep dyslexia, and letter-by-letter reading, defined by reading patterns, are viewed as distinct and as characterisations of different individuals. These approaches are implicit tendencies rather than explicit stances; however, see Coltheart (1980a) for an exemplification. We believe that the data in the present Chapter indicate that the different reading patterns that constitute the definitions of the different acquired dyslexias can occur simultaneously in a single patient and be caused by a common deficit. Indeed, not only does R.F. produce letter-by-letter reading, surface dyslexic reading, and semantic errors and circumlocutions, she also produces neologisms that are probably due to a conflation of different strategies.

Second, in much of the current literature, it is implied that particular syndromes are directly produced by, and directly reflect, deficits in the functional architecture of information-processing modules. We believe our data support the view that the patterns of reading observed may also reflect the operation of alternative strategies or biases *as responses to* a deficit in information processing, in order to meet the demands of a task. Thus, inability to access complete lexical phonology from a printed word may lead to attempts to use: (1) sub-lexical orthographic-phonological correspondences; (2) the names or phonological values of single letters; (3) semantic circumlocution or semantically based single-word guesses (semantic errors); or (4) phonological self-cueing, as in tip-of-the-tongue phenomena. The one which will be used on a particular trial may be due to attentional bias to, or predominance of, one type of knowledge or processing approach, or they may be combined. Thus one patient may combine elements of deep dyslexia, surface dyslexia, and letter-by-letter reading. Conversely, when a patient displays, say, deep dyslexic performance, it may be more appropriate not to say that the patient *is* a deep dyslexic, but that she or he has responded to a deficit in a deep dyslexic fashion. Descriptions of behaviour must not be mistaken for descriptions of deficits nor for descriptions of people.

ACKNOWLEDGEMENTS

Special thanks to our colleagues Drs. Frances Friedrich, Christine Glenn, Michael Posner, and John Walker for their helpful comments. Dr. Margolin was a recipient of the NIH Individual Research Service Award F32 NS 06788.

REFERENCES

Albert, M. L., Yamadori, A., Gardner, H., & Howes, D. (1973). Comprehension in alexia. *Brain,* **96,** 217–328.

Baddeley, A. D. (1979). Working memory and reading. In P. A. Kolers, M. E. Wrolstad, & H. Bouma (eds.), *Processing of Visible Language Vol. 1.* New York: Plenum Press.

Baron, J., & Strawson, C. (1976). Use of orthographic and word-specific knowledge in reading words aloud. *Journal of Experimental Psychology, Human Perception and Performance,* **2,** 386–393.

Beauvois, M.-F. (1982). Optic aphasia: A process of interaction between vision and language. *Philosophical Transactions of the Royal Society of London,* **B298,** 35–47.

Becker, C. A. (1976). The allocation of attention during visual word recognition. *Journal of Experimental Psychology, Human Perception and Performance,* **2,** 556–566.

Butterworth, B. (1979). Hesitation and the production of verbal paraphasias and neologisms in jargon aphasia. *Brain and Language,* **8,** 133–161.

Caramazza, A., & Berndt, R. S. (1978). Semantic and syntactic processes in aphasia: A review of the literature. *Psychological Bulletin,* **85,** 898–918.

Carr, T. H., McCauley, C., Sperber, R. D., & Parmalee, C. M. (1982). Words, pictures, and priming: On semantic activation, conscious identification, and the automaticity of information processing. *Journal of Experimental Psychology: Human Perception and Performance*, **8,** 757–776.

Coltheart, M. (1980a). Deep dyslexia: A review of the syndrome. In M. Coltheart, K. Patterson, & J. C. Marshall (eds.), *Deep Dyslexia*. London: Routledge & Kegan Paul.

Coltheart, M. (1980b). The semantic error: Types and theories. In M. Coltheart, K. Patterson, & J. C. Marshall (eds.), *Deep Dyslexia*. London: Routledge & Kegan Paul.

Coltheart, M., Besner, D., Jonasson, J. T., & Davelaar, E. (1979). Phonological recoding in the lexical decision task. *Quarterly Journal of Experimental Psychology*, **31,** 489–507.

Coltheart, M., Patterson, K., & Marshall, J. (eds.) (1980). *Deep Dyslexia*. London: Routledge & Kegan Paul.

Cox, D. R. (1970). *Analysis of Binary Data*. London: Methuen, pp. 35–40.

Dunn, L. M. (1959). *Peabody Picture Vocabulary Test*. Circle Pines, Minn.: American Guidance Service Inc.

Ellis, A. W., Miller, D., & Sin, G. (1983). Wernicke's aphasia in normal language processing: A case study in cognitive neuropsychology. *Cognition*, **15,** 111–144.

Glushko, R. J. (1979). The organization and activation of lexical knowledge in reading aloud. *Journal of Experimental Psychology: Human Perception and Performance*, **5,** 674–691.

Goodglass, H. (1980). Disorders of naming following brain injury. *American Scientist*, Nov–Dec, 647–655.

Goodglass, H., & Kaplan, E. (1972). *The Assessment of Aphasia and Related Disorders*. Philadelphia: Lee & Febiger.

Green, D. W. (1977). The immediate processing of sentences. *Quarterly Journal of Experimental Psychology*, **29,** 135–146.

Henik, A., Friedrich, F. J., & Kellogg, W. A. (1983). The dependence of semantic relatedness effects upon prime processing. *Memory & Cognition*, **11,** 366–373.

Johnson, N. F. (1980). Part-whole relationships in word processing: Psycholinguistics of the eyeball. Paper presented at the Midwestern Psychological Association, St. Louis, Mo.

Kapur, N., & Perl, N. T. (1978). Recognition reading in paralexia. *Cortex*, **14,** 439–443.

Kay, J., & Marcel, A. (1981). One process, not two, in reading aloud: Lexical analogies do the work of non-lexical rules. *Quarterly Journal of Experimental Psychology*, **3A,** 397–413.

Keele, S. W., & Neill, W. T. (1978). Mechanisms of attention. In E. C. Carterette, & M. P. Friedman (eds.), *Handbook of Perception*, Vol. 9. New York: Academic Press.

Kleiman, G. M. (1975). Speech recoding and reading. *Journal of Verbal Learning and Verbal Behaviour*, **14,** 323–339.

La Pointe, L., & Horner, J. (1979). *Reading comprehension battery for aphasia*. C.C. Publications, Inc., P.O. Box 23699, Tigard, Or. 97223.

Larsen, S., & Hamill, D. (1976). *Test of Written Spelling*. Calif.: B. L. Winch & Assoc.

MacKinnon, A. R. (1959). *How Do Children Learn to Read?* Vancouver: Copp Clark.

Marcel, A. J. (1980). Surface dyslexia and beginning reading: A revised hypothesis of the pronunciation of print and its impairments. In M. Coltheart, K. Patterson, & J. C. Marshall (eds.), *Deep Dyslexia*. London: Routledge & Kegan Paul.

Marcel, A. J. (1983). Conscious and unconscious perception: An approach to the relations between phenomenal experience and perceptual processes. *Cognitive Psychology*, **15,** 238–300.

Marshall, J. C., & Newcombe, F. (1973). Patterns of paralexia: A psycholinguistic approach. *Journal of Psycholinguistic Research*, **2,** 175–199.

McClelland, J. J., & Rumelhart, D. (1981). An interactive activation model of context effects in letter perception: Part 1. *Psychological Review*, **83,** 375–407.

Meyer, D. E., & Schvaneveldt, R. W. (1971). Facilitation in recognising pairs or words: Evidence of a dependence between retrieval operations. *Journal of Experimental Psychology*, **90,** 227–234.

Midgley-West, L. (1977). Unpublished PhD dissertation, Birkbeck College, London University.

Morton, J., & Patterson, K. E. (1980). A new attempt at an interpretation, or, an attempt at a new interpretation. In M. Coltheart, K. Patterson, & J. C. Marshall (eds.), *Deep Dyslexia*. London: Routledge & Kegan Paul.

Newcombe, F., & Marshall, J. C. (1980). Transcoding and lexical stabilization in deep dyslexia. In M. Coltheart, K. Patterson, & J. C. Marshall (eds.), *Deep Dyslexia*. London: Routledge & Kegan Paul.

Paivio, A. (1971). *Imagery and Verbal Processes*. New York: Holt, Rinehart & Winston.

Paivio, A., Yuille, J. C., & Madigan, S. A. (1968). Concreteness, imagery, and meaningfulness values for 925 nouns. *Journal of Experimental Psychology*, Monograph Suppl. **76** (1), part 2.

Patterson, K. E. (1978). Phonemic dyslexia: Errors of meaning and the meaning of errors. *Quarterly Journal of Experimental Psychology*, **30**, 587–607.

Patterson, K. E. (1979). What is right with "deep" dyslexic patients? *Brain and Language*, **8**, 111–119.

Patterson, K. E. (1981). Neuropsychological approaches to the study of reading. *British Journal of Psychology*, **72**, 151–174.

Patterson, K. E. (1982). The relation between reading and phonological coding: Further neuropsychological observations. In A. W. Ellis (ed.), *Normality and Pathology in Cognitive Functions*. London: Academic Press, pp. 77–111.

Posner, M. I. (1978). *Chronometric Explorations of Mind*. New Jersey: Lawrence Erlbaum Associates Inc.

Potter, M. C., & Faulconer, B. A. (1975). Time to understand pictures and words. *Nature*, **253**, 437–438.

Raven, J. C. (1960). *Guide to the Standard Progressive Matrices*. London: H. K. Lewis.

Schwartz, M. F., Saffran, E. M., & Marin, O. S. M. (1980). Fractionating the reading process in dementia: Evidence for word-specific print-to-sound associations. In M. Coltheart, K. Patterson, & J. C. Marshall (eds.), *Deep Dyslexia*. London: Routledge & Kegan Paul.

Shallice, T. (1981). Neurological impairment of cognitive processes. *British Medical Bulletin*, **37**, 187–192.

Shallice, T., & Warrington, E. K. (1980). Single and multiple component central dyslexias. In M. Coltheart, K. Patterson, & J. C. Marshall (eds.), *Deep Dyslexia*. London: Routledge & Kegan Paul.

Shallice, T., Warrington, E. K., & McCarthy, R. (1983). Reading without semantics. *Quarterly Journal of Experimental Psychology*, **35A**, 111–138.

Smith, P. T., & Groat, A. (1979). Spelling patterns, letter cancellation and processing of text. In P. A. Kolers, M. Wrolstad, & H. Bouma (eds.), *Processing of Visible Language*, Vol. 1. New York: Plenum.

Thorndike, E. L., & Lorge, I. (1944). *The Teacher's Word Book of 30,000 Words*. New York: Columbia University.

Vallar, G., & Baddeley, A. D. (1984). Phonological short-term store, phonological processing and sentence comprehension: A neuropsychological case study. *Cognitive Neuropsychology*, **1**, 121–141.

Warrington, E. K. (1975). The selective impairment of semantic memory. *Quarterly Journal of Experimental Psychology*, **27**, 635–657.

Warrington, E. K., & Shallice, T. (1979). Semantic access dyslexia. *Brain*, **102**, 43–63.

Wechsler, D. (1958). *The Measurement and Appraisal of Adult Intelligence*, 4th ed. Baltimore: Williams & Wilkins.

Woodcock, R. W. (1976). *Goldman–Fristoe–Woodcock Auditory Skills Test Battery Technical Manual*. Minnesota: American Guidance Service Inc.

APPENDIX I
Spelling Tasks (January/February)
Spelling to Dictation

Oral Spelling		Written Spelling	
Target	*Response*	*Target*	*Response*
up	+	that	thate
it	+	bed	peade
dog	+	this	+
had	hade	him	+
plant	plante	trip	tripe
left	leaft	went	+
when	wan	spring	springe
spend	speand	next	+
storm	storme	pile	+
strong	+	hardly	haley
shake	+	able	aple
forty	+	strange	+
tardy	+	expect	expet
signal	cide	hospital	+
section	sexshon	district	districk
salute	celote	legal	leagle
political	politecal	entire	indire
institution	instareson		

Errors in Written Naming

Semantic Errors		Other Errors	
truck	→car	*Unrelated*	
rake	→garage	spring	→weight
wheel	→car	anchor	→time
vest	→shirt		
keys	→car	*Incomplete*	
iron	→heat	thread	→cli
queen	→woman		
duck	→bird	*Omissions*	
butterfly	→flower	web	
parachute	→fly	waterfall	
		lobster	
		Semantic plus Misspelling	
		crib	→sleap
		necklace	→julery

APPENDIX I—*continued*
Spelling of Non-words to Dictation

Acceptable Spellings	R.F.'s Spelling	Acceptable Spellings	R.F.'s Spelling
1. nad	nade	28. groy, groi	grogh
2. bab	cages	29. quib, kwib	quape
3. tash	tash	30. fubwit	fungewete
4. wess, wes, whess, whes	west	31. yoy, yoi	youghey
5. ab	ape	32. jesh	keathes
6. chad	chage	33. abfim (-phim, -phym)	apfeaurn
7. gog	goge	34. imbaf, imbaff	empgh
8. nid	negage	35. quibbest, quibest	quibest
9. ift, iffed	iftage	36. wush, whush	watches
10. chid	chage	37. ull	alouegh
11. nen	nanged	38. shenning	shagenhing
12. shiff, shif	shagh	39. bofmib, boffmib	bobthmide
13. hess, hes	hagges	40. etbom, etbomb	aletmome
14. unhip	upnighe	41. wifyep (wiff-. whif-, whiff-)	witchfepeg
15. lev	lenye	42. febmifsack (-miff-; -sak, -sac)	fedmistsaf
16. plen	plenged		
17. besh	patash	43. zeepstoll (-stol, -stall)	segbstal
18. poe, po	poe	44. depnonlel, depnonlell	septnonlaye
19. und, unned	under	45. veese, veece	feast
20. stabe, staib	stafbe	46. woff, whoff	wapcy
21. esh	esagh	47. wotfob, whotfob	watfod
22. kug, cug	cageagh	48. bafmotbem, baffmotbem	patchmompen
23. ain, ane, aine	anade		
24. friz	frageze	49. gacked, gackt	gatche
25. smakes	smake	50. laifed, lafed, laift	leafth
26. spong	sponge		
27. lenny, lennie	latenny		

APPENDIX II
Reading Errors Resulting in Real Words (Paivio et al. List—January/February)

Target	Response	Target	Response	Target	Response
thought	telegraph	amount	appoint	death	dead
earth	eyes	factory	vital	hillside	half side
fox	fan	direction	driving	footwear	foot year
snake	stack	forethought	for	newspaper	new paper
table	top	theory	theorize	ice box	ice pack
coin	can	competence	competitive	soul	salt
portal	bottle				

APPENDIX III
Reading of Non-words (January/February)

Stimulus	Response	Stimulus	Response
1. dee	–	21. floke	/flaki/
2. ap	/æd/	22. pell	/pɪl/
3. nay	+	23. plad	/pleɪd/
4. bim	+	24. nile	/nɛkɪl/
5. rayed	/reɪbɛd/	25. whie	/waɪtʃ/
6. kack	+	26. hets	/hits/
7. ziz	/zaɪz/	27. fime	/faɪmi/
8. shum	+	28. sirk	/ʃrik/
9. cag	/kædz/	29. wosh	/wɪʃ/
10. len	+	30. lundy	/leɪzud/
11. weet	+	31. hode	/hɒdi/
12. hend	+	32. cheb's	/tʃɛbriz/
13. fing	/fink/	33. toaf	/tooki/
14. neap	/neɪp/	34. rembay	/rimbi/
15. wuff	/wɪf/	35. yev	/jɛks/
16. suss	/ʃoʃ/	36. ying	/mjɛnt/
17. fy	/fʌni/	37. spoze	/ʃʌbɪri/
18. twib	/twib/	38. gocks	/gooʃi/
19. yox	+	39. reth	/ritɛbætʃ/
20. rhunk	/ribɛnkɪk/	40. baim	/beɪ·ɪm/

+ = correct; – = no response.

APPENDIX IV
"Surface" Reading Errors (Coltheart et al. Words—August/September)

Stimulus	Response	Stimulus	Response
build	/bjuld/	democracy	/di'mɔrɪdʒ/
subtle	/'sʌbtəl/	castle	/'kæstəl/
pint	/pɪnt/	abyss	/'æbɪst/
kept	/kipt/	circuit	/'sərkɪs/
equity	/'ikwɪt/	protein	/'prootaɪn/
move	/'muvi/	average	/'ævərdʒ/
gang	/grɛŋ/	amount	/æmutɪv/
journal	/'dʒɔrəl/	idea	/'ɪndɪə/
gauge	/dʒæg/	sequel	/'sʌkwɪl/
profile	/'proo·vɪl/	fallacy	/fɔlʌsi/
prove	/prɒ vaɪd/	strewn	/strooʊn/
borough	/barooz/	pine	/pæn/
scarce	/skarʃ/	reason	/'risɛnt/
lose	/lɔf/	promise	/proo mɪs/
sword	/sword/		

APPENDIX V

Convergence of Responses in Naming and Reading (August/September)

Target	Responses to Picture	Responses to Word
1. vase	Flowers, you plant things in it, you put flowers in it.	It has flowers in it . . .
2. newspaper	It costs you money and it comes everyday in the mail . . .	It costs you money, Oregonian (a newspaper) . . .
3. elephant	He's in the zoo.	You can see him at the zoo . . .
4. coin	Money, that's not really paper, its other monies . . .	Money, how many do you have . . .
5. barber	Hairdresser, you pay him to cut your hair.	Oh, he cuts your hair.
6. chimney	Where the heat of my stove comes out of . . .	I had my stove . . .
7. safe	You keep safety deposit things in these and money, or people will rob you, safety deposit box.	I just called the bank today because of the safety . . .
8. lobster	It's in, you get them in the ocean and you eat them . . .	I know what this is, I cook with it, it's very expensive . . .
9. logs	Wood, burning wood, tree wood.	Oh, I know what that is, I use them with that thing I cut . . .
10. prisoner	He's in prison, he's a robber (pause) no, they got out, I don't know what they're called.	. . . they were very bad and they were taken back to jail . . . if you're bad that's what you become . . .

APPENDIX VI

Reading Errors Demonstrating Comprehension But Incorrect Phonology

Word	Response	Reading Attempts
January 1982		
1. gentleman	If you were a rich man I'd put this on you ...	/æntɪlmæn/
2. city	Oh, I know this one, it's like over town, it's in Portland ...	/kæts/
3. flower	I know what it says, it's outside ...	/faɑl/
4. railroad	If I went in that I'd be out of town ...	/rilreɪt/
5. machine	That's in your car ...	/maɪkənəl/
August/September 1982		
1. key	How drive your car and get in your home when you lock the door ...	/keɪ/
2. cigarette	You smoke these ...	/streɪks/
3. telephone	You can make long distance calls on this ...	/tɛl poɷn/ /tɛl foɷn/ /tɛl li foɷn/ /tɛl ə foɷn/ /tɛl ə foɷn/
4. baby	... at the hospital you have them ... little teeny children ...	/baɪ bi/ /beɪ bi/
5. pen	You are writing with it ...	/paɪn/
6. apple	I just froze these ... I cut them off the tree ... to make pie ...	/eɪpəlz/
7. elephant	You can see them at the zoo ...	/ilɛ pɛnt/
8. prisoner	... they were very bad and they were taken back to jail ... if you're bad that's what you become ...	/praɪzənɪrz/

APPENDIX VII

Effects of Task Demands on Reading (August/September)

Stimulus	Unconstrained Response	Constrained Response
cherry	I'm going to plant a tree like that in my backyard. I'm going to plant apples, pears, cherry, that's what it is.	tree
pear	I just said it, it was a tree too, cherry, apple, it's the peach, pear that's the one it is.	tree
pants	Jeans, ants, no, its what I'm saying, men wear them.	jeans
banana	Those are in Hawaii, you buy them at . . . any store, they're on sale this week . . .	banana
bus	That's what I ride to college.	Trimet (name of bus company)
train	Arlington (a city), its no longer there where it used to go . . .	rain
table	That's what we eat on at home, in the kitchen . . .	table
horse	You pay money, big money, when they win . . . race horse . . . horse.	horse
bed	Sleep, bed.	sleep
apple	That's the apple, that's the one.	apple
fed	F-e-d-, I don't know what that is.	animals
car	Ron Tonkin built car (a Television commercial slogan).	car
boat	Yacht . . . boat.	boat
desk	I don't know what that is, d-e-s-k, /ɛsk/, dress.	d-e-s-k
chair	I know what that is—I gave him (her son) 2 antique chairs, and that's the word.	(pointed to a chair in the room)
dog	That's Pumpkin Puss (her dog), that's the dog.	dog

APPENDIX VII—*continued*

Stimulus	Unconstrained Response	Constrained Response
cat	That's Tabby Two (her cat), that's the cat.	cat
bear	That's there (points to her ear). Beer? no, it's like Pumpkin, it's like Tabby, it's like animal.	air
hat	I bought that for my Dad last Christmas.	hat
shirt	Blouse, jacket, where did you buy, I bought Billy (her son) 3 shirts.	shirt

7 Word Comprehension in Surface Dyslexia

M.-C. Goldblum

INTRODUCTION

The existence of spelling–sound correspondences is, by definition, the basis of alphabetic writing systems. It is this regularity in transcoding that gives the user of these codes the ability to read most, if not all, real words of his language and a potential ability to read all non-words that conform to the structure of the same language. The obviousness of this fact does not mean, however, that phonological recoding is required in order to achieve the lexical level and that in alphabetical systems written words cannot be treated as symbols much as they are in other writing systems, like Chinese or Japanese (kanji).

A large number of experiments have established that even in alphabetical writing systems subjects are in many cases achieving lexical access without pre-lexical phonological recoding (see Coltheart, 1978, for a review), and most accounts of normal reading assume that two routes are available for lexical access corresponding to these two procedures (Coltheart, 1978, 1980; Meyer et al., 1974). In the direct, visual, lexical route, words are identified as familiar sequences of graphemes. For the non-lexical route, words are processed by means of spelling–sound conversion rules before identification and comprehension.

The use of one route, rather than the other, appears, however, to be variable and to be highly dependent on strategies. These strategies are influenced by task demands or contextual setting as well as by the structure of the stimuli (Baron, 1976; Baron & Strawson, 1976; Coltheart, 1978; Martin, 1982; Meyer et al., 1974; Shulman et al., 1978).

One cause of these strategic variations can be easily detected in languages like French (or English) in which there is an inherent limitation to the efficiency of the phonological recoding procedure.

In French, as in English, the spelling–sound correspondence rules are complex. For example, in French *emps, an, ant, and, ans, ang, eant, amp, eng, ent, end, ens, en, ean, aon, aen, anc*, together with plural forms in some cases, are all possible spellings of the phoneme /ã/. This happens to be the case for most French phonemes so that, for instance, phonological recoding alone of the two sentences: "les pins sont près du port" and "les pains sont près du porc," leads to ambiguity. Moreover, the rules contain a great number of exceptions and inconsistencies. The sequence of graphemes *aon*, for example, is in some instances rendered as /ã/ (as in *faon, paon, taon, Laon* . . .) and in some instances rendered as /aɔ̃/ (as in *Raon, Pharaon, Lycaon* . . .). Homophony, irregularity, as well as the reading of symbols and abbreviations like M., Mme, Dr., Cie, etc., &, $, are clear instances where correct lexical access cannot be achieved through phonological recoding and where the direct visual route has to be used.

In the past 10 years, neuropsychological reports of dyslexic patients for whom the phonological route is not available as a result of brain damage have produced considerable support for the existence of the direct access route (Marshall & Newcombe, 1973; Patterson & Marcel, 1977; Saffran & Marin, 1977; Shallice & Warrington, 1975). They have also provided the interesting possibility of further investigating the reading process that occurs when the direct visual route is operating in isolation. However, this last assumption has been challenged by the fact that there are two categories of such patients.

Some of them, labelled "deep dyslexics" after Marshall and Newcombe (1973), present a virtually total inability to read non-words or to match printed non-words in terms of rhyme or homophony. These characteristics, which establish that the patients cannot derive phonology through the use of spelling–sound correspondence rules, are accompanied by a relatively well-preserved ability to read isolated words. This preserved reading ability of deep dyslexics is, though, also markedly dependent on some parameters: concreteness, imagery, part of speech; and when incorrect, the patients' misreadings are often semantic or visual paralexias.

These particularities have led to considerable theoretical reflexions (see Coltheart, Patterson & Marshall, 1980). Some of the first explanations proposed (Marshall & Newcombe, 1973; Saffran & Marin, 1977; Saffran, Schwartz & Marin, 1976) had a more or less unitary approach to deep dyslexic symptoms, and were particularly adapted to account for the occurrence of semantic errors. They assumed that there is a natural imprecision within the semantic system, at least when it lacks convergent phonological information.

Such an explanation, presupposing basically normal operation of the direct route, encounters, however, many difficulties. It does not explain the visual errors, and it has difficulties with the fact that normal Chinese or Japanese readers do not seem to produce semantic paralexias in reading ideographic characters, although they have to use the direct route. Another apparently strong argument against it comes from the description of phonological alexia (Beauvois & Derouesné, 1979; Shallice & Warrington, 1980).

In this syndrome, as well as in deep dyslexia, the phonological recoding route is impaired, but this impairment does not result in the same pattern of word reading as is observed in deep dyslexia. One important difference is the absence of semantic paralexias. The existence of this other, obviously purer syndrome, implies that the lack of the phonological recoding route cannot explain the semantic errors of deep dyslexics, and therefore these errors do not reveal the natural instability of semantics. It suggests that one (at least) other additional deficit within the direct route is responsible for semantic errors. There are many possibilities currently being discussed for disruptions at various stages along the direct route that could give rise to semantic errors (Friedman & Perlman, 1982; Morton & Patterson, 1980; Shallice & Warrington, 1980).

These possible disruptions of the direct route are of considerable importance for the understanding of surface dyslexia. This reading impairment appears to be a mirror image of phonological alexia because it is characterised by a preserved ability to read non-words and regular words, together with a striking inability to read irregular words that are "regularised." To stay within two-route models, one has to conclude then that surface dyslexia reflects a preservation of the pre-lexical phonological route, and that the disorder is a selective impairment within the lexical direct route. As has already been mentioned when discussing deep dyslexia, there are various stages at which the visual direct route can be impaired, and therefore one can expect that, excluding the representational semantic level—as we are concerned only with specifically dyslexic disorders—there can be at least two different categories of surface dyslexia. A "semantic access deficit" surface dyslexia would correspond to a pre-semantic impairment, and a "word retrieval" surface dyslexia to a post-semantic impairment.

Most of the relatively few reported cases (Coltheart et al., 1983; Marshall & Newcombe, 1973; Shallice & Warrington, 1980; Shallice, Warrington & McCarthy, 1983) belong to the first category. In these cases the pre-semantic or semantic locus of disruption is made clear by the patient's incorrect interpretation of words for which the application of spelling–sound rules can produce a phonological code that corresponds to another lexical entry, as in the example provided by Marshall and Newcombe (1973) of *listen* read "*Liston* ... the boxer." Only one case of surface dyslexia, in which irregular words that are regularised when read aloud are still *sometimes* understood, has been described already by Deloche et al. (1982). On a simple version of current models of visual word recognition and production, the effect of a post-semantic retrieval deficit should not be confined to the retrieval of output lexical phonology in reading tasks. The same deficit should be apparent in spontaneous speech and object-naming tasks. This is indeed the case for Deloche et al.'s patient, who is described as presenting with severely disordered naming.

In this chapter I report another case of the second category of surface dyslexia, in which semantic access is preserved. However, in this patient difficulty of word retrieval appears to be restricted to reading, and therefore cannot be attributed to failure of the semantic system to activate lexical output phonology.

This dissociation, in which word retrieval from semantics, and pre-lexical, spelling-to-sound rule-based phonology are both preserved, is not accounted for by two-route models in which retrieval of lexical output phonology is necessarily mediated by semantics. It is better accounted for by models of reading (like Morton's logogen model; see Morton & Patterson, 1980), which contain a reading route that allows output phonology to be activated directly by visual lexical inputs, and separately from semantic processing (Funnell, 1983; Schwartz et al., 1980). If this were the case, the interpretation of deep dyslexia and phonological alexia, particularly in relation to the idea of an "intrinsic instability of semantics," needs to be reconsidered.

CASE REPORT

B.F. is a right-handed, 32 year-old woman who entered the neurosurgery ward on 22 February 1978 having sustained an embolic cerebrovascular accident. On neurological examination she presented with a right inferior quadrantanopia and no evidence of motor or sensory deficit. A CT scan performed on 4 November 1978 revealed the presence of an irregular zone of hypodensity that involved the temporo-parieto-occipital region of the left hemisphere. On neuropsychological examination she had no apraxia or agnosia.

At the time of the stroke she had severe language disturbances that resembled pure word deafness, which then turned into a conduction aphasia. The findings reported here were collected at a time when her aphasia had resolved to a considerable extent. She had very occasional word-finding problems and, though her spontaneous speech was fluent, it was occasionally interrupted by paraphasias. These included phonologically similar word substitutions, and phonemic paraphasias. Her execution (thus comprehension) of verbal commands was 78% for auditory and 96% for visual (written) verbal commands, on the standard examination used in our laboratory (Hécaen & Boller, 1979). The high incidence of errors in the auditory version of the test essentially resulted from a misunderstanding of the function word in commands such as "put the glass beside the pencil"; B.F. responded to the various function words as if they all meant "on."

Her repetition performance has been described in separate papers as an auditory analogue to deep dyslexia (Goldblum, 1979, 1980). She had severely disturbed repetition of non-words and, though her word repetition was relatively spared, she produced many phonological and some semantic errors. Her ability to do mental calculation and arithmetic was severely disturbed. Auditory–verbal short-term memory was limited to four digits.

B.F.'s naming abilities were rather well preserved but will be described in more detail in the following section. Her reading was impaired and much more so when words to be read were exception words or were irregular. Additional data on B.F.'s reading behaviour can be found in Kremin (1980). Her writing was impaired in a very interesting way. In both spontaneous writing and writing to dictation she presented elements of both surface and deep dysgraphia, as well as paragrammatism. This complex picture, which should take into account her "deep" dysphasia and her "surface" dyslexia, is not discussed here.

READING EXAMINATION

General Findings

B.F. was presented with a list of 180 written items, half words and half non-words. The list was originally developed as a control for the repetition task. Thus, words were not selected in terms of irregularity/regularity—this distinction being meaningless in the auditory modality—and the length of the stimuli was determined by the number of syllables, at the level of production and not according to the number of letters. As a result there is not total agreement between the number of items when the stimuli are analysed separately for one or the other criterion.

The word list contained 70 content words (10 monosyllables, 30 bisyllables, 30 trisyllables) and 20 function words (10 monosyllables and 10 bisyllables). The 90 non-words were constructed from the 90 preceding words, by substitution or inversion of some phonemes.

As one can see from Table 7.1, B.F.'s word-reading scores are not affected by length (in terms of number of syllables) nor by part of speech—at least as concerns the contrast between content and function words. Content word reading, however, is superior to (corresponding) non-word reading. This effect could show that B.F. uses lexical information for reading. It could also reflect only a facilitation of word *production* over non-word *production*.

SD–G*

TABLE 7.1
Reading Scores on Words and Non-words: Influence of the Number of
Syllables in the Oral Response

		Words				Non-words	
		Number of Syllables	% Correct			Number of Syllables	% Correct
Content words	N = 10	1	90	Derived from content words		1	70
	N = 30	2	80			2	57
	N = 30	3	80			3	50
Function words	N = 10	1	90	Derived from function words		1	90
	N = 10	2	90			2	80

To try to evaluate further, at the input level, the influence of length of stimuli on reading of words versus non-words, the responses were analysed according to the number of letters within the targets. The 90 words and (corresponding) non-words were separated into three classes: two to five letters, six to eight letters, and nine or more letters. Results of this analysis are presented in Table 7.2.

Contrary to the preceding analysis there is an effect of number of letters in (content) word reading. However, B.F. makes less errors on words of any length than on non-words. This advantage for words seems to support the hypothesis that B.F. uses some lexical information for word reading (at least for short ones). Two further analyses were carried out on B.F.'s content word reading, to try to see if any of the parameters that are known to have some influence on (lexical) word reading were involved in B.F.'s successes or failures.

Influence of Word Frequency

Among the 70 content words, 11 were contained in the band 9–10–11 (frequency superior to 256/125,000) and were classified as high frequency, and 21 from the band 0 (frequency = 1/125,000) were classified as low frequency (Vikis-Freiberg, 1974). Results are presented in Table 7.3. On this small sample of words, B.F.'s scores were 86% on low-frequency words and 91% on high-frequency words.

Influence of Abstractness

Ten judges were asked to categorise the 70 content words as "abstract" or "concrete." Twelve words for which there was no agreement between judgements were then removed from this analysis. Results for the 24 abstract

TABLE 7.2

Reading Scores on Words and Non-words: Influence of the Number of Letters in the Stimulus

| | Number of Letters | | | | | | | | |
| | 2-5 | | | 6-8 | | | 9-12 | | |
	Correct	Incorrect	% Correct	Correct	Incorrect	% Correct	Correct	Incorrect	% Correct
Content words (N=70)	19	3	86	31	8	80	6	3	66
Non-words (N=70) derived from content words	11	9	55	22	16	58	6	6	50
Function words (N=20)	14	1	93	4	1	80	—	—	—
Non-words (N=20) derived from function words	13	2	87	4	1	80	—	—	—

TABLE 7.3

Reading Scores on Words: Influence of the Frequency and Abstractness/Concreteness of the Stimuli

	Number of Letters									Total %
	2–5			6–8			9–12			
	Correct	Incorrect	% Correct	Correct	Incorrect	% Correct	Correct	Incorrect	% Correct	
High-frequency words (N = 11)	5	1	83	5	0	100	—	—	—	91
Low-frequency words (N = 21)	10	1	91	8	2	80	—	—	—	86
Concrete words (N = 34)	7	1	87	16	5	76	3	2	60	76
Abstract words (N = 24)	2	1	66	14	3	82	3	1	75	79

and 34 concrete words are presented in Table 7.3. On the whole, B.F. had a similar score (76–79% correct) on the two types of words.

By contrast, B.F.'s failures seemed to be clearly related to a difficulty in assigning the correct phonology to words that contained a letter, or a sequence of letters, for which the spelling–sound correspondence rules are variable, like: *ien* in *chrétienté* /kretjẽte/ that she read /kretjãte/ (as in *impatienté* /ɛ̃pɑsjãte/); or the sequence *mn* in *automne* /otɔn/ that she read /otɔm/.

To assess this possibility, B.F.'s responses to words and non-words were analysed separately according to the presence or absence in the stimuli of letters, or sequence of letters, for which there is an inconsistent pronunciation. Nineteen out of the 70 content words contained such an ambiguity, and were classified as inconsistent words. Within the 19 words no distinction has been made between words that have an inconsistent but regular pronunciation and those that have an irregular pronunciation in terms of grapheme–phoneme correspondence (GPC) rules, although this distinction could in principle give very valuable information concerning B.F.'s difficulties. The words and non-words of the list were not originally selected for reading, but repetition; therefore their structure was not a priori controlled for a particular level of regularity in spelling–sound correspondence.

When trying to classify words unselected on this dimension, one is immediately confronted by the fact that in French, strict GPC rules are rather infrequently in accord with none the less regular spelling–sound correspondences. This is partly due to the usual complex written representation of a single phoneme, in French, but also to the presence of other contextual rules. For instance the two words *faim* and *fin* both have the same pronunciation /fɛ̃/. If one admits GPC rules like *ai* /ɛ/ (that one should admit if only to account for cases like *ou* /u/ where there is no other simple correspondence), these words are perfectly regular because they obey a rule of nasalisation of the vowel before a *final* nasal consonant. There are many other rules like deletion of the final *e*, or final consonant, that raise problems for a description of regular spelling–sound correspondences in French. The two words *marc* and *parc* are an example of inconsistency for the sequence *arc*: *parc* /park/ is regular in terms of GPC "rules" but irregular concerning the other rules of deletion of final consonant; the reverse is true for *marc* /mar/. Even considering that simple GPC rules are not the basis for regularity of spelling–sound correspondences in French, many problems will remain because in some cases there is a conflict between two perfectly "clear" rules, like in words such as *anguille* /ãgij/ and *aiguille* /egɥij/. In this couple *aiguille* may appear to be more regular in terms of GPC rules, but actually one has to recognise that *aiguille* is related to *aigu* and *anguille* cannot be related to *angu* (non-word) to give each word its correct pronunciation.

This problem can be irremediable in two words like *aigue* (feminine of *aigu*—acute) in which only the final *e* is regularly not pronounced, and *aigue* (meaning water, as in *aigue-marine, aigue-morte*), in which the *u* is also regularly not pronounced but signals the hardening of the *g* that otherwise would correspond to /ʒ/ as in *linge, lange, mange*, etc.

As concerns non-words, 26/70 items contained ambiguous letters, or sequence of letters, which were classified as inconsistent non-words. There are no normative data concerning the way in which inconsistent non-words are read in French, and there is a priori no reason to reject one of the possible readings of an inconsistent non-word. However, for reasons related to what has been briefly mentioned previously about rules for word reading, some responses were classified as incorrect although they correspond to apparently correct application of GPC rules.

For instance, a response like /tiksimym/ for *tiximum* was scored as an error. This non-word was derived from the word *maximum* /mɑksimɔm/. We considered that two possibly acceptable readings existed for this non-word, /tiksimɔm/ (as in *maximum, helium*, etc.) and /tiksimœ̃/ (as in *parfum*), because the rule to derive /ym/ from written information is only applied to a sequence like "-*um* + vowel" (as in *albumine* or *parfume* or *tiximume*). The strict GPC rule *um*→/ym/ in final position cannot be realised in French, because the rule is to nasalise the vowel followed by a nasal consonant (*m* or *n*) in final position.

As was said before, we lack any normative data that could possibly show that non-words are read by the use of *simple* GPC rules, even if they actually contradict other very general and frequent rules in word reading. As a consequence of this possibility, and as B.F. was very sensitive to the similarity of non-words to words of the stimuli (see Lexical Decisions), this criterion might have resulted in overestimating her errors on inconsistent non-word reading. B.F.'s responses on the two types of stimuli are presented in Table 7.4.

B.F. had higher scores on consistent words (86% correct) than on inconsistent words (63%) and on consistent non-words (66%) than on inconsistent non-words (38% correct). Although there is a strong effect of consistency, there is also a strong effect of lexicality: consistent words are better read than consistent non-words, and inconsistent words better than inconsistent non-words.

As we had observed in the previous analysis a possible effect of length for word reading, we divided the consistent and inconsistent stimuli into short (two to five letters) and long (five and more letters) items. Results of this comparison (Table 7.4) show that the length effect for words disappears. The previously obtained superiority for reading short words could possibly be due to a tendency in the sample for short words to be more consistent than long ones.

As there was a general facilitating effect of lexicality, we tried to see if the

TABLE 7.4
Reading Scores on Words and Non-words: Influence of the Consistency
versus Inconsistency and Length of the Stimuli

	Consistent % Correct			Inconsistent % Correct		
	Total (N=51)	Short (N=18)	Long (N=33)	Total (N=19)	Short (N=4)	Long (N=15)
Words (N=70)	86	94	82	63	50	67
	(N=44)	(N=15)	(N=29)	(N=26)	(N=5)	(N=21)
Non-words (N=70)	66	60	69	38	40	38

frequency or abstractness/concreteness of the stimuli had any influence on the occurrence of errors, considering consistent and inconsistent words separately. The distribution of errors (Table 7.5) appears to be equal for the two types of words. But it should be noticed that none of the high-frequency words were inconsistent and that abstract words tended to be more frequently inconsistent than concrete words.

Lexical Decisions

Two days after she had done the reading test, B.F. was given the same list of 180 items for visual lexical decisions. She made 7 misses on the 90 words (3 on the 16 words she had read incorrectly and 4 on the 74 she had read correctly). On the 90 non-words, she made 4 false–positive resonses (1 on the 34 incorrectly read items and 3 on the 56 correctly read items).

TABLE 7.5
Reading Scores on Consistent and Inconsistent Words: Effect
of Word Frequency and Concreteness versus Abstractness of
the Stimuli

	Consistent Words		Inconsistent Words	
	Correct	Incorrect	Correct	Incorrect
High frequency (N=11)	10	1	—	—
Low frequency (N=21)	15	0	3	3
Concrete (N=34)	24	4	3	3
Abstract (N=24)	13	2	6	3

In summary, B.F.'s notable difficulty with inconsistent words, together with the nature of her misreadings, indicated a surface dyslexic pattern of performance. Although her reading performance suggested a lexical involvement, as has already been discussed in Marcel (1980, pp. 235–236), the length, concreteness/abstractness, and frequency of words per se did not appear to be important compared to the consistency/inconsistency dimension. However, one has to bear in mind that high-frequency words tend to be short, consistent, and concrete, and low-frequency words tend to be long, inconsistent, and abstract, and that these interactions may have some functional significance.

Reading of Inconsistent Words

To investigate B.F.'s difficulties with spelling–sound correspondences further, she was given two lists of inconsistent words. The basic principle was to find pairs of words with a contrast in pronunciation of the same sequence of letters, as is the case in *anguille* /ãgij/ versus *aiguille* /egɥij/, or *meule* /møl/ versus *seule* /sœl/. All the words that we have used have a unique correct pronunciation. Some words were included although they do not form a "minimal pair." They are words that cannot be derived by simple spelling–sound rules, for instance English words integrated into French, or French words for which we could not find (at that time) a contrasting instance; for instance only *faon* /fã/ is in the list (and not *pharaon* /faraõ/). The first list of 30 words was presented to B.F. in May 1978, the second list of 60 words in October 1978.

This second list has been presented to five control subjects whose mother tongue was French, and to two bilinguals who were very fluent in French but whose mother tongue was not French. Their error rates were, respectively, 7% and 12%.

On the first list B.F. read correctly 18/30 words (60%): the stimuli, and the misreadings, are reported in Table 7.6 in their order of presentation. In only one case did she produce a grapheme–phoneme confusion that was totally inappropriate (first attempts at *steak*→/strak/). She made one clear visual error: *anguille*→"aiguille." In another instance—*noyau*→/nwajõ/—one could also detect a visual error (*Noyon*, the name of the city where she lives). All the other errors are confusions between different spelling–sound correspondence possibilities.

Although her language condition had improved greatly between May and October, she had the same difficulties with the second list (see Table 7.7). She was correct on only 31/60 words (52%). She made two possibly visual errors: *fuel*→"ruelle" and *saoul*→"raoul." She also made some grapheme–phoneme confusions, like /l/→/r/ in *cholesterol* or /i/→/y/ in *hymne*. But errors on the 31 words that were incorrectly read all involved the use of an inappropriate spelling–sound correspondence rule beside these errors.

TABLE 7.6
Reading of 30 Inconsistent Words (May 1978)

Stimulus	Correct Pronunciation	B.F.'s Oral Reading
faon	/fã/	/fɔ̃/ ... enfin, .. +
subtil	/sybtil/	+
choléra	/kolera/	/ʃolera/
rayon	/rɛjõ/	+
talus	/taly/	+
anguille	/ãgij/	aiguille ... aiguille ... /ãgyij/
chorizo	/ʃoritso/	/ko/ ... +
coeur	/kœr/	+
aiguille	/eguij/	/egij/
oignon	/ɔnjõ/	+
faience	/fajãs/	+
poële	/pwal/	/po-ɛl/ ... /poɛl/
steak	/stɛk/	/strak ... strak/ ... /steak/ .. oui, c'est un steak
choriste	/korist/	/ʃorist/
science	/sjãs/	+
lien	/ljɛ̃/	/ljã/ ... /ljã/? ...
paien	/pajɛ̃/	/paj ... pajã ... pjã ... P.I.A. ... pajã/
sole	/sɔl/	+
môle	/mol/	+
aôut	/ut/	+
persil	/pɛrsi/	+
bonus	/bonys/	+
meule	/møl/	+
seule	/sœl/	+
noyau	/nwajo/	/nwajõ/
Joël	/ʒoɛl/	+
Caen	/kã/	/kaã/ ... /ka-ã/ ... /kaã/
méandre	/meãdr/	+
toast	/tost/	/toast/, non ... /toast/ ... ah ... +
choeur	/kœr/	... +

From Table 7.6, one can see that B.F.'s successes are not limited to words in which the correct spelling of the ambiguous letters corresponds to GPC rules: *talus, oignon, Août, persil, meule* were all read correctly although they do not respect strict GPC rules. B.F.'s failures also do not always correspond to regularisations in terms of GPC rules, in many cases like, for example, *faon, aiguille, lien, paien,* and *Caen.*

In the second list (Table 7.7) as well, failures and successes are not related to the use of one single strategy that would consist of applying GPC rules. She uses simple rules sometimes, for example: *Caen*→/kaɛn/, but for the same word she had previously used a more complex though incorrect rule

TABLE 7.7
Reading of 60 Inconsistent Words (October 1970)

Stimulus	Correct Pronunciation	B.F.'s Oral Reading
phénix	/feniks/	+
chocolat	/ʃokola/	+
albumine	/albymin/	/albinyn ... albynil/ ... mine
voix	/vwa/	+
science	/sjãs/	+
chorus	/korys/	/ʃ ... ʃ/ +
aiguille	/egɥij/	+
voeux	/vø/	+
album	/albɔm/	/albyl/
agneau	/anjo/	+
paien	/pajɛ̃/	+
stagner	/stagne/	/stra-nje/
ration	/rasjɔ̃/	+
sas	/sas/	+
rhume	/rym/	+
anguille	/ãgij/	/egwij/
Caen	/kã/	/kaɛn/
lien	/ljɛ̃/	/ljã/
noeud	/nø/	+
faience	/fajãs/	+
onyx	/oniks/	+
rhum	/rɔm/	/rym/ (rhume)
bénitier	/benitje/	/bəni-tje/
dompteur	/dɔ̃tœr/	/dɔ̃p-tœr/
condamné	/kɔ̃dane/	+
initier	/inisje/	/initje/
bosse	/bɔs/	+
hymne	/imn/	/yn/ (une)
fosse	/fos/	/fɔs/
taon	/tã/	/taɔ̃/
cation	/katjɔ̃/	/kasjɔ̃/
saoul	/su/	/raul/ ... (Raoul) ... /rul/ (roule)
flemme	/flɛm/	/flam/ ... (flamme)
quotient	/kɔsjã/	/kotjɛ̃/
Raoul	/raul/	+
chrétien	/kretjɛ̃/	+
femme	/fam/	+
maintien	/mɛ̃tjɛ̃/	/masjɛ̃ ... mɛ̃tj.../, oui, /mɛ̃sjɛ̃/
martien	/marsjɛ̃/	/mar-tjɛ̃/
tas	/tɑ/	/tas/ ... (tasse)
chrysanthème	/krizãtɛm/	+
faon	/fã/	+
opium	/opjɔm/	/omjom ... opjom/
poèle	/pwal/	/pwɛl/
automne	/otɔn/	/otɔm/
compteur	/kɔ̃tœr/	/kɔ̃p-tœr/

TABLE 7.7   cont.
Reading of 60 Inconsistent Words (October 1970)

Stimulus	Correct Pronunciation	B.F.'s Oral Reading
moelle	/mwal/	/mo-ɛl/
Joël	/ʒɔɛl/	+
rien	/rjɛ̃/	+
cholestérol	/kolɛsterɔl/	/ʃorɛstərɔl ... terɔl, ʃ ... Korɛstərɔl/
toast	/tost/	/toast/
Noël	/nɔɛl/	+
prompte	/prɔ̃t/	/prɔ̃pt/
Léon	/leɔ̃/	+
steak	/stɛk/	/strak/ ... /steak/
Moise	/moiz/	m ... +
élection	/elɛksjɔ̃/	+
régner	/renje/	+
fuel	/fjul/	/ryɛl/ ... (ruelle) ... /fɥɛl/
escroc	/ɛskro/	+

/kaã/. She read *taon* as /taɔ̃/ and not /taɔn/, but later read correctly *faon* as /fã/, although on the preceding list she read it as /faɔ̃/. She read *automne* as /otɔm/ and not /otɔmm/, for *hymne* /imn/, which is regular according to GPC rules, she produced /yn/ in which the sequence *mn* is given its irregular correspondence. *Flemme* was not read correctly (and regularly) as /flɛm/ but rather as /flam/'. She applied, correctly this time, the same correspondence rule later when reading *femme* /fam/.

On the first list B.F. made two particularly interesting responses. She read the word *Caen* as /kaã/; when asked if she knew what it meant she said: "/kaã/? (Yes, what is it?) /kaã/ it is kaã/ ... /kaã/ (Is it an object?) ... (shook her head) ... (a country?) ... (shook her head) une v ... (the beginning of a city—une ville) ... /kaã/ ? /kaã/? (Do you know this word?) /kaã/ it is ... there was someone, but who is it now? /kaã/ is it the lady? it is ... it is the same one, isn't it? /kaã/." She nearly said that it was a city (une v ...) but stopped and began wondering if this was not the name of someone from Hécaen's laboratory,[1] even though she knew very well that Hécaen's name is pronounced /ekã/ and not /ekaã/.

With *steak* /stɛk/ she first produced /strɑk/, then /steak/, which is a regularisation error. When asked if she knew the word she answered: "Yes, it is a /stɛk/." But when asked, immediately after that answer, to read the word again she produced exactly the same incorrect reading.

In the second list she read *fuel* /fjul/ as *ruelle*, then /fɥɛl/. After completing reading the list she was asked again what the word was. She read it: "/fjœl/

---

[1] H. Hécaen was the director of the Neuropsychology Unit, at that time.

c'est du ... c'est du /mɑ-ut/ du! (what is it?) mazout (a form of fuel) ... (and this one is?) ...; this time she produced correctly /fjul/. Among other things, these examples show that B.F. can understand some words for which she has the incorrect phonology.

Our clinical impression was that B.F. had no difficulty in understanding the meaning of misread inconsistent words; this impression was based on two facts. First, on many previous testing sessions she used to mention when (on very few occasions) she did not "understand"—she would say: "I do not even know it." Second, occasionally, during her various unsuccessful attempts to read inconsistent words, she produced the correct word in a low voice as if to guide the selection of spelling–sound correspondence rules to read it. Not only did comprehension appear to be spared, but it also seemed to be quite separate from, and of little assistance for, reading aloud. For these reasons, B.F. was asked about the meaning of the words, while reading this particular list, only on the exceptional occasions when we had the impression that maybe she did not understand the word.

Comprehension of Inconsistent Words

We tried to assess B.F.'s comprehension of misread inconsistent words more formally in a word association test. Thirty inconsistent words for which she had previously produced misreadings were selected. For each word a multiple choice of four written words was constructed. Among the four words, one had a semantic relationship to the target; for example, *anguille* (eel): *fenêtre*, poisson, *coudre, église* (the full set of choices is presented in Appendix I). B.F. was first asked to read aloud the target word. This word was then removed from her vision but presented again in the (rare) cases when she asked to see it again. She was then asked to point to the word that had a meaning relationship to the target.

The associate to the stimulus was a synonym or a near synonym (*échalotte–oignon*) in 15 cases; a superordinate (*cheval–rosse*) in 6 cases; a subordinate (*médecine–science*) in one case; an antonym (*savoir–ignorer*) in one case. The relationship between the two words was more loose (*planète--martien*) in the other 7 cases.

Results

As was the case with the previously used lists of inconsistent words, B.F.'s reading score was 60% correct; by contrast her mean score on the association test was 80% (see Table 7.8). This value was obtained by the use of a rather severe criterion, and underestimates B.F.'s comprehension of written words. In one of the six failed associations, when *super* was read correctly as /sypɛr/ she first pointed correctly to *meilleur*, but she then retracted and said she was not sure, because the word meant "some sort of fuel" and that she "did not

TABLE 7.8

Scores on the Association
Test According to Reading
Scores

Reading	Association	
	Correct	*Incorrect*
Correct	14	4
Incorrect	10	2

see something really related to it." In another case, after *rhum* was read incorrectly with a regularisation error /rym/, resulting in another lexical form *rhume*, she spent some time hesitating between the associate to *rhum* (*antillais*) and a word (*lit*) which could be considered an associate of her oral response, *rhume*. When asked to make a final decision she opted for the wrong associate of the lexical entry *rhume*. Even considering those two responses as incorrect, her score on association, which presumably reflects comprehension, is superior to her reading score.

Reading and comprehension appear to be separate in this patient: Whether or not she could read a word correctly was statistically independent of whether she chose the correct association for it. However, this statement needs some comments, as concerns B.F.'s performance on the association test for correctly read inconsistent words as opposed to incorrectly read inconsistent words. The nature of the oral reading errors (see Table 7.9) indicates that, at least for the 12 incorrectly read words in this test, the spelling–sound process (or route) has been used to read aloud. Her ability to choose the correct association for those words that she read aloud wrongly was far above chance, as she scored 10/12 here (chance = 3/12, binomial $p = .00004$). This indicates also that the use of the spelling–sound correspondence process for reading aloud does not arise only because of a deficit in semantic representation or because of a deficit in visual access to semantics. Possibly it could arise from a post-semantic (word retrieval) deficit affecting these words specifically.

The fact that a number of inconsistent words (60%) are correctly read could possibly be explained by the same relatively simple interpretation: their correct reading could be attributed to the use of the direct semantic route. The implication of this position would be that the direct semantic route in B.F. suffers only a *partial* post-semantic impairment.

However, one should notice that B.F.'s success in reading inconsistent words is fairly constant (between 50 and 60%) both over lists and over time, although her success or failure on the same item is highly variable. The two lists used were both constructed using (mainly) pairs of words with a similar

TABLE 7.5
Reading Responses for Correct Associations and Incorrect Associations

Stimulus	Correct Pronunciation	Correct Associations		Correct Choice
		Responses	Reading	
science	/sjãs/		+	médecine
ration	/rasjɔ̃/		+	part
album	/albɔm/		+	livre
choléra	/kɔlera/		+	maladie
bastion	/bastjɔ̃/		+	caserne
agneau	/anjo/		+	mouton
chorizo	/ʃoritso/		+	saucisson
oignon	/ɔnjɔ̃/		+	échalotte
rose	/roz/		+	fleur
voix	/vwa/ᵃ		+	parole
voeux	/vø/ᵃ		+	souhaits
quotient	/kɔsjã/	/kɔsjɛ̃ ... ko/ ... un *quotient*	+	division
paien	/pajɛ̃/	un /pajã/ ... un *paien*	+	incroyant
damné	/dane/	/damne/, *damné*	+	enfer
saoul	/su/ᵃ	/saul/ ... /sul/ᵃ (*saoule*)	−	ivre
stagner	/stagne/	/sta ... stanje/	−	croupir
anguille	/ãgɥij/	aiguille ... /ãgɥij ... ãgi/ ...	−	poisson
poêle	/pwal/ᵃ	/po-ɛl/	−	radiateur
martien	/marsjɛ̃/	/marsjã/	−	planète
rosse	/rɔs/	/rɔs/	−	cheval
fosse	/fos/ᵃ	/rɔs/ᵃ (*rosse*) ... /fɔs/	−	creuser
fuel	/fjul/	/fyɛl/ ... un /fjɔl/ ... un /fyɛl/ ... /fjɔl/ ... /fyɛl/ ... /fyɛl/ ... un /fjɔl/ (*fiole*)	−	mazout
hymne	/imn/	/ym ... im ... ymᵃ/ (*hume*)	−	cantique
tas	/tɑ/	/tas/ᵃ (*tasse*)	−	amas

Incorrect Associations

Stimulus	Correct Pronunciation	Responses	Reading	Correct Choice	Incorrect Choice
ignorer	/iɲɔre/		+	savoir	permettre
super	/sypɛr/		+	meilleur	?
compteur	/kɔ̃tœr/ᵃ	/kastɛm/ … un /kɔ̃stœr/ … /kɔ̃/ un /kɔ̃tœr/ᵃ (correct for *conteur*)			
opium	/opjɔm/	/op … opo … opo/ … *opium*	+	numéro	cirque
rhum	/rɔm/ᵃ	/rym/ᵃ (*rhume*)	+	droguer	balle
initier	/inisje/	/inisjɑ̃/	−	antillais	lit
			−	introduire	cuire

ᵃIn "Correct Pronunciation," this signals the existence of a homophone. In "Responses," this signals that the incorrect reading has a lexical entry, noted in parentheses.

spelling pattern of different pronunciation, so that this value of approxima-tely 50% correct *could* be due to the use of a simple consistent GPC strategy that would fit half of the words of the lists. Examination of the stimuli and of the responses in failed or passed items, however, does not favour this explanation. In both cases B.F. used various different reading strategies, including but not restricted to application of simple GPC rules. She read *tien* as both /tjɛ̃/ and /sjɛ̃/ but assigned these two pronunciations to the wrong words in *martien* and *maintien*; she also read *ien* as both /jɛ̃/ and /jɑ̃/ and assigned the two pronunciations to the correct words *paien* and *faience*. She read *aen* as both /aen/ and /aɑ̃/, and *gui* as /gi/, /gɥi/ and even /gwi/, etc. Then her nearly chance level in reading inconsistent words seems to be more in line with the suggestion that B.F. was reading these words by non-lexical spelling–sound correspondences (not necessarily GPC rules) that she, how-ever, applied randomly.

According to this position, one could still argue that in 14 correctly associated words, out of the 18 correctly read ones, the meaning could have been accessed through pre-lexical phonological recoding. One has first to consider that 2/12 correctly read and associated words (*voix* /vwa/ and *voeux* /vø/) have homophones (*voie–voit, veut*). Second, analysing the 10 incorrect readings when correct association was achieved appears to give little support to the importance of pre-lexical phonological recoding for lexical access in B.F. One instance—*saoul*—is not pertinent to this question. Though possibly due to application of spelling–sound correspondence rules, the phonologi-cally incorrect form has a lexical entry which is semantically and morpholo-gically close to the target—/sul/ *saoule* is the feminine of /su/ *saoul*.

In the other nine cases, the phonology obtained by application of spelling–sound correspondence rules cannot be the base of the correct semantic interpretation of the written stimulus. The errors resulting from "regularisation" on *stagner–poêle–martien–rosse–fosse* (see Table 7.9) have no lexical entry. More important, the errors on *anguille–fuel–hymne–tas* all result in a phonological form that corresponds to a lexical entry that is very different in meaning.

The incorrect responses for these nine words show clear confusions between alternative possible spelling–sound correspondences; but beside these errors, they contain also in some cases possible "visual errors" such as *fuel→fiole, anguille→aiguille, hymne→hume*. In these instances the *written* stimulus was understood (as shown by the correct association). This fact makes it difficult to account for at least these particular "visual" errors in terms not only of input logogen failure, but also of semantic (access or representation) failure (Shallice & Warrington, 1975).

I would rather propose that at least these three errors result from misselection in the output phonological lexicon. Some support for this suggestion and its implications in accounting for visual errors in dyslexic syndromes in general is presented later.

I have presented some evidence for the parallel use of a largely preserved phonological route and a largely preserved direct semantic route (at least as far as semantic representation), as well as of the relative independence of these two processes in B.F. A number of problems still remain. First, although B.F.'s understanding of inconsistent words was quite good, she failed the association test on six items. Moreover, four of these failures were on correctly read words. This suggests that there is some representational semantic deficit in this patient.

Of the six words two were, in fact, at least partially understood (*rhum* and *super*); two other failures were on abstract verbs (e.g. *initier* and *ignorer*); and we wonder about the concreteness of *opium* for our patient. The final error is on a phonologically ambiguous word /kɔ̃tœr/ meaning *compteur* or *conteur* for which she chose an associate corresponding to the meaning of *dompteur* (visual error).

We cannot totally exclude a semantic deficit that may be more important for abstract words. Those failures could also be the result of other artefacts. For example, *ignorer* associated to *savoir* is the only instance in which antonymy has been used, and the relationship between *initier* and its associate *introduire* is unclear (both words have many abstract meanings and at least one concrete meaning). It is anyway difficult to draw any causal relationship between this hypothetical semantic deficit and the dominant use by this patient of spelling–sound correspondence rules in reading inconsistent words.

A second question is raised by her strange preference for the obviously inefficient spelling-to-sound process for reading inconsistent words. Before trying to answer this problem, one has to consider that maybe B.F. used the spelling–sound correspondence process in reading because she had a post-semantic word retrieval deficit. One example cited before suggested that this was not very plausible. On the contrary, the good production of *steak* when commenting on the meaning of the written word indicated that it was easier for B.F. to name it than to read it. However, a careful scrutiny of her naming performance was in order.

NAMING

B.F. was submitted to a routine naming test for 20 objects and 20 pictures on 26 September 1978. Two of the pictures (microscope and diapason) were not recognised by the patient and have been left out of the analysis. Her responses to the remaining 38 items have been classified as correct if the words were produced without any hesitation or preceding error. B.F.'s correct score was 27/38 (71%). The incorrect responses are reported below:

fer à cheval (horseshoe)→"fer (quelle sorte?) à cheval."

moulin à vent (windmill)→"moulin (quelle sorte?) à vent."

bague (ring)→"une /gɑp/, une ! . . . bague."

thermomètre (thermometer)→"un thermo . . . un /bɛrmo/ un ter-mètre (un?) thermomètre."

seringue (syringe)→"nəʒɛ̃/ . . . une seringue."

robinet (tap)→"/torɔbinɛ/ . . . /torɔbin/ . . . (un?) un robinet."

boîte d'allumettes (matchbox)→"des /ɛgɥi/ . . . des allumettes, mais c'est une . . . boîte d'allumettes."

chaine (chain)→"une /gɛ/ une gaine (sheath), non! (une?) une ch . . . une chaine."

briquet (lighter)→". . . (qu'est-ce que c'est?) une gaz, mais c'est pas ça . . . un briquet."

chaussure (shoe)→"des, des gants . . . ou des bottes . . . pas des bottes . . . des souliers . . . des souliers."

bateau (boat)→" un battoir? (beater) un bat . . . oui, c'est ça . . . un bateau."

All the incorrect responses end with the correct word, and the two first incorrect instances should perhaps in fact be taken as totally correct. Four other responses indicate a *post* word-retrieval deficit of *production*.

There are still five cases (out of 38) in which, although the correct response is available and is produced, a word retrieval deficit is possible. Two of these contain clear phonological errors (chaine→"gaine," bateau→"battoir". Indeed, had the visual task been reading, these could have been taken as "visual" errors. One case (boîte d'allumettes→/ɛgɥi/) is not really classifiable.

Only two responses include semantic errors. The final answer to *chaussure* ("des souliers") is, strictly speaking, incorrect, but an acceptable response because normal control subjects do produce it. They improve it sometimes by "well . . . *one* shoe." *Des* souliers like *des* lunettes, *du* pain, *du* gaz, is the categorical name.

In the *briquet* example, B.F. did not answer "du gaz" but "*une* gaz." We transcribed the word as *gaz* because of the obvious semantic relationship between *briquet* (*à gaz*) and *gaz*. However, this last word could be understood as *gaze* (gauze), and B.F. did put an article before the noun that corresponds to this last interpretation (une gaze). Genuine semantically based activation of the word should have been *un* or *du gaz*. This last example indicates the need for a much more sophisticated model of word retrieval, even for object naming, than simple activation of phonology (output logogens) by semantics.

We will only consider here the fact that B.F. has no word-retrieval problem in 87% of the naming test responses, and that this score is very much better than her irregular word-reading ability.

DISCUSSION

As noted in the introduction to this chapter, most published cases of surface dyslexia involve either a visual word comprehension disorder or a severe naming disorder, the ability to use spelling–sound correspondences being relatively unimpaired. These cases can be described entirely on the basis of a dual-route model of reading.

In B.F., written word comprehension is largely preserved (or at least superior to her ability to read aloud) as are her naming abilities. This patient's reading of inconsistent words is, nevertheless, impaired, and shows errors typical of surface dyslexia. It suggests that such a case of surface dyslexia is the result of damage to another route for reading than the two usually considered ones.

I assume that this route, which allows reading of inconsistent (as well as consistent) lexical units, is based on direct correspondence between visual inputs (input logogens) and phonological outputs (output logogens). I suggest here that it is damage to this route which, in a patient with a preserved ability to realise spelling–sound correspondences, is a sufficient source of surface dyslexic reading performance. Such damage does not of course exclude the possibility that some additional pre-semantic, semantic, or post-semantic deficit can also be present.

A pre-semantic or semantic deficit in itself may *not* be sufficient to cause surface dyslexia. This has been demonstrated by the observation of a demented patient W.L.P., who could read irregular words that she could not understand (Schwartz et al., 1980). However, as observed in W.L.P. and even more dramatically in the patient M.P. (Bub, Cancellière, & Kertesz, Chapter 1 in this book), the ability to read words via the direct lexical (non-semantic) process appears to be restricted to words of high or at least moderate frequency. On lower-frequency words, such a patient may be forced to rely on spelling–sound correspondences for oral reading and will therefore make surface dyslexic errors on low-frequency irregular words.

That a post-semantic (word-retrieval) deficit—a deficit of activation from semantics of intrinsically preserved output phonology—is in itself not sufficient to give rise to surface dyslexia cannot be easily demonstrated, and in fact this is an interpretation offered by Kay and Patterson (Chapter 4 in this book) for their patient E.S.T. The pattern of B.F.'s scores in reading versus naming, however, suggests that such an interpretation cannot always be appropriate. I have already mentioned that one of the difficulties lies in the possibly greater complexity of naming performance than is usually supposed.

A unique post-semantic locus for word-retrieval deficit is indeed once again dependent on the number of "routes" involved in models of word processing. If, as suggested by Wernicke in 1874, not only repetition but also, though to a lesser degree, naming and spontaneous speech use a "route" linking "auditory word images" (auditory input logogens) directly to "articulatory word images" (output logogens), *together with* a route from "concept associations" (semantics), there is no unique locus for naming deficits to arise. However, if a word-retrieval deficit (caused by post-semantic disruption of the semantic route) was a sufficient condition for surface dyslexia to arise, it should be a symptom constantly associated with at least one type of anomia. Neuropsychological studies of reading in anomic patients could help to answer this question, but I do not know of any systematic investigation into irregular word reading in anomic patients.

The hypothesis for the existence of a lexical non-semantic route of reading has been suggested in other studies of dyslexia (Coltheart et al., 1983; Friedman & Perlman, 1982; Funnell, 1983; Kremin, 1982; Morton & Patterson, 1980; Saffran & Marin, 1977; Schwartz et al., 1980). This possibility is contained in some normal word-processing models, like Morton's logogen model (1979), and some experiments with non-brain-damaged subjects also support its existence. For instance, Potter and Faulconer (1975) present results indicating that reading words is faster than naming corresponding pictures, but that understanding (category matching) is, on the contrary, slightly faster for pictures than for words. This pattern of results suggests, at least, that normal reading and comprehension of words are two separate processes.

A critical point for this issue lies in studies of the different reading codes such as Chinese or Japanese kanji symbols. Two-route models assume—and the question is open for three-route models—that ideograms are read by a visual *semantic* route. Results from an experiment by So et al. (1977), similar to the previously mentioned one by Potter and Faulconer, suggest on the contrary that in non-brain-damaged Chinese subjects, reading of isolated ideograms may rely on the direct lexical (but not semantic) connection from visual input to output phonology.

The type of process that this "route" involves is labelled here "phonological" and "direct". By "direct" I mean that the transcoding applies to larger stored units (maybe words) than the units dealt with by the other spelling-to-sound transcoding "route." These two phonological "routes" can possibly be only extremes of one single complex process, or of two processes that are progressively integrated. The apparent independence between the two phonological routes could then be an artefact of brain lesions, that would give clear pictures only at end points of this, or these, process(es). Glushko (1979), Marcel (1980), and Shallice and Warrington (1980) have all proposed views that could be compatible with this assumption. With reference to dementia, in order to explain the absence of surface dyslexia in Schwartz et al.'s (1980) patient, who could read irregular words that she could not understand, Shallice and Warrington (1980) also propose that phonological transcoding at the level of large units is the first mechanism to suffer from brain damage. They propose that, as the deterioration increases, the various levels of phonological correspondences would be destroyed, until the neural bases for phonological transcoding at the smallest level are also impaired (see also Shallice & McCarthy, Chapter 15 in this book).

The study of patients with focal brain damage does not contradict this possibility but shows that the two extremes of phonological recoding can be impaired separately (large units in surface dyslexia—small units in phonological alexia). It is proposed that in B.F. the lexical non-semantic route is severely damaged, and it is assumed also that this route is normally the most efficient one for reading aloud single words, even though the other routes do contribute to normal reading. The pattern of errors produced by B.F. indicates that she primarily relies on the spelling–sound correspondence route to produce a response; however, some errors suggest that although the lexical route is damaged, it may have been used, and may be responsible for the incorrect responses. It is proposed that "phonological" but lexical errors like *aiguille→anguille* typically reflect the disturbance in the lexical non-semantic route. Some degree of preservation in this route could perhaps explain the general lexical superiority effect found in B.F.'s reading of the first unselected list of words and non-words. According to this position, what is sometimes interpreted as a "cut" in a route of a model should rather be viewed as a dysfunction in a process, yielding errors rather than, or as well as, "no responses."

One could argue that although these errors indicate a lexical involvement in B.F.'s word reading, they could be classified as visual (input) errors rather than phonological (output) errors. Being devoted to surface dyslexia, this chapter has been using French language irregularity or inconsistency for convenience. This emphasis should not make us forget that, even in a complex and relatively incoherent spelling–sound correspondence system like French, the phonological correspondence is basic, and works at least approximately for most words. Most French words that share some phonemes will very probably be visually similar. Given this relation, it is a priori difficult to disentangle visual from phonological factors. (See also Chapter 16, by Derouesné and Beauvois, for a discussion of visual and/or phonological errors.) In this chapter I have been reluctant to call errors like *aiguille→anguille* or *fuel→fiole* simply "visual," because they were not associated with a visual semantic access deficit. They were indeed also present in object naming and, although very infrequently, in spontaneous speech. It is therefore obviously difficult to judge them as visual on the basis that, in a reading task, the stimulus is visual. In B.F. these errors may be attributed more plausibly to a level before, but very close to, the level of output phonology.

If, as I assume, the lexical non-semantic route is not only a tool for the neuropsychologist working on "surface dyslexia" but represents a largely dominant process for oral reading, one needs to consider its significance in other dyslexic syndromes such as "deep dyslexia" and "phonological alexia." To put it simply, I assume that it is, not necessarily entirely, but largely preserved in many phonological alexic patients and very impaired in deep dyslexic patients. Some indication of impairment to this route could, I think, be sought in relationship to the occurrence of so-called "visual errors" in these syndromes. Indeed, so-called "visual" errors I would rather propose generally to call phonological errors (although some of them, of course, may actually be visual).

Japanese, which uses different types of orthography, appears once again to give information critical to this issue. The nature of kanji symbols makes it improbable that two words that share features in output phonology will also be visually similar. On the contrary there must be eventually a tendency for maximum distinctiveness. Conversely, two visually similar symbols are unlikely to be phonologically similar. This situation should then offer the possibility to detect unmistakable "visual" errors. When discussing the peculiarities of Japanese dyslexic syndromes, Sasanuma (1980, pp. 84–85) underlines the fact that, contrary to what is observed in English-speaking dyslexics, Japanese patients make very few "visual" errors in general. She notes also that "visual" errors occur more frequently in kana word reading, which uses phonological recoding by means of character-to-syllable correspondence rules, than in kanji word reading. It is also mentioned that the visual errors that affect kana word reading may represent also phonological (output) confusions.

Sasanuma proposes that part of the explanation for this difference between Japanese- and English-speaking dyslexics lies in the greater distinctiveness of kanji symbols. This notion of distinctiveness may reflect the law of "maximum contrast," which is a principle of every spoken and written language. This principle, however, does not prevent some signs from being visually similar, and potentially confusable, in Japanese as well as in other writing systems.

According to the position that in B.F. the lexical non-semantic route is severely, if not totally damaged, this patient is left with two other possibilities for oral reading. It is not my aim here to prove that these two other reading possibilities (or routes) are both perfectly spared, but merely that for B.F. they are both more efficient than the damaged lexical route.

Our results indicate that, being left with a "choice" between these two other routes, B.F. relies rather on spelling-to-sound recoding, even when reading inconsistent words for which this recoding is unreliable, though she could produce a response by use of semantics. She uses semantics to activate the names of objects and pictures and produces very few (5%) semantic errors. Any impairment that she has in the semantic route is surely not sufficiently serious to *force* reliance on spelling-to-sound recoding. Her *preference* for the recoding routine might be based on two facts, which are not mutually exclusive. First, this preference could indicate that the semantic route is fundamentally inadequate to reading aloud. The semantic route is used for and adapted to understanding, which is the basic aim in the normal situation, namely silent reading, or to activate a phonological code in situations like spontaneous speech and (not frequently outside the laboratory) naming from confrontation. These situations do not necessarily require a perfect match to a target, as is the case in oral reading. Second, and as a consequence of this proposal, the fundamental coherence between orthography and phonology, although imperfect, represents a possible bias for the choice of the spelling-to-sound transcoding "route" instead of the semantic "route" when the direct lexical (non-semantic) "route" is damaged in French-speaking patients. It is proposed that in B.F. these two possibilities could explain why she *reads* words by spelling–sound correspondence, even in cases when she could have *said* the word (as she did in the *steak* example) via the comprehension of its meaning. As concerns comprehension in B.F. it is not meant here that it was totally preserved. Actually some words were not understood in the association test, and although she could match written function words on the basis of antonymy she had a severe comprehension deficit of the same words when used in a sentence.

It might also be of some interest to mention that, although B.F. could often choose the correct semantic associate for an incorrectly read inconsistent word, when she was first presented with the task she protested that she would be unable to do it, and had to be encouraged to try. She was surprised to discover that she could do it rather easily and was particularly puzzled in some cases when she read incorrectly both the target and the associate to which she correctly pointed. For instance, she read *stagner* /stɑgne/ as /stɑnje/ (meaningless) and correctly associated it to *croupir* that she read /krupje/ (croupier); she read *martien* /marsjɛ̃/ (martian) as /marsjɑ̃/ and correctly associated it to *planète* (planet) that she read /platɛn/. In both cases she commented that "she did not even know these ones" (the associates). She systematically confused "to know" and "to pronounce correctly." Actually, although her performance gave some evidence to the contrary, B.F. was convinced that phonological (re)coding was a necessary step to achieve comprehension of the written words.

To summarise, B.F.'s deficit is characterised here as a dysfunction in a process that maps word-specific visual inputs to phonology. This direct, lexical phonological process is also considered to be dominant in normal oral reading, although the other spelling-to-sound phonological recoding procedure may (indeed has been shown to) participate in reading in non-brain-damaged subjects (Treiman et al., 1983).

Damage to the direct lexical mapping process, caused by a brain lesion, is assumed to be marked by some characteristic "phonological" output errors. I further proposed that a certain proportion of errors, formerly called "visual," in other dyslexic syndromes could be "phonological" errors, and then reflect damage, to various degrees, to this process in these syndromes.

When this mechanism is severely but selectively impaired, as in B.F., the other spelling-to-sound phonological recoding process is used as an alternative strategy, and the reading deficit results in surface dyslexia. The mechanisms that underlie comprehension of written information are considered here as structurally independent of those that underlie oral reading. The fact that semantic mediation is not typically used by B.F. as an alternative strategy in word reading did not appear to be the consequence of a pre-semantic, representational, or post-semantic deficit, but rather suggests that the semantic route may not be well adapted for oral reading.

Reading by semantics is observed in other dyslexic conditions in which no phonological code (whether obtained by word-specific or spelling–sound correspondences) is available, such as deep dyslexia in alphabetical writing systems, deep and surface dyslexia in Japanese kanji. According to this view, deep dyslexia is considered as being basically a combination of surface dyslexia plus phonological alexia.

Deep dyslexic patients, however, are characterised by a great variability in their general word-reading ability. Moreover, there also seems to be a great variability in the relative frequency of occurrence of visual versus semantic errors within this category of patients. Usually these errors are taken to indicate an additional deficit in the semantic route. However, it was proposed here that "visual" errors should not necessarily be attributed to a semantic access failure. With regard to semantic errors, one should also consider the possibility that, even if there is a *structural* independence between phonological recoding(s) and semantic processing, this does not mean, necessarily, that there is a *functional* independence between the two processes. On the contrary, it is possible that, even if the structure of the semantic "route" is intact, with the exception of some words (concrete, imageable, etc.), both the access to, and maintenance of, an internal phonological representation are necessary to guarantee complete semantic access and processing.

ACKNOWLEDGEMENTS

I thank the editors of this book, and especially K. E. Patterson, for their helpful comments and criticisms. I am also grateful to J. Morton and T. Shallice for their useful criticisms and help in the translation of the French text. I also wish to thank G.

Gosnave for the support that his discussing of some of the ideas presented in this paper provided to me.

REFERENCES

Baron, J. (1976). Mechanisms for pronouncing printed words: Use and acquisition. In D. Laberge, & S. J. Samuels (eds.), *Basic Processes in Reading: Perception and Comprehension*. Potomac, Md.: Lawrence Erlbaum Associates Inc.

Baron, J., & Strawson, C. (1976). Use of orthography and word specific knowledge in reading words aloud. *Journal of Experimental Psychology: Human Perception and Performance, 2*, 386–393.

Beauvois, M. F., & Derouesné, J. (1979). Phonological alexia: Three dissociations. *Journal of Neurology, Neurosurgery and Psychiatry, 42*, 1115–1124.

Coltheart, M. (1978). Lexical access in simple reading tasks. In G. Underwood (ed.), *Strategies of Information Processing*. London: Academic Press.

Coltheart, M., Patterson, K. E., & Marshall, J. C. (eds.) (1980). *Deep Dyslexia*. London: Routledge & Kegan Paul.

Coltheart, M., Masterson, J., Byng, S., Prior, M., & Riddoch, J. (1983). Surface dyslexia. *Quarterly Journal of Experimental Psychology, 35A*, 469–495.

Deloche, G., Andreewsky, E., & Desi, M. (1982). Surface dyslexia: A case report and some theoretical implications to reading models. *Brain and Language, 15*, 12–31.

Friedman, R. B., & Perlman, M. B. (1982). On the underlying causes of semantic paralexias in a patient with deep dyslexia. *Neuropsychologia, 20*, 559–568.

Funnell, E. (1983). Phonological processes in reading: New evidence from acquired dyslexia. *British Journal of Psychology, 74*, 159–180.

Glushko, R. J. (1979). The organization and activation of lexical knowledge in reading aloud. *Journal of Experimental Psychology: Human Perception and Performance, 5*, 674–691.

Goldblum, M. C. (1979). Auditory analogue of deep dyslexia. *Experimental Brain Research.* Suppl. *II: Hearing Mechanisms and Speech*, 397–405.

Goldblum, M. C. (1980). Un équivalent de la dyslexie profonde dans la modalité auditive. Numéro spécial des Annales de l'Université de Toulouse Le Mirail. *Grammatica, I*, 158–176.

Hécaen, H., & Boller, F. (1979). L'évaluation des fonctions neuropsychologiques. Examen standard de l'Unité de Recherches Neuropsychologiques et Neurolinguistiques (U-111) de l'INSERM. *Revue de Psychologie Appliquée, 29*, 247–266.

Kremin, H. (1980). Deux stratégies de lecture dissociables par la pathologie: Description d'un cas de dyslexie profonde et d'un cas de dyslexie de surface. *Grammatica, VII* (1), 131–156.

Kremin, H. (1982). Alexia: theory and research. In R. N. Malatesha, & P. G. Aaron (eds.), *Reading Disorders, Varieties and Treatments*. New York: Academic Press.

Marcel, T. (1980). Surface dyslexia and beginning reading: A revised hypothesis of the pronunciation of print and its impairments. In M. Coltheart, K. E. Patterson, & J. C. Marshall (eds.), *Deep Dyslexia*. London: Routledge & Kegan Paul, pp. 197–226.

Marshall, J. C., & Newcombe, F. (1973). Patterns of paralexia. *Journal of Psycholinguistic Research, 2*, 175–199.

Martin, R. C. (1982). The pseudohomophone effect: The role of visual similarity in non-word decisions. *Quarterly Journal of Experimental Psychology, 34A*, 395–409.

Meyer, D. E., Schvaneveldt, R. W., & Ruddy, M. G. (1974). Functions of graphemic and phonetic codes in visual word recognition. *Memory and Cognition, 2*, 309–321.

Morton, J. (1979). Facilitation in word recognition: Experiments causing change in the Logogen Model. In P. A. Kolers, M. E. Wrolstad, & H. Bouma (eds.), *Processing Visible Language*. New York: Plenum.

Morton, J., & Patterson, K. (1980). A new attempt at an interpretation or an attempt at a new interpretation. In M. Coltheart, K. Patterson, & J. C. Marshall (eds.), *Deep Dyslexia*. London: Routledge & Kegan Paul, pp. 91–118.

Patterson, K., & Marcel, A. J. (1977). Aphasia, dyslexia and the phonological coding of written words. *Quarterly Journal of Experimental Psychology, 29*, 307–318.

Potter, M., & Faulconer, B. A. (1975). Time to understand pictures and words. *Nature, 253*, 437–438.

Saffran, E., & Marin, O. S. M. (1977). Reading without phonology: Evidence from aphasia. *Quarterly Journal of Experimental Psychology, 29*, 515–525.

Saffran, E. M., Schwartz, M. F., & Marin, O. S. M. (1976). Semantic mechanisms in paralexia. *Brain and Language, 3*, 255–265.

Sasanuma, S. (1980). Acquired dyslexia in Japanese: Clinical features and underlying mechanisms. In M. Coltheart, K. E. Patterson, & J. C. Marshall (eds.), *Deep Dyslexia*. London: Routledge & Kegan Paul, pp. 48–90.

Schwartz, M. F., Saffran, E. M., & Marin, O. S. M. (1980). Fractionating the reading process in dementia: Evidence for word-specific print-to-sound associations. In M. Coltheart, K. E. Patterson, & J. C. Marshall (eds.), *Deep Dyslexia*. Routledge & Kegan Paul, pp. 259–269.

Shallice, T., & Warrington, E. K. (1975). Word recognition in a phonemic dyslexic patient. *Quarterly Journal of Experimental Psychology, 27*, 187–199.

Shallice, T., & Warrington, E. K. (1980). Single and multiple component central dyslexic syndromes. In M. Coltheart, K. E. Patterson, & J. C. Marshall (eds.), *Deep Dyslexia*. London: Routledge & Kegan Paul, pp. 119–145.

Shallice, T., Warrington, E. K., & McCarthy, R. (1983). Reading without semantics. *Quarterly Journal of Experimental Psychology, 35A*, 111–138.

Shulman, H. G., Hornak, R., & Sanders, E. (1978). The effects of graphemic, phonemic and semantic relationship on access to lexical structures. *Memory and Cognition, 6*, 115–123.

So, K. F., Potter, M. C., & Friedman, R. B. (1977). Reading in Chinese and English: Naming versus understanding. Unpublished manuscript.

Treiman, R., Freyd, J. J., & Baron, J. (1983). Phonological recoding and use of spelling-to-sound rules in reading of sentences. *Journal of Verbal Learning and Verbal Behavior, 22*, 682–700.

Vikis-Freiberg, V. (1974). *Frequence d'usage des mots au Québec*. Montreal: Les Presses de l'Université de Montréal.

Wernicke, C. (1874). *Der Aphasische Symptomencomplex*. Breslau: M. Cohn & Weigert.

APPENDIX I

Stimulus in Order of Presentation	Semantic Relationship	Multiple Choice			
		1	*2*	*3*	*4*
science	subordinate	*médecine*	volonté	cendrier	hachoir
ration	synonym	partir	*part*	verre	carton
voix	synonym	chose	permis	décence	*parole*
stagner	synonym	*croupir*	vouloir	fermeté	bossu
saoul	synonym	*ivre*	long	plante	pieu
hymne	synonym	filament	*cantique*	fleur	plage
album	synonym	danger	*livre*	mot	stylo
quotient	associative	menu	trouble	*division*	cinéma
tas	synonym	raison	pâte	sincère	*amas*
choléra	superordinate	*maladie*	cuisine	ours	bonbon
anguille	superordinate	fenêtre	*poisson*	coudre	église
opium	associative	pinson	dignité	*drogue*	baille
païen	synonym	*incroyant*	tiroir	fumigène	serpent
bastion	superordinate	*caserne*	pensée	fossile	machine
agneau	superordinate	bague	lanterne	*mouton*	tasse
poêle	synonym	baguette	soufre	chaise	*radiateur*
chorizo	synonym	maladie	*saucisson*	arbre	bastion
voeux	synonym	ration	ivre	vache	*souhaits*
compteur	associative	*numéro*	rosse	gazelle	cirque
martien	associative	commerçant	*planète*	rusé	vendu
rhum	associative	saison	*antillais*	bracelet	lit
damné	associative	boisson	claque	rosace	*enfer*
oignon	synonym	misère	cruche	*échalotte*	crayon
fuel	synonym	fièvre	leçon	*mazout*	sable
rose	superordinate	légume	*fleur*	mer	ciel
initier	synonym	*introduire*	fermer	lancer	cuire
rosse	superordinate	laitue	animal	*cheval*	bouteille
ignorer	antonym	chanter	*savoir*	permettre	jouer
fosse	associative	trouble	lapin	*creuser*	meuble
super	synonym	signer	blond	court	*meilleur*

Numbers in the multiple choice indicate the spatial arrangement: 1, upper left; 2, upper right; 3, down left; 4, down right. Words in italic are the correct associated words.

III   SURFACE DYSLEXIA IN VARIOUS ORTHOGRAPHIES

III Introduction

One of the perspectives available for drawing distinctions between different patterns of dyslexia, whether acquired or developmental, is to consider which properties of written stimuli affect reading success and which do not. Patterson (1981) illustrates this approach by pointing out that, in deep dyslexia (Coltheart, Patterson, & Marshall, 1980), the likelihood of a stimulus being read correctly depends on its semantic properties (concrete words being read better than abstract words), its syntactic properties (content words being read better than function words), and its lexical properties (stimuli having no lexical entries, i.e. non-words, cannot be read at all). In phonological dyslexia (e.g. Funnell, 1983) only the last of these variables has a consistent effect on reading. In pure alexia or letter-by-letter reading (e.g. Patterson & Kay, 1982) it is an orthographic variable—the number of letters in the stimulus—that is most strongly associated with the likelihood that stimuli can be read, because stimuli with many letters are less likely to be read correctly than stimuli with few letters. Finally, in surface dyslexia, it is the correspondence between orthography and phonology that is important: words containing correspondences that are the standard ones (i.e. regular words) are read better than words containing non-standard correspondences (i.e. irregular words).

One of the virtues of this perspective on dyslexia is that it makes clear the fact that there must be various dependencies between patterns of dyslexia, on the one hand, and varieties of writing system, on the other. These dependencies have been discussed by Marshall (1976) and by Coltheart (1984); one or two examples will be given here. In the logographic writing system of Chinese, there are no orthographic elements corresponding to letters, so one could not observe any form of dyslexia in which reading success depended upon the number of letters in the stimulus. Furthermore, pronounceable non-words cannot (as far as we know) be written using the Chinese writing system, so one could not observe phonological dyslexia in Chinese either. In syllabic writing systems such as kana, one of the two Japanese writing systems (which are described by Sasanuma, 1980), there are no elements corresponding to letters, so nothing corresponding exactly to letter-by-letter reading as seen in readers of alphabetic scripts could be seen in kana reading.

It is with surface dyslexia, of course, that considerations of the nature of writing systems are of most importance, because the property of regularity of spelling–sound correspondence, so influential in surface dyslexia, is specifically a property of writing systems. If one were to define the disorder as a selective difficulty in reading words with irregular correspondences between graphemes and phonemes, one might then conclude that surface dyslexia could exist for only a relatively small number of languages, namely those whose writing systems are such that irregular words exist. One could have surface dyslexia in English or French, for example, but not in Spanish, Italian, Chinese, Japanese, or Indian languages, such as Kannada.

However, this is too superficial a view of the relationship between surface dyslexia and writing systems. The reason is that, where the appropriate tests have been carried out, many surface dyslexic patients show three symptoms additional to that of difficulty with irregular words. First, in oral reading of polysyllabic words with one or more stressed syllables, patients may assign stress incorrectly (e.g. reading *oboe* as /ə'boɷ/). Second, many patients make homophone confusions in reading comprehension (e.g. defining the printed word *pane* as "to feel distress"). Third, patients often make spelling errors that are phonologically plausible (e.g. spelling "cough" as *coff*). It follows that, when one is considering the relationships between the properties of surface dyslexia and the properties of writing systems (and of specific languages within writing systems), it is not sufficient to consider whether the language in question permits irregular words. One must also consider whether it permits (a) a variety of syllabic stress patterns, (b) the existence of homophones with different spellings, and (c) different orthographic representations of a particular phonological segment. Only where the latter condition holds are phonologically acceptable spelling errors possible. As noted in the introduction to Part I of this book, Luria (1960) was perhaps the first to draw attention to the relationship between the properties of writing systems and the possible forms of spelling impairments.

The chapter by Masterson, Coltheart, and Meara describes investigations of a language whose writing system does not permit the occurrence of irregular words, but *does* permit the occurrence of homophones and of phonological spelling errors, the language in question being Spanish. A (developmental) case of surface dyslexia in Spanish is described—a case in whom homophone confusions in silent reading comprehension of Spanish, and phonological spelling errors in writing Spanish to dictation, were prominent. The subject could also read and write in English: and he was surface dyslexic in English as well as Spanish.

In Italian, there are no irregular words, no homophones (words with the same pronunciation but different spellings), and no options in the assignment of an orthographic representation to a phonological segment. Thus an Italian reader with a reading impairment cannot display difficulty with irregular words (since there are none), cannot confuse homophones (since there are none), and cannot make phonologically acceptable spelling errors (since there is, in Italian, only one correct way to spell each phoneme). Stress errors are, however, possible in Italian. In Italian polysyllabic words, stress is typically on the penultimate syllable; but there are some words and, in particular, names which depart from this standard pattern. For example, it is the second syllable in Teroldego (a wine name) that is stressed. Correct stress assignment for all Italian polysyllabic words therefore requires lexical access, and accordingly surface dyslexia in Italian can be revealed by stress errors in oral reading.

In summary, considering alphabetically written languages, we find a spectrum of possible patterns of these four surface dyslexic symptoms. At one extreme, English and French permit all four symptoms; towards the other extreme, Italian permits only one of the four. If there existed an alphabetically written language with perfectly consistent grapheme–phoneme and phoneme–grapheme correspondences which furthermore had no variability in stress patterns, then none of the four symptoms could occur.

If we consider syllabic writing systems, here the Japanese language and many Indian languages are important. Karanth describes in her chapter the syllabic writing system used for the Indian language Kannada. This system is one in which none of the symptoms of surface dyslexia could occur. The reason for this is that oral reading, and also spelling to dictation, can be error-free even if they are entirely performed non-lexically, and reading comprehension can be error-free even if it is entirely performed via an intermediate phonological recoding of the written stimulus. These two statements are true by virtue of the facts that: (1) the mappings of syllabograph to syllable and syllable to syllabograph are one-to-one and invariant in Kannada; and (2) there are no exceptions to a general system for assigning stress to polysyllabic words, the system being that all syllables are equally stressed. The writing system of Kannada does not rule out the possible occurrence of deep dyslexia, nor phonological dyslexia; and as for pure alexia (letter-by-letter reading), Karanth describes one form this disorder might take in Kannada.

Japanese is written using a mixture of syllabic and logographic writing systems. The question of whether one can think of surface dyslexia as occurring when a writing system is logographic was discussed by Coltheart

(1982). At first thought, the answer is no, because the only way to read a logograph aloud, or to comprehend it, is to process it lexically: any abolition of specifically lexical processing of written language will therefore simply *abolish* oral reading, spelling, and comprehension of logographs, rather than yielding such errors as homophone confusions and regularisations. However, in cases of surface dyslexia in English, some errors are observed in which it appears that lexical *phonology* has been accessed correctly from print without direct access from print to lexical *semantics*. In such cases, comprehension of print will be indirect (achieved via phonology), but what is important is that the intermediate phonological recoding is obtained *lexically*. One infers that this has happened when one observes homophone confusions with irregular words (e.g. *bury*→"it's a fruit on a tree"). Here the semantics are wrong yet the phonology must have been obtained via lexical processing. This kind of error *can*, in principle, occur in logographic writing systems, provided that there exist pairs of homophones that are written differently; this is abundantly true of Chinese, and of the Japanese logographic system kanji.

Unfortunately, homophone confusions in dyslexic reading of Chinese or of kanji have not yet been investigated. In the chapter by Sasanuma, however, other aspects of surface dyslexia are discussed in relation to the dual-writing system of Japanese. A disturbance of lexical processing of print, at any stage between written input and spoken output, with relative preservation of non-lexical processing, should in Japanese yield poorer reading of kanji than kana, in contrast to Japanese cases of deep dyslexia (Coltheart, 1980; Sasanuma, 1980) where it is kanji that is spared relative to kana. One such case of selective sparing of kana is reported by Sasanuma (1980), and another is reported by Sasanuma in Chapter 9. Her patient S.U. achieved normal accuracy in reading, spelling, and comprehending words written in kana, but was decidedly impaired in all three of these tasks when kanji was used. This pattern represents a selective disturbance of lexical processing in reading and spelling, and hence may correspond to surface dyslexia and dysgraphia in alphabetic scripts.

However, S.U. made semantic errors in reading and writing of kanji. Such errors are not reported in cases of surface dyslexia and dysgraphia in readers of alphabetic scripts. Does this raise doubts about treating S.U.'s disorder as corresponding to some form of surface dyslexia? Not at all; it merely reinforces the point, made by various authors in this book, that there are various loci, within the sequence of stages constituting the lexical system for processing print, at which a processing impairment will generate surface dyslexic symptoms. A defect at that lexical stage which recognises the visual forms of printed words is present in some cases of surface dyslexia; see Coltheart et al. (1983), and especially, Table 4.2 of Chapter 4 by Kay and Patterson, where this defect is demonstrated by impaired lexical decision performance when words are irregular and non-words are pseudohomophones. But S.U.'s lexical defect was not at this stage, because his lexical decision performance with kanji was of normal accuracy. A defect at the stage of output phonology was clearly present for S.U. (the patient exhibited severe anomia and fluent paraphasia) and this would impair the oral reading of kanji. However, the *comprehension* of kanji would not be impaired by such a defect. As comprehension of kanji was, however, also impaired, S.U. must have had, in addition to the output impairment, an impairment of access from kanji to semantics—a "semantic access dyslexia" (Warrington & Shallice, 1979)—which would compromise comprehension of kanji and could generate semantic errors in oral reading. Why postulate an access disorder rather than a disorder within the semantic system itself? The answer is because comprehension of words written in kana was preserved.

The three chapters in Part III illustrate two general points. First, the psycholinguistic analysis of dyslexias (and dysgraphias) enables one to make explicit the relationships between the forms taken by dyslexias and dysgraphias and the properties of the writing systems employed by people exhibiting these disorders. Such psycholinguistic analysis facilitates the investigation of dyslexias and dysgraphias in various orthographies, and the comparison of these disorders across orthographies. Second, this kind of analysis allows one to explore the extent to which models of reading and writing developed initially in relation to alphabetic writing systems can be appropriately applied to other types of writing system. As it happens, the theoretical framework used by Sasanuma to interpret her Japanese case is very similar to that used by Kay and Patterson to interpret their English case.

REFERENCES

Coltheart, M. (1980). Deep dyslexia: A review of the syndrome. In M. Coltheart, K. Patterson, & J. C. Marshall (eds.), *Deep Dyslexia*. London: Routledge & Kegan Paul.

Coltheart, M. (1982). The psycholinguistic analysis of acquired dyslexias: Some illustrations. *Philosophical Transactions of the Royal Society, B298*, 151–164.

Coltheart, M. (1984). The right hemisphere and disorders of reading. In A. Young (ed.), *Functions of the Right Cerebral Hemisphere*. London: Academic Press.

Coltheart, M., Masterson, J., Byng, S., Prior, M., & Riddoch, J. (1983). Surface dyslexia. *Quarterly Journal of Experimental Psychology, 35A*, 469–495.

Coltheart, M., Patterson, K., Marshall, J. C. (eds.) (1980). *Deep Dyslexia*. London: Routledge & Kegan Paul.

Funnell, E. (1983). Phonological processes in reading: New evidence from acquired dyslexia. *British Journal of Psychology, 74*, 159–180.

Luria, A. R. (1960). Differences between disturbances of speech and writing in Russian and in French. *International Journal of Slavic Linguistics and Poetics, 3*, 13–22.

Marshall, J. C. (1976). Neuropsychological aspects of orthographic representation. In R. J. Wales, & E. Walker (eds.), *New Approaches to Language Mechanisms*. Amsterdam: North Holland.

Patterson, K. E. (1981). Neuropsychological approaches to the study of reading. *British Journal of Psychology*, *72*, 151–174.

Patterson, K. E., & Kay, J. (1982). Letter-by-letter reading: psychological descriptions of a neurological syndrome. *Quarterly Journal of Experimental Psychology, 34A*, 411–422

Sasanuma, S. (1980). Acquired dyslexia in Japanese: Clinical features and underlying mechanisms. In M. Coltheart, K. Patterson, & J. C. Marshall (eds.), *Deep Dyslexia*. London: Routledge & Kegan Paul.

8 Surface Dyslexia in a Language Without Irregularly Spelled Words

J. Masterson, M. Coltheart, P. Meara

INTRODUCTION

The symptom of surface dyslexia that has attracted most theoretical interest so far is a selective difficulty in the reading aloud of words with irregular relationships of spelling to sound. This effect was first explicitly documented by Shallice and Warrington (1980), using a set of 39 regular and 39 matched irregular words published by Coltheart, Besner, Jonasson, and Davelaar (1979). One of the patients they described, R.O.G., correctly read 36/39 of the regular words and 25/39 of the irregular words. The other patient, E.M., read 28/39 regular words and 5/39 irregular words. Data from other surface dyslexics to whom this set of words was administered are provided by Coltheart (1982), and further data are provided in the chapters by Saffran and by Kay and Patterson in this book.

Associated with this effect in surface dyslexics is a specific type of reading error—the "regularisation error": when an irregular word is misread, the incorrect response often takes the form of assigning to each grapheme of the stimulus the phoneme that is most commonly associated with it—the "regular pronunciation" of that grapheme. Hence *sew* is read as /sju/ (cf. *new, few, chew, crew*, etc.), *sword* as /swɔd/, *yacht* as /jætʃt/, and so on. By definition, regularisation errors can only be made in response to irregular words: the regular pronunciation of regular words is the correct pronunciation.

Poorer performance with irregular than with regular words, and the occurrence of regularisation errors, are central to the description of surface dyslexia. Both symptoms depend on the presentation of irregular words to the patient. There are languages in which irregular words do not exist, languages for which a system of grapheme–phoneme correspondences exists that is not violated by any word in the language. Examples of such languages are Spanish, Italian, Finnish, and Hungarian; in contrast to these are languages such as English, French, and Danish, in which there are numerous irregularly spelled words.

How are we to think about surface dyslexia in relation to languages with no irregular words? Whatever form or forms of brain damage produce acquired surface dyslexia in readers of English, French, or Danish must also occur in readers of Spanish, Italian, Finnish, or Hungarian: but what consequences will these patterns of brain damage have for reading if, because of the nature of the language involved, effects associated with irregular words cannot be observed? Surface dyslexia occurs as a developmental reading disorder also (Holmes, 1973; Coltheart, Masterson, Byng, Prior, & Riddoch, 1983). Its aetiology is unknown; but whether the disorder is a constitutional or an environmental one, the aetiology must surely be something to which the reader of an entirely regular language could be exposed. What consequences, if any, would such exposure have for such a reader?

One approach to this issue is to study dyslexia in those bilinguals whose two languages are such that one language possesses irregular words whereas the other does not. If such a person exhibits surface dyslexia in the former language, what will reading in the latter language be like? We present such a case; the two languages involved are English and Spanish.

The spelling system of Spanish is perfectly regular; that is, there exists a system of spelling–sound rules that correctly describes the pronunciation of all written words in Spanish, and so no irregular words exist. However, the language is not regular with respect to sound–spelling rules, at least as far as Latin American Spanish is concerned, because there are certain phonemes that can be spelled in more than one way. The letters *b* and *v* are pronounced identically; initial *h* is not pronounced; and the letters *s*, *z*, and *c* (when followed by *e*) are pronounced identically.

The importance of this feature of Spanish is that, although difficulties with irregular words and regularisation errors cannot occur in Spanish, other symptoms of surface dyslexia can—homophone confusions in reading comprehension, and phonological errors in spelling. Coltheart et al. (1983) showed that in the two cases of surface dyslexia they studied, a written homophone was often comprehended as its mate (e.g. *mown* understood as "to complain"), and there was a spelling disorder in which most misspellings of words preserved the phonology of the target word (e.g. "familiar" spelled to dictation as *fermillyer*). The features of the Spanish writing system to which we have just referred are such that these symptoms are permitted to occur in Latin American Spanish; because *haza* (a field for crops) is identical in pronunciation to *asa* (handle), one could observe the error of defining *haza* as "handle," and this would be a homophone confusion in reading comprehension. Similarly, because *z* and *s* are pronounced identically, writing *hasa* in a writing-to-dictation task where the stimulus is "haza" would be a phonological spelling error, exactly like writing *fermillyer* for "familiar" in English.

These considerations set Spanish aside from languages such as Italian. Both languages have no irregularly spelled words, in other words there is a universally applicable system of grapheme–phoneme rules in each of these languages. However, Italian is unlike Spanish in possessing also a universally applicable system of phoneme–grapheme rules; that is, for every Italian phoneme there is only one possible grapheme. Hence homophones do not exist in Italian (that is, homophones with different spellings); nor is it possible to spell a word wrongly while preserving its phonology, because the new spelling will have a new pronunciation. An English–Italian bilingual dyslexic who is surface dyslexic in English would thus be of great interest. Also interesting, however, is the English–Spanish bilingual. If surface dyslexia is present in the reading of English, will the reading of Spanish also demonstrate impairments, and will the impairment in Spanish correspond to surface dyslexia insofar as the Spanish language permits this?

CASE REPORT

F.E. is a right-handed male, born on 18 December 1953. He comes from a middle-class family who live in Colombia, South America, and who are Spanish-speaking. F.E. was born and lived in Colombia until the age of 18, when he came to England. There is no history of any birth trauma. Developmental milestones were normal and he has not had any serious physical illnesses. He learned English at school in Colombia from the age of 8 years onwards. He has lived and studied in England since 1973, sharing accommodation with English and foreign students, and pursuing a course in business studies. He has one brother and one sister. His brother and two cousins are left-handed. All other members of the family are right-handed. His mother, brother, and sister all have difficulty with spelling (in Spanish). F.E. also has spelling difficulty in English. He has not received any remedial therapy for this problem, but, shortly before the investigations to be reported in the next section were carried out, he approached his GP about his difficulty because it was feared that his poor spelling might prevent him from passing his final examinations.

On 4 May 1981 the Wechsler Adult Intelligence Scale (WAIS) was administered to F.E. and he obtained the following scores:

Verbal IQ	100
Performance IQ	119
Full-scale IQ	112
Verbal Subtests	
Information	12
Arithmetic	8
Similarities	13
Digit span	7
Performance Subtests	
Picture completion	14
Picture arrangement	12
Block design	13
Coding	11

His IQ was also assessed on this occasion on Raven's Standard Progressive Matrices and he achieved a score equivalent to an IQ of 125, which corresponds to the superior level. There is a discrepancy between his performance on non-verbal and verbal tests, however. His performance on the Digit Span Subtest of the WAIS reflects a verbal short-term memory deficit.

On 18 March 1981 the Schonell Reading Test was administered and F.E. obtained a score of 79/100 correct (equivalent to a reading age of 12.3 years). The Schonell Spelling Test was administered on 11 February 1981 and he scored 49/100 correct (spelling age = 9.9 years). The spoken version of the English Picture Vocabulary Test was administered on 18 February 1981 when F.E. obtained a score of 105/125 correct (equivalent to a vocabulary age of 16.7 years).

TESTING IN ENGLISH

Reading Regular and Irregular Words

The 39 regular and 39 matched irregular words published in Coltheart et al. (1979), typed individually in lowercase on index cards, were presented one at a time to F.E., and he was asked to read each one aloud. He took 310 seconds to read this set of words; he made errors with 15 of the irregular words and 8 of the regular words. This difference, using McNemar's Test, is significant only by one-tailed test ($\chi^2 = 2.88$, $\chi^2_{.10} = 2.71$). Eight regularisation errors were observed: *sew*→/su/, *broad*→/brooɑd/, *subtle*→/sʌbtəl/, *bury*→/bʌri/, *borough*→/'bɒroɑ/, *sword*→/swɔd/, *circuit*→/'sə:kwɪt/, and *yacht*→/jætʃt/.

Spelling to Dictation

As already mentioned, F.E. made 51/100 errors when the Schonell Spelling Test (Form A) was administered. In six cases no spelling was attempted. The remaining 45 errors are shown in Table 8.1. It can be seen that more than half of F.E.'s spelling errors preserve phonology. In addition, his non-phonological spelling errors sometimes show the influence of *Spanish* phoneme–grapheme rules: for example, "avoid"→*aboid* reflects the fact that the graphemes *b* and *v* are pronounced identically in the form of Spanish spoken by F.E. Hence these, and other comparable, examples are also phonologically correct, with reference to Spanish rather than English spelling rules.

Comprehension of Written Homophones

One hundred pairs of homophones were selected, plus a spoken definition of one member of each pair of homophones. The way in which a comprehen-

TABLE 8.1
Errors Made on the Schonell Spelling Test

"talk"	→*tolk*	"spare"	→*spear*
"ground"	→*graund*	"daughter"	→*doughter*
"brain"[a]	→*brein*	"edge"	→*age*
"write"	→*rate*	"search"[a]	→*serch*
"noise"	→*noice*	"concert"[a]	→*consert*
"freeze"	→*frese*	"financial"[a]	→*finantual*
"avoid"	→*aboid*	"capacity"[a]	→*capasity*
"duties"	→*deatis*	"surplus"	→*surplese*
"recent"[a]	→*reasent*	"exceptionally"[a]	→*exceptionaly*
"instance"[a]	→*instanse*	"successful"[a]	→*suxesfull*
"liquid"	→*liquet*	"colonel"	→*carnel*
"readily"[a]	→*redilly*	"approval"[a]	→*appruval*
"guess"[a]	→*gess*	"accomplished"[a]	→*acomplished*
"attendance"[a]	→*attendanse*	"remittance"	→*remetanse*
"welfare"	→*welthfear*	"referring"[a]	→*refering*
"various"[a]	→*verious*	"courteous"	→*carties*
"genuine"	→*genuing*	"affectionately"	→*afectionally*
"interfere"[a]	→*interfear*	"definite"[a]	→*defenit*
"accordance"[a]	→*accordanse*	"guarantee"[a]	→*garantee*
"mechanical"[a]	→*mecanical*	"anniversary"[a]	→*aniversary*
"anxious"	→*angeous*	"irresistible"	→*erresistable*
"cough"[a]	→*coff*	"hydraulic"[a]	→*highdrolic*
"fitted"	→*feated*		

[a] Errors that we would claim to be phonologically correct spellings of the stimulus word.

sion test was devised from these will be illustrated with reference to the sample homophone pair *peel/peal*. The definition was "rind of a fruit," and our wish was to measure the extent to which reading comprehension was phonologically mediated: such mediation would be indicated by the subject, confronted with the two printed words *peel* and *peal*, choosing the latter as the word corresponding to the spoken definition "rind of fruit." Because such a choice might instead be a visual error, or a random response, additional foil items are needed. What is needed first is a foil item which resembles *peel* visually as much as *peal* does: we chose *feel*. If these three items only were presented, the subject might settle on the strategy of choosing *peel* because it is visually similar to both *peal* and *feel*, which are less similar to each other. Therefore a fourth item is needed, which is as similar to *peal* as *feel* is to *peel*: we chose *peat*.

The task, then, consisted of hearing a spoken definition and selecting the correct word from a set of four: the correct item (*peel*), its homophone (*peal*), a word visually similar to the correct item (*feel*), and a word visually similar to the homophonic foil (*peat*). The occurrence of at least some degree of phonological mediation of reading comprehension would be indicated if, when an incorrect response is made, the homophone *peal* is chosen more often than the other two incorrect items.

In this task, F.E. made 41/100 errors. Of these, 10 were failures to respond. Of the remaining 31 responses, 20 were choices of the homophone of the correct response. By chance one would expect $31/3 = 10.3$ choices of the homophone, and 20 choices is significantly greater than chance ($\chi^2 = 13.69$, $p < .001$). Thus F.E. shows a strong, though far from complete, tendency to read via an intermediate phonological encoding.

Summary of English Testing

With respect to English, F.E. is a developmental dyslexic by the conventional criteria: he is of above-average intelligence, there is no evidence of neurological abnormality, and spoken vocabulary is at an adequate level, whereas reading and spelling are both severely impaired. We claim specifically that F.E., with respect to English, exhibits the developmental form of surface dyslexia, the evidence being: (1) that oral reading is worse for irregular than regular words (although this difference was significant only on a one-tailed test); (2) that spelling errors are, in the majority of cases, phonologically correct renderings of the stimulus word; and (3) that reading comprehension is sometimes mediated by intermediate phonological recoding, as shown by the frequent occurrence of homophone confusions in reading comprehension.

TESTING IN SPANISH

Reading Aloud

Single words

The 78 regular and irregular words from Coltheart et al. (1979) used to test reading aloud in English were translated into Spanish, and presented for reading aloud under the same conditions as those for the English words. All 78 were correctly read.

Connected Text

A 500-word passage of continuous Spanish prose was presented for reading aloud. Three errors were made by F.E. The name *Budi* was read as "Dudi" (which, presumably used here as a name, is not a word in Spanish); *acerceban* (they were approaching) was read as "creaban" (they were creating); and *y a* (and to) was read as "los" (the).

Non-words

A set of 74 pronounceable and orthographically legal non-words was created by changing single letters in 74 genuine Spanish words, and these non-words were presented to F.E. one at a time for oral reading. Only three of these non-words were misread: *techer*→/tɛtʃə/ (which is the pronunciation of *teche*, the subjunctive of the verb *techar*, meaning "to put a roof on": the correct response to the non-word is /tɛtʃɛr/); *gonar*→"gomar" (not a word in Spanish); *teller*→"taller" (not a word in Spanish).

These tests indicate that, as far as reading aloud is concerned, F.E. is not dyslexic in Spanish—his performance on the three oral reading tasks is essentially normal. Intact oral reading is not, however, inconsistent with the presence of surface dyslexia in Spanish, as we have noted. An over-reliance on grapheme–phoneme rules (which is a common theoretical description of surface dyslexia—see Coltheart et al., 1983) would not have observable effects on oral reading in Spanish, because all words can be read aloud correctly using such rules.

Reading Comprehension

Over-reliance on grapheme–phoneme rules would, however, impair reading comprehension in Spanish provided that one tests comprehension of homophones. We therefore did so, selecting 20 pairs of homophones, 40 words in all, and presenting them as single printed words that F.E. was asked to define. This test occupied two sessions, several weeks apart, and the two members of any homophone pair never occurred in the same session. Of these 40 items, 16 were correctly defined, 2 were wrongly defined and the error was not a homophone confusion, 10 elicited the response "don't know," and 12 resulted in homophone confusions.

Spelling to Dictation

Twenty-four words were dictated to F.E. by another native speaker of Latin American Spanish (we thank Dr. M. Wyke for these data). Fourteen of these words were wrongly spelled. Nine of the misspellings were phonologically correct (e.g. "avanzando"→*abansando*, "hallazgos"→*allasgos*). There was one letter deletion, and four instances where the response was correct except for the omission or addition of a stress-marking accent. Accent errors in spelling are common for normal Spanish spellers.

CONCLUSIONS

In dealing with English, F.E. was poor at reading irregular words aloud (and when doing so made regularisation errors); he confused homophones, and he made spelling errors in which phonologically correct spellings predominated. In other words, he exhibited the major symptoms of surface dyslexia as summarised by Coltheart et al. (1983).

In dealing with Spanish, the same pattern emerged, to the extent to which the Spanish spelling system permits: although reading aloud was unimpaired, the reading comprehension test revealed the presence of homophone confusions, and spelling was poor, with a predominance of phonologically correct misspellings.

Thus F.E. was surface dyslexic in both English and Spanish, despite the large differences between the spelling systems of the two languages, and despite differences between his experiences with the two languages (he learned Spanish some years before learning English). It is possible that this co-occurrence of surface dyslexia in the two languages is fortuitous (although we think this unlikely, especially as the other bilingual surface dyslexic we have studied—the developmental case, C.D., described by Coltheart et al. (1983)—was surface dyslexic in both her languages, these being English and French). If it is accepted that this co-occurrence is not simply coincidental, one asks why it is that in both languages F.E. shows an over-reliance on reading via grapheme–phoneme rules, with selectively impaired ability to recognise words via a direct orthographic route: that is, why the dyslexias in the two languages are the same variety of dyslexia.

One possibility, which requires much more investigation before it can be anything more than speculation, is that the component of the reading system that subserves direct orthographic word recognition is not language specific in polyglot readers, but instead is used for reading any alphabetically written language for which such a polyglot has some reading competence. If this is so, a developmental impairment of this component would result in a developmental surface dyslexia affecting all the languages that such a person had learned to read. What might one expect, however, if one of these languages were one that in principle could be read aloud, comprehended, and spelled perfectly without requiring anything other than use of phoneme–grapheme and grapheme–phoneme rules—Italian, for example? And what might one expect if one of these languages was not alphabetic at all—Chinese, for example?

Investigations of these kinds of bilingual cases allow one to assess hypotheses concerning just how such languages are read. As reading and spelling Italian can be based entirely on rule use and do not *need* reference to word-specific knowledge, one would like to know whether such knowledge *is* used by skilled readers and spellers of Italian. As reading and writing Chinese cannot be rule-based and must depend upon word-specific knowledge, one would like to know whether the cognitive component used for word-specific (orthographic) recognition in reading an alphabetic language is the same as, or separate from, the component used for word-specific (ideographic) recognition in reading Chinese.

REFERENCES

Coltheart, M. (1982). The psycholinguistic analysis of acquired dyslexias: Some illustrations. *Philosophical Transactions of the Royal Society of London, B298*, 151–164.

Coltheart, M., Besner, D., Jonasson, J. T., & Davelaar, E. (1979). Phonological recoding in the lexical decision task. *Quarterly Journal of Experimental Psychology, 31*, 489–508.

Coltheart, M., Masterson, J., Byng, S., Prior, M., & Riddoch, J. (1983). Surface dyslexia. *Quarterly Journal of Experimental Psychology, 35A*, 469–495.

Holmes, J. M. (1973). Dyslexia: A neurolinguistic study of traumatic and developmental disorders of reading. Unpublished PhD thesis, University of Edinburgh.

Shallice, T., & Warrington, E. K. (1980). Single and multiple component central dyslexic syndromes. In M. Coltheart, K. E. Patterson, & J. C. Marshall (eds.), *Deep Dyslexia*. London: Routledge & Kegan Paul.

9 Surface Dyslexia and Dysgraphia: How Are They Manifested in Japanese?

S. Sasanuma

INTRODUCTION

In certain cases of dyslexia in speakers of Indo-European languages (notably in English and French), orthographically regular words are more likely to be read aloud correctly than irregular words. Coltheart, Masterson, Byng, Prior, and Riddoch (1983) suggest that this single symptom, of nine they examined, "may be considered necessary and sufficient for the diagnosis of surface dyslexia."

Japanese is written in a mixture of two scripts, the ideographic kanji script and the syllabic kana script; a brief description of the characteristics of this dual-writing system is found in Sasanuma (1980a) and Morton & Sasanuma (1984). If the kanji script represents "the ultimate case" of orthographic irregularity (Henderson, 1982) while the kana script represents the opposite pole of this regularity dimension, the Japanese counterpart of surface dyslexia may be characterised by a greater number of errors in reading aloud kanji than in reading aloud kana. This is exactly what has been found in the patient K.K., whose symptom complex was analysed by Sasanuma (1980a) and judged to represent a Japanese form of surface dyslexia. In other words, the cardinal feature of the symptom complex exhibited by this patient was a severe impairment in reading aloud kanji in contrast to a marked sparing of kana.

This study presents another case of surface dyslexia in a Japanese patient, whose oral reading of kanji is selectively impaired. Three main issues of our concern are: (1) what are other prominent features of the reading and writing impairment exhibited by the patient?; (2) how do these features compare with those of surface dyslexia manifested in speakers of Indo-European languages

225

(English and French)?; and (3) what are some possible explanations for these patterns of impairment?

CASE REPORT

The subject S.U., a 46-year-old qualified interior designer with 14 years of education, was first seen at the Tokyo Metropolitan Geriatric Hospital in May 1981. At this time he had had a 27-month history of aphasia due to CVA, followed by an operation to remove a haematoma in the subcortical region of the left temporal lobe. A neurological examination had disclosed nothing remarkable. A CT scan performed 18 months post onset had indicated a well-defined low density area in the temporo-parieto-occipital region (involving the angular and supramarginal gyri) of the left hemisphere, with a moderate enlargement of the left ventricle.

The evaluation of S.U.'s linguistic impairment using the Roken Test of Differential Diagnosis of Aphasia (Sasanuma, 1978) at the time of this investigation (from September through October 1981) essentially showed a pattern of Wernicke's aphasia characterised by fluent but paraphasic speech. On the test of confrontation naming of 100 daily objects, he made correct and prompt responses on 20 items; 29 of his responses were correct but delayed (response latencies of over 6 seconds). Of 51 errors, 7 were semantic associations (e.g. shirt→"sweater"), 31 were circumlocutions (e.g. pigeon →"It's bigger than a sparrow"), 2 were phonological approximations (e.g. /kagi/ (*key*)→/kaki/), and the rest were either irrelevant or "don't know" responses. In short, the majority of errors were semantic approximations of the targets. He retained his auditory comprehension for isolated words (no errors on either 10 high-frequency or 10 low-frequency words) but showed increasing difficulty in understanding longer and more complex sentences (6/ 10 errors on sentences given in a form of verbal command). His auditory retention span (pointing span) dropped to four for digits and to three for object names.

Severe impairment appeared in S.U.'s reading and writing performances disproportionately in kanji as compared to kana processing.

INVESTIGATION OF READING AND WRITING ABILITIES

The following battery of tests was given to S.U. to delineate the pattern of his impairment in processing written language and to suggest the underlying mechanisms of such processing:

1. Oral reading of 300 isolated words in kanji or kana.
2. Lexical decision tests with kanji and kana strings.
3. Reading comprehension of a subset of the single words in kanji and kana used in test 1.
4. Writing to dictation of the same 300 isolated words in kanji or kana used in test 1.
5. Kana-to-syllable and syllable-to-kana conversions.

All the tests were administered under no time pressure in two to three sessions a week over the span of several weeks. Three normal adults with no history of brain damage served as control subjects. Their ages and educational levels were matched with those of S.U.

In the following sections each test is introduced, followed by the results and discussion.

1. Oral Reading of 300 Isolated Words

We asked S.U. to read aloud a total of 300 isolated words in kanji or kana in various syntactic classes (nouns, verbs, adjectives, and function words) and with different abstractness levels and frequencies of usage. With the exception of function words, which are written only in kana, these test words normally appear in kanji in adult literature. However, non-brain-damaged literate adults can always read the kana versions of the test words.

Reading Aloud Concrete Versus Abstract Nouns in Kanji and Kana

The kanji version of the test employed a set of 20 single-character "concrete" nouns and another set of 20 single-character "abstract" nouns. They were taken from Kitao et al.'s (1977) list of the 881 kyoiku kanji characters rated by 1000 college students in terms of concreteness (C), hieroglyphicity (H), and familiarity (F); the concrete words were those 20 kanji with the highest C-values in the list, while the abstract words were those 20 with the lowest C-values. The F-values of the abstract and concrete words were equivalent.

The same 20 concrete and 20 abstract words written in kana with two to four characters per word constituted the kana version of the test.

Reading Aloud Verbs and Adjectives in Kanji and Kana

A set of 20 single-kanji, high-frequency verbs with inflectional endings (infinitive forms) in kana, and a set of 20 single-kanji, high-frequency adjectives formed by the addition of kana suffixes were employed, along with kana versions of the same sets, with two to four characters per word.

Reading Aloud "Function" Words in Kana

The test consisted of 40 kana function words, two to four characters in length. They included conjunctions, interrogative words, particles, demonstratives, and others.

Reading Aloud Words from the Modified Peabody Test

This test used a set of 50 words transcribed in kanji and kana from the Modified Peabody Test (described later in this chapter) as stimuli. All but five (which were verbs) were nouns, drawn from a wide range of frequency of usage and abstractness levels. Word length was also varied in terms of the number of characters (one to three for words in kanji and one to six for words in kana) as well as of moras (one to six).

The results summarised in Table 9.1 show that S.U. obtained perfect or near perfect scores in all of the kana versions of the tests, with only one error on a function word (あるいは *or* /aruiwa/→ あるいた *walked* /aruita/), which was interpreted to be an instance of visual paralexia.

In contrast, his performances on the kanji versions of the same tests were markedly inferior, with better performance on concrete nouns (55% correct responses) than on any other set of words. Word length, either in terms of the number of characters or of moras, did not seem to affect his performances.

TABLE 9.1
Performance of S.U. (Percentage Correct) on the Oral Reading of Isolated Words

	Concrete Nouns (N=20)	Abstract Nouns (N=20)	Adjectives (N=20)	Verbs (N=20)	Function Words (N=40)	Modified Peabody (N=50)
Kanji	55.0	15.0	20.0	15.0	—	10.0
Kana	100.0	100.0	100.0	100.0	97.5	100.0

Table 9.2 presents the distribution of different types of errors S.U. made in reading aloud kanji. As shown, the greatest number of errors were irrelevant responses—substitutions of words that have no relationship with the target words (47), followed by circumlocutions (22), semantic errors (15), neologisms (14), and *on/kun* confusions (3). (The *on/kun* distinction is discussed further later.) There were no instances of visual or phonological errors. Interestingly, semantic errors did occur (14.9% of all paralexic errors) across the different syntactic classes. Some examples are now shown; those marked with asterisks might have a visual component:

TABLE 9.2
Types of Errors Made by S.U. in the Oral Reading of Isolated Words in Kanji

	Concrete Nouns (N=20)	Abstract Nouns (N=20)	Adjectives (N=20)	Verbs (N=20)	Peabody (N=50)	Total (N=130)
Visual	0	0	0	0	0	0
Phonological	0	0	0	0	0	0
Semantic	3	3	4	1	4	15
Circumlocution	1	1	1	1	18	22
Irrelevant	5	12	2	7	21	47
Neologistic	0	0	7	7	0	14
On/Kun	0	0	2	1	0	3
No response	0	1	0	0	2	3
Total errors	9	17	16	17	45	104

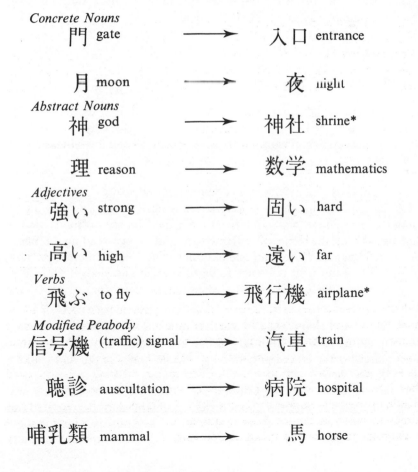

Concrete Nouns

門 gate ⟶ 入口 entrance

月 moon ⟶ 夜 night

Abstract Nouns

神 god ⟶ 神社 shrine*

理 reason ⟶ 数学 mathematics

Adjectives

強い strong ⟶ 固い hard

高い high ⟶ 遠い far

Verbs

飛ぶ to fly ⟶ 飛行機 airplane*

Modified Peabody

信号機 (traffic) signal ⟶ 汽車 train

聴診 auscultation ⟶ 病院 hospital

哺乳類 mammal ⟶ 馬 horse

In addition, S.U. made a sizeable number of circumlocution errors (21.8% of all paralexic errors), especially on abstract, low-frequency words in the Modified Peabody Test, indicating that as words become more abstract and less familiar S.U. had greater difficulty accessing more than the appropriate "sphere" or "field" of the target word's meaning. For example,

恐怖	fear	⟶	"When one dies, or . . ."
裁判官	a judge	⟶	"Punishes a bad guy . . ."
退屈	boredom	⟶	"There is nothing to do."
曲芸	(acrobatic) feats	⟶	"He climbs and everybody looks at him."

This pattern of S.U.'s error responses on kanji suggests that his kanji processing strategy was undoubtedly "lexical."

Another finding of interest is S.U.'s neologistic responses which occurred only on some adjectives and verbs, where kanji (representing the root or free morpheme of the word) and kana (representing the suffix or bound morpheme of the word) are concatenated, for example, 話す *to talk*, 細い *narrow*. Predictably, he could read the kana part of all these words correctly, but his readings of the kanji component of many of these words (14/40) were far from the target pronunciations, or were substituted by the *on*-readings of the character (e.g. 洗う *to wash* /ara-u/→/seN-u/; 重い *heavy* /omo-i/→/choo-i/), thus yielding meaninginless sound strings.

Most kanji characters have several alternative readings, i.e. both an *on*-reading (Sino-Japanese reading derived from the Chinese pronunciation of the characters at the time of borrowing), and a *kun*-reading (a native Japanese reading), or more than one of either kind. These different readings are assigned to kanji with reference to word-specific knowledge. Thus in 洗う *to wash*, the *kun*-reading /ara/ should be used for 洗, the correct response being /ara-u/; instead, S.U. assigned the *on*-reading /seN/, responding /seN-u/. Similarly, *heavy* was read as /choo-i/ rather than /omo-i/; /choo/ is the *on*-reading for 重 while /omo/ is the *kun* reading, which is correct here.

The occurrence of these *on/kun* confusions may reflect that S.U.'s oral reading is mediated by internal phonological representations derived without semantic access. That is, he assigned one of the several readings for these kanji without reference to word-specific meaning. The presence of kana suffixes concatenated with kanji roots in these words might have had a triggering effect on the use of this non-semantic strategy for the kanji part of the words as well.

2. Lexical Decision

Having established that S.U.'s oral reading of kanji is selectively impaired, the next question has to do with possible loci of the malfunction along the lexical route from print to phonology. The first candidate, access to lexical orthography, or "visual input logogens" (Morton & Patterson, 1980) can be examined by means of lexical decision tasks with kanji and kana.

The kana version of the task consisted of 40 three-character strings: 20 high-frequency real words and 20 non-word kana strings. The kanji version of the test consisted of 40 two-character strings: 20 high-frequency words and 20 non-words. To produce non-words, we combined pairs of high-frequency kanji characters in such a way that no meaning could be derived from the compound thus synthesised.

The results summarised in Table 9.3 reveal that S.U.'s performance on both kanji and kana was as accurate as that of the normal controls, although his response latencies (i.e. the time interval between the presentation of each stimulus word and his response) for kanji and kana, words and non-words, were significantly longer than the corresponding times for the normal control who was slowest in his responses (t values from 4.19 to 15.5, p values from < .01 to < .001). Furthermore, S.U.'s mean response latency for kana non-words was significantly longer than that of all three other sets of stimuli ($p < .01$). Taken together, we interpret these findings as indicating that for kanji, access from the visual information to the lexical orthography, or the

TABLE 9.3
Performance of S.U. on Lexical Decision Tasks (Chance Level=50.0%)

	S.U.				Controls			
	Kanji		Kana		Kanji		Kana	
	%	(sec.)	%	(sec.)	%	(sec.)	%	(sec.)
Words	90.0	(5.0)	100.0	(3.7)	100.0	(0.7)	100.0	(1.2)
Non-words	100.0	(4.0)	100.0	(10.5)	86.7	(2.0)	96.7	(1.4)
					(R:80.0–100.0)		(R:95.7–100.0)	

visual input logogens, was functional.[1] Long latencies might indicate some kind of functional inefficiency at this level, although it could arise at a later stage of processing as well. The next question, then, is to what extent these kanji strings recognised as words can be comprehended or matched with their semantic representations.

3. Reading Comprehension of Single Words

Word–Picture Matching Test Adapted from the Peabody Picture Vocabulary Test

We modified the Peabody Picture Vocabulary Test (PPVT) (Dunn, 1965) in such a way that we could require S.U. to match each word written in kanji or kana with one of the four pictures in a display. Moreover, the test was compressed into one-third of the original length (i.e. into 50 words of increasing difficulty) in order to avoid fatigue on the part of patients.

The results are summarised in Table 9.4, and presented together with the results of the performance of the control subjects. For the sake of comparison, the results of S.U.'s oral reading (cf. p. 228) and auditory comprehension of the same set of 50 words are also listed. S.U. had a 98% correct response rate on the kana version of the matching task, which is well within the normal range, just as was his performance on the oral reading test of the same words. His comprehension of kanji (78% correct responses), on the other hand, was inferior to the normal level of performance but markedly superior to his oral reading performance on the same set of words (only 10% correct responses), indicating a clearcut dissociation between comprehension and oral production. In other words, S.U. was able to correctly read aloud only 5/39 kanji on which he demonstrated "comprehension" by matching pictures to them, but failed to correctly produce the remaining 34 words. Words not "comprehended" were never read aloud correctly, suggesting that S.U. did not, or could not, use the direct route from print to lexical phonology bypassing semantics as far as these 50 words in kanji are concerned. His mean response latencies for both kanji and kana in the comprehension tasks were again significantly longer than those of the normal controls (t = 6.94 and 9.62, $p < .001$ in each case), and furthermore his mean response latencies for kana were significantly longer than those for kanji

---

[1] We do not know exactly what level(s) of processing is being tapped by the lexical decision task in general, although it appears relatively safe to assume that a given stimulus has to reach at least as far as the orthographic lexicon in order to be or not to be recognised as a word. When the subject is a brain-damaged patient like S.U., however, the test is given under no time pressure (that is, the patient can have each stimulus in his view as long as he wishes), and thus there may be a possibility that he uses a strategy of consulting not only his orthographic lexicon but also his semantic lexicon in order to judge whether a given stimulus is a word or not. Because we are not sure about the latter possibility, however, we have given S.U. a separate test for comprehension.

TABLE 9.4

S.U.'s Reading Comprehension of 50 Single Words in the Modified
Peabody (Chance Level=25%) in Relation to His Oral Reading and
Auditory Comprehension of the Same Words

	S.U.		Controls	
	Kanji %	Kana %	Kanji %	Kana %
Reading comprehension	78.0 (4.7)[a]	98.0 (8.9)	100.0 (1.4)	98.3 (1.1) (R:95.0–100.0)
Oral reading	10.0	100.0	97.3 (R:92.0 100.0)	100.0
Correct on both comprehension and reading	10.0	98.0		
Correct on comprehension only	68.0	0		
Correct on reading only	0	2.0		
Auditory comprehension	96.0 (5.1)		100.0	
Correct on auditory comprehension only	20.0	0		

[a]Figures in parentheses are comprehension latencies in seconds.

$(t = 5.15, p < .001)$.

How do we interpret these findings? The results indicate that information
from lexical orthography for these 34 words has reached semantics, but that
this information is blocked from gaining access to lexical phonology. In
other words, the functional locus of impairment responsible for S.U.'s
inability to read aloud some kanji seems to originate at the level of access to
lexical phonology or the phonological lexicon itself.

This interpretation appears to be quite plausible because lexical phonology is required not only for reading "irregular" words such as kanji but also
for object naming and word recall in spontaneous speech, which were
markedly impaired in S.U.

It is also possible, however, that S.U.'s access to the semantic representation of some kanji words was not complete or specific enough to retrieve
the words' exact phonological addresses. Obviously, "comprehension" as
measured by a word–picture matching task does not guarantee retrieval of
the full semantic representation of any given word, especially when semanti-

cally related distractors are not systematically included in the non-target alternative pictures in the matching test, as is the case with the PPVT. To explore this point further, we gave two additional tests to S.U.

Detection of Semantically Related Kanji Words

S.U. was shown a list of three words in kanji (e.g. *typhoon, thunder, wind*) and was asked to point to the one item from a display of three other words in kanji (e.g. *winter, rain, water*) that he thought was most closely related to the three words in the first list. There were 20 items in the test, of which S.U. responded correctly to only 12 or 60% (the chance level = 33%), whereas the mean of correct responses by normal controls was 98.3%.

Classification of Kanji Words into Superordinate Categories

There were four tasks in this test. In each task, S.U. was asked to classify 25 words in kanji (each printed on an index card) according to their five superordinate categories, for example, food, animals, furniture, weather, and plants. A different set of 25 kanji words and 5 superordinate categories was used in each task. The results showed that S.U. was able to classify correctly only 50/100 words, or 50% correct responses (chance level = 20%), whereas control subjects made no errors.

These findings obtained from the two additional tests can indeed be interpreted as indicating a certain malfunction in S.U.'s retrieval of the full semantic description for kanji. The question of whether he also had some deficit in the internal organisation of semantic memory itself cannot be answered definitively as we did not give him equivalent tests through other modalities, namely with kana or with auditory presentation.

4. Writing 300 Single Words to Dictation

S.U. was asked to write to dictation the same 300 single words that he read aloud in test 1.

Writing Concrete Versus Abstract Nouns in Kanji and Kana

The same sets of words used in the first part of test 1 (20 single-character "concrete" nouns in kanji and kana and 20 single-character "abstract" nouns in kanji and kana) were used in this test.

Writing Verbs and Adjectives in Kanji and Kana

The same sets of words used in the second part of test 1 were employed, that is, a set of 20 high-frequency verbs and a set of 20 high-frequency adjectives transcribed in kanji (with kana endings) and in kana.

Writing "Function" Words in Kana

The same set of 40 function words in kana employed in the third part of test 1 were used as the stimuli.

Writing Words in the Modified Peabody Test

S.U. wrote the same set of 50 words in kanji and kana in the Modified Peabody Test used in the final part of test 1.

Table 9.5 summarises the performance of S.U. and that of the control subjects on these tests. The control subjects earned perfect scores on all the tests except one—the kanji version of 50 words in the Modified Peabody Test—on which they achieved a mean correct response rate of only 74%, indicating that even the normal control subjects make errors in writing low frequency words in kanji. On the other hand, S.U.'s overall pattern of performance showed a striking similarity to that of his performance on the oral reading tasks. In other words, S.U. had perfect or near perfect scores on all of the kana versions of the tests, but made a large number of errors on the kanji versions of the same tests, with better performance on concrete nouns as compared to all other forms.

Table 9.6 shows an analysis of the types of errors made by S.U. in writing single kanji words to dictation. It can be seen that the errors made by the normal controls were centred on two types of paragraphic responses, namely graphic errors (e.g. 供 → 烘) and graphically incomplete responses

(e.g. 輪 → 車), plus "don't know" responses. These types of para-

TABLE 9.5

Performance of S.U. (Percentage Correct) on Writing Isolated Words to Dictation

	Concrete Nouns (N=20)	Abstract Nouns (N=20)	Adjectives (N=20)	Verbs (N=20)	Function (N=40)	Peabody (N=50)
Kanji	70.0	10.0	10.0	35.5	—	8.0 74.0[a]
Kana	100.0	100.0	95.5	95.5	100.0	100.0

[a] The mean performance of the control subjects for kanji.

TABLE 9.6
Types of Errors Made by S.U. in Writing to Dictation of Isolated Words in Kanji

	Concrete Nouns (N=20)	Abstract Nouns (N=20)	Adjectives (N=20)	Verbs (N=20)	Peabody (N=50)	Total (N=130)
Graphic	0	0	0	1	1 (7)[a]	2
Incomplete	0	0	0	0	3 (3)[a]	3
Homophonic	0	0	0	1	0	1
Semantic	3	0	4	2	4	13
Irrelevant	0	3	2	2	0	7
Neologistic	0	0	5	1	0	6
Others	0	2	1	1	3	7
No response	3	13	6	5	35 (3)[a]	62
Total errors	6	18	18	13	46 (13)[a]	101

[a]The mean performance of the control subjects.

graphic errors take place exclusively in kanji, not in kana, and tend to constitute the majority of errors made by the normal subjects (Sasanuma & Fujimura, 1972).

In S.U., on the other hand, graphic errors (聞く *to hear*→ 開く *to open*)

and graphically incomplete responses (鋸 *saw* → 釒，天文台 *astronomical observatory*→天 台) constituted only a small portion (5/101 or 5%) of his total errors. Instead, S.U. exhibited, in addition to a large number of "don't know" responses (62 in all), a sizeable number of semantic errors (13 or 33.3% of all the paragraphic responses), followed by irrelevant responses—substitutions of words that have no relationship to the target words (7)—and neologistic responses (6).

The following are some examples of S.U.'s semantic errors in writing:

Concrete Nouns

月   moon   ⟶   星   star

店   shop   ⟶   屋   house

Adjectives

広い   wide   ⟶   厚い thick

冷たい   cold   ⟶   温い warm

Verbs

笑う   to laugh ⟶ 泣く to cry

話す   to speak ⟶ 読む to read

Modified Peabody

矢   arrow ⟶ 弓   bow

背広   business ⟶ 服   dress
    suit

線路   railway ⟶ 鉄   iron

These errors indicate that S.U.'s strategy in processing kanji in writing was clearly lexical, as was the case with his oral reading of kanji.

How do we interpret these error patterns? S.U.'s close to normal performance on the auditory comprehension task with 50 words in the Modified Peabody Test (90% correct responses) might be interpreted as indicating that auditory information for the majority of test words has reached semantics, but this information has failed to be encoded into the appropriate orthographic form. In other words, the functional locus of malfunction can be identified at the stage of access to lexical orthography or the graphic output logogen (Morton, 1980). Additionally, there is a possibility of a problem at the level of access to semantics, which may make the retrieval of a semantic representation for some words somewhat incomplete or underspecified, as was discussed earlier with regard to the impaired oral reading of kanji. If this is the case, then, a less-than-complete retrieval of the semantic code for some kanji may affect the retrieval of their precise orthographic representation, particularly when there is no means of segmental translation from sound to print to double-check the responses.

As for the six neologistic responses occurring exclusively in adjectives and verbs, they can be interpreted as representing a reversed version of the neologistic readings produced by S.U. in the oral reading of adjectives and verbs in kanji–kana concatenations (cf. p. 230). In other words, these writing errors are characterised by the correctly written kana suffix concatenated with the incorrect kanji, which is homophonic to the pronunciation of the kanji root of the target word, but irrelevant in terms of the meaning of the word (e.g. 切る /ki-ru/ *to cut* → 木 (ki) *tree* plus る /ru/-suffix.

It appears as if he bypassed semantics and converted phonological segments of the heard word into a kanji-plus-kana sequence, where one of the many readings of the kanji corresponds to that phonological segment represented by the kanji in the target word, but is orthographically irrelevant to the word's meaning.

Taken together, these findings indicate that S.U.'s overall pattern of writing impairment is surprisingly similar to that of his reading performance, with highly selective impairment of kanji processing. On the other hand, the relative distribution of the types of errors he exhibited on kanji in writing was only partially similar to that in reading. For instance, the proportion of "no responses" was far greater in writing, whereas the proportion of "irrelevant responses" was much greater in reading, and so was the proportion of "neologistic responses." "Circumlocutions" were characteristic errors only for reading.

It appears as if the task of writing had the effect on S.U. of suppressing those circumlocutions or irrelevant and neologistic responses that he produced freely in the oral reading task. The finding is of interest because, with the surface dysgraphic patient T.P. (Hatfield & Patterson, 1983) the major proportion of her reading errors were real words rather than neologisms, whereas no parallel phenomenon occurred in her spelling errors. In fact, the majority of the latter errors were phonologically plausible non-words that are homophonic to the target. Similar findings are reported by Coltheart et al. (1983) and by Kremin (Chapter 5 in this book) for writing errors in their respective cases C.D. and H.A.M. Hatfield and Patterson (1983) suggest as an explanation of this difference in error types between reading and spelling that in phonological spelling the target word is typically comprehended before the response code is generated, that is, comprehension of the stimulus words typically precedes code translation from phonology to orthography with little or no motivation to generate "meaningful" responses, whereas in surface dyslexia comprehension of the stimulus word typically follows code translation from graphemes to phonology.

If we use a similar line of reasoning, S.U.'s neologistic responses in reading kanji might have been due to the fact that he understood the meanings of the test words prior to reading them aloud and had little motivation to make his oral responses acceptable to his phonological lexicon. His relatively high performance rate (78% correct responses) for even low frequency kanji words in the Modified Peabody test will support this speculation.

5. Kana–Syllable and Syllable–Kana Correspondence

From the foregoing tests it was suggested that the knowledge of both kana–syllable and syllable–kana correspondence rules might be well preserved in S.U. To confirm this point, we examined his phonological coding in a context in which the possible effects of the lexical-semantic system were eliminated.

Reading Aloud Nonsense Kana Strings

A set of 20 non-words was constructed by changing the sequential order of the characters, or replacing one kana character with another character, in each of 20 two-character high-frequency real words. S.U. was then asked to read aloud this set of kana strings.

Writing Nonsense Kana Strings to Dictation

S.U. was asked to write to dictation the same set of 20 kana strings.

The results showed that S.U. performed 100% correctly on both tests indicating that his kana–syllable and syllable–kana conversion rules are well preserved.

GENERAL DISCUSSION

The prominent features of S.U.'s symptomatology uncovered in the present study can be summarised as follows:

1. There was a clearcut dissociation between kanji and kana processings, that is, a severe impairment in kanji processing in contrast to a marked preservation of kana processing.
2. This dissociation between kanji and kana processing was observed not only in S.U.'s oral reading of isolated words but also in his writing these words to dictation.
3. The majority of paralexic as well as paragraphic errors on kanji were "lexical," including a substantial number of semantic errors (14.9% of paralexic and 33.3% of paragraphic errors) and circumlocutions (21.8% of paralexic errors).
4. In kana processing, on the other hand, no phonological errors (in the sense of misapplication of kana–syllable and syllable–kana correspondence rules) were observed.
5. Comprehension of words in kanji, when measured in the word–picture matching paradigm, was significantly better than oral reading as well as writing to dictation of the same set of words.

How do these patterns of dyslexia and dysgraphia shown by S.U. compare with the symptom patterns generally observed among the surface dyslexic users of alphabetically written languages?

Coltheart et al. (1983) presented an interim list of nine symptoms of surface dyslexia based on their findings from their studies of two surface dyslexics:

1. Regular words are more likely to be read aloud correctly than irregular words.

2. Incorrect readings of irregular words are often regularisations.
3. Incorrect readings of polysyllabic words are sometimes correct except for being wrongly stressed.
4. Silent homophone matching is more accurate with regular words, next best with non-words, and worst with irregular words.
5. Silent reading comprehension is often mediated by prior phonological recoding; this is always the case when the phonological recoding is incorrect.
6. Homophone confusions occur in silent reading comprehension.
7. Even when speech comprehension is otherwise intact, when a word is spelled aloud to the surface dyslexic (the task being to say or understand the word) the same errors occur as are seen in reading aloud.
8. "Orthographic" errors (letter additions, alterations, omissions, or transpositions) occur in reading aloud, and impair the reading of non-words as well as the reading of words.
9. Spelling is defective, with the majority of spelling errors being phonologically correct.

They consider the first of these symptoms to be necessary and sufficient for a diagnosis of surface dyslexia; symptoms 2, 3, and 4 are parasitic to the first symptom (they occur whenever the first symptom occurs); symptoms 5 and 6 are not inevitable (they do not occur in some cases); it has yet to be determined whether the last three symptoms, 7–9, occur invariably or not.

With reference to this list, the first and second features exhibited by S.U.—a selective deficit on kanji in reading as well as in writing—would correspond to the first symptom in the list, constituting a sufficient condition for a diagnosis of surface dyslexia as it is manifested in Japanese. We should not forget, however, that this correspondence is based on an assumption that kanji, which is a logographic code, not a phonological one, represents the "ultimate" form of orthographic irregularity. In other words, the tendency of "regularisations," which is the second symptom in the list, is simply impossible in principle in reading kanji.

On the other hand, the third feature demonstrated by S.U.—appearance of semantic errors on kanji in both reading and writing tasks—does not have a counterpart in the list, and thus requires some explanation for the possible reasons for the discrepancy. The same is true with the fourth feature—an almost error-free performance on kana processing—which does not seem to correspond to any of these symptoms, either. Finally, the fifth feature—the reasonably well-preserved comprehension of kanji in contrast to severely impaired oral reading (with little indication of phonologically based comprehension errors)—corresponds to the absence of symptoms 5 and 6 on the list, which does not preclude the diagnosis of surface dyslexia; in fact, there are reports of a few cases of surface dyslexia in which these symptoms are characteristically absent (Goldblum, Chapter 7; Kremin, Chapter 5; Kay & Patterson, Chapter 4; Margolin, Marcel, & Carlson, Chapter 6; all in this book).

What about the remaining symptoms 3, 4, and 7–9 in the list? Are they manifested in S.U.'s symptomatology, and if they are, in what forms? Symptom 3—errors of stress— may be roughly equivalent to errors of "word accent" in Japanese. However, these were not observed in S.U.'s oral reading of kana words, although there were instances of letter-by-letter reading with reduction of fluency on some low-frequency polysyllabic words. Of course, there were no instances of this kind in his reading of kanji. As for symptom 4, it is obvious again that there are no homophonic regular (kana) words in Japanese; the task of silent homophone matching with kanji was almost impossible for S.U.,[2] as was predicted. Symptom 7 will not occur in Japanese for the obvious reason that spelling is neither used nor necessary in dealing with kana or kanji, since symptom 7 concerns *alphabetic* spelling of words. Occurrence of symptom 8—orthographic errors—was not observed in S.U.'s kana reading, but it could occur in a future case where the functional integrity of the phonological route is less spared than it is with S.U. As for symptom 9—phonologically correct spelling errors—again these will not occur in Japanese, because of the same reasons cited for symptom 7. However, S.U. showed severe impairment in writing kanji to dictation, the underlying mechanism of which is quite different from that of the spelling problem.

This brief comparison of salient features shown by S.U. with representative symptoms of surface dyslexia listed by Coltheart et al. (1983) reveals some basic correspondences as well as some important discrepancies. A closer look at some of these discrepancies seems to be in order.

Semantic Errors for Kanji

S.U. made not only a substantial number of circumlocutions but also a number of semantic errors in his oral reading and writing to dictation of kanji words of various syntactic classes, which is evidence for at least in-field comprehension of these words. A smaller proportion of semantic errors was also committed by a surface dyslexic Japanese patient, K.K., in his oral

---

[2]We gave S.U. a set of 20 kanji words (10 single and 10 compound kanji words) and for each word asked him to point to one kanji word out of four in a display, which sounded the same as the stimulus word. The four kanji in the display consisted of one semantic foil, one phonological foil, one visual foil, and a homophone that was the target. S.U. responded correctly only on three items (15%), which is below the chance level (25%). A vast majority of S.U.'s error responses (14/17) were semantic, with two phonological errors and one visual error, respectively. Incidentally, this homophone matching task with kanji has proved to be extremely difficult not only for another surface dyslexic patient K.K. (Sasanuma, 1980a) but for our deep dyslexic patients Y.H. (Sasanuma, 1980a) and S.N. (Sasanuma, 1980b) as well.

reading of kanji (Sasanuma, 1980a). However, semantic errors rarely occur in surface dyslexic (and dysgraphic) users of alphabetical scripts. In fact, Coltheart, Patterson and Marshall (1980) consider the presence of semantic errors to be a sufficient basis for the diagnosis of deep dyslexia.

A major source of this discrepancy can be found in the basic difference in the nature of the orthographic codes used. The ideographic nature of kanji, and their close association with lexical/semantic representation, suits them for gaining direct access to meaning from print and for using this semantic specification for the retrieval of output phonology in the case of oral reading (and output orthography in the case of writing). In other words, the most likely route of access to output phonology for kanji is lexical–semantic, notwithstanding a partial malfunction at some point along the way, with little means to provide a phonological check for possible misreadings, viz. semantic errors. When the orthography of the surface dyslexic and dys-graphic is English or French, on the other hand, partially or totally spared segmental translation from print to phonology and from phonology to print may serve as a backup code, thus preventing the production of semantic errors. The fact that no kanji words were read correctly without comprehension (Table 9.5) would indicate that a so-called third route, or direct lexical but non-semantic access from print to whole-word phonology, did not seem to be of help to provide a backup code for reading aloud kanji, either.

Kana Processing

The test results of S.U.'s reading and writing kana (regular) words revealed only a few errors (1/300 words in reading and 2/300 words in writing). The error rate in reading kana words of various syntactic categories for another Japanese surface dyslexic patient, K.K. (Sasanuma, 1980a), was quite low also (5%). On the other hand, surface dyslexic users of alphabetically written languages such as English and French—E.S.T. (Kay & Patterson, Chapter 4), B.F. (Goldblum, Chapter 7), C.D. (Coltheart et al., 1983), and R.O.G. (Shallice & Warrington, 1980)—tend to show somewhat higher error rates on reading aloud regular words: 31%, 12%, 10%, and 8%, respectively. Multiple factors may contribute to this tendency (e.g. specific lists of "regular" words used, relative severity of impairment in each patient, etc.) but differences in the relative complexity of the print–sound correspondence rules between these languages and Japanese may be a partial explanation. In other words, the transparency of the print–sound correspondences for kana in Japanese, along with the extremely simple syllabic structures, makes such a script highly suited for segmental coding.

Conversely, S.U.'s low error-rate performance data offer little information as to the specific type of segmental strategies he might have adopted for the oral reading of kana words, for example whether it is a kana–syllable conversion procedure, and if so, whether it is guided, or not guided, by lexical constraints (Glushko, 1979; Marcel, 1980). Furthermore, it might not be totally inconceivable that he used a non-segmental visual strategy for some kana words just as he did for kanji.

This brings us directly to the issue of a lexical access code for kana. What type(s) of strategies did S.U. use? As far as kanji processing is concerned, this study has already provided strong indications that S.U. must have used a visual (or orthographic) code to access lexical semantics. Did he ever use the same strategy for the kana words? S.U.'s mean response latency calculated from his reading comprehension of 50 single words from the Modified Peabody Test (see Table 9.4) was significantly longer than that for kanji (8.9 sec vs. 4.7 sec), suggesting that the mode of access to meaning for kana is clearly different from that used for kanji.[3] On the basis of these data it is tempting to speculate that S.U.'s comprehension of these kana words was based on his phonological recoding of these words, whereas access to semantics for kanji was obtained directly through lexical orthography.

Additional and more compelling data were obtained from a deep dyslexic patient Y.H. (Sasanuma, 1980a), showing that her phonological recoding route was almost totally non-functional and that the visual route, which was relatively unimpaired, could not provide lexical access to kana with only a few exceptions of very high-frequency words. This indicates that it is less likely for kana to gain direct access to the internal lexicon, except perhaps in the case of very high-frequency words, perhaps because the access code for kana words is phonological.

However, a somewhat different sort of information is available from S.U.'s lexical decision test performance. As shown in Table 9.3, the accuracy of his decision was 100% for kana words and non-words, and a comparably good performance was obtained for kanji words and non-words. In addition, his mean response latency for kana words (3.7 sec) was as short as those for kanji words (5.0 sec) and non-words (4.0 sec), but his mean response latency for kana non-words (10.5 sec) was significantly longer than those of all three other sets of the test items. Given that frequency of usage of both kana and kanji test words used was very high in contrast to the frequency of the Peabody words used for the comprehension task, and that the nature of the task was essentially word recognition, it is perfectly possible for S.U. to have relied on a lexical strategy of mapping the familiar visual form of the kana word directly onto lexical orthography (and possibly onto semantics). How-

---

[3]S.U.'s response latencies for reading aloud 50 words in kana from the Modified Peabody Test ranged from 0.8 sec to 13.0 sec with a mean of 5.0 sec, which were significantly slower than the corresponding scores for a control subject, which ranged from 0.7 sec to 2.0 sec with a mean of 1.7 sec. As S.U. did not have any articulatory problems, the possible cause for these long latencies for the oral reading of words in kana should be sought elsewhere.

ever, the same strategy will not work with unfamiliar kana strings or non-words, thus S.U. had to switch to an alternative strategy of phonological recoding in order to be able to judge that these kana strings were indeed non-words.

There is another source of evidence supporting the possibility that high-frequency kana words do achieve direct access via graphic form to the lexicon. This evidence comes from a clinical study of another Japanese deep dyslexic patient, T.O. (Hayashi, Ulatowska, & Sasanuma, in press) whose overall symptom picture is surprisingly similar to that of Y.H., a deep dyslexic patient reported by Sasanuma (1980a), with one important exception. In Y.H. both oral reading and reading comprehension of kana words were profoundly impaired whereas in T.O. a marked dissociation between the two tasks was observed. Although T.O. made no correct responses in reading aloud a set of 29 kana words (these were all original Japanese words or loan words, which can be expressed only in kana), she earned a score of 100% correct responses on a word–picture matching test with the same set of kana words as stimuli. In this matching task, pictorial stimuli were composed of three different line drawings (one correct match to the target, one semantic foil, and the third, which was irrelevant to the target). A similar but less striking dissociation between reading aloud and comprehension of kana words was reported in yet another deep dyslexic patient, S.N., with 8% of correct oral reading of 50 kana words in contrast to 52% correct comprehension of the same set of words (Sasanuma, 1980b).

How do we interpret these findings? Because the kana–syllable conversion route in both of these patients, T.O. and S.N., appeared to be severely impaired, it is quite probable that they used a visual access route for the retrieval of semantics for high-frequency kana words. It is intuitively plausible that the need for phonological recoding of kana words might be much less for gaining lexical access to semantics than it is for finding their pronunciations. In other words, there is a strong likelihood that optional use has been made of alternative strategies depending on the particular demand of the situation, namely, one for the oral reading task and the other for the comprehension task.

In Terms of a Processing Model and of Strategies

Given the specific pattern of symptoms exhibited by S.U., what are the possible explanations in terms of a processing model? In some recent versions of the standard model of reading alphabetic scripts, three routes or procedures to retrieve the phonology of printed words are assumed:

1. A route that makes use of visual information to specify an entry into the lexical semantics from which word phonology is retrieved.

2. A route for phonological recoding by segmenting the printed word into segments of various sizes and assigning phonology to these segments with, or without, reference to word-specific knowledge.
3. A route that gives direct access from visual information to word-specific phonology, independent of semantics.

With reference to this model, S.U.'s selective impairment in reading aloud kanji words can be interpreted to indicate reduced functional integrity of the first route and his resulting reliance primarily on the second route. Whether this phonological recoding of kana words was achieved by application of non-lexical kana–syllable conversion rules or with reference to orthographic analogy will not be determined on the basis of the performance data obtained from S.U. in this study.

On the other hand, S.U.'s relatively well-preserved reading comprehension of the test words (including those kanji that he failed to read aloud correctly), along with his near normal lexical decisions on both kana and kanji, clearly indicate that impairment of the first route is far from total.

Similar findings of reasonably good lexical decisions and reading comprehension are reported for surface dyslexic users of English and French, namely E.S.T., B.F., and H.A.M., studied by, respectively, Kay and Patterson (Chapter 4), Goldblum (Chapter 7), and Kremin (Chapter 5) (in this book). These findings taken together indicate that comprehension of visual word information is not necessarily based on phonological recoding in all surface dyslexic patients but that visual access from print to semantics is preserved in various degrees in some patients and for some types of tasks. In the case of Japanese orthography, kanji makes an inevitably good candidate for visual access to semantics, but in addition, high-frequency kana words may also find direct access to semantics without the mediation of phonological recoding, as is suggested by the test data. In other words, it looks as if optional use is made of these alternative routes or procedures depending on the relative degree of malfunction in either of these routes in a given patient as well as on the nature of the task demand and/or types of test words used (viz. kanji vs. kana, high- vs. low-frequency words, etc.).

How, then, did information from those kanji that reached semantics fail to access their phonological representations? The first possibility may be that of functional independence between the semantic lexicon and the phonological lexicon, with the locus of dysfunction located at the point of access to phonology or at the phonological lexicon itself. Another possibility may be a malfunction at the level of semantic access with a reduction in specificity for visual information to achieve exact semantic representations, which in turn affects the retrieval of exact phonological representations. Emergence of a substantial number of semantic errors as well as circumlocutions in oral reading of kanji in S.U. may partially support this second possibility, although we would assume, at the same time, that visual access to lexical semantics tends to be an intrinsically inexact procedure, leading to the activation of a semantic network rather than a single lexical representation, and thus needs to be counteracted by some means so as to prevent possible errors. In a patient like S.U., however, these means will be extremely limited, because there is no way of providing a phonological check in the case of kanji, and because the so-called third route, which gives direct access from print to phonology, is not functional.

As for the third route, there seems to be no reason why Japanese kanji should not be processed through this route; kanji can be translated directly into phonology without prior access to semantic representation. In fact, a meticulous search by Hagiwara (1982) uncovered three cases in Japanese neurological literature in which some evidence of oral reading of kanji not mediated by semantics can be detected.

The first case, reported by Fujii and Morokuma (1959), was a 30-year-old man afflicted with acute encephalitis who had an episode of recurrent tonic convulsion lasting 3 hours at 4 months post onset. A language evaluation performed at 5–8 months post onset disclosed an overall pattern of Gogi (word-meaning) aphasia, or the mixed form of transcortical aphasia. The defining feature of this syndrome is marked impairment in reading and writing kanji with relative preservation of kana processing in the context of fluent oral repetition, but profound difficulty in comprehension as well as in word retrieval. According to the report, this patient retained the ability to read aloud some kanji without comprehension, and among the examples of the patient's responses cited by the authors there are at least two unambiguous instances of correct oral reading of the test words in kanji (a single kanji meaning "fan" and a three-character compound kanji meaning "ostentatious person") which were not accompanied by comprehension: the patient mumbled to himself "What is 'fan'?" immediately after his correct oral reading of the first word; and when asked to explain the meaning of the second word he read aloud correctly he answered, "To make something like 'haiku' (a Japanese 17-syllabled poem), isn't it?"

The second case was a 56 year-old driver with a diagnosis of transcortical sensory aphasia at $2\frac{1}{2}$ months post onset of right hemiparesis and right hemianopia (Kurachi & Takekoshi, 1977). Characteristic features of this syndrome again include severe impairment of comprehension and word retrieval, combined with relative sparing of fluent oral repetition. As for reading, the test findings reported by the authors indicate that the patient was able to read aloud five test words (*coin, watch, eyeglasses, key, and pencil*) written in kanji as well as in kana accurately as well as fluently, but failed to match these words with target objects. This dissociation, however, was only transient, disappearing completely at $4\frac{1}{2}$ months post onset, at which time the second evaluation was performed.

The third case with suspected dissociation between oral reading and comprehension of kanji was reported by Hirose (1949). This patient was a 36-year-old policeman with two episodes of CVAs, 2 years and 7 months, respectively, prior to a detailed neuropsychological evaluation. The overall pattern of linguistic impairment disclosed was that of sensory aphasia characterised by fluent but paraphasic speech, marked deficits in auditory comprehension and in word retrieval as well as in oral repetition, combined with profound impairment of reading and writing kanji. Kana processing, on the other hand, was only moderately impaired. His performance in reading kanji was somewhat different from the previous two cases in that he had a conspicuous tendency to read aloud some kanji using the correct *on*-reading (47/204 single kanji in the first test; and 19/107 single kanji and 10/80 compound kanji in the second test) but without accompanying comprehension (although no mention is made by the author as to the method of testing comprehension).

It will be apparent from these brief case histories that salient features shared by all three cases include better performance with kana than kanji, marked impairment in comprehension (both auditory and visual) as well as in word finding/naming, combined with fluent but paraphasic (sometimes incoherent) speech. In other words, it appears as if this particular dissociation between oral reading and reading comprehension for kanji tends to take place only in the context where severely compromised semantic processing is combined with marked sparing of phonological processing. There is a surprising similarity between the general picture of the three cases above and that of a case of pre-senile dementia, W.L.P. (Schwartz et al., 1980), in whom evidence for word-specific print-to-sound associations was first established.[4] Taken together these findings would suggest the importance of the overall context of linguistic deficits, with reference to which the reading impairment in question emerges.

Final Remarks

The general conclusion drawn from the present study on the reading impairment of S.U. appears to be in support of a more recent version of the standard model of reading, in which relative independence of three routes is assumed. However, in view of the possibility that the degree of dysfunction in a given system will seldom be all-or-none and that dynamic reorganisation processes may be taking place in the recovering organism, it is highly probable that interactions among these systems are far more active than has generally been assumed on the basis of such a model. The nature and extent

---

[4]The final diagnosis for the second of these three cases turned out to be pre-senile dementia, or Pick's disease (personal communication with Dr Kurachi).

of these interactions may be investigated more profitably in a future study if linguistic deficits in modalities other than those in reading are also taken into account, in such a way that interactions among different modalities as well as different systems in a given modality can be pursued in a broader perspective.[5]

ACKNOWLEDGEMENTS

The author is deeply indebted to Dr Yoko Fukusako of the Tokyo Metropolitan Geriatric Hospital and Ms Shuko Murakami of the Tokyo Metropolitan Institute of Gerontology for their cooperation in conducting this research.

REFERENCES

Coltheart, M., Masterson, J., Byng, S., Prior, M., & Riddoch, J. (1983). Surface dyslexia. *Quarterly Journal of Experimental Psychology*, *35A*, 469–495.

Coltheart, M., Patterson, K., & Marshall, J. C. (eds.) (1980). *Deep Dyslexia*. London: Routledge & Kegan Paul.

Dunn, L. M. (1965). *Expanded Manual for the Peabody Picture Vocabulary Test*. Circle Pines: American Guidance Service.

Fujii, K., & Morokuma, O. (1959). Gogi shitsugoshoo no ichi shoorei. (A case of word-meaning (Gogi) aphasia). *Seishin Igaku [Clinical Psychiatry]*, *1*, 431–435.

Funnell, E. (1983). Phonological processes in reading: New evidence from acquired dyslexia. *British Journal of Psychology*, *74*, 159–180.

Glushko, R. J. (1979). The organization and activation of orthographic knowledge in reading aloud. *Journal of Experimental Psychology: Human Perception and Performance*, *5*, 674–691.

Hagiwara, H. (1982). Dissociations between syllabic and ideographic script processing in Japanese brain-damaged patients. Thesis submitted to the Faculty of Graduate Studies and Research in partial fulfilment of the requirements for the degree of Master of Arts, University of Montreal.

Hatfield, F. M., & Patterson, K. E. (1983). Phonological spelling. *Quarterly Journal of Experimental Psychology*, *35A*, 451–468.

Hayashi, M. M., Ulatowska, H. K., & Sasanuma, S. Subcortical aphasia with deep dyslexia: A case study of a Japanese patient. (In press.)

Henderson, L. (1982). *Orthography and Word Recognition in Reading*. London: Academic Press.

Hirose, M. (1949). Kankakusei Shitsugo no sai ni okeru shitsudoku [Dyslexia in the case of sensory aphasia]. *Shinri [Psychology]*, *5*, 42–50.

Kitao, N., Hatta, T., Ishida, M., Babazono, Y., & Kondo, Y. (1977). Concreteness, hieroglyphicity and familiarity of kanji (Japanese form of Chinese characters). *Japanese Journal of Psychology*, *48*, 105–111 (in Japanese).

Kurachi, M., & Takekoshi, T. (1977). Shojishoogai no keido na kankaku shitsugo—Sokuhukukekkoono chomei na ichirei—[Sensory aphasia with relative preservation of writing ability: Collateral flow from the frontal to the middle cerebral artery]. *Noo to Shinkei [Brain and Neurology]*, *29*, 1085–1091.

---

[5]Some of the work reported in this chapter is also discussed in Sasanuma (1984).

Marcel, T. (1980). Surface dyslexia and beginning reading: A revised hypothesis of the pronunciation of print and its impairments. In M. Coltheart, K. Patterson, & J. C. Marshall (eds.), *Deep Dyslexia*. London: Routledge & Kegan Paul.

Morton, J. (1980). The logogen model and orthographic structure. In U. Frith (ed.), *Cognitive Processes in Spelling*. London: Academic Press.

Morton, J., & Patterson, K. (1980). A new attempt at an interpretation, or, an attempt at a new interpretation. In M. Coltheart, K. Patterson, & J. C. Marshall (eds.), *Deep Dyslexia*. London: Routledge & Kegan Paul, pp. 91–118.

Morton, J. & Sasanuma, S. (1984). Lexical access in Japanese. In L. Henderson (ed.), *Orthographies and Reading*. London: Lawrence Erlbaum Associates Ltd.

Sasanuma, S. (1978). *Roken Test of Differential Diagnosis of Aphasia*. Tokyo: Yaesu Rehabilitation Ltd (in Japanese).

Sasanuma, S. (1980a). Acquired dyslexia in Japanese: Clinical features and underlying mechanisms. In M. Coltheart, K. Patterson, & J. C. Marshall (eds.), *Deep Dyslexia*. London: Routledge & Kegan Paul, pp. 48–90.

Sasanuma, S. (1980b). Patterns of kanji/kana impairment in aphasia: A study of eight cases. *Neurological Medicine, 13*, 206–212 (in Japanese).

Sasanuma, S. (1984). Can surface dyslexia occur in Japanese? In L. Henderson (ed.), *Orthographies and Reading*. London: Lawrence Erlbaum Associates Ltd.

Sasanuma, S., & Fujimura, O. (1972). An analysis of writing errors in Japanese aphasic patients: Kana vs. kanji in visual recognition and writing. *Cortex, 8*, 265–282.

Schwartz, M. F., Saffran, E. M., & Marin, O. S. M. (1980). Fractionating the reading process in dementia: Evidence for word-specific print-to-sound associations. In M. Coltheart, K. Patterson, & J. C. Marshall (eds.), *Deep Dyslexia*. London: Routledge & Kegan Paul, pp. 259–269.

Shallice, T., & Warrington, E. K. (1980). Single and multiple component central dyslexic syndromes. In M. Coltheart, K. Patterson, & J. C. Marshall (eds.), *Deep Dyslexia*. London: Routledge & Kegan Paul, pp. 119–145.

10 Dyslexia in a Dravidian Language

P. Karanth

The study of aphasiological disorders in Dravidian languages, though having a short history of less than a decade, shows promise of interest for aphasiologists the world over. Of these disorders the dyslexias, both acquired and developmental, hold special interest because of the unique characteristics of the orthographic systems of the Dravidian languages. This chapter illustrates the quasi-syllabic orthography of Kannada, one of the major Dravidian languages, presents data from dyslexia in Kannada, and discusses the implications that these data hold for current classifications of dyslexia.

THE PHONOLOGY OF KANNADA

Vowels

The basic Kannada vowel system consists of five long and five short vowels. Vowels like /æ/ and /ɔ/ exist in only a few loan words and have no grapheme in the writing system. Dipthongs /ai/ and /aɷ/ also occur, each having its own grapheme.

Consonants

The basic Kannada consonant system consists of 34 consonants.

Syllables

Any monosyllable of Kannada consists of a vowel preceded by zero, one, two, or three consonants; that is, the possible syllable structures are V, CV, CCV, and CCCV. It must be noted that CCCV syllables are rare in Kannada and are generally to be found in loan words. Further, though the number of possible CCV syllables is more than 1000, only about 300 geminations and CCV clusters occur in Kannada. For example, the syllables /jmɑ/, /vgɑ/, and /sdɑ/ are not to be found in Kannada words.

THE ORTHOGRAPHY OF KANNADA

For each of the 10 vowels there are two characters, a primary form and a secondary form. In order to write a syllable that consists of a vowel and no consonant, the primary form is used. To write a syllable in which the vowel is preceded by one or more consonants, the secondary form is used (see later). The primary and secondary written forms for a vowel in general look quite different: for example, the primary form for /ɑ/ is ᘉ but its secondary form is ᘈ. Similarly, the dipthongs /ai/ and aɷ/ also have their primary and secondary forms in written Kannada.

Consonants

The consonants also possess primary and secondary written forms. The primary form is used for writing the first consonant of a syllable. The secondary form is used for writing the second or third consonant of any syllable that begins with a consonant cluster (see later). Written representations of consonants without vowels are possible but are rarely found in Kannada writings. They are generally found in grammar texts illustrating morphophonemic rules, or in writing loan words. To write a consonant without an accompanying vowel, the symbol ᘈ is written above the consonant cluster.

In addition to characters representing the basic Kannada vowels, dipthongs, and consonants, there are a few additional characters, generally used to accommodate Sanskrit loan words:

1. Two additional graphemes are used to accommodate the vocalic /r/ found in Sanskrit loan words, in its primary and secondary forms.
2. The symbol : (called "visarga") is included to accommodate Sanskrit words; it represents a glottal fricative before a consonant.
3. The symbol O (called "anusvaara") can replace the nasals like ṅ, ñ, ṇ, n, and m. It can replace the nasals ṅ, ñ, ṇ, and n before a homorganic consonant and can replace m before any consonant or in the word-final position.

Syllables

1. V Syllables

As described earlier, a syllable that is just a vowel is written using the primary orthographic form of the vowel.

2. CV Syllables

If the primary orthographic form of a consonant is written down, this is read not as a consonant phoneme, but a CV syllable, the vowel being the vowel /ɑ/. This is why something needs to be changed in the consonant character if it is to be read as a single consonant phoneme (as described earlier). If one wishes to write a CV syllable where the vowel is not /ɑ/, then the secondary form of this vowel character must be added to the primary orthographic form of the consonant character. These various possibilities are illustrated in Table 10.1.

TABLE 10.1
Examples of Writing V and CV Syllables in Kannada

Phonemic Representation	Orthographic Representation
/a/	ಅ
/u/	ಎಐ
/k/	ಕ್
/ka/	ಕ
/ku/	ಕು

The only exception to this rule is the addition of /i/ where the primary orthographic form of the consonant itself undergoes some change, for example /ki/ - ಕಿ .

3. CCV Syllables

With two exceptions (described later), one writes CCV syllables as follows: the first consonant is written in its primary form, and *below* this the second consonant is written in its secondary form, the vowel character being indicated by the first consonant; for example, bhaktha (devotee) (masc.) ಭಕ್ಥ; bhakthe (devotee) (fem.) ಭಕ್ಥೆ .

There are two exceptions to this principle. First, if the first member of the consonant cluster is O, representing the nasals, the second consonant is written in its primary form and immediately following (not under) the O, for example manga (monkey) ⊒ロ . Second, if /r/ occurs as the first member of a consonant cluster, as in some Sanskrit loan words, then the primary form of the second consonant is written immediately preceding (not under) the allograph of /r/, for example Suurya (sun) ᴙᴐᴑᴇ .

4. CCCV Syllables

CCCV syllables are not common in Kannada and are generally to be found in loan words. In these cases the first consonant is written in its primary orthographic form with appropriate indicators of the final vowel. The secondary form of the second consonant is written immediately below this and the secondary form of the third consonant is written further below as in shaastra (scripture) ᴚᴃ ; shaastri (pundit) ᴚᴃ , where ᴐ is the secondary form of /t/ and ᴑ is the secondary form of /r/.

The two exceptions described above with reference to CCV syllables hold true here too.

The Kannada Writing System: Syllabic or Alphabetic?

Kannada writing, like all other Indian modes of writing, is semi-syllabic. In other words, it takes as the written unit not the simple sound or phoneme but the syllable (aksara) and further as the substantial part of the syllable, the consonant or the consonants that precede the vowel—the latter being merely implied or being written by a subordinate sign attached to the consonant. The primary form of the vowel is used only when it forms a syllable by itself as in the morpheme *aa* (that), or when it is not combined with a preceding consonant, that is, when it is in the word-initial position. When more than one consonant precedes the vowel, forming with it a single syllable, their characters must be combined into a single compound character.

Although it is true that all the CV syllables of a particular consonant in Kannada will have something in common, it must be remembered that the Kannada reader does not learn the consonant component and the vowel component separately and then combine it to form a syllable. Instead, having first learned the basic syllabary with the primary forms of the vowels and the consonants in combination with the vowel /a/, the reader is taught the entire syllabary containing all possible CV combinations. The separate components of each phoneme in a written syllable are not dealt with independently except at a much later stage in grammar school. (Attempts are now being made, however, to teach Kannada writing to children by introducing their component elements.)

Further, most of the CCV syllables in Kannada are geminated, the non-geminated CCV and CCCV syllables primarily occurring in loan words from Sanskrit. It is likely that the method of compounding complex syllables, which is not really essential for Kannada (which is basically a CVCVCV language), is itself borrowed from Sanskrit to accommodate Sanskrit loan words. It is relevant that all Indian scripts, be they of languages of Indo-Aryan origin such as Devanagari or those of Dravidian origin such as Kannada, have originated from the Brahmi script with a comparatively short evolutionary history, so that the basic system is common to all of them.

Not all of the subtypes of dyslexia that have been identified so far in alphabetic scripts are likely to be found in Dravidian languages such as Kannada. Surface dyslexia, for instance, wherein the major criterion for the diagnosis is the patient's selective difficulty in reading irregular words, will not be observed in Kannada, which does not contain irregular words. Parallels for surface dyslexia in languages like Spanish, which do not contain irregular words but do have homophones by virtue of having identical pronunciations for different letters, are cited in Chapter 8 of this book. The homophone confusions, as well as the phonological spelling errors seen in the writing of these patients, are said to be symptomatic of surface dyslexia. However, in languages that not only lack irregular words, but in which alternative spellings of a sound or word are not possible, surface dyslexia cannot be observed. Irregular words cannot be found in Dravidian languages like Kannada, where the semi-syllabic orthography bears a perfect correspondence to the phonology of the language. Further, the homonyms that are found in Kannada are both homophones and homographs. Finally, the stress errors observed in surface dyslexic readers of languages such as English (e.g. reading *oboe* as /ə'boɷ/) cannot occur in Kannada because all syllables in Kannada words are given equal stress.

Hypothetically, only one indication of surface dyslexia in Kannada can be seen, the possibility having occurred to me while analysing some data on developmental dyslexia in Kannada (Rama, unpublished). Errors such as letter reversals and confusions arising from graphemic and phonemic similarity that are reported in Western literature on developmental dyslexia are found in developmental dyslexics reading Kannada. The group of errors that concerns us here is that involving the O (anusvaara), where the child has difficulties in arriving at its phonemic realisation. The anusvaara is the one grapheme in Kannada which represents more than one phonemic value, being representative of /m/, /ṅ/, /ñ/, /n/, and /ṇ/, its value in individual instances being determined by its phonemic context. Whether there is a category of adult dyslexics who would experience difficulties with this particular grapheme is something to be looked for in the future. (N.R., the visual dyslexic described in the following section, could read this character correctly.)

ILLUSTRATIVE DATA

The data on which the present discussion of dyslexia in Dravidian languages, such as Kannada, is based are drawn from an adult aphasic with a very circumscribed language disorder centring mainly around reading.

The case (Karanth, 1981) is that of N.R., a 57-year-old male aphasic who was multilingual and literate in both Kannada and English. He had a naming difficulty, a moderate degree of constructional apraxia, and a mild colour agnosia. The details of his reading assessment and recovery have been given earlier (Karanth, 1981) and will not be repeated here, except to list the major highlights and discuss these in terms of current classifications of dyslexia. N.R.'s major difficulty was in reading. He complained that he could see words and sentences but that they did not make any sense to him. When asked to read, he traced individual letters with his finger, and having thus identified the letters "spelled" out the word and only then comprehended it. Sentences were read similarly by laboriously first identifying each word character-by-character. Reading, when achieved in this fashion, was error-free with good comprehension. N.R. found it more difficult to read Kannada than English and took more time to read Kannada. The ability to recognise orally spelled words was good in both Kannada and English, including irregularly spelled words like "laugh." His spontaneous writing was charac-terised by a few paraphasic errors, which he failed to recognise as he was unable to read what he himself had written. Although he wrote well to dictation, he found it extremely difficult to copy both print and script, the latter being more difficult. He was unable to maintain a horizontal line.

N.R.'s strategy of reading through deciphering by sequential "spelling" worked differently in English and Kannada. In English he traced the letter, *named* each letter, and then used these letter names to identify the word. On the other hand, in Kannada, because the letter name is also the letter sound, by merely identifying the letters of a word the patient arrived at the phonological form of the word. In other words, in reading Kannada words N.R. uttered a sequence of *syllables*, each syllable corresponding to one of the characters in the word's printed form and, of course, to one of the syllables in the word's spoken form. In view of the additional stage of processing in reading English, one might have expected N.R. to find Kannada easier to read than English. His greater difficulty in reading Kannada is probably to be ascribed to the greater number of visual symbols employed in Kannada, with the finer visual discrimination that this entails. Irrespective of the relative degree of difficulty in the two orthographies

(English and Kannada), it is clear that in the latter case, the script itself precludes the (relatively) clear distinction that can be made in English between surface dyslexics and letter-by-letter readers (in the sense of Patterson & Kay, 1982).

DISCUSSION

N.R. has several parallels with the cases of Sasanuma (1974) and Warrington and Shallice (1980). In particular, N.R. and the patient reported by Sasanuma share such features as intact spoken language, including spontaneous speech; repetition of sentences and auditory comprehension are intact. Both patients had slight difficulties in naming objects, colour naming, and visuo-constructional abilities. More importantly, both patients had a severe reading difficulty with fairly well-preserved writing; their reading of syllabically written words was characterised by slow, error-free reading generally aided by the tactic of finger tracing. Further, their recovery patterns ran in parallel. Both patients had two orthographic systems available to them, and the efficacy of their reading abilities in the two systems differed significantly. Whereas Sasanuma has used her data to highlight the different modes of operations that are used in the process of reading syllabic orthographies such as kana (graph→sound→meaning) and that employed in ideographic symbols such as in kanji (graph→meaning), N.R. highlights the differences in reading syllabic orthographies such as Kannada and alphabetical orthographies such as English.

The patients reported by Warrington and Shallice (1980) also share features with those reported by Sasanuma (1974) and Karanth (1981), the most important of which is their slow, halting, character-by-character reading along with relatively well-preserved writing. Based on their extensive experimental investigations Warrington and Shallice reject several possible causal factors in this type of reading disorder, and conclude that the disorder is due to an impairment of a visual word-form system; they consequently label the condition "word-form dyslexia." Warrington and Shallice contend that by letter spelling their patients reconstruct the words presented to them visually from the auditory names of the letters, and thus overcome the impairment of a visual word-form system. My own interpretation of the reading disorder seen in these patients, however, is closer to the suggestion of Newcombe and Marshall (1981) that letter naming may serve "to direct the patient's attention to the visual stimulus." Support for this interpretation can be drawn from the data of Sasanuma and my own data, as well as from some of the experimental results of Warrington and Shallice themselves. To begin with, all four patients read through the process of identification of individual letters and stringing these together to form words, often tracing the letters before naming them. Oral reading achieved in this manner was error-free, and all four patients easily comprehended what they read. All four patients could copy reasonably accurately, though slowly. These factors, coupled with the subjective observations of the patients themselves (for instance, N.R. said he could see the print but that it did not make sense; R.A.V. reported that he could no longer see words as blobs of meaning), are in line with the experimental results of Warrington and Shallice that factors such as selective attention and visual span of apprehension are reasonably normal. However, it is doubtful whether this necessarily means that the perception of the constituent parts of a word is normal. Even without visual-field defects, difficulty in selective attention, or impaired span of visual apprehension, one could still have difficulty in discriminating between visual symbols that look alike such as b, d, p, q, g, j in English and ಐ, ಚ, ಛ, and ಜ in Kannada. Evidence for such an interpretation comes from the relative ease with which N.R. read English as compared to his native Kannada. Though the reading strategy (letter-by-letter reading) was the same in both English and Kannada, the patient found Kannada much more difficult. Suppose that N.R. did in fact have no difficulty in identifying letters but only had a deficit in the word-form system that was bypassed by use of an oral spelling strategy (in which N.R., like the others, was good). In this case, Kannada, wherein the letter name and the letter sound are the same, should have been much easier to read, for the processes of letter-by-letter reading and phonological "reading" are more or less identical in Kannada. For instance, the Kannada word /vimaana/ (aeroplane) would be read by an English letter-by-letter reader as /vi/.../ai/.../em/.../ei/.../ei/.../en/.../ei/→/vimaana/, whereas N.R. read this word thus: /vi/.../maa/.../na/→/vimaana/.

Consequently, the greater difficulty that N.R. faces in a syllabic orthography like Kannada can only be explained in terms of the greater number of graphemes and their relative complexity, which call for finer discriminations. The tactile or kinaesthetic cues employed by these letter-by-letter readers can be seen as an additional aid to the process of letter identification.

Looking at the data in terms of the block diagram on the classification of acquired dyslexias given by Newcombe and Marshall (1981), I suggest that the affected level in these patients can be located within the box labelled "visual analysis." A difficulty in visual analysis is generally eliminated on two grounds, either by ruling out visual and perceptual factors (as Warrington and Shallice attempt) or on the basis of the fact that at least some of these patients do not make errors in letter reading. As stated earlier, even in the absence of factors such as a visual-field defect, difficulty in selective attention, and impaired visual span of apprehension, one could still have difficulty in discriminating between letters. Familiarity with a script may heighten one's sensitivity to the differentiating features of that particular script. One could "see" an unfamiliar script and yet not perceive the specific features and contrasts, which are acquired over a period of time. It is possible that this sensitivity is what is disturbed in these patients, who seek to overcome it by focusing on the letter and/or by finger tracing. Having identified the letters either through tactual cues or by focusing on and naming them, the patient can then read and comprehend the word; in other words, all the possible routes to comprehension and pronunciation are then available.

In ideographic scripts such as the Japanese kanji, the existence of a very large number of different characters will mean that any reading disorder in which there is difficulty in discriminating between characters (whether these be letters if the script is alphabetic, syllabographs if it is syllabic, or ideographs if it is ideographic) will be especially severe. Also, because an ideographic character cannot be identified by piecemeal analysis of its parts, there will be no means of overcoming reading difficulties caused by inability to identify whole characters. Thus, as Sasanuma (1980) observes, her patient could read some kanji words instantaneously (implying that the defect at the visual analysis level was not total) but, where this instantaneous reading did not occur, the character could not be identified at all. Moreover, Sasanuma's examples of the errors in reading kanji are indicative of a partial visual identification with the patient probably guessing the rest.

ACKNOWLEDGEMENTS

The grant of a travel allowance from the Commonwealth Foundation to enable my participation in the seminar on "Surface Dyslexia" held at Oxford, 22–25 September 1982, is gratefully acknowledged. My very sincere thanks to Dr John C. Marshall for having made all of it possible.

REFERENCES

Karanth, P. (1981). Pure alexia in a Kannada-English bilingual. *Cortex, 17*, 187–198.

Newcombe, F., & Marshall, J. C. (1981). On psycholinguistic classifications of the acquired dyslexias. *Bulletin of the Orton Society, 31*, 29–46.

Patterson, K. E., & Kay, J. (1982). Letter-by-letter reading: Psychological descriptions of a neurological syndrome. *Quarterly Journal of Experimental Psychology, 34A*, 411–441.

Rama, S. (1980). Diagnosis and remediation of dyslexia: An attempt. PhD. thesis, in preparation, University of Mysore.

Sasanuma, S. (1974). Kanji versus Kana processing in alexia with transient agraphia: A case report. *Cortex, 10*, 89–97.

Sasanuma, S. (1980). Acquired dyslexia in Japanese: Clinical features and underlying mechanisms. In M. Coltheart, K. Patterson, & J. C. Marshall (eds.), *Deep Dyslexia*. London: Routledge & Kegan Paul.

Warrington, E. K., & Shallice, T. (1980). Word-form dyslexia. *Brain, 103*, 94–112.

IV SURFACE DYSLEXIA AND THE DEVELOPMENT OF READING

IV Introduction

A basic theme of much of this book, and of its sister volume *Deep Dyslexia* (Coltheart, Patterson, & Marshall, 1980), is that an understanding of acquired disorders of reading can be achieved by interpreting such disorders in relation to information-processing models of normal reading. Such models conceive the mental system we use when we read as consisting of a set of independent information-processing modules; the models also specify routes by which information is passed from module to module. The set of preserved and impaired reading abilities exhibited by any person with an acquired dyslexia is ascribed to a particular pattern of impairments of the modules, or of the pathways connecting them, or both.

This approach to acquired dyslexia from cognitive psychology has enjoyed a certain success in recent years. As a consequence, the approach has been taken up by those interested in developmental dyslexia. The simplest way of doing this is to ask which, if any, of the varieties of acquired dyslexia also occur as developmental dyslexias. For example, Marshall (1984) describes six forms of acquired dyslexia and discusses the likelihood that developmental analogues of each could occur. He concludes that this is at least possible in all six instances, although not all of the six patterns have in fact been observed in developmental dyslexics. The most convincing analogue is developmental surface dyslexia, first described by Holmes (1973) and later by Coltheart (1982), Coltheart, Masterson, Byng, Prior, and Riddoch (1983), and Job, Sartori, Masterson, and Coltheart (1984). A developmental disorder analogous to phonological dyslexia has been described by Temple and Marshall (1983) and Temple (1984); and there are recent claims for the existence of developmental deep dyslexia (Johnston, 1983) and developmental spelling dyslexia, or developmental letter-by-letter reading (Prior & McCorriston, 1983).

The rationale for this application of the methods used for the information-processing analysis of acquired dyslexia to the study of developmental dyslexia is made clear by Marshall (1984):

> I shall assume (I hope uncontroversially) that the syndromes of developmental dyslexia must be defined over *a* functional architecture of visible language processing. But I shall further speculate that *the* relevant functional architecture is the one that correctly characterizes the normal, fluent, adult reading system. The syndromes of developmental dyslexia will accordingly be interpreted as consequent upon the selective failure of a particular adult component (or components) to develop appropriately, with relatively intact, normal (adult) functioning of the remaining components (p. 46).

The chapter by Temple exemplifies this sort of approach. Temple offers a particular model of the adult procedures for reading aloud, and uses it to interpret four developmental and two acquired cases of dyslexia.

This approach to developmental dyslexia is challenged in the chapter by Frith. Although she concurs with Marshall that it is likely to be profitable to interpret cases of developmental dyslexia in relation to normal reading, her contention is that it is a model of the *acquisition* of reading, not a model of the normal, fluent, adult reading system, that should be used for interpreting developmental dyslexia.

Why this might be so can be illustrated with reference to the model of learning to read and to spell described by Frith. This model involves a sequence of three stages of learning to read. There is an initial stage at which children identify single words by specifically visual properties such as the presence of particular graphic features, or overall word shape; this she refers to as the *logographic stage*. At the next stage, children are capable of using procedures for mapping letters onto sounds, and so may be able to recognise unfamiliar words by translating them into phonological form and recognising the resulting phonological representation: this is the *alphabetic stage*. The last stage is the *orthographic* stage: here the young reader identifies words via analysis of their abstract orthographic structure. This procedure for word identification differs from the logographic procedure in that words are analysed in more detail and in terms of abstract-orthographic properties, not concrete visual properties. The procedure differs from the alphabetic procedure in that the recognition of the word can follow directly from the orthographic analysis, without requiring an intermediate phonological translation. Further discussions of this type of model, and of its application to the analysis of individual cases of developmental dyslexia, may be found in Seymour and MacGregor (1984).

Now, if this is an appropriate account of the development of reading, and if the first of Frith's stages must be negotiated successfully for normal, adult, fluent reading to be acquired, there is an important implication. The logographic processing of words (in the sense that Frith uses the term) would be an essential component of learning to read; but it apparently is not relevant to skilled adult reading (because there is no evidence, at least for single isolated words viewed without time constraint or visual degradation, that skilled adult readers identify words by using idiosyncratic visual features such as word shape or the presence of individual letters). If this is so, then a developmental dyslexia involving impairment of the logographic stage could *not, contra* Marshall, "... be interpreted as consequent upon the selective failure of a particular adult component (or components) to develop appropriately." In other words, the type of approach to developmental dyslexia from acquired dyslexia considered by Marshall would be at best of limited applicability. In general, then, to the extent that there are aspects of the process of learning to read which have no counterpart in the process of normal skilled reading, there will be patterns of developmental dyslexia that have no counterpart among the acquired dyslexias. Only future work can provide us with evidence as to whether this is so.

A quite separate objection which can be raised to any attempts to map acquired dyslexic syndromes onto developmental dyslexic syndromes is the objection to the concept of syndrome itself. There is no doubt that the use of this concept has assisted initial progress in the study of acquired dyslexia from the information-processing perspective. Several varieties of acquired dyslexia, differing greatly from each other, have been identified and labelled, and thus the gross heterogeneity of unselected cases of acquired dyslexia has been explicitly acknowledged.

Within any one syndrome, however, heterogeneity also exists, because the same symptom can be caused by different types of impairment within the information-processing system used for reading; for example, as is discussed in various places in this book, regularisation errors in reading aloud can arise for any of several different reasons. If it is tenable to take the view that the study of acquired dyslexia has reached the stage where thinking in terms of a small number of basic syndromes (such as surface dyslexia or phonological dyslexia) may no longer much assist progress, then clearly one may no longer wish to ask questions as general as: "Does surface dyslexia exist as a developmental dyslexia?" or "Do surface dyslexics read like young normal readers?" (Marcel, 1980).

Data suggesting the inappropriateness of such questions are provided in the chapter by Masterson. The two cases of surface dyslexia she describes, a developmental case and an acquired case, had in common an impaired ability at reading non-words aloud. Now, first of all this is not true of all surface dyslexics (for example, it was not true of the patient described by Bub, Cancelliere, and Kertesz in Chapter 1, nor, as Masterson's normative data on non-word reading show, of the patient, H.T.R., described by Shallice, Warrington, & McCarthy, 1983). Second, though Masterson's two cases shared the symptom of impaired non-word reading, they differed in the *kind* of non-word reading deficit they had. The acquired case, E.E., produced mainly errors that violated common English grapheme–phoneme correspondence rules. In contrast, the developmental case, C.D., did not: most of her erroneous responses were "graphic errors," that is, orthographic approximations to the stimulus. Furthermore, Masterson shows not only that E.E. and C.D. differed from each other, but also that neither produced a pattern of non-word reading errors resembling the pattern yielded by young normal readers.

This heterogeneity is also demonstrated in the chapter by Temple. All six cases she describes, two acquired and four developmental, were surface dyslexic in the sense that they had difficulties in reading irregular words and produced regularisation errors when reading aloud such words. Their ability to use orthographic-phonological correspondences to read words that they failed to "recognise as wholes," however, varied from very good (N.G.) to extremely poor (M.S.); furthermore, the cases in whom this ability was impaired were distinctly heterogeneous with respect to the *type* of impairment evident. Despite this heterogeneity, it was possible for Temple to offer a theoretical interpretation of the reading impairments of every case using a single (albeit multi-stage) model of the processes involved in reading aloud via orthographic-phonological correspondences.

This illustrates an alternative to the use of the concept of syndrome. If one relinquishes the idea that there is a relatively small number of basic syndromes, to one of which every patient is to be assigned, the question of how to generalise from present to future patients is raised; and one answer to this question is that one can attempt to interpret every patient in terms of a single model of the reading system (rather than in terms of a single fixed set of acquired dyslexic syndromes). Even if no two patients ever exhibit identical constellations of syndromes, this would not rule out the possibility of interpreting all patients with reference to a single model.

In the case of developmental rather than acquired reading disorders, it may be a model of *learning* to read that should be used for interpretation, as Frith argues. However, the point remains that even if all developmental dyslexics are treated as individual cases, and even if each case is unlike all others, this does not imply that it will be impossible to interpret all such cases with reference to just one model of the acquisition of reading. As Frith demonstrates in her chapter, developmental impairments at various points within the sequence of stages she proposes as underlying learning to read and to spell would generate various different patterns of disordered reading, various different patterns of disordered spelling, and various combinations of dyslexias with dysgraphias. Hence a very large number of different symptom patterns would be expected if even this relatively simple model were appropriate. Of course, there are also many symptom patterns that would never be observed if the model were an appropriate one, and the search for such patterns is one of the ways in which one can seek to falsify any such model.

REFERENCES

Coltheart, M. (1982). The psycholinguistic analysis of acquired dyslexia: Some illustrations. *Philosophical Transactions of the Royal Society*, *B298*, 151–164.

Coltheart, M., Masterson, J.C., Byng, S., Prior, M., & Riddoch, J. (1983). Surface dyslexia. *Quarterly Journal of Experimental Psychology*, *35A*, 469–495

Coltheart, M., Patterson, K., & Marshall, J. C. (eds.) (1980). *Deep Dyslexia*. London: Routledge and Kegan Paul.

Holmes, J. (1973). Dyslexia: A neurolinguistic study of traumatic and developmental disorders of reading. Unpublished PhD. thesis, University of Edinburgh.

Job, R., Sartori, G., Masterson, J., & Coltheart, M. (1984). Developmental surface dyslexia in Italian. In R. N. Malatesha, & H. A. Whitaker (eds.), *Dyslexia: A Global Issue*. The Hague: Martinus Nijhoff.

Johnston, R. S. (1983). Developmental deep dyslexia? *Cortex*, *19*, 133–193.

Marcel, A. J. (1980). Surface dyslexia and beginning reading: A revised hypothesis of the pronunciation of print and its impairments. In M. Coltheart, K. Patterson, & J. C. Marshall (eds.), *Deep Dyslexia*. London: Routledge and Kegan Paul.

Marshall, J. C. (1984). Toward a rational taxonomy of acquired dyslexias. In R. N. Malatesha, & H. A. Whitaker (eds.), *Dyslexia: A Global Issue*. The Hague: Martinus Nijhoff.

Prior, M., & McCorriston, M. (1983). Acquired and developmental spelling dyslexia. *Brain and Language*, *20*, 263–285.

Seymour, P. H. K., & MacGregor, C. J. (1984). Developmental dyslexia: A cognitive experimental analysis of phonological, morphemic and visual impairments. *Cognitive Neurpsychology*, *1(1)*, 43–82.

Shallice, T., Warrington, E. K., & McCarthy, R. (1983). Reading without semantics. *Quarterly Journal of Experimental Psychology*, *35A*, 111–138.

Temple, C. M. (1984). Developmental analogues to acquired phonological dyslexia. In R. N. Malatesha, & H. A. Whitaker (eds.), *Dyslexia: A Global Issue*. The Hague: Martinus Nijhoff.

Temple, C. M., & Marshall, J. C. (1983). A case study of developmental phonological dyslexia. *British Journal of Psychology*, *74*, 517–533.

11 Surface Dyslexia: Variations Within a Syndrome

C. M. Temple

The term "surface dyslexia" was first used by Marshall and Newcombe (1973) to refer to a patient who appeared to rely on the phonological recoding of words to read and understand. The patient did not recognise words holistically but tended to "sound them out" to obtain their pronunciation and meaning. Particular difficulty was encountered reading words with irregular spelling-to-sound patterns. Homophonic words, e.g. *sale* and *sail*, also tended to be confused (Coltheart, 1981). The most prevalent theoretical explanation of surface dyslexia has been expressed in terms of a dual- or triple-route model of the reading process. In a dual-route model there are two ways in which a word might be read aloud: via the semantic system or else via an abstract set of grapheme–phoneme rules (Fig. 11.1). Triple-route models include an additional system where a route goes directly from word detectors to phonological output, bypassing semantics. This route deals with whole-word correspondences (Fig. 11.2). These three routes are called, respectively, the "semantic route," the "phonological route," and the "direct route." Surface dyslexia may be considered as a disorder in which there is over-reliance on the phonological route to reading, the other two having been disrupted by pathology. In addition, the phonological reading route that is used may itself be partially impaired.

Since the original description of Marshall and Newcombe (1973), a number of cases of surface dyslexia have been described. However, it has become apparent that although the term "surface dyslexia" was originally used to refer to a single symptom complex, the term is now used to cover a variety of different disorders. These disorders are all surface dyslexias in that

269

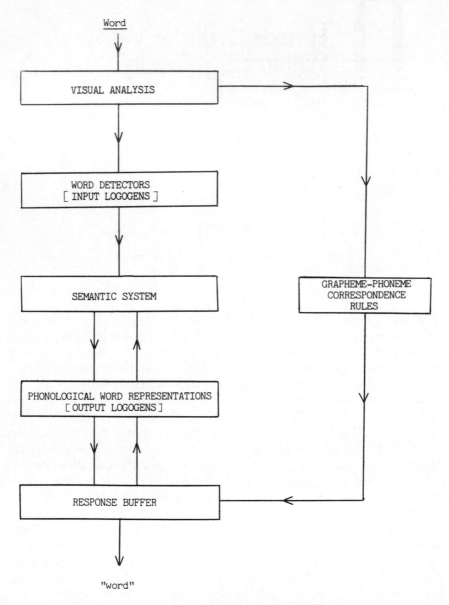

Word

VISUAL ANALYSIS

WORD DETECTORS
[INPUT LOGOGENS]

SEMANTIC SYSTEM

PHONOLOGICAL WORD REPRESENTATIONS
[OUTPUT LOGOGENS]

RESPONSE BUFFER

GRAPHEME-PHONEME
CORRESPONDENCE
RULES

"word"

FIG. 11.1.   A dual-route model of reading.

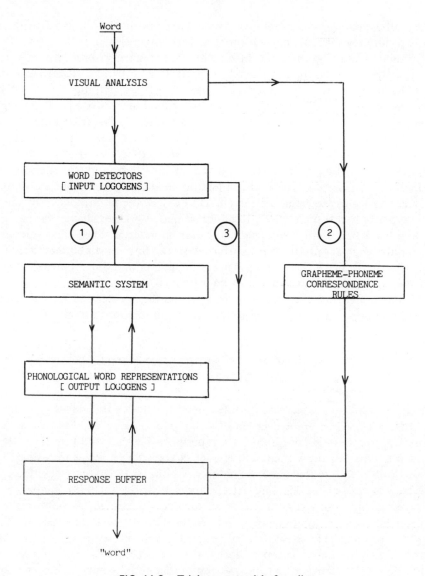

Word

VISUAL ANALYSIS

WORD DETECTORS
[INPUT LOGOGENS]

①   ③   ②

SEMANTIC SYSTEM

GRAPHEME–PHONEME
CORRESPONDENCE
RULES

PHONOLOGICAL WORD REPRESENTATIONS
[OUTPUT LOGOGENS]

RESPONSE BUFFER

"word"

FIG. 11.2.   Triple-route model of reading.
1 = The Semantic Route.
2 = The Phonological Route.
3 = The Direct Route.

they all appear to result from an over-reliance on a phonological reading route, but they differ from each other in various ways.

Shallice, Warrington, and McCarthy (1983) have chosen recently to restrict the term "surface dyslexia" to patients who exhibit disturbance in grapheme–phoneme correspondence rules themselves, making errors of the sort *recent*→"rissend." When correct rules are used in the wrong context, e.g. *phase*→"face," they call the syndrome "semantic dyslexia." Rather than dividing the old surface dyslexias into new surface dyslexias and semantic dyslexias, it may be more useful and less confusing to retain the term "surface dyslexia" as a cover term for a group of disorders and to attempt to subclassify this group. One of the difficulties in attempting to subclassify the surface dyslexias has been that, in current models, the phonological reading route has only one main stage. It is represented as a letter string that passes into a black box, "grapheme–phoneme correspondence rules," and emerges as a phonological output. Many surface dyslexics have partial impairment in this system. If the surface dyslexias are to be differentiated the representation of the system, in our models, must be expanded.

This chapter outlines such an expansion and then presents details of cases of surface dyslexia that may be distinguished, in terms of the new model.

AN EXPANSION OF THE REPRESENTATION OF THE PHONOLOGICAL ROUTE

A new view of the phonological route is incorporated in the model presented in Fig. 11.3. When a word is read by this phonological reading route the following process is envisaged. After peripheral visual analysis the letter string is input to the parser. The parser is responsible for segmenting the word into orthographic units or chunks. Coltheart (1978) has described a system of graphemic parsing based upon Venezky's (1970) analysis of English orthography. In this, a string of letters is turned into a string of graphemes, where "grapheme" is defined as the written representation of a single phoneme. This definition of grapheme will also apply here. So the graphemic parsing of sheep is sheep→⟨sh⟩ + ⟨ee⟩ + ⟨p⟩. The system of chunking differs from graphemic parsing in that chunks may be bigger than graphemes. A "chunk" is defined as the written representation of p phonemes where $0 < p < N$, and N is the number of phonemes in a word. Thus for example: station→⟨st⟩ + ⟨a⟩ + ⟨tion⟩.

A word may be parsed in a number of different ways. The preferred parsing will depend on the experience of the reader. As contact with the printed word increases parsing rules are internalised. A young beginning reader tends to parse into smaller chunks than an experienced adult reader. The smallest chunk size is the single letter. A fluent adult reader may be able

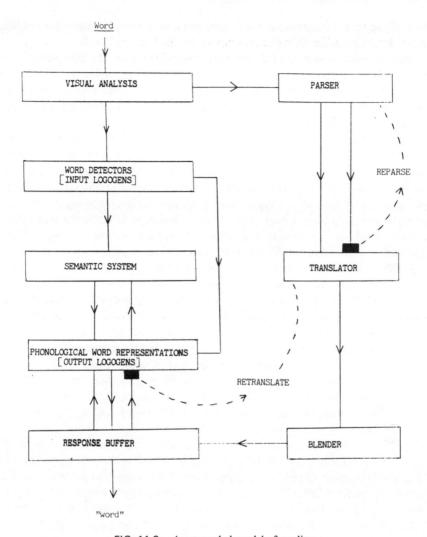

FIG. 11.3.   An amended model of reading.

to use polygraphemic chunks. The reader will initially parse into the largest chunks his system can deal with. An extreme version of this hypothesis would be that a fluent adult reader could use morphemic chunks and that, thus, the direct route would be incorporated into the phonological route rather than existing as a separate entity. Indeed, Shallice and Warrington (1980) do abandon the direct route. However, the expansion of the phonological route envisaged here does not necessitate such action and in this model the direct route will be left as it stands. It will be assumed in the discussions that follow that the phonological route cannot process whole words in unity. If it could, the definition of a chunk would have to alter so that $0 < p \leqslant N$.

After parsing of the letter string the chunks are input to the translator. The translator differs from previous representations in that not only can it translate chunks of larger size, but also it has multiple potential translations. A number of different *phonological* forms can be assigned to any one *orthographic* chunk. Thus, just as the translator of languages may have a variety of different alternatives from which to select his or her preferred equivalent, so the translator of chunks may have alternatives to choose from. Once again experience will have affected this system. The fluent reader will have more alternatives to choose from than the beginner. Readers of English will have more alternatives to choose from than readers of Italian. All the alternatives from which the selection is to be made are valid in the sense that such a translation would be appropriate for some word in the language. The alternatives are graded. That of highest token frequency is most likely to be tried first. If this does not work, the next most frequent may be tried. Thus the translation $ch \rightarrow$ /tʃ/ is more probable than the translation $ch \rightarrow$ /k/. When dealing with a chunk like *oll* both /ɒl/ and /oɔl/ are probable translations (see Chapter 14 for further discussion of this). Recent prior activation will increase the probability that a particular translation will be selected. This accounts for the findings of Kay and Marcel (1981), who observed that in reading a list of stimuli the pronunciation of a segment in a nonsense word was affected by the way that the same segment was pronounced in a word that had been read immediately previously. The selected phonological segments pass to the blender where they are combined and a phonological output emerges.

Two feedback loops act as checks for the system. First, if the translator has no representation to translate a chunk it has been sent, a feedback demand will be made for reparsing. The word will then be parsed into smaller chunks. Second, if, after blending, the output is not a word, a feedback system may demand retranslation. The blended phonological output is held in the response buffer while a check is made in the phonological word representations to see if there is a matching word. If there is no match, there is a feedback demand to the translator. A properly functioning highly developed system is likely to demand more retranslations than an impaired or a poorly developed system. This feedback system enables the alternative translations available to the translator to be used and enables appropriate output selection. Thus, for example, if

$$pint \rightarrow \langle p \rangle \langle int \rangle \rightarrow /p/ \ /ınt/ \rightarrow /pınt/,$$
$$\text{parser} \quad \text{translator} \ \text{blender}$$

then there will be no match in the phonological word representations for /pınt/ and there will be a retranslation demand; in other words, there is a lexical checking system. Some retranslation demands are clearly under cognitive control. If the stimulus is short and there is confidence about the response, or the subject is told that the stimulus is a nonsense word, then there may be no retranslation demand and a neologism may be produced.

To illustrate the system and its limitations, the reading of three irregular words, *deaf, dread*, and *bread*, will be outlined. The system cannot process the word *deaf* in unity. The first parsing is into the largest chunk possible.

1. *deaf*→⟨d⟩⟨eaf⟩→"no translation"→REPARSE.
2. *deaf*→⟨d⟩⟨ea⟩⟨f⟩→/d/ /i/ /f/→/dif/
        parser   translator   blender
     →"no word"→RETRANSLATE.
     lexical
     check
3. *deaf*→⟨d⟩⟨ea⟩⟨f⟩→/d/ /ɛ/ /f/→/dɛf/
        parser   translator   blender
     →"OK"   →"deaf".
     lexical
     check

Deaf is a difficult word for the system to cope with. It will only be read correctly if the system is sufficiently developed that the alternative translation *ea*→/ɛ/, which occurs in about 60 words, has been internally coded.

dread→⟨dr⟩⟨ead⟩→?
         parser   translator
bread→⟨br⟩⟨ead⟩→?
         parser   translator

The translation of the letter combination *ead* poses a problem for the translator because it may take a translation as in *mead, bead, plead* or as in *head, dead, instead, dread, thread*. If the translation /id/ is chosen for *dread*, the lexical check system should detect that the output is not a word and demand a correct retranslation. However, if the translation /id/ is chosen for *bread*, the lexical check system will detect no difficulty as "breed" is a word. *Bread* may then be misread as "breed." If *dread* is being read in a mixed list of words and non-words then misreading may also occur since the lexical check system will be inoperative. Thus the envisaged system can read a number of irregular words that cannot be read by the phonological reading route of Coltheart (1978). However, words like *bread* will still have a high risk of being read incorrectly by the system and words like *yacht* will never be read correctly by it.

Different malfunctions in the system will produce different symptoms of disorder. When the parser is not functioning properly but the rest of the system is intact, one may see an error of the sort *cheat*→/kəhɛæt/, that is, *cheat*→⟨c⟩⟨h⟩⟨e⟩⟨a⟩⟨t⟩ instead of *cheat*→⟨ch⟩⟨ea⟩⟨t⟩; or *station*→ /steɪtəɔn/, that is, ⟨st⟩⟨a⟩⟨t⟩⟨i⟩⟨on⟩ instead of *station*→⟨st⟩⟨a⟩⟨tion⟩. These types of error are called "chunking errors." The first is also an error of graphemic parsing. The second is a failure to parse into a chunk bigger than a grapheme. When the translator is not functioning properly two different types of error may result. If the ability to utilise alternatives or the ability to correctly select between alternatives is lost, one may get an error of the sort *low*→/laɔ/. This type of error is called a "valid translation error." Many, but not all, of these errors will be regularisations. If, alternatively, the malfunction of the translator produces mismatches between chunks and phonological segments one may get errors of the sort *table*→"pable." This error is called an "invalid translation error." These errors will often produce nonwords. Other researchers have interpreted these errors as resulting from an earlier processing stage. It is clear that if a misparsing has occurred and the translator is intact, valid translation errors will nevertheless result. All parsing errors produce mistranslations. But mistranslations may also occur in the absence of a misparsing. Thus, for example, the error *cheat*→/kəhɛæt/ is a parsing error that produces a resultant valid mistranslation. In contrast, the error *rough*→/roɔ/ is a valid translation error that has not resulted from a misparsing: *rough*→⟨r⟩⟨ough⟩, the correct parsing. This is the correct parsing because it is into the largest chunks below the level of the whole word, for which translations are available. However, the selected value of translation for *ough* is inappropriate but not invalid (cf. *ough* in *dough*).

The most probable type of error to result from malfunction of the blender is the omission or repetition of one of the phonological segments. The blender is more likely to have difficulty with long series of segments than with short ones. It is possible that in reality this is a simplification and the blender is capable of more severe perturbations, but for the moment these will be ignored. It is a theoretical possibility that omissions also occur in the parsing process. This is clearly an empirical issue but omission errors are restricted to the blender here because of the personal observation in both children and adults that surface dyslexics can be heard to systematically sound out detached parts of a word. Yet when attempting to blend them into a word, bits seem to disappear. It may be that a poor short-term memory reduces the efficiency of the blender.

Surface dyslexics may thus vary on at least four dimensions: in their chunking skills, in their ability to choose from multiple valid translations, in their ability to use only valid translations, and in their ability to blend.

Surface dyslexia has been described as both an acquired and a developmental disorder (Coltheart, 1982; Coltheart, Masterson, Byng, Prior, & Riddoch, 1983; Holmes, 1973). Both types of case show regularity effects and homophone confusions. Details of a number of cases of surface dyslexia will now be presented, and an attempt will be made to explain their differences and similarities in terms of the expanded model. Both developmental and acquired cases will be described. This is not to say that reading breakdown is always regression (Holmes, 1978), but that in the case of surface dyslexia, the patterns of reading disability in the two groups are so similar that the same model can elucidate both.

CASE REPORTS

Case 1: M.S.

M.S. is a 22-year-old male who was involved in a traffic accident at the age of 18. A CT scan indicated "slight generalised atrophy of the whole left hemisphere, in particular the left temporo-parietal region, and of the right temporal region." Perimetry revealed a dense, right homonymous hemianopia. Tested by Dr Freda Newcombe in May, June, and November 1981 he attained a score of 52/57 on Ravens Progressive Matrices, equivalent to an IQ greater than 117. On the Wechsler Adult Intelligence Scale his verbal IQ was 79 and his performance IQ 90. Schonell single-word reading age was 5.5 years; Schonell spelling age (written) was 6.5 years. There was also evidence of "gross memory impairment." More extensive background information and details on this patient are presented elsewhere (see Chapter 2 in this book), so discussion here will be restricted to an outline of reading skills.

M.S. no longer retains even the most fundamental chunking skills. Parsing is at a single-letter level. Even the digraphs *th* and *sh* have been lost. He never reads *th* as /θ/ or /ð/ and he never reads *sh* as /ʃ/. Thus we find errors such as: *these*→"tihessey" /təhɛseɪ/, *them*→"tihem" /təhɛm/, *either*→"e-it-her" /ɛ/-/ɪthər/, *shone*→"sihonney" /sə/ /hɒneɪ/. Invariably, each grapheme in a double consonant is assigned its own phonological translation. Thus we find errors such as: *press*→"piresisi" /pərɛsɛsɛ/, *mattress*→"mate tir esisi" /meɪt/ /tər/ /ɛsəsə/.

M.S. no longer retains even the most fundamental chunking skills. Parsing is at a single-letter level. Even the digraphs *th* and *sh* have been lost. He never reads *th* as /θ/ or /ð/ and he never reads *sh* as /ʃ/. Thus we find errors such as: *these*→"tihessey" /təhɛseɪ/, *them*→"tihem" /təhɛm/, *either*→"e-it-her" /ɛ/-/ɪthər/, *shone*→"sihonney" /sə/ /hɒneɪ/. Invariably, each grapheme in a double consonant is assigned its own phonological translation. Thus we find errors such as: *press*→"piresisi" /pərɛsəsə/, *mattress*→"mate tir esisi" /meɪt/ /tər/ /ɛsəsə/.

Having parsed at the single-letter level M.S. almost always assigns a valid translation. However, even where the single-letter parsing is correct, valid translation errors may be produced when vowels are involved. M.S. has difficulty determining whether the translation of a vowel should be short or long. Thus we find: *hid*→"hid or hide," *mop*→"mop or mope," *rip*→"ripe or rip."

Only one type of invalid translation error now occurs. *B–d* confusions were present, but a recent mnemonic taught by Dr Freda Newcombe to the patient seems to have been largely effective in eliminating these. Previously, responses occurred such as:

debt → "bedit" /bɛdət/

or "debit" /dɛbət/

knob → "kinobby" /kənɒbə/

or "kinoddy" /kənɒdə//

The invalid translations remaining occur as the result of the use of letter names. Thus we find: cold→"C, old" /si/ /oᴐld/, clue→"C, louis" /si/ /lui/, mimic→"mimi C" /mɪmɪsi/. It is clear from a number of the foregoing examples that M.S. also tends to insert schwas in consonant clusters. Some of these are presumed to be produced as a result of the limitations of the vocal tract, which cannot utter some digraphs without schwas, for example *bt* in *debt*.

To summarise, M.S. is a surface dyslexic with very extensive impairment in the semantic and direct routes. His primary disorder in the phonological route is an ability to parse into chunks. He can only parse at a single-letter level. In addition, he makes invalid translation errors resulting from the use of letter names.

Case 2: N.G.

N.G. is a 13-year-old, left-handed boy from Tanzania who came to England at the age of 3. He is the youngest of six children. All education has been given in English and N.G.'s siblings have had no school difficulties. More extensive details of this case are to be found in Temple (1984).

At 18 months N.G. had his first generalised tonic-clonic seizure. At age 9 he developed complex partial seizures, which by the age of 11 had become longer in duration. They have further developed recently and now consist of partial onset with secondary generalisation into a convulsion followed by prolonged post-ictal confusion. EEG investigations show diffuse slowing of basic rhythms and independent spike discharges in the right anterior temporal and left anterior to mid-temporal areas, that on the left tending to be more active. CT scan is normal and the cause of the seizure disorder is unknown.

Tested by Mr Ralph Burland, Chief Clinical Psychologist at the Park Hospital for Children, Oxford, in September 1982, on the Wechsler Intelligence Scale for Children (WISC), a large verbal performance discrepancy was apparent. Verbal IQ was 69 (vocabulary subtest score = 1), performance IQ was 106. This 37-point difference is highly significant (Wechsler, 1974). The short WISC, which is thought to yield a purer verbal performance picture (Maxwell, 1956), yields a verbal IQ of 59 and a performance IQ of 135. A poor vocabulary score is also found on the Peabody Picture Vocabulary Test, which is performed at the 6 year 10 months level. The verbal/non-verbal discrepancy apparent on the WISC scores is also present on memory tests (Baxter–Burland battery, unpublished). There is a severe deficit in auditory comprehension. Bishop's Test of the Reception of Grammar is performed at the 8-year level. Auditory comprehension deficits are also noticeable in conversation with N.G. Reading and spelling are impaired although they are better than might be expected on the basis of his low verbal IQ. The Schonell single-word reading age is 11 years 6 months and the Schonell spelling age is 11 years 1 month. The Neale Analysis of Reading yields an accuracy score of 10 years 6 months and a comprehension score of 6 years 11 months. Thus the auditory comprehension deficit is mirrored in a reading comprehension deficit. In terms of the model in Fig. 11.3, N.G.'s functional lesion may be in the semantic system itself.

The qualitative nature of N.G.'s reading pattern is that of surface dyslexia. He shows consistent regularity effects and homophone confusions. For example, on the Coltheart list (Coltheart, Besner, Jonasson, & Davelaar, 1979) N.G. reads 20/39 irregular words and 39/39 regular words ($\chi^2 = 22.54$, $P < .001$). All of the errors are valid translation errors. Some are regularisations, e.g. *pint*→/pɪnt/, *steak*→/stik/, *subtle*→/sʌbtəl/. Others are not. Errors made to words containing the consonant cluster *ough* cannot be regularisations as there is no regular translation of *ough*. There are, however, many valid translations, for example translations in *rough, cough, through, thorough, hiccough, bough, dough, bought*. Three of the errors on the Coltheart list involved the consonant cluster *ough*. However, in each case, a valid translation was selected: *borough*→[⟨b⟩⟨or⟩⟨ough⟩]→"borrow" (*ough* as in *dough*); *thorough*→[⟨th⟩⟨or⟩⟨ough⟩]→/θɒroʊ/ (*ough* as in *dough*); *trough* ₁ →[⟨tr⟩⟨ou⟩⟨gh⟩]→/trɑɒf/ (*ou* as in *sound*, *gh* as in *rough*). The third of these errors, in addition to being a valid translation error, is also a parsing error because *ough* should have been parsed as one chunk, as the system is based upon parsing into large chunks first.

There is a further error, which is both a valid translation error and a parsing error: *circuit*→⟨c⟩⟨ir⟩⟨c⟩⟨ui⟩⟨t⟩→/kəkjut/. The letters *ci* should have been parsed as one chunk, in order to produce a soft translation of the *ci* as /sə/ rather than as /kə/. This is another case of inappropriate parsing leading to a valid translation error. However, errors that are both chunking errors and valid translation errors are fairly rare in the corpus of N.G.'s errors. Most errors are valid translation errors alone.

I have suggested that malfunction of the blender might produce omission or repetition of one of the phonological segments. This is the only other type of error made by N.G. and it occurs only with very long stimuli and even then rarely. N.G. was asked to read aloud the 20 words on Nelson's regular word list (Nelson & O'Connell, 1978). These are 9–14 letters in length and the words are of rapidly declining frequency. N.G. read 16/20 correctly. Three of the errors were blender errors involving omission of a syllable: *tipularian*→"tipulian" /təpjuləæn/, *individual*→"invidual" /ɪnvɪdjuəl/, *organisations*→"organations" /ɔgæneɪʃənz/.

To summarise, N.G. is a surface dyslexic whose phonological route produces valid translation errors. These result from limited development of the translator. Occasionally the valid translation errors are induced by chunking errors but in general chunking skills are well developed. When very long stimuli are attempted the blender may malfunction and omission errors result.

The impairment of N.G.'s phonological route is very slight. There are no invalid translation errors (unless the omission errors are to be interpreted in this way), and chunking skills are good. Reading of non-words is extremely good, for example 20 non-words of up to eight letters in length were all read aloud correctly. N.G.'s pattern of performance closely parallels that of the patient of Bub, Cancelliere, and Kertesz (Chapter 1) and is similar to the performance of W.L.P. (Schwartz, Saffran, & Marin, 1980) in the later stages of assessment.

Case 3: Ph.B.

Ph.B. is a 12-year, 9-month old boy. He was a late walker and is clumsy. He has no neurological abnormality and is right-handed, right-footed and right-eyed. On the Wechsler Intelligence Scale for Children, his verbal IQ is 134 and his performance IQ is 111. His score on the Peabody Picture Vocabulary Test is at the 16th percentile for his age. On the Neale Analysis of Reading his accuracy score is 9 years 10 months and his comprehension score is 11 years 8 months. On the Salford Reading Test his reading age is 9 years 5 months. His Schonell spelling age is 8 years 8 months. Ph.B. is a developmental surface dyslexic. He shows consistent regularity effects. For example, Ph.B. was presented with a list of 52 words constructed by the author. Half were regular and half were irregular and the two groups were balanced for imageability, frequency, and length in letters. The words were presented individually for reading aloud. Ph.B. read correctly 25/26 regular words and 17/26 irregular words ($\chi^2 = 6.07$, $P < .05$). The impairment of Ph.B.'s phonological route is not severe. Non-words are read with good accuracy.

Ph.B.'s chunking skills are well developed. For example, he can correctly process the string of letters *ight* in words and also *tion*. Those errors that result from the malfunctioning of the phonological route are predominantly translation errors. Some are valid translation errors, for example *elite*→"eel-ight" /ilaɪt/, *holy*→"holly", *cliche*→"clitchey" /clɪtʃeɪ/. More are invalid translation errors, for example *patient*→"pardent" /pɑdənt/, *influence*→"in-fusence" /ɪnfjusəns/, *design*→"desite" /dəsaɪt/. There is a tendency with longer stimuli to omit a phoneme or phonemes, for example *average*→"av-age" /æveɪdʒ/, *variation*→"varation" /veɪreɪʃən/, *ambition*→"abition" /æbɪʃən/. This may reflect a malfunction of the blender. Any of the errors that are the same as the foregoing, and are also words, can be interpreted as visual paralexias resulting from disorder elsewhere in the system. However, the neologistic responses must result from the phonological route.

To summarise, Ph.B. has only a mildly impaired phonological route. Chunking skills are good. Both valid and invalid translation errors occur and longer stimuli produce omission errors in the blender.

Case 4: S.L.

S.L. is a 12-year-old developmental surface dyslexic. He is of average intelligence. On the Wechsler Intelligence Scale for Children, his verbal IQ is 91 and his performance IQ is 105. Tested by Judith Hockaday, Consultant in Paediatric Neurology at the John Radcliffe Hospital, Oxford, no neuro-logical abnormality was found. Minor features on examination were right/left confusion and mild dyspraxia on sequential finger movements. Reading and spelling are severely impaired. Schonell single-word reading age is 7 years 8 months. Schonell spelling age is 7 years.

S.L. has a much less well-developed system of chunking than Ph.B. and N.G., although he is above the single-letter level of M.S. He is able to translate the digraphs *th*, *ch*, and *sh*. The letters *c* and *g* are not parsed with the following vowel and thus tend to be translated in hardened form, for example *digest*→/dəgəst/, *fancy*→/fænkeɪ/, *influence*→/ɪnfələŋk/. The letter combination *tion* is never parsed as one chunk and translated correctly as /ʃən/, for example *ration*→ræton/, *station*→stæton/, *nation*→næton/, *motion*→/mɒtɪŋ/. About half of S.L.'s errors are valid translation errors: *biscuit*/bɪskjut/, *chemist*→/tʃemɪst/, *debt*→/debət/.

There are also many invalid translation errors: *neighbour*→"nedgibor" /nɛdʒɪbɒr/, *health*→"thereth" /θeɪrəθ/, *disgrace*→"diskung" /dɪskuŋ/. Several of the invalid translations result from vowel difficulties: *both*→

"bath", *cheat*→"chate" /tʃeɪt/. Omission of word segments, interpreted as blender errors, occur rarely: *strict*→/strɪk/. Even invalid error responses tend to be of the same length as the stimulus.

To summarise, S.L. is a developmental surface dyslexic with impairment in the parser and the translator. Blender errors are rare.

Case 5: P.B.

P.B. is a 10½-year-old developmental dyslexic of average intelligence. On the Wechsler Intelligence Scale for Children his verbal IQ is 95 and his performance IQ is 101. In addition to reading and spelling difficulties, P.B. has associated problems. He cannot tell the time or discriminate left from right. He can recite neither the alphabet nor the months of the year. He cannot say what month the year begins with, what month Christmas is in, or what month it was at the time of testing. His three attempts to copy a picture of a cube are shown in Fig. 11.4. At the time of testing his Neale reading age was 8 years 7 months, his Salford reading age was 8 years 5 months, and his Schonell spelling age was 6 years 8 months. He also had severe difficulties with arithmetic.

Regularity effects are marked in P.B.'s reading. He is able to read almost no irregular words. For example, on the balanced list of 52 words referred to earlier, P.B. read 15/26 regular words but only one irregular word ($\chi^2 = 15.25$, $P < .001$). Chunking skills are around the same level as those of S.L. Digraphs *ch*, *sh*, *th* can be processed but little beyond this level is mastered. Even these can produce errors, for example *either*→"eat her" /it/ hə/. However, it is difficult to determine exactly how P.B. parses many words because the majority of his errors are invalid translation errors. Only about one in ten errors are valid translation errors, for example *talk*→/tælk/, *war*→/wə/ /ær/. The invalid translation errors range from slight violations of validity to gross deviations. Examples of gross deviations are: *clear*→ "slurch" /slʌrtʃ/, *secretary*→"sencharet" /sɛntʃərɛt/, *health*→"hallit" /hælət/. Sections of words were often omitted, interpreted as blender errors: *purchase*→"purchs" /pʌrtʃəz/, *stomach*→"stomch" /stɒmtʃ/, *solemn*→ "somee" /sɒmi/, *digest*→"jest".

Of the dyslexics discussed, P.B. has the most widespread impairment in his phonological route. Malfunction is apparent in each of the systems previously outlined. There are parser errors, valid translation errors, invalid translation errors, and blender errors. Invalid translation errors are particularly prominent.

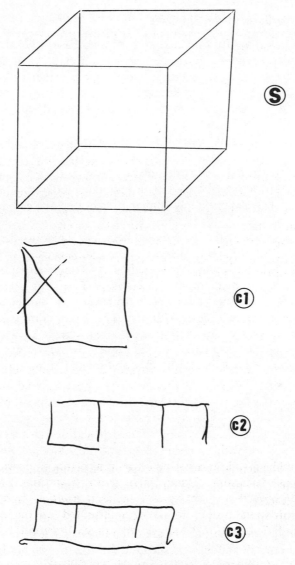

FIG. 11.4.   Attempts at cube copying by P.B.

Case 6: A New Look at an Old Case

J.C. was first described by Marshall and Newcombe in 1973. He is now 58 and retired. Prior to the war he trained as an electrician. At the age of 20, he sustained a severe penetrating missile wound (for further case details, see Marshall & Newcombe, 1973). Although a severe reading and spelling deficit has remained for 37 years, J.C. retained the ability to read blueprints after his injury and worked successfully as an electrician until his recent retirement. His current Schonell reading age is 8 years 4 months and his Schonell spelling age is 7 years.

Extensive data on J.C. were presented by Holmes (1973). It was she who first suggested that some children with developmental dyslexia had a pattern of reading performance strikingly similar to acquired surface dyslexics like J.C.

In terms of the cases already presented here, J.C.'s reading performance is closest to that of S.L. Like S.L., J.C.'s chunking skills are less well developed than those of Ph.B. and N.G., but are above the single-letter level of M.S. J.C. is able to process the digraphs *th*, *ch*, and *sh*. The letter *g* tends not to be parsed with the following vowel and is translated in hardened form, for example *image*→/ɪmeɪg/, *digest*→/dɪgəs/. The letter combination *tion* is rarely parsed as one chunk and translated as /ʃən/. As with S.L., the translation /tɔn/ is popular, for example *nation*→næton, *portion*→ /poωətɔn/, *motion*→moωtɔn/. Both valid and invalid translation errors are plentiful:

shiny→/ʃɪneɪ/ and *purchase*→ /pɔsʤə/
shady→/ʃædeɪ/   *strange*→/stɛrɪʤ/
choir→/tʃoωə/.

Marcel (1980) has discussed the errors of J.C. and concludes that "the notion of failed or misapplied grapheme–phoneme rules cannot alone account for the data." It is of interest to see whether his criticisms can be answered within the amended model. Marcel points out that for J.C. the phonetic values given to graphemes are often inconsistent from one word to the next. The current model can account for this by suggesting that the mechanism in the translator, which enables the correct selection between valid alternatives, has been lost. Selection becomes to an extent random and inconsistencies result. Marcel also notes that omissions may occur of syllables, for example *banishment*→"banment", and of single-letter realisations, for example *guest*→"just." These may be accounted for in the current model by positing a blender impairment producing loss of phonological segments during blending.

A number of more severe perturbations are reported in paralexic responses. There are two possible explanations within the current model. Many paralexic responses may not result from processing in the phonological route at all; rather they may result from imperfect analysis in the partially preserved semantic or direct routes. Even in the severe case of M.S., some sight vocabulary remains and thus there is some preserved processing capacity in these routes. Alternatively, the stimulus may be processed via the phonological route and a neologistic response may be produced. If the system of feedback for retranslation is impaired, and yet J.C. knows that he is seeking a word not a neologism, he may use what neologistic phonological information he has to access an entry with some similarity among the phonological word representations (see Fig. 11.3). As most paralexic responses are more similar to the original stimulus in the first few letters than in the last, it may be that the selection from feedback to the phonological word representation is particularly based on initial rather than terminal sounds.

Even when responses are neologistic there are occasions when phonemes or phoneme clusters appear to be added to the stimulus. To account for these errors one must clarify the possible range of invalid errors. In other words, invalid errors may produce a phonological output inappropriate to the chunk size of the input, for example:

strange→⟨st⟩⟨r⟩⟨ange⟩   parser
          ↓   ↓   ↓
       →/stɛ/ /r/ /ɪdʒ/   translator
       →/stɛrɪdʒ/   blender.

Alternatively, or additionally, one might wish to posit a further way in which the translator may malfunction. Specifically, it may occasionally output a phoneme or phoneme cluster that was not supposed to be activated, for example:

strange→⟨st⟩⟨r⟩⟨ange⟩
       →/st/ /ɛ/ /r/ /ɪdʒ/
       →/stɛrɪdʒ/.

Certain circumstances might make these interjections more probable. Thus the occurrence of a consonant cluster might increase the possibility of an interjected vowel.

To conclude, as Marcel (1980) pointed out, misapplied grapheme–phoneme rules cannot account for all the data of J.C. Nor can they account for the data of many other surface dyslexics. However, impairment considered in terms of an expanded phonological route of parser, translator, and blender can account for the pattern of deficit observed in J.C. and the range of different disorders found in the surface dyslexias.

SUMMARY

"Surface dyslexia" is a term used to cover a range of different acquired and developmental reading disorders, all of which are characterised by regularity effects, homophonic confusions, and an observable tendency to "sound out" words to attain their pronunciation and meaning. Many theoretical interpretations of the disorder suggest that there is over-reliance on a phonological route to reading, other route(s) having been disrupted by acquired pathology or having failed to develop. In addition, the phonological route is itself often impaired in surface dyslexia, although the nature and severity of the impairment varies from patient to patient. In order to understand these variations an expanded model of the phonological route has been presented. This consists of three main stages: parser, translator, and blender. The parser divides the letter sequence into a number of segments or chunks. The smallest chunk is the grapheme. Larger chunks are polygraphemic. In the translator, each chunk is assigned to one of several valid phonological segments. These are combined in the blender. Disorder at each of these stages produces a different type of error.

Details of a number of cases of surface dyslexia have been presented and their characteristics explained in terms of the expanded model. Some cases represent relatively pure disorders with impairment at only one stage; for example M.S. has an impaired parser. Others have more widespread impairment (Table 11.1).

TABLE 11.1

Site of Impairment and Prevalence of Different Error Types for Six Surface Dyslexics

| | Site and Error Type | | | |
| | Parser | Translator | | Blender |
Case	Chunking Errors	Valid Errors	Invalid Errors	Omission and Repetition Errors
M.S.	+ + +	+ + +	+ (only from the use of letter names)	−
N.G.	−	+ + +	−	−
Ph.B.	−	+ +	+ +	+ (Long stimuli— omissions)
S.L.	+	+ +	+ +	−
P.B.	+ +	+	+ + +	+ +
J.C.	+	+ +	+ +	+

− = very few; + = some; + + = many; + + + = almost all.

The surface dyslexias may thus be ranked both quantitatively, in terms of the overall severity of the disorder of their phonological route, and qualitatively in terms of the particular subsystems involved. The performance of each subsystem may also be assessed quantitatively producing a number of dimensions across which the surface dyslexias may vary.

ACKNOWLEDGEMENTS

I am grateful to Dr. Judith Hockaday, Consultant in Paediatric Neurology at the John Radcliffe Hospital, Oxford, for the referral of S.L.; to Dr. G. Stores, Consultant Neuropsychiatrist and to Mr. Ralph Burland, Senior Clinical Psychologist, at the Park Hospital for Children, Oxford, for referral of N.G. and permission to report medical and psychological test results obtained by them. I would also like to thank Mrs. Ursula Pearce and Mrs. Wendy Gilmour of the New Reading Centre, Oxford, for all their help and cooperation and for providing extended opportunities to work with Ph.B. and P.B. Dr. Freda Newcombe kindly provided access to J.C. and M.S. Thanks also to the editors for their many constructive comments on an earlier version of this chapter. This work was supported by an MRC studentship.

REFERENCES

Coltheart, M. (1978). Lexical access in simple reading tasks. In G. Underwood (ed.), *Strategies of Information Processing*. London: Academic Press.

Coltheart, M. (1981). Disorders of reading and their implications for models of normal reading. *Visible Language*, *15*, 245–286.

Coltheart, M. (1982). The psycholinguistic analysis of acquired dyslexias: Some illustrations. *Philosophical Transactions of the Royal Society London*, *B298*, 151–164.

Coltheart, M., Besner, D., Jonasson, J. T., & Davelaar, E. (1979). Phonological recoding in the lexical decision task. *Quarterly Journal of Experimental Psychology*, *31*, 489–508.

Coltheart, M., Masterson, J., Byng, S., Prior, M., & Riddoch, J. (1983). Surface dyslexia. *Quarterly Journal of Experimental Psychology*, *35A*, 469–495.

Holmes, J. (1973). Dyslexia: A neurolinguistic study of traumatic and developmental disorders of reading. PhD. thesis, University of Edinburgh.

Holmes, J. (1978). "Regression" and reading breakdown. In A. Caramazza, & E. B. Zurif (eds.), *Language Acquisition and Breakdown*. Baltimore: Johns Hopkins University Press.

Kay, J., & Marcel, T. (1981). One process, not two, in reading aloud: Lexical analogies do the work of non-lexical rules. *Quarterly Journal of Experimental Psychology*, *33A*, 397–413.

Marcel, T. (1980). Surface dyslexia and beginning reading: A revised hypothesis of the pronunciation of print and its impairments. In M. Coltheart, K. E. Patterson, & J. C. Marshall (eds.), *Deep Dyslexia*. London: Routledge & Kegan Paul.

Marshall, J. C., & Newcombe, F. (1973). Patterns of paralexia: A psycholinguistic approach. *Journal of Psycholinguistic Research*, *2* (3), 175–199.

Maxwell, A. E. (1956). A factor analysis of the Wechsler Intelligence Scale for Children. *Journal of Educational Psychology*, *29*, 237–241.

Nelson, H. E., & O'Connell, A. (1978). Dementia: The estimation of premorbid levels using the new adult reading test. *Cortex*, *14*, 234–244.

Schwartz, M. F., Saffran, E. M., & Marin, O. S. M. (1980). Fractionating the reading process in dementia: Evidence for word-specific print-to-sound associations. In M. Coltheart, K. E. Patterson, & J. C. Marshall (eds.), *Deep Dyslexia*. London: Routledge & Kegan Paul.

Shallice, T., & Warrington, E. K. (1980). Single and multiple component central dyslexic syndromes. In M. Coltheart, K. E. Patterson, & J. C. Marshall (eds.), *Deep Dyslexia*. London: Routledge & Kegan Paul.

Shallice, T., Warrington, E. K., & McCarthy, R. (1983). Reading without semantics. *Quarterly Journal of Experimental Psychology*, *35A*, 111–138.

Temple, C. M. (1984). Surface dyslexia in a child with epilepsy. *Neuropsychologia*, **22**, 569–576.

Venezky, R. L. (1970). *The Structure of English Orthography*. The Hague: Mouton.

Wechsler, D. (1974). *Manual of the Wechsler Intelligence Scale for Children*. New York: Psychology Corporation.

12 On How We Read Non-Words: Data From Different Populations

J. Masterson

In the original theoretical account of surface dyslexia, Marshall and New-combe (1973) interpreted the disorder as arising from damage to the pathway between visual and semantic addresses. Such damage forces the patient to resort to a process of grapheme–phoneme conversion for reading aloud. In addition, Marshall and Newcombe described various kinds of reading errors in their surface dyslexic patients J.C. and S.T., which were interpreted as indicating that the patients were imperfect at applying grapheme–phoneme rules, in addition to their impairment of the pathway from visual to semantic addresses.

Models of reading of the kind proposed by Marshall and Newcombe and others (e.g. Coltheart, 1980; Morton & Patterson, 1980) postulate that there are two independent routes for reading aloud—a "direct" or "lexical" route and a rule-based non-lexical route. Surface dyslexia arises when there is damage to the lexical route. If the routes are independent, such damage need not entail any impairment of the non-lexical route. Therefore, if every surface dyslexic patient resembled J.C. and S.T. in exhibiting impaired use of both routes, one would begin to be uneasy about a fundamental assumption of dual-route models: the independence of the two routes. This independence assumption obviously implies that it is possible for surface dyslexics to exhibit intact use of the non-lexical route.

More recently, at least two cases of surface dyslexia, H.T.R. (Shallice, Warrington, & McCarthy, 1983) and M.P. (see Bub, Cancellière, & Kertesz, Chapter 1 in this book), have been reported whose reading of non-words was good (implying that the non-lexical route was functioning well). However, the percentages of non-words read correctly by these patients were less than 100; for example, H.T.R. read 84% of a set of non-words correctly.

Whether this might be regarded as intact use of the non-lexical route is the first issue with which this chapter is concerned. We know from the error rates in non-word reading by normal readers reported by Calfee, Venezky, and Chapman (1969) that we cannot make the assumption that normal readers will score 100% correct when reading non-words aloud without time pressure; we therefore cannot assume that the failures of H.T.R. and M.B. to achieve such a score implies impairment of the non-lexical route in these patients.

For those surface dyslexics such as J.C. and S.T. in whom an impairment of the non-lexical route was evident, a second issue arises: is their non-word reading qualitatively different from that of normal readers, or is the difference simply quantitative? To answer this question, an analysis of the types of errors made in non-word reading by normals and by surface dyslexics is needed.

The third and final issue with which this chapter is concerned is the relationship between the young normal reader and the surface dyslexic. Marcel (1980) has argued that both types of reader exhibit a limitation in the number of orthographic lexical addresses available in the reading system, and has suggested that there are many similarities in the kinds of reading errors made by these two types of reader. Because, in the model of reading proposed by Marcel (1980) and by Kay and Marcel (1981), even non-words are read via access to the orthographic lexical addresses of words, Marcel's account of surface dyslexia predicts that the way surface dyslexics read non-words will resemble the way non-words are read aloud by young normal readers. The work reported in this chapter explores these issues by comparing the non-word reading of two surface dyslexics, a group of skilled adult readers, and a group of young normal readers of varying ages. Previous work reporting non-word reading by surface dyslexics, adults, and children does not permit such comparisons very readily because there are no previous studies in which the same non-words were given to the different groups.

The stimulus material used was a set of 120 orthographically legal non-words varying in length from four to six letters. This set included numerous examples of all three of the types of letter–sound correspondence distinguished by Calfee et al. (1969). These types are:

1. Invariant correspondences (e.g. $d \rightarrow$ /d/ as in *dack*).
2. Variant but predictable correspondences (e.g. $c \rightarrow$ /k/ before *a*, *o*, and *u* and $\rightarrow$ /s/ before *e*, *i*, and *y*, as in *centle* and *cipe*).
3. Unpredictable correspondences (e.g. $ch \rightarrow$ /tʃ/ or $\rightarrow$ /k/ or $\rightarrow$ /ʃ/, as in *chone*).

The subjects were two surface dyslexics (a developmental case, C.D., described in detail by Coltheart, Masterson, Byng, Prior, & Riddoch, 1983, and an acquired case, E.E., briefly discussed by Coltheart, 1982) and four groups of normal readers of varying ages: a 7-year-old group (N = 6), a 9-year-old group (N = 6), a 16-year-old group (N = 6), and an adult group (N = 14) with an age range of 18–30 years. All subjects were asked to read the 120 non-words aloud, without time pressure, and their responses were phonetically transcribed for subsequent analysis.

WHAT IS "NORMAL" PERFORMANCE?

In order to determine how accurately skilled adult readers read these non-words, one needs first to determine what the correct response is for each non-word. There is no entirely non-arbitrary way of doing this, but two procedures suggest themselves. The first is to define, as the correct response to any non-word, that response which was made by the largest number of subjects in the adult group of normal readers. The second is to define the correct response as that which is prescribed by the correspondence rules given in Wijk (1966) and Venezky (1970).

Table 12.1 shows just how frequent the most frequent response was for the 120 non-words. For only 46 non-words were the 14 adult readers unanimous; for 14 non-words only two different responses were chosen; and so on, down

TABLE 12.1
Frequency Distribution of the Number of Times the
Most Popular Response Occurred for Each Non-word

Number of Subjects (Maximum = 14) Giving the Most Frequently Given Response	Frequency Within the Set of 120 Non-words
14	46
13	14
12	16
11	13
10	4
9	8
8	4
7	6
6	2
5	3
4	2
3	1
2	1
1	0
0	0

to the non-word yielding the least agreement across subjects, *omage*, for which the largest number of subjects giving the same response was two. Table 12.2 shows the distribution of the number of different responses given to each non-word. The maximum was, again, for the non-word *omage*: 10 different responses were produced by the 14 subjects.

If we define as the correct response that made by the largest number of subjects, then the mean percentage of correct responses averaged across subjects was 83%. This figure is reduced if we define as the correct response that which agrees with the correspondence rules given by Wijk (1966) and Venezky (1970), because for several non-words the most popular response was not the response specified by these rules (e.g. *cloum*→/klum/ occurred seven times while *cloum*→klaɔm/ occurred only twice). On the Wijk–Venezky definition of correct response, the mean percentage of correct responses was 79%.

These percentages are very similar to the non-word reading levels reported (for different sets of non-words) from the patients H.T.R. (Shallice et al., 1983) and M.B. (Bub, Cancellière, & Kertesz, Chapter 1). If one can assume comparability of the different sets of non-words, then this is evidence in support of the view that there was no impairment of the non-lexical route in these two surface dyslexic patients. However, as is seen shortly, the two surface dyslexics described in this chapter were certainly far worse than normals at non-word reading.

TABLE 12.2
Frequency Distribution of the Number of Different
Responses Occurring to Each Non-word

Number of Different Responses Given to the Non-word (Maximum = 14, Minimum = 1)	Frequency Within the Set of 120 Non-words
1	46
2	33
3	19
4	11
5	5
6	1
7	0
8	4
9	0
10	1
11	0
12	0
13	0
14	0

QUALITATIVE COMPARISONS

In order to compare non-word reading across groups in a qualitative as well as a quantitative way, reading responses need to be categorised. A classification system was used that was based on the descriptions of both Marshall and Newcombe (1973) and Coltheart et al. (1983) of the types of error made by surface dyslexics. This was necessary in order to detect the kinds of errors made by normal readers when they are forced to rely on phonological processing. If normal readers also make the alteration, addition, deletion, and position change errors described by Coltheart et al. or, similarly, if they violate correspondence rules in their non-word reading, then we must conclude that these errors are a normal consequence of relying on phonologically mediated reading and are not due to an additional impairment as a consequence of brain damage.

The classification scheme used is outlined in Table 12.3 where examples of error in different categories can also be found. It can be seen from Table 12.3 that two main categories of error ("graphic" and "rule") were delineated. The "graphic" error category contains errors that appear to have resulted from the alteration, deletion, addition, or positional change of one or more letters of the stimulus, whereas the "rule" section contains instances of violation of correspondence rules according to Wijk (1966) and Venezky (1970). A response that consisted of use of a less frequent correspondence rule than the one specified by Wijk and Venezky was not counted as an error; for example, the response /kloɒm/ for *cloum* was not counted as an error because *ou*→/oɒ/ occurs in *soul* etc., even though the major correspondence listed by Wijk and Venezky for this vowel digraph is /aɒ/. The errors that are included in the rule section, then, consist of instances where the context in which the grapheme occurs had not been taken into account in converting it into a phoneme, and the correspondence rule has been violated. Table 12.4 represents the results of the analysis of errors.

Consider first the comparison of errors made by the acquired surface dyslexic, E.E., and the overall results obtained for the adult readers. It is clear that E.E. made *substantially* more errors in reading non-words than did the normal adults. Therefore his non-lexical reading routine must be impaired. Thus E.E. resembles the surface dyslexics J.C. and S.T. described by Marshall and Newcombe (1973) in that his reading disorder includes an impairment of grapheme–phoneme rule application.

Turning next to a comparison of E.E.'s performance with that of the 7-year-olds, we can see that there is a similar incidence of errors in the graphic category but not in the rule category, as E.E. makes many more rule errors than even the youngest children do. As discussed earlier, the views of Marcel (1980) would lead one to expect similarities between the reading of non-words by the 7-year-olds and by E.E. However, his explanation of these

TABLE 12.3
Categories of Error and Examples for Each

A. Graphic Errors

1. Single-letter errors, e.g.
   (i)   Substitution   *thase*→/tʃeɪs/ (chase)
   (ii) Deletion   *nood*→/nɒd/ (nod)
   (iii) Addition   *sorage*→/stɔrɪʤ/ (storage)
   (iv) Position change   *girn*→/grɪn/ (grin)

2. Combinations of 1. (i)–(iv), e.g.
   (i) and (iv)   *castop*→/kɒstɪp/

3. Combinations of more than two errors per word, e.g.
   (i) and (ii) and (iv)   *geniar*→/sɪnʤə/

4. Errors involving more than one letter, e.g.
   (i)   *cade*→/geɪb/

5. Errors involving more than one letter in combination
   with other errors, e.g. 1.(i) and (ii)   *lurge*→/ləd/

B. Rule Errors

1. One error per word, e.g.
   (i)   Realising final *e*   *sile*→/saɪli/
   (ii) Ambiguous consonant error   *cipe*→/kaɪp/
   (iii) Vowel–vowel digraph error   *nauge*→/neɪjuʤ/
   (iv) Lengthening single vowel   *pleck*→/plik/
   (v)   Vowel error in vowel + *r*   *girter*→/gɪɒtə/
   (vi) Vowel realised incorrectly
         with final *e*   *spage*→/spɔʤ/

2. More than one error per word, e.g.
   (i) and (ii)   *tuice*→/tjukə/

C. Combinations of One Graphic and One Rule Error, e.g.

A. (i) and B. (iii)   *coab*→/koɑɪb/

D. Combinations of More Than One of the Above, e.g.

A. (ii) and (iii) and B. (ii)   *cactul*→/sæstru/

similarities does not predict that they should be confined to the graphic error
category as they appear to be. This is because Marcel accounts for errors of
this nature as an attempt to make (aural–oral) lexical sense of the stimulus.
However, when subjects are reading a set of stimuli that they know are all
non-words, there is no reason for them to attempt to make lexical sense of
any of them.

The results could be incorporated, however, into the following account of
phonological processing. Suppose that non-words can be read either by

TABLE 12.4
Error Data Summary. Mean for Six Normal Readers at Four Age Levels (Standard Deviations are in Brackets) Together with Total Error in Each Category for E.E. and C.D.

	7 years	9 years	16 years	Adults	E.E.	C.D.
A. Graphic Errors						
1. One per word						
(i) Substitution	9.0	4.5	1.5	0.33	8	26
	(7.29)	(3.78)	(1.76)	(0.52)		
(ii) Deletion	4.17	2.0	1.17	0.17	3	10
	(2.04)	(0.89)	(1.17)	(0.41)		
(iii) Addition	3.33	2.33	0.17	0.00	4	12
	(3.27)	(3.50)	(0.41)			
(iv) Position	0.83	0.67	0.17	0.17	2	7
	(1.33)	(1.21)	(0.41)	(0.41)		
2. Two+ per word	4.0	1.0	0.00	0.17	4	12
	(3.74)	(1.26)		(0.41)		
3. Multi-letter	2.0	1.0	0.00	0.17	0	4
	(2.45)	(1.09)		(0.41)		
Total Means Graphic	23.33	11.5	3.00	1.01	21	71
	(16.44)	(10.56)	(3.22)	(0.93)		
B. Rule Errors						
1. One per word						
(i) Realising final e	0.5	0.67	0.00	0.83	12	0
	(0.55)	(1.63)		(1.33)		
(ii) Ambiguous consonant error	4.83	1.83	1.33	1.5	1	0
	(2.13)	(2.31)	(1.97)	(2.34)		
(iii) Vowel–vowel digraph error	0.83	0.67	0.17	0.67	8	0
	(1.60)	(0.52)	(0.41)	(0.82)		
(iv) Lengthening single vowel	1.00	1.00	0.17	0.5	12	1
	(1.55)	(1.26)	(0.41)	(0.55)		
(v) Vowel error in vowel + r	0.67	0.17	0.17	0.33	0	0
	(1.03)	(0.41)	(0.41)	(0.82)		
(vi) Vowel realised incorrectly with final e	0.33	0.67	0.00	0.00	0	0
	(0.52)	(0.82)				
2. Two+ per word	0.00	0.00	0.00	0.00	5	0
Total Means Rule	8.16	5.01	1.84	3.83	38	1
	(3.61)	(4.73)	(2.56)	(3.87)		
C. Combinations of Graphic and Rule Errors						
	4.17	1.0	0.17	1.17	8	5
	(2.23)	(1.55)	(0.41)	(2.40)		
Mean Total Errors	35.66	17.51	5.02	4.67	67	77
	(18.24)	(11.11)	(5.44)	(4.37)		

resort to a set of grapheme–phoneme correspondence (GPC) rules or by resort to a lexically based method of processing that operates in the following manner. When a non-word is encountered, the set of lexical orthographic entries is searched for a close match to the stimulus based on a criterial set of features. If a match is found, the orthographic entry is altered to correspond to the stimulus by means of grapheme–phoneme conversion involving the substitution of one or more of the graphemes in the accessed orthographic entry with another grapheme or graphemes. Subjects' own observations support the notion of a lexical analogy strategy, augmented by grapheme–phoneme conversion as an alternative way (to the use of grapheme–phoneme rules alone) of deriving the pronunciations of non-words. Thus, even though the information was not requested by the experimenter during testing, subjects would often make comments such as the following (from an adult normal reader who had responded /noɔl/ for the non-word *noal*) "I thought of 'coal' and changed the 'C' to an 'N'."

Both types of processing (grapheme–phoneme based or lexically based) would take time but one type of processing may be quicker for some items than others. The outcome of the faster mode of processing for a particular item would be given as the response.

This hypothesis can be applied to the present results as follows. If the grapheme–phoneme type processing operates more slowly than the lexical method in beginning readers and in E.E., then the outcome of the lexically based method of processing will more often be given as a response by them. If, in addition, both have a limited capacity store in which to hold the outcome of these operations before a response is made, then the response will very often not "match" the stimulus exactly, thus resulting in "graphic errors." The scant evidence for this hypothesis is as follows. If digit span can be taken to reflect the capacity of the store required to hold the outcome of phonological processing in any way, then the beginning readers do show evidence of a reduction in the capacity of this store since they have a reduced digit span compared to normal adult readers. A reduced digit span has been described in all the surface dyslexics for which reports of memory performance exist (Coltheart et al., 1983; Marshall & Newcombe, 1973; also Goldblum, Chapter 7, and Kremin, Chapter 5, both in this book) and was found in all four surface dyslexics (E.E. being one of these) specifically tested for this by Masterson (1983). A further line of evidence for this hypothesis comes from examination of Table 12.5, which gives the proportions of lexicalisations for the different error categories (i.e. instances where the response was a word rather than a non-word). From this we can see that lexicalisations are more likely to arise as a result of graphic errors than as a result of rule errors. Although Marcel (1980) and others have argued against the approach of inferring modes of normal processing from errors supposedly made when using that method of processing, it is tempting to argue that

TABLE 12.5
Percentage of Lexicalisations According to Type of Error (Based Upon
Only Those Responses in Which a Single Graphic or Rule Error Was Made)

	7 years	9 years	16 years	Adults	E.E.	C.D.
Graphic errors	37.86	29.8	50.00	25.00	35.3	63.6
Rule errors	14.28	20.0	27.3	4.5	3.1	a

a Only one rule error made.

the higher incidence of lexicalisations in the graphic error category reflect a breakdown in the processing that should convert the phonology obtained via access to a lexical orthographic entry into a response appropriate for a non-word.

The results concerning incidence of rule errors can perhaps be explained in the following way. When using rule-based processing to pronounce non-words, the complex nature of grapheme–phoneme rules in English again places a strain on the limited capacity store of the beginning reader, and the parsing mechanism responsible for marking letters into units suitable for conversion into phonemes breaks down (so that, for example, the rule that specifies whether initial c should be /s/ or /k/, depending on what the next letter is, cannot be properly used). Because this limitation of processing capacity does not exist in adult reading, such rules can be more easily accommodated.

In E.E., the operation of the rule system is prone to error in the first place because of the limitation in processing capacity shared with the beginning readers, but also because the rules themselves have been distorted as a result of brain damage.

In the light of the foregoing argument that lexicalisations reflect the lexically based method of processing, it seems strange that rule errors should ever result in a lexicalisation, because the locus of these errors has been ascribed to faults in the operation of an entirely non-lexical system. However Shallice et al. (1983) point out that lexicalisations can arise by chance through a purely non-lexical phonological process.

Although evidence for the hypothesis is extremely scant, it seems to be the only one that can help to explain the results obtained in reading the same set of non-words by C.D., the developmental dyslexic. Table 12.4 shows that she made a total of 77 errors, 71 of which were graphic errors. The proportion of lexicalisations made is 63.6% for graphic errors but 100% for rule errors. Further examination of the result demonstrates that only one response was made in the single errors rule section, from which the lexicalisation rate is derived. The stimulus in this case is the non-word *clim* and C.D.'s response was /klaɪm/. This has been classified as a rule error (also for the 7- and 9-

year-olds who committed the same error) because of a strict adherence to the classification scheme, which meant that wherever a single vowel not in the context of the final *e* was lengthened, the error was assigned to rule error 1 (iv); however, it seems likely that *clim*→/klaɪm/ could in fact be an instance of a graphic error. This would mean that no single rule errors were made by C.D., and this contrasts sharply with E.E.'s pattern of results where the majority of errors are in the rule category. (There are four instances of rule error, however, in the combined graphic and rule errors (category C) for C.D.)

One way of explaining this is to say that C.D.'s rule system works extremely slowly, even more slowly than that of E.E. and the 7-year-olds, and this results in the outcome of the lexical-orthographic mode of processing being given as a response more often than the outcome of a rule-based system for processing.

As mentioned earlier, the evidence for the hypothesis is extremely limited; for the moment, therefore, all we can say with some degree of certainty is that the non-word reading of the two surface dyslexics E.E. and C.D. is similar to that of beginning readers in that they make many errors, resulting in a response that shares a visual similarity with the stimulus. (This type of error has been called a "visual error" in relation to real-word reading.) The fact that this type of error, rather than a rule error, is more likely to result in a real word being given as a response suggests that graphic errors have some other locus than errors based on faulty GPC rules.

Our own studies and others of non-word reading in surface dyslexics show that there is considerable heterogeneity among patients. Some surface dyslexics may be normal or nearly so at non-word reading. Neither of our patients was normal, but they showed different patterns of abnormality, E.E. frequently violating GPC rules and C.D. rarely, if ever, doing so. Although there was some quantitative resemblance between young normal readers and these dyslexics, neither of the dyslexics yielded a pattern qualitatively resembling what one sees with young normal readers. Hence our results do not support the view that surface dyslexia is functionally similar to young normal reading.

Finally, the problems inherent in reading English via non-lexical procedures (that is, because of the variable nature of the relationship between print and sound in English) are attested to by the lack of agreement among normal readers as to how certain non-words should be pronounced and by the following quote from C.H., an acquired surface dyslexic, when trying to read the word *bury*: "/bʌri/ ... /bjuri/ ... it could be anything unless you know it, what is it?" (J.M. tells him.) "In that case there should be an 'E' there then I'd say /bɛri/ every time!"

REFERENCES

Calfee, R. C., Venezky, R. L., & Chapman, P. S. (1969). *Pronunciation of Synthetic Words with Predictable and Unpredictable Letter–Sound Correspondences.* Technical Report No. 71 from the Project on Language Concepts and Cognitive Skills Related to the Acquisition of Literacy. University of Wisconsin.

Coltheart, M. (1980). Reading, phonological recoding, and deep dyslexia. In M. Coltheart, K. Patterson, & J. C. Marshall (eds.), *Deep Dyslexia.* London: Routledge & Kegan Paul.

Coltheart, M. (1982). The psycholinguistic analysis of the acquired dyslexias: Some illustrations. *Philosophical Transactions of the Royal Society of London, B298,* 151–164.

Coltheart, M., Masterson, J., Byng, S., Prior, M., & Riddoch, J. (1983). Surface dyslexia. *Quarterly Journal of Experimental Psychology, 35A,* 469–495.

Kay, J., & Marcel, A. J. (1981). One process, not two, in reading aloud: Lexical analogies do the work of nonlexical rules. *Quarterly Journal of Experimental Psychology, 33A,* 397–413.

Marcel, A. J. (1980). Surface dyslexia and beginning reading: A revised hypothesis of the pronunciation of print and its impairments. In M. Coltheart, K. Patterson, & J. C. Marshall (eds.), *Deep Dyslexia.* London: Routledge & Kegan Paul.

Marshall, J. C., & Newcombe, F. (1973). Patterns of paralexia. *Journal of Psycholinguistic Research, 2,* 175–199.

Masterson, J. (1983). Unpublished PhD. thesis, University of London.

Morton, J., & Patterson, K. (1980). A new attempt at an interpretation, or, an attempt at a new interpretation. In M. Coltheart, K. Patterson, & J. C. Marshall (eds.), *Deep Dyslexia.* London: Routledge & Kegan Paul.

Shallice, T., Warrington, E. K., & McCarthy, R. (1983). Reading without semantics. *Quarterly Journal of Experimental Psychology, 35A* (1), 111–138.

Venezky, R. L. (1970). *The Structure of English Orthography.* The Hague: Mouton.

Wijk, A. (1966). *Rules of Pronunciation for the English Language.* London: Oxford University Press.

13 Beneath the Surface of Developmental Dyslexia

U. Frith

ARE COMPARISONS BETWEEN DEVELOPMENTAL AND ACQUIRED DISORDERS MEANINGFUL?

It seems straightforward to define developmental dyslexia as a disorder in which reading skills have never been gained and acquired dyslexia as a disorder in which reading skills have been lost. The questions that these particular definitions pose are whether the affected skills in the two disorders are comparable, and whether the remaining intact skills, as well as any compensatory strategies, are similar. It also seems straightforward to answer these questions empirically—without too much prior concern for the under-lying nature of the skills that are being compared. However, the recent progress in our understanding of acquired dyslexia was due *not* to such collections of empirical data, but rather to the fruitful application of detailed information-processing models to reading failure. Just as it was necessary to make explicit certain theoretical assumptions about the *nature of skilled reading* in order to advance in the empirical study of acquired dyslexia, so it may well be necessary to make explicit assumptions about the *nature of reading development* in order to advance our understanding of developmental dyslexia.

A developmental model has certain requirements that are not met by a structural model of skilled reading. Above all, it needs to explain how the various strategies that are mastered by the skilled reader come into being. If one ignores the question of acquisition then one is forced to make some rather odd assumptions. Presumably one would have to believe that the skills that are seen as components of the end-state of reading mastery have always

301

been there. For instance, one would have to believe that the brain is equipped from birth with a grapheme-to-phoneme converter. If there were an innate deficiency in the brain structure underlying a specific skill, one would then expect a particular type of reading failure. This would be directly comparable to acquired reading failure. At the price of faith in predestination this theory essentially dispenses with developmental factors. Thus, it ignores not only maturational processes and their complex interaction with the environment, but also social, cultural, and educational factors that influence the acquisition of literacy. Given the fact that the majority of the world's population do not read at all and that the majority of literate people read in non-alphabetic scripts, one might wish to view the acquisition of literacy by the English-speaking schoolchild in a more relative light.

Nevertheless, it is reasonable to assume that there are certain brain structures corresponding to basic cognitive processes that are necessary for literacy skills to develop. If these are impaired at an early age, then this would result in problems of literacy acquisition. On the other hand, it is theoretically possible that a defect exists that interferes with developmental processes, be they maturational or experiential, while the basic cognitive processes are intact. A third and perhaps most likely possibility is that there is an interaction with impairments in basic cognitive processes and developmental ones. If we take this possibility seriously then it is necessary to face some very complex issues that are intrinsic to developmental psychology in general: for instance, what are developmental factors, and how do they interact with basic cognitive processes?

The simplest model of developmental change is one of a steady and gradual improvement over time. Thus, a child might become faster and faster at decoding words phonemically until in the end the process is so fast that it seems to be instantaneous. Likewise, with time, the entries in the internal lexicon might become so numerous that every single word is present and can be "looked up." Unfortunately, this simple model has to be rejected because it cannot account for the phenomenon of "dips and drops" in development (Bever, 1981; Bower, 1974; Strauss, 1982). Also, it cannot account for differences in speed of acquisition, which range from sudden insight-type improvements to very slow changes and apparent plateaux. It is possible to explain these phenomena if we view the acquisition of skills as a sequence of steps. A step forward in the sequence is identified with the adoption of a new strategy. Thus sudden improvement is allowed for by the move from one step to the next higher (cf. Bryan & Harter, 1899). A fall-off in performance is also allowed for, because, by applying a new unpractised strategy in place of a well-practised old one, performance may initially drop. This model of developmental change seems applicable to reading acquisition: a child learning to read shows plateaux, sudden improvements, gradual increases, and drops in performance (Downing & Leong, 1982). We can therefore assume that for reading there is a developmental sequence of steps, with new strategies introduced at different points in the sequence. At the same time it is reasonable to assume that there are connections, however complex, between earlier and later phases of acquisition. Clearly, the "outcome" of the developmental sequence is the skilled reader. Structural models of skilled reading are therefore helpful when considering developmental models and vice versa.

It must be emphasised that a developmental approach implies special awareness of the interaction of constitutional and environmental factors. This is not a notable feature of structural approaches. Perhaps environmental factors are less important when one is dealing with highly skilled readers. After all, at that stage automatic processes are operating, and these are by definition under rigid internal control. This is not the case with developing readers. Here, for example, the influence of school and home can plainly be seen in what, why, and how they read (Clark, 1976; Entwisle, 1979; Francis, 1982; Seitz, 1977).

Clearly, the use of a developmental model for the study of developmental dyslexia does not rule out a comparison with acquired dyslexia. Indeed, it is my contention that such a comparison can only become meaningful if the differences between structural and developmental approaches are made explicit, and their complementary nature is made apparent.

WHAT IS A DEVELOPMENTAL DISORDER?

In a major textbook on child psychology Rutter (1976) describes developmental disorders as "an important group of conditions in which there is a specific delay in the emergence of a biologically impaired function (p.695)." Developmental speech/language disorder is diagnosed "by a delay in the development which is out of keeping with the child's general level of intelligence, which is not associated with a gross hearing loss or any overt neurological condition, and which is associated with a normal social usage of the language available to the child (p.699)." This definition focuses on the discrepancy between expected and actual attainment. Useful as it is in initially establishing what kind of children one might be talking about, it has very limited explanatory value. The term "delay" is of rather questionable use here, as it is entirely unspecified. Thus, it is uncertain whether or not it should be contrasted with "deviance." Delay is commonly interpreted as a merely quantitative difference and deviance as a necessarily qualitative difference. However, it has not yet been established whether such a dichotomy is actually applicable. In any case, today's qualitative difference is often tomorrow's quantitative one, depending on theory and refinement of measuring instruments. In order not to prejudge this issue I would like to use the term "delay" *when development is slow and eventually catches up* and "deviance" *when there is a life-long handicap.* Only in the latter case would it seem justified to talk of a developmental *disorder*.

The lack of a clear concept of developmental disorders has not helped the still faintly burning controversy as to whether developmental dyslexia exists, although there are other reasons for the controversy as well (Frith, 1981). The discrepancy definition, as applied to reading failure by Rutter and Yule (1975) and Rutter (1978), is useful in order to distinguish specific and general deficits. But it is not without problems. Thus, it excludes children who, despite a specific deficit, manage to gain a normal score on a reading test by using effective compensatory strategies. Similarly, it can falsely include children who fail, for instance, because of erratic school attendance. While a discrepancy definition remains at best descriptive, it is possible to move towards a more explanatory definition by applying a developmental framework. In this framework *developmental disorder can simply be seen as a persistent failure to advance to the next step in the normal acquisition process.*

The contrast to a developmental disorder is a disorder acquired in childhood not resulting in developmental arrest. It seems highly likely that just as adults can acquire various forms of dyslexia through specific brain accidents, so can children. This should be an equally rare occurrence in both cases, and there is no reason to expect it to be differentially distributed as to sex, except insofar as sex differences may exist for brain accidents in childhood. Clearly, the relatively high frequency of developmental dyslexia (see Tansley & Panckhurst, 1981, for a review of prevalence studies) and also its highly asymmetrical sex ratio suggest a different category of disorder. In what way the categories of developmental disorders and childhood brain trauma should be distinguished in terms of intact, faulty or compensatory strategies is an empirical question; and, of course, whether or not identical trauma in adult and child will have identical psychological consequences is precisely the kind of question addressed by a developmental approach.

The new definition of developmental dyslexia as developmental arrest has some important implications. It allows the possibility that a child fails to advance normally from step 1 to 2, or from 2 to 3, and so on. Hence it is rational to expect that each point marks a particular type of dyslexia. We can postulate as many types of dyslexia as we postulate steps in acquisition. At the same time we rule out the possibility that skills higher in the normal developmental sequence are intact when earlier ones are missing or incomplete by the normal criteria. We do not rule out that the child is continuing to improve his reading skill. Indeed, *after the point of arrest in the normal sequence the child would be expected to go on to develop compensatory strategies.* These strategies may be teacher induced or spontaneously adopted ones. They might well mimic normally used strategies, but they would be different in the way they arose and in the way they are used. In practice, differences might be demonstrated using measures of automaticity, for example latency and variability of responses. Thus, we have a new definition of developmental *deviance* in contrast to developmental *delay*. The child who shows delay is expected to develop strategies as they arise in the normal sequence, but at a slower pace. The child who shows deviance develops abnormal or compensatory strategies after the point of failure. At the same time any strategies he or she had acquired before the arrest will be available as normal. No such constraints exist for post-developmentally acquired disorders. Components of a previously completed system might become impaired independently of each other, and regardless of their order of acquisition.

In order to implement a developmental approach it is necessary to find a theory that would help us to envisage the sequence of normal reading acquisition. The value of such a theory is of course determined by its power to fit the known facts as well as to predict new ones. In the present context, however, the main requirement is that the theory should allow us to interpret facts already known about developmental reading disorders.

A THEORY OF READING ACQUISITION

There are few satisfactory theories of literacy acquisition, but Marsh and his colleagues (1977, 1980, 1981, 1983) have presented a cognitive developmental theory that is admirably suited for the present purpose. They postulate four stages in the development of reading in terms of four learning strategies with specific predictions for reading unknown words and reading known words in isolation and in context. Moreover, they provide empirical evidence for the existence of the four stages and their successive emergence over the school years. Briefly, *rote learning* is the first strategy for learning new words. This is complemented by so-called *linguistic guessing*, that is, a child often tries to predict a word from context. At stage 2, for the first time guesses are based on *visual letter cues* as well as linguistic context. At stage 3, *sequential decoding* in letter-by-letter and phoneme-by-phoneme fashion is introduced. At stage 4, *hierarchical decoding* appears, that is, the interpretation of each phoneme becomes dependent on its letter context (for example the pronunciation of *c*). Lastly, at this stage, the *analogy* strategy first appears, which from then on is used more and more for the successful reading of new words. Evidence from reading and spelling errors supports this model very well, as do observational studies of young readers (Biemiller, 1970; Francis, 1982; Soderbergh, 1971; Weber, 1970).

Marsh's cognitive developmental theory can be adapted so as to provide links to current models of skilled reading. My own preferences for the way this theory might be modified are expressed below. The development of reading is divided into three phases identified with three strategies. Let us call these "logographic," "alphabetic," and "orthographic."

The Three Strategies

The terms "logographic" and "alphabetic" cover the same processes respectively as Marsh et al.'s rote learning and sequential decoding strategies. The term "orthographic" replaces their analogy strategies. Their hierarchical decoding can either be considered orthographic, or an advanced form of the alphabetic strategy.

Logographic skills refer to the instant recognition of familiar words. Salient graphic features may act as important cues in this process. Letter order is largely ignored and phonological factors are entirely secondary, in other words the child pronounces the word after he or she has recognised it. If the child does not know the word, he or she will refuse to respond. However, the child will often be prepared to guess on the basis of contextual or pragmatic cues.

Alphabetic skills refer to knowledge and use of individual phonemes and graphemes and their correspondences. It is an analytic skill involving a systematic approach, namely decoding grapheme by grapheme. Letter order and phonological factors play a crucial role. This strategy enables the reader to pronounce (not necessarily correctly) novel and nonsense words.

Orthographic skills refer to the instant analysis of words into orthographic units without phonological conversion. The orthographic units ideally coincide with morphemes. They are internally represented as abstract letter-by-letter strings. These units make up a limited set that—in loose analogy to a syllabary—can be used to create by recombination an almost unlimited number of words. The orthographic strategy is distinguished from the logographic one by being analytic in a systematic way and by being non-visual. It is distinguished from the alphabetic one by operating in bigger units and by being non-phonological.

The three strategies, defined in this way, can readily be related to components in current models of skilled reading (Morton & Patterson, 1980; Shallice, Warrington, & McCarthy, 1983). For example, word-form analysers might be derived from early logographic skills; grapheme-to-phoneme skills would need to have been constructed out of alphabetic knowledge; lastly, word-component analysers, as postulated by Shallice & McCarthy (Chapter 15 in this book) could be readily traced to orthographic skill acquisition.

The present model leaves open the possibilities of how the initially acquired strategies are continued in skilled reading. Thus, they may remain available at all times, such that in case of need a reader can "fall back" on earlier strategies. On the other hand, once the orthographic strategy has become established, the previous strategies might be less accessible: it is possible that they cannot be used later without special retraining or in special (e.g. experimental) circumstances.

The Sequence

At present no more than a basic outline of a three-phase theory of reading acquisition can be provided. The aforementioned three strategies are hypothesised to follow each other in strict sequential order. Each new strategy is assumed to "capitalise" on the earlier ones. The logographic strategy might be thought of as capitalising on the basic (and impressive) memory skills that the child brings with him or her when starting to learn to read. Nevertheless, the child has to apply these basic skills to the written word. This is acknowledged by the "look-and-say" method. The logographic strategy is assumed to dominate the first phase of reading acquisition allowing a sizeable sight vocabulary to develop. This assumption is supported by evidence from many observational studies (see Torrey, 1979, for a review).

At the next phase the alphabetic strategy is adopted. Observational and some experimental evidence supports this assumption (Condry et al., 1979; Pick et al., 1978). It is generally agreed that a *"phonics"* stage in reading is of great importance and cannot simply be skipped (Chall, 1967). Here, at least some explicit instruction would seem to be necessary. This must be so if one accepts the notion that the alphabetic system is arbitrary and constitutes a relatively recent cultural invention (cf. Gleitman & Rozin, 1977). During this second phase conversion rules for sounds and letters are acquired; first simple rules, then so-called context-sensitive rules (soft *c* rule, silent *e*; Marsh et al., 1981).

Finally, the child will adopt the orthographic strategy. That this strategy can be differentiated from the logographic one, and also that it appears at a later stage of development, is consistent with findings by McCaughey et al. (1980). Abstract orthographic, as opposed to visual logographic and phonological alphabetic knowledge, was shown to exist by a reading age of 7 (Snowling & Frith, 1981). Whereas for the orthographic strategy there is no catchy label from teacher usage, it is clear that teachers in fact do employ methods to promote orthographic skills as defined in the present context. For instance, Stern and Gould (1965) emphasise the use of morphemes in teaching what they call *"structural reading."* Similarly, the well-known Gillingham–Stillman method (1956) stresses the synthesis of phonemic elements into meaningful units and the knowledge of syllable structure.

For a long time there has been controversy over the developmental succession of visual and phonological reading strategies. This could be because differences between logographic and orthographic strategies have been largely ignored and either one has been assumed to represent a visual strategy. The three-phase model offers potentially a reconciliation. Although in its present form the model does not incorporate mechanisms of change, a particular suggestion is presented later in this chapter, where the three-phase model is modified, and becomes a six-step model.

From 0 to Phase 1

Even before phase 1 is entered the child has in some sense started to learn to read. The earliest attempts at reading and writing, however, do not imply sufficient linguistic awareness to qualify to be called logographic skills. Perhaps they are better described as symbolic skills. During this phase a child has to acquire some understanding of such difficult metalinguistic terms as "word" and "sentence." Work in this area has been reviewed recently by De Goes and Martlew (1983). Metalinguistic awareness of written language cannot be taken for granted in beginners and develops in an orderly fashion. This is vividly documented by Ferreiro (1978).

Given that a child has mastered the symbolic pre-literacy phase, he or she is ready to enter the *logographic phase*. When this happens is very hard to predict and shows immense individual variation (Francis, 1982). Children often spontaneously acquire an impressive sight vocabulary. Soderbergh (1971), reports that her 3-year-old child acquired in this fashion 120 words within 3 months. This may be an exceptional case, but it may turn out that this sort of achievement is not uncommon among 4- and 5-year-olds (cf. Smith, 1971). Interestingly, adults often do not credit this skill as "reading." In common usage reading is often identified with decoding or recognising unfamiliar words. This, however, presupposes the next phase of reading acquisition.

From Phase 1 to Phase 2

It is popularly assumed that the look-and-say strategy is abandoned when the storage has reached a critical limit and visually similar words become confused. This contention is an example of the many *post-hoc* hypotheses that attempt to explain the mechanism of developmental change. One suggestion for the transition to phase 2 that needs to be taken seriously is the appearance of phoneme awareness (Gleitman & Rozin, 1977; Liberman et al., 1977). The work by these authors makes clear the radical nature of the change from logographic to alphabetic principles. A detailed discussion of this important work is beyond the scope of this Chapter.

From Phase 2 to Phase 3

The same principles are assumed to operate as with previous transitions. As with the introduction of the alphabetic strategy, the introduction of the orthographic strategy might result in apparent setbacks in performance.

Thus "good," phonetically plausible spellings may disappear and become "bad" errors. These would be bad only in the sense that they disregard phonology, but good in the sense that they apply orthographic units, even if an inappropriate one was chosen. The work of Smith (1983) and Sterling (1983) suggests that morphological knowledge, which may well be the hallmark of orthographic skill, can be clearly demonstrated in children's spellings.

Once the three phases have been passed through one could consider the essential period for literacy acquisition to be completed. However, at least a *Phase 4* is conceivable where the independence of written from spoken language is achieved and written language is handled as a system in its own right. Too little is known about this further development of functional literacy, but it need not concern us here, because not reaching a higher level of skill than Phase 3 is not usually regarded as failure.

The Principles of Change

Reading performance, assessed in terms of reading age, increases roughly as chronological age increases. Whereas this may be true for a group of children as a whole, an individual child would not be expected to show a smooth and gradual increase. Exactly when and how rapid spurts, decreases, plateaux, and slow gradual increases in performance occur is a matter of empirical investigation. The present theory aims to provide a framework for explaining these surface changes in terms of underlying step-wise improvements in skill. These step-wise changes of course are part of a complex developmental process about which we know hardly anything. I would like to suggest that we leave unexplained for the moment the maturational and educational factors, which we recognise as the necessary triggers of change, and instead focus on what it is that they trigger. It is clearly not enough to assume that at point one the logographic strategy is adopted by the child, at point two the alphabetic one, and so forth. If this was the case, then strategies would either replace each other, each starting again from zero, or be run in parallel. Neither of these possibilities allows for the type of change where there appears to be a sudden "breakthrough" in reading competence.

I would like to hypothesise that a breakthrough to the next phase of development would only occur if there is a merging of the old and new strategy. Certain components of the old strategy might be retained because they enhance the new strategy. Thus, it may be crucial that the "goal" of instant word recognition (which is established in the logographic phase) is preserved while the child gets to grips with grapheme-by-grapheme conversion. For the orthographic strategy it is easy to imagine that there must be a merging of instant recognition and piecemeal analytic skills, each of which is assumed to be predominant at an earlier phase. My hypothesis then requires that what is triggered by developmental factors is a process of "merging." Vague as it is, this hypothesis would immediately explain why it is that children apparently "choose" their own time to apply taught knowledge. It seems that they have to wait until everything is right for the old and new to merge together. This is consistent with recent explanations of developmental change using the concept of "success" of earlier strategies (Karmiloff-Smith, 1979, 1984), or the notion of agreement between old and new strategies (Bryant, 1982). If this particular developmental process fails we would expect that the child would simply not move on to the next step in normal development. In no way could drill in the new strategy by itself reinstate the normal progress, and I think that this is exactly what we find with many well-tutored dyslexics. Thus we are not surprised that a teacher complains that "Johnny knows all the rules of phonics, but he doesn't apply them." Furthermore, the hypothesis would give a rationale for teaching compensatory strategies even though one would not expect them to be as efficient as normal strategies.

We now have to consider *how* a child might move from one step to the next. What provides the impetus for the adoption of the various strategies?

FROM THREE-PHASE TO SIX-STEP MODEL

In the basic outline of the three-phase model a general literacy skill, for example reading age, was the target variable. Clearly this is not satisfactory, and instead a number of specific variables that are all performance aspects of literacy could be considered. In particular, there is *the* major division of literacy skills into input and output components, word recognition (reading), and word production (writing). It is this division that I would like to use in order to redesign the basic model. I have argued previously (Frith, 1979, 1980) that writing and reading skills will sometimes show dissociations in development. The hypothesis I would like to put forward now is simply that *normal reading and writing development proceeds out of step*. This hypothesis results in a noticeable modification of the acquisition model, as shown in Table 13.1. Table 13.1 shows that each phase is divided into two steps with either reading or writing as the pacemaker of the strategy that identifies the phase. The division into steps also allows a differentiation in terms of level of skill in a particular strategy, here symbolised by number subscripts. Level 1 would imply that the skill is present in very basic form only; level 2, that it is more advanced, and so on. Thus one might postulate that only when logographic skill has reached level 2 in reading is it ready to be adopted for writing.

The alphabetic strategy is first adopted for writing, whereas the logographic strategy is continued to be used for reading, perhaps at an even more

TABLE 13.1
The Six-step Model of Skills in Reading
and Writing Acquisition

Step	Reading	Writing
1a	*logographic* $_1$	(symbolic)
1b	logographic$_2$	logographic$_2$
2a	logographic$_3$	*alphabetic*$_1$
2b	alphabetic$_2$	alphabetic$_2$
3a	*orthographic*$_1$	alphabetic$_3$
3b	orthographic$_2$	orthographic$_2$

advanced level 3. Only when the alphabetic strategy reaches level 2 will it be adopted for reading. The rationale for the antecedence of writing here is provided by the idea that the alphabet is tailor-made for writing rather than for reading (Frith & Frith, 1980). Thus it is easy to learn to write using the relatively small set of letters. At the same time the limited number of symbols creates ambiguities when translation into sound is required. Although observational and experimental evidence needs to be collected to test this feature of the present model, it would provide an explanation for the finding (see Part I Introduction) that in acquired disorders phonological (i.e. alphabetic) reading is always accompanied by phonological spelling, but not vice versa.

Phase 3 again shows reading as the pacemaker resulting in step 3a. Orthographic knowledge at level 1 is presumed to be weak—sufficient to be used in recognising words, but not to be used in guiding the writing of words. Level 2 would imply that orthographic representations are now precise enough to be useful for spelling. It is plausible to assume that they would then be "transferred" to the spelling output system. The highly skilled reader/speller requires internal representations that are exact in terms of letter-by-letter detail.

In summary, the theory now states that at each phase there is a first step involving a divergence between strategies used for reading and writing, then a step involving convergence. Developmental progress is envisaged as an alternating shift of balance between reading and writing. Reading is the pacemaker for the logographic strategy, writing for the alphabetic strategy, and reading again for the orthographic one.

While this model is as yet purely speculative, it suggests numerous experiments that may either change or disprove it.

SOME TESTABLE PREDICTIONS

The internal representation of words acquired during the logographic phase might well resemble memory images for other types of graphic stimuli. Because there is as yet no proper guiding principle for the analysis of a written word, it is reasonable to suppose that the child selects the graphic features that are salient to him and uses them as critical identifiers. Thus, the x in Alex, the exclamation mark after the word bang! may be of special significance to a child. This child might say "Alex" when seeing the word Max and "bang" when seeing the word big! In attempts at writing the child would be expected to preserve the x and the ! and to omit those features that are not salient to him or her. Matching to sample or sorting techniques would be useful for investigating salient features. Stimuli would have to be prepared with systematic graphic variations. Presumably, the child would class together stimuli that seem similar, that is, share the same internal representation. Certain changes of graphic features, for example letter type, may signal changes of word identity, even if the orthographic sequence remains intact. On the other hand, changes in orthographic sequence would be readily tolerated, because there is no commitment to sequential order. (The opposite would be predicted for children at the orthographic phase.)

It would be possible to test the hypothesis that at first the most important cues might come not from the written stimulus but from the situational context. It remains to be seen to what extent semantic or episodic context support is crucial in this process and exactly what it contributes to word recognition. Clearly, the more a child relies on cues from the word rather than context, the more efficient, and of course, situationally independent, his word recognition should become. One very important cue in this respect is the first letter of a word. It is known that sounding out the first letter acts as a powerful cue for recognition, so that the remaining letters in the word need not be sounded out at all (Marsh et al., 1981). This is one way through which the logographic strategy might become viable for quite advanced reading.

The suggestion that spelling practice will be more important to the acquisition of the alphabetic principle than reading practice can be readily tested. It is conceivable that it is the orderly sequential production of letters when writing which might be "copied," even unnecessarily, for word recognition. Thus, the piecemeal left-to-right decoding of a word might first make sense to a child as a deliberate reflection of the first-to-last writing process. This then would become the guiding principle of analysis that was missing before. When a child has learned to spell a word (oral or written spelling) then he or she may realise that what is important is temporal order rather than salient graphic features. The first letter of a word is both prominent in the spelling sequence and graphically salient. This may be an example of a merging of components of two strategies.

The orthographic strategy is postulated to differ from the logographic strategy, being based on segmentation into letter-by-letter units. This claim is also amenable to experimental investigation. The theory would predict, perhaps counterintuitively, that a child at phase 1 could not recognise words embedded in words. Thus words inside the word *scared*, such as *car*, *care*, *red*, *scar*, *ed*, *are*, some of which are likely to be highly familiar, would not be "seen" unless the irrelevant letters are actually blocked out. The process involved in seeing the embedded word *car* might at this stage be similar to seeing *ear* in *scared*, because commitment to fixed letter order is lacking. In contrast, a child at phase 3 should see *car* more readily than *ear*. Furthermore, this child would automatically give prominence to morphologically salient units, for example he or she might be quicker at finding *scare-* and *-d* compared to *car-* and *-red*. Perhaps these latter solutions might occur more readily to the child using an alphabetic strategy. This child might always specially attend to the first two or three letters, regardless of their morphological relevance, because they come first in the left-to-right sequential decoding process.

Predictions can also be made for the different strategies in spelling a completely unfamiliar word. Use of the logographic strategy would mean that the word cannot be written at all. Use of the alphabetic strategy in basic form would mean that individual phonemes are converted into individual graphemes and strung together ("frend" for *friend*, "gust" for *just*). When this strategy is more advanced, then context-sensitive rules are used, and errors such as "gust" for *just* would no longer be made. Use of the orthographic strategy would mean that instantly segmented units are matched with internally represented units. Hence an unfamiliar word will be spelled by using components of familiar words ("inteligents" for *intelligence*). As a result a good speller can spell nonsense words apparently "in analogy" with existing words, regardless of whether a so-called regular or irregular spelling is present (Campbell, 1983). Different types of otherwise phonetically acceptable spelling errors would therefore be predicted to occur at the different phases of acquisition. For example, the unfamiliar word *traction* might be spelled "trackshen," or "trackshun" at phase 2. At phase 3, however, instant segmentation would take place, which entails that the first segment of the word can be spelled with regard to an existing unit, say *track*, and the ending can be spelled as a known morpheme such as "sion" or "tion." A misspelling might thus be "tracksion." Similarly, if the target word is *generally*, then it might well be misspelled as "genralee" at phase 2, and as "genraly" at phase 3. The classification of spelling errors according to the extent to which they preserve morphemes or small orthographic units (ght, ou, or, etc.) would thus be of interest. Longitudinal studies of individual children would certainly provide tests of the usefulness of the present model.

An Explanation of Reading–Spelling Dissociations

Apart from a number of testable predictions the model can neatly account for the three types of reading/spelling dissociations that have been described in normal schoolchildren. These are Read's (1971, 1980) pre-school orthographers, Bryant and Bradley's (1980; Bradley & Bryant, 1979) first-year readers, and Frith's (1980) type-B spellers of secondary-school age.

Read's (1971, 1980) pre-school orthographers show the beginning of an alphabetic writing strategy, without having yet applied this strategy to reading (phase 2a). Thus, they cannot read back later what they themselves have written. Although in these studies there is no documentation either way as regards logographic word recognition skills, it would have to be assumed that such children were able to recognise at least some words by sight. For the reasons already mentioned such skill, if it existed, may well have been disregarded as not proper reading.

Bradley and Bryant's (1979) and Bryant and Bradley's (1980) beginning readers showed that they were able to recognise some words. This is likely to have been a result of applying a logographic strategy. Some of the words they recognised were highly irregular (*school*, *light*) and could thus not have been tackled by alphabetic strategies. On the other hand, the same children were able to spell correctly some words that showed simple phoneme–grapheme relationships (*bun*, *mat*) presumably by applying an alphabetic strategy, and these they were not necessarily able to recognise. This pattern fits perfectly with phase 2a. However, Bryant and Bradley's work also extends to phase 2b. They demonstrated that the children could be given a "set" to use the alphabetic strategy for reading, and then were able to read such words as *bun*, *mat*, *leg*, on which they previously failed. In view of the model's claim for the antecedence of the alphabetic strategy in writing, it is important supportive evidence that the children succeeded with the alphabetic strategy in reading certain words—only if they were also able to succeed in writing these words. Exactly this would be expected in phase 2b.

Frith's (1980) type-B spellers belong to phase 3a, whereas type-A spellers would belong to phase 3b. Type-B spellers can use an alphabetic strategy as shown by their phonetically acceptable spelling errors. However, when reading, their strategy seems to be orthographic. This dissociation is shown strikingly by their ability to distinguish correctly between homophones (e.g. *their–there*) in recognition, an ability which they seem to lack when writing these words. Type-B spellers are characterised by persistent difficulties. However, even a very cursory glance at the reading and spelling performance of normal children in the later years of primary school suggests that there are differences in strategies for these two activities. It is typical, for example, at that stage (presumably phase 3a) that a child often has to construct a word from laborious phoneme-to-grapheme rules when writing, but effortlessly recognises the word in question when reading.

POSSIBLE OUTCOMES OF DEVELOPMENTAL
READING FAILURE

Although both the basic and modified version of the theory are only rough sketches and would need to be elaborated in more detail, they do provide a guide for looking at developmental reading disorders.

Given our previous definition of developmental reading disorder, it is clear that we can theoretically distinguish at least between arrest at phase 1 and arrest at phase 2. Obviously we cannot decide what the arrest is due to, because we are far from penetrating into the complexities of maturational and environmental causes of change. It would, however, already be useful to establish whether it is possible to accommodate some of what is known about developmental dyslexia within the present framework.

Failure of the Logographic Principle

It is theoretically possible that a child fails to acquire any sight vocabulary, but in practice such cases are conspicuously rare. What is striking is the ability to acquire a respectable sight vocabulary even when there is severe mental retardation (O'Connor & Hermelin, 1963) and at very young ages (Doman, 1965). From this it seems that it is unlikely to be a major factor in accounting for developmental dyslexia. If such cases occur they should be especially evident with logographic scripts, and this would be interesting to establish.

Boder's (1973) dyseidetics might perhaps be cases in point. These are rare children who are said to show some knowledge of letter–sound correspondences but little ability to recognise words instantly, and who apparently cannot rely on good memory images when spelling words. However, this pattern does not necessarily implicate logographic failure. Even with intact logographic skills, relatively poor spelling is only to be expected, because of the absence of sequential order as a guiding principle. Evidence for logographic failure in reading would be, for instance, that words with striking visual features are recognised no more readily than those with unremarkable ones.

Failure of the Alphabetic Principle

Suppose a child fails to advance from phase 1 to phase 2. Of course, this child will not, therefore, be at a standstill. He or she will continue to improve in logographic skills and the child's reading age will still increase, if slowly. Difficulty in grasping and applying the alphabetic principle will mainly be obvious in the child's unsuccessful attempts at writing, and at sounding out and "blending" letters in reading (decoding) unfamiliar words. Unfortunately, this sort of difficulty often attracts the verdict "unable to read," because logographic skills are frequently not given any credit. Rozin, Poritsky, and Sotsky (1971) have shown that young children in socially adverse circumstances, who failed to learn to read in the normal school environment, were able to learn a set of 30 Chinese symbols with only 2–5 hours' tutoring. From this success we must infer that a logographic strategy was available. Why then was it not used in their reading of English words? The children experienced continuous failure in trying to grasp the alphabetic strategy. Here they may have been so poorly motivated in normal reading tasks that they would not even use the strategy that they were able to master. In the case of these children there may have been delay rather than deviance. What happens, however, when the alphabetic strategy presents an insurmountable barrier to normal progress?

The hypothesis I would like to propose here is that a developmental "arrest" at phase 1 characterises classic developmental dyslexia. From then on the sequence of literacy development would be abnormal. Usually when a child fails to progress there is intervention. Ideally, everything possible is done to promote advance to the next phase, namely the alphabetic one. With drill in "phonics" certainly a resemblance of alphabetic skills can be achieved. These skills, however, would never become automatic enough to be applied effortlessly. On the other hand, other compensatory strategies might be developed; perhaps there is also extended use of logographic skills. A further prediction from the model is that the normal effortless mastery of the orthographic strategy should be just as impossible as effortless mastery of the alphabetic strategy. Yet, again a resemblance of this skill might be found with specific training in orthographic segmentation. This is suggested by the work of Scheerer-Neumann (1981), who showed that a striking poverty in the utilisation of intra-word structure could be overcome by placing gaps between segments and by specific training in syllable segmentation.

Miles' (1982) study of 300 cases leaves no doubt that it is perfectly possible for a developmental dyslexic to become, on the surface, a good reader. It would be predicted that such a person used strategies that differ from those acquired in normal development. From the sparse evidence so far one can quote two pertinent observations: on "bad days" the painfully acquired reading competence can be seemingly lost again (Simpson, 1980); a variety of cognitive dysfunctions (involving phonological coding, see later) can still be uncovered by sensitive tests (Ellis & Miles, 1981; Miles & Ellis, 1981). The first observation implies that the skills are not automatic, the second, that improvement in reading is due to "symptomatic" treatment, but does imply that the underlying deficit has not been removed.

Sensitive test material is provided by non-words. It is strongly predicted that, even in "ex"-dyslexics, word-recognition skill in terms of speed and accuracy will be way ahead of non-word skills. Although logographic recognition shows improvement, and reading age as measured by such word recognition tests as the Schonell, goes up, performance with non-words shows very little improvement with reading age (Snowling, 1981). Baddeley et al. (1982) found that older, well-tutored dyslexic boys with a reading age of 10 years read fewer non-words correctly than controls of the same reading age. The significance of this result in the light of related work has been discussed by Snowling (1983). Seymour and MacGregor (1984) have found poor non-word skills relative to word skills in almost all their individually studied adolescent and adult dyslexic readers. Naidoo (1972), in her extensive description of 98 dyslexic boys, found that their main problems were those of sounding out and blending letters, typical alphabetic skills. The finding that dyslexic children with good word-recognition skills showed no spelling-regularity effect and a hugely increased word–non-word effect (Frith & Snowling, 1983) would be consistent with the notion that words are not recognised by phonological piecemeal analysis, but by logographic strategies.

Some important confirmation for the developmental sequence of strategies and the effect of arrest comes from a study of children with serious speech problems by Snowling and Stackhouse (1983). These children were able to acquire a considerable sight-word vocabulary, but, when compared with normal children from the same school who had a similar sight vocabulary, showed a greatly impaired phonetic spelling strategy. Relevant to this question is the often-quoted (Makita, 1968) absence of classic developmental dyslexia in Japan. This could readily be explained by the fact that the Japanese script involves logographic and syllabic but not alphabetic skills.

The Phonological Dysfunction Hypothesis and Classic Developmental Dyslexia

If we accept the identification of developmental arrest at phase 1 with classic developmental dyslexia, it is tempting to speculate on a reason for this arrest. It seems to me that at this stage the attractively simple hypothesis of a basic phonological dysfunction deserves the most serious consideration. Independent authors with very different experimental approaches have provided evidence that seems to converge on this possibility. As far as the three-phase model is concerned, it is clear that phase 2 is the only one where a connection to phonological processes is required. If there is a basic cognitive deficit in this area this would be most detrimental at the point of transition to phase 2, and may well go unnoticed.

The hypothesis assumes that the problem exists in speech regardless of whether reading is acquired or not. Reading failure would be seen as an artefact of alphabetic writing systems. Thus it is crucial to demonstrate that developmental dyslexics show specific impairments on non-reading tasks involving phonological processing. Some such demonstrations are now listed:

1. Retrospective reports of delayed speech acquisition (Fundudis et al., 1979; Ingram, 1962, 1969; Ingram et al., 1970; Mason, 1967; Naidoo, 1972; Rutter et al., 1970).
2. Prospective studies relating poor sound categorisation skills (rhyming, alliteration) to later reading backwardness (Bradley & Bryant, 1983).
3. Difficulties in orally repeating unfamiliar words (Godfrey et al., 1981; Miles, 1974, 1982; Snowling, 1981).
4. Phonological inaccuracies in paired associate learning with nonsense words (Done, 1982).
5. Slowness in picture naming (Denckla & Rudel, 1976).
6. Slowness in name-code as opposed to physical-code matching (Ellis, 1981).
7. Poor awareness of position of articulatory organs during phoneme production (Montgomery, 1981).
8. Poor speech acoustic-cue discrimination abilities (Tallal, 1980; Tallal & Stark, 1981).

These examples implicate a large variety of so-called auditory-verbal dysfunctions. In contrast, so-called visual-perceptual dysfunctions, another "old favourite" among causal explanations of dyslexia, have not fared very well in recent years (Bradley & Bryant, 1981; Hulme, 1981; Vellutino, 1979). Vellutino (1979) in particular has made a strong case for a verbal-processing dysfunction in dyslexia. Certainly among the most reliable findings in this area are deficits in the recall of phonologically structured lists, such as digits, multiplication tables, the alphabet, months of the year, etc. (Ellis & Miles, 1981). Apart from evidence from outside the reading task, there is also some evidence from reading and spelling errors that would support the hypothesis of a phonological dysfunction. Nelson and Warrington (1974) and Frith (1980) found that misspellings in dyslexic children betray phonological problems. For instance, dyslexic children fail, more often than controls, to preserve the number of syllables let alone phonemes (Farnham-Diggory & Nelson, 1983).

Despite the support that can be derived from recent studies the phonological dysfunction hypothesis is of rather limited use in its present form. It still remains to be specified how phonological skills affect the acquisition of alphabetic skills, and what aspect is the most critical, be it phonemic segmentation, phonological assembly, articulatory programmes, or meta-linguistic skills.

Failure of the Orthographic Principle

The theory states that phase 2, identified by the adoption of alphabetic strategies, is only an intermediate step towards phase 3. It was hypothesised that a merging of instant recognition and analytic sequential skills would result in the breakthrough to this last phase, where orthographic units are employed in reading rather than salient graphic features or grapheme–phoneme correspondences. Again, we have to consider what the failure to achieve this particular transition might mean: we would expect pronounced reliance on the alphabetic principle together with a lack of orthographic skills, whereas logographic skills should be intact. If over-reliance on alphabetic strategies is the hallmark of acquired surface dyslexia, then this failure constitutes a developmental analogue. However, there might be differences in terms of intactness and accessibility of logographic skills. As a preliminary term for developmental arrest at phase 2 I would suggest "developmental dysgraphia." This distinguishes it from "dyslexia," which was defined as arrest at phase 1, and further points to a striking problem associated with this condition, namely *spelling* so-called irregular words. These words would always tend to be regularised according to phoneme–grapheme rules. On the other hand, *reading* irregular words would only be a problem if the logographic strategy has been discouraged (which does happen). Regular words, by definition, would be spelled and read correctly, simply by application of the alphabetic strategy. Compensatory strategies would again be expected.

Children arrested at phase 2 are probably those that Naidoo (1972) and Nelson and Warrington (1974) identified and described as spelling-only retardates. These children were separable from classic dyslexic children on a number of tests. Their reading skill was generally more advanced and they made significantly fewer phonetically inaccurate errors. Also, unlike dyslexics, they showed no impairments on any language tests. The present theory-imposed categorisation into two types of developmental reading disorder accords well with the main findings from these two studies. In both studies large groups of children diagnosed as reading retarded were scrutinised with the purpose of finding distinct subgroups. Interestingly, both studies turned up only two subtypes, and the same ones, although this was *not* specifically predicted in either case. The frequent failure to find evidence for a large variety of subtypes in developmental dyslexia cannot be ignored and constitutes a glaring difference to studies in acquired dyslexia.

Nevertheless, it is generally acknowledged that children with developmental reading disorders are anything but a homogeneous group. The present theory attributes some heterogeneity to the underlying deficits, but most of it to the development of abnormal or compensatory strategies. These would be expected to be very diverse indeed. Classification according to development subsequent to the point of arrest in the normal developmental sequence would of course also be possible, but this is another matter and needs to be kept separate.

Having identified just two points of developmental arrest, one at phase 1, the other at phase 2, it remains to be seen if it would be possible to identify arrest within phases, namely at steps 1a, 1b, 2a, 2b, etc. This would imply that each of the three basic strategies might be applied to reading/or writing exclusively without transfer from one activity to the other. This one might consider very unlikely. However, just such a case may be presented by the type-B speller.

A Selective Failure of the Orthographic Strategy and Type-B Spellers

Type-B spellers were previously described as poor spellers who are at the same time good readers. It was shown (Frith, 1979, 1980, 1982) that spelling errors in these cases were such that good alphabetic skills must be presupposed. Of course, the alphabetic strategy is never very efficient for reading, and when the children were forced to use it, for instance when reading nonsense words, or reading phonetically rendered text, then they were much less successful than when they could read using orthographic skills. However, whereas orthographic skills seemed strong in reading (e.g. correct identification of homophones) they seemed weak in spelling (confusion of homophones). Thus, type-B spellers could read their own misspelled words rather less well than type-A spellers could read theirs. Exactly this pattern of results would be expected for developmental arrest at step 3a and is different from arrest at step 2b, as in dysgraphia.

What failure can we suppose to underlie this persistent reading/spelling dissociation? Clearly, a hypothesis is required that allows the orthographic principle to be grasped fully and applied with consummate skill for reading, yet explains why this principle fails for spelling. Although the notion of separate orthographic output logogens (Morton, 1980) fits extremely well with this phenomenon, the puzzle remains of how faulty output logogens came about in the first place.

It has already been argued that the power of orthographic strategies for spelling eventually depends on the precision of the internal representation of the hypothesised orthographic units. At step 3a, representations may still be imprecise (level 1). This is not necessarily detrimental to reading, but very much so for spelling. For this reason spelling will still have to rely on alphabetic strategies, and lag behind reading.

I previously put forward the hypothesis that precise orthographic representations (whether or not they are separated for purposes of input and output) are acquired as the result of a reading strategy that gives equal attention to all letters in a word. This was supported by some experiments

(Frith, 1980, 1983). Such a strategy would therefore involve more work than was just necessary and sufficient for word recognition. It is conceivable that individual differences exist in terms of willingness/capacity to adopt such a wastefully inelegant strategy, and this would provide an explanation for arrest at this point in the sequence.

AN e-CANCELLATION EXPERIMENT WITH TYPE-B SPELLERS

To inquire further into this attention-to-detail hypothesis Dolores Perin and I carried out an e-cancellation experiment. We chose e-cancellation as just the sort of task to discriminate people who did and did not habitually pay attention to letter-by-letter detail. We hoped that the type of e that was missed would give us clues as to exactly which detail was likely to be *not* represented in imprecise internal orthographic images. Previously (Frith, 1979) I found it useful to distinguish important and unimportant es in words on the basis of whether they are necessary for identification of a word. For instance, *lift.d* can be identified as "lifted" without the missing letter e; *l.ft* cannot be identified as "left", unless there is an e, otherwise, it could be "lift" or "loft." Whether or not an e is important can be easily established by this guessing technique. Important es are usually in stressed syllables, mostly at the beginning or in the middle of a word and are clearly pronounced. Unimportant es are usually in unstressed syllables, often near the end, and are usually schwa sounds or completely silent. I found that normal adults tend to miss more of the unimportant than the important es in an e-cancellation task.

The distinction between important and unimportant es makes sense insofar as it helps us to hypothesise what detail in a word may be skipped without penalty. This can be called "reading by partial cues." With an orthographic reading strategy that is just sufficient for recognition (but not for building up precise representations and hence *not* sufficient for word production) one could afford to skip unimportant es but not important ones. This may be then what type-B spellers do. Certainly, in spelling it is precisely with schwa sounds that type-B spellers have particular trouble. They often do not know if it is *independent* or *independant*; *existance* or *existence*. Perhaps this difficulty stems from a relative neglect of these letters. Further, if these letters are neglected, then they are not internally represented. If they are not represented, then they might not be noticed during the cancellation task. The strong prediction can therefore be made that type-B spellers, who are equal to type-A spellers when cancelling important es, should show more misses than type-A spellers for unimportant es.

We used a sample of fourth-formers (aged 14) from five Inner London schools. All spoke English as a first language and all were assessed on the

Spar Reading Test which involves sentence completion with multiple choice (jet planes fly *fairy–farm–finish–fast*...) and a dictation test based on 30 regular and irregular words from Schonell's lists (1942). We initially selected 14 type-A spellers. These showed ceiling performance on both the reading and spelling test. There were also 12 type-B spellers who performed at ceiling (95–100% correct) when reading and much less well (42–65%) when spelling. The final selection of the subjects was based on their *e*-cancellation performance.

We presented two ordinary typed A4 pages each with 170 words, containing the letter *e* just once, intermixed with 130 words without any letter *e*. On one page, *e*-words had mainly important *e*s, on the other page, mainly unimportant ones. The order of presentation was balanced, each subject receiving both pages.

The two groups were matched in terms of the number of misses of important *e*s. The range was from 4 to 15 misses in this category. This matching procedure left nine subjects in each group. The results are shown in Table 13.2. They bear out the prediction that type-B spellers miss more unimportant *e*s than type-A spellers, even though they miss just as few important *e*s as type-A spellers ($z = 1.90$, $p = .023$). This supports the hypothesis that habitual attention to letter-by-letter detail in type-A spellers is superior compared to that in type-B spellers. Furthermore, it suggests quite concretely that neglect of schwa vowels may be a feature of imprecise orthographic images. If equal attention to all letters including schwa vowels is an essential requirement for skilled use of the orthographic strategy in spelling, then this aspect of skill seems to be inadequate in type-B spellers.

We still have the problem of explaining the persistent use of imprecise orthographic representations in spelling but not in reading. It seems reasonable to assume that type-B spellers who become truly excellent readers in the end do manage to build up precise orthographic input representations. Indeed, this must be so if they do not confuse homophones. Why then do they not use these excellent input-specific representations to modify their poor output-specific ones? One possibility is that modification is very

TABLE 13.2
Results of *e*-Cancellation Task:
Number of *e*s Missed (out of 170)

	Important *es*		Unimportant *es*	
	Mean	SD	Mean	SD
A (N = 9)	7.44	(2.55)	12.56	(7.55)
B (N = 9)	7.11	(3.30)	17.56	(12.69)

difficult once automatic output programmes have been established. Their output programmes may have been established prematurely, that is, at a point before the input representations have reached the critical level 2. In normal development the trigger for moving forward from step 3a to step 3b would be the time when level 2 orthographic representations are available. A type-B child, on the other hand, might not reach this critical level for a very long time, and hence—perhaps in the way of compensation—will use level 1 orthographic representations, imprecise as they are, as the basis for spelling output programmes.

This hypothesis would derive support if it could be shown that spelling errors in type-B individuals exhibited undeniable orthographic elements (besides the already demonstrated alphabetic ones), such as morpheme preservation, or graphemic elaboration that is superfluous to the phonetic rendering of the word (*wright* for "write").

SUBTYPES OF DEVELOPMENTAL AND ACQUIRED READING AND WRITING DISORDERS

Developmental disorder was defined as a failure to advance normally from one phase to another. This contrasts with post-developmental disorder where there can be a loss of skill at whatever phase it was acquired. With a simple framework of three phases of literacy acquisition we can therefore distinguish two types of developmental but six types of post-developmental disorder. These are illustrated in Table 13.3. Types 1 and 2 are the only ones that should be quite closely comparable for both groups. A type 0 is conceivable where even the logographic principle fails. This, however, I

TABLE 13.3
Schematic Representation of Subtypes of Dyslexia According to Strategy
Available (+) or Not Available (−)

	Subtypes of Developmental Disorder		Subtypes of Post-developmental Disorder					
	1	*2*	*1*	*2*	*3*	*4*	*5*	*6*
Logographic strategy	+	+	+	+	+	−	−	−
Alphabetic strategy	−	+	−	+	−	+	−	+
Orthographic strategy	−	−	−	−	+	−	+	+

would consider to be likely only in the context of severe subnormality or severe brain damage.

Patterson (1981) has used a similar format for the schematic representation of different types of acquired dyslexia. Her dimensions of classification, however, were expressed in terms of reading performance rather than in terms of underlying skills. It is very easy to draw the two together. The logographic strategy would be characterised in terms of a strong word/nonword effect, a content/function effect, and imageability/concreteness effect. The last two effects could both be considered to reflect an underlying age of acquisition effect. Thus, content words and concrete words are acquired earlier and are therefore likely to have been part of the early logographic representations. Deep dyslexic patients, given the present classification, would correspond to type 3. Type 1 may conceivably be another variant of deep dyslexia where orthographic skills are severely impaired in addition to alphabetic ones. The word length and the spelling regularity effect are characteristic of alphabetic skills, and if these are intact, as in types 2, 4, and 6, we can speak of variants of surface dyslexia.

If the present definition of developmental disorder is accepted, then there will always be more types of acquired disorder, however much one refines the theory of acquisition and however many subtypes of developmental failure one might identify.

SUMMARY AND CONCLUSIONS

The subtypes of developmental reading and writing failure that are suggested by the present theory can now be summarised.

Classic developmental dyslexia is the failure of alphabetic skills. It corresponds to arrest at phase 1 in the normal developmental sequence. One explanation of the failure that is favoured by a number of recent studies is in terms of a disorder of the phonological system. The theory predicts that dyslexic children are able to use logographic skills. This strategy is assumed to be characteristic of phase 1 in the young beginning reader. Nevertheless, dyslexic children do not necessarily resemble beginners because they also develop compensatory strategies. With time they can gradually improve in the use of logographic skills way beyond the level reached by young children and can build up a good sight vocabulary. Second, we know that dyslexic children are often especially drilled in "phonics" with the result that they do acquire alphabetic skills to a certain extent. This is not akin to normal developmental breakthrough, however, as they always have to spend more effort using this strategy than normal children. Typically, they are slower, more variable, and cannot always maintain the effort under stress. In contrast, the effortless automatic use of the skill is typical of normal readers.

Developmental dysgraphia is the failure of orthographic skills and corresponds to arrest at phase 2. If children find it difficult to handle these particular skills, then they are expected to continue to rely on alphabetic (and, if encouraged, logographic) skills. This is characteristic of phase 2b in normal literacy acquisition, and probably also of some cases of acquired surface dyslexia. Again, it needs to be added that compensatory strategies can lead to a reasonable degree of competence. Dysgraphic children (sometimes called spelling-only retardates) are not as severely handicapped as dyslexic children, because their developmental failure occurs later in the developmental sequence.

A variant of developmental dysgraphia at a more advanced phase of acquisition (phase 3a), and therefore a still milder handicap, is found in the *type-B speller*. This disorder implies a failure of the orthographic principle for spelling but not for reading, and results in the initially surprising combination of excellent reading and atrocious spelling. In the case of type-B spellers, orthographic representations for spelling production may have been established prematurely on the basis of still imprecise orthographic representations for word recognition. An experiment using *e*-cancellation illustrated that attention to letter-by-letter detail, which may be crucial for increasing the precision of representations, can be taken for granted in type-A spellers, but not in type-B spellers.

It would be paradoxical if the developmental approach to developmental disorders ignored developmental processes subsequent to the point of arrest in the *normal* sequence. Indeed it needs to be emphasised that we *expect* at least some improvement in literacy skills after such arrest. There is likely to be progress in earlier strategies that have been mastered normally. There may also be compensatory strategies. Hence, the present theory has no provision for "stagnation." Following arrest, therefore, we would not expect to find exactly the same picture in a dyslexic or dysgraphic child as in a normal child who is at that phase of acquisition where the arrest occurred.

The present framework may allow a fresh approach to comparisons between developmental and acquired reading disorders. It seems important to acknowledge that developmental disorders are not simply disorders occurring in childhood. The aetiology of developmental disorders must be located in the developmental process whereas brain trauma can occur at any time. In order to contrast these two types of problems it was suggested that a developmental disorder is defined as arrest at a particular phase in the developmental sequence. With an acquired disorder, a loss of a strategy may occur regardless of the order of acquisition. The patient may still retain a strategy that previously had been built up on the one he or she lost. A developmental disorder rules out such a case.

One major aim for research is to discover what it is that actually goes wrong when there is an arrest in development. There is the possibility that a defect in underlying factors, for example, a phonological dysfunction, may prevent normal progress. There is the possibility that strategies fail to be merged together. As was briefly suggested earlier, one outstanding feature of normal development is the ability to pool strategies belonging to different phases. Thus, an arrest in the normal sequence can be seen perhaps as an inability to merge strategies rather than as an inability to acquire new ones.

Although much has still to be worked out to make the present model credible, it may have served a purpose in alerting us to the fallacy that developmental and acquired disorders are one and the same. Perhaps it has made the point that the already existing *structural model*, useful as it is in describing the skilled reading process, needs to be complemented by a *developmental model* in order to make sense of the varieties of developmental dyslexia.

ACKNOWLEDGEMENTS

While making extensive revisions to this chapter I have been greatly helped by the editors' questions and criticisms. I am especially grateful, for their many helpful suggestions and clarifications, to John Morton, Maggie Snowling, Lindsay Evett, Alan Leslie, and Chris Frith.

REFERENCES

Baddeley, A. D., Ellis, N. C., Miles, T. R., & Lewis, V. J. (1982). Developmental and acquired dyslexia: A comparison. *Cognition, 11*, 185–199.

Bever, T. G. (ed.) (1981). *Regressions in Development: Basic phenomena and theoretical alternatives.* Hillsdale, NJ: Lawrence Erlbaum Associates Inc.

Biemiller, A. J. (1970). The development of the use of graphic and contextual information as children learn to read. *Reading Research Quarterly, 6*, 75–96.

Boder, E. (1973). Developmental dyslexia: A diagnostic approach based on three atypical reading-spelling patterns. *Developmental Medicine and Child Neurology, 15*, 663–687.

Bower, T. G. R. (1974). Repetition in human development. *Merrill Palmer Quarterly, 20*, 303–319.

Bradley, L., & Bryant, P. E. (1978). Difficulties in auditory organization as a possible cause of reading backwardness. *Nature, 271*, 746–747.

Bradley, L., & Bryant, P. E. (1979). Independence of reading and spelling in normal and backward readers. *Developmental Medicine and Child Neurology, 21*, 504–514.

Bradley, L., & Bryant, P. E. (1981). Visual memory and phonological skills in reading and spelling backwardness. *Psychological Research, 43*, 193–199.

Bradley, L., & Bryant, P. E. (1983). Categorizing sounds and learning to read: A causal connection. *Nature, 301*, 419–421.

Bryan, W. L., & Harter, N. (1899). Studies on the telegraphic language. *Psychological Review, 6*, 345–375.

Bryant, P. E. (1982). The role of conflict and of agreement between intellectual strategies in children's ideas about measurement. *British Journal of Psychology, 73*, 243–251.

Bryant, P. E., & Bradley, L. (1980). Why children sometimes write words which they do not read. In U. Frith (ed.), *Cognitive Processes in Spelling*. London: Academic Press.

Campbell, R. (1983). Writing nonwords to dictation. *Brain and Cognition, 19*, 153–178.

Chall, J. (1967). *Learning to Read: The great debate*. New York: McGraw-Hill.

Clark, M. M. (1976). *Young Fluent Readers*. London: Heinemann.

Condry, S. M., McMahon-Rideout, M., & Levy, A. A. (1979). A developmental investigation of selective attention to graphic, phonetic and semantic information in words. *Perception & Psychophysics, 25*, 88–94.

Denckla, M. B., & Rudel, R. (1976). Naming of object drawings by dyslexic and other learning disabled children. *Brain & Language, 3*, 1–15.

De Goes, C., & Martlew, M. (1983). Young children's approach to literacy. In M. Martlew (ed.), *The Psychology of Written Language—Developmental and Educational Perspectives*. Chichester: John Wiley & Sons.

Doman, G. J. (1965). *Teach your Baby to Read*. London: Jonathan Cape.

Done, J. (1982). *Age of acquisition effect, name latency and dyslexia*. Paper presented at BPS Developmental Section, Annual Conference, Durham.

Downing, J., & Leong, C. K. (1982). *The Psychology of Reading*. London: Collier Macmillan.

Ellis, N. (1981). Visual and name coding in dyslexic children. *Psychological Research, 43*, 201–218.

Ellis, N. C., & Miles, T. R. (1981). A lexical encoding deficiency I: Experimental evidence. In G. T. Pavlidis, & T. R. Miles (eds.), *Dyslexia Research and Its Applications to Education*. New York: Wiley.

Entwisle, D. R. (1979). The child's social environment and learning to read. In T. G. Waller, & G. E. Mackinnon (eds.), *Reading Research: Advances in Theory and Practice*, Vol. 1. New York: Academic Press.

Farnham-Diggory, S., & Nelson, B. (1983). Microethology of spelling behaviour in normal and dyslexic development. In D. R. Rogers, & J. A. Sloboda (eds.), *The Acquisition of Symbolic Skills*. New York: Plenum.

Ferreiro, E. (1978). What is written in a written sentence? A developmental answer. *Journal of Education, 160*, 25–39.

Francis, H. (1982). Learning to read. *Literate Behaviour and Orthographical Knowledge*. Hemel Hempstead: George Allen & Unwin.

Frith, U. (1979). Reading by eye and writing by ear. In P. A. Kolers, M. Wrolstad, & H. Bouma (eds.), *Processing of Visible Language, I*. New York: Plenum Press.

Frith, U. (1980). Unexpected spelling problems. In U. Frith (ed.), *Cognitive Processes in Spelling*. London: Academic Press.

Frith, U. (1981). Experimental approaches to developmental dyslexia: An introduction. *Psychological Research, 43*, 97–109.

Frith, U. (1982). Specific spelling problems. In R. N. Malatesha & H. A. Whitaker (eds.), *Dyslexia: A Global Issue*. The Hague: Martinus Nijhoff.

Frith, U. (1983). The similarities and differences between reading and spelling problems. In M. Rutter (ed.), *Developmental Neuropsychiatry*. New York: Guilford Press.

Frith, U., & Frith, C. D. (1980). Relationships between reading and spelling. In J. F. Kavanagh, & R. L. Venezky (eds.), *Orthography, Reading and Dyslexia*. Baltimore: University Park Press.

Frith, U., & Snowling, M. (1983). Reading for meaning and reading for sound in autistic and dyslexic children. *British Journal of Developmental Psychology, 1*, 329–342.

Fundudis, T., Kolvin, I., & Garside, R. F. (1979). *Speech Retarded and Deaf Children*. London: Academic Press.

Gillingham, A., & Stillman, B. W. (1956). *Remedial Training for Children with Specific Disability in Reading, Spelling, and Penmanship*. Cambridge, Mass.: Educators Publishing Service.

Gleitman, L. R. & Rozin, P. (1977). The structure and acquisition of reading, I: Relations between orthographies and the structure of language. In A. S. Reber, & D. L. Scarborough (eds.), *Towards a Psychology of Reading*. Hillsdale, NJ: Lawrence Erlbaum Associates Inc.

Godfrey, J. J., Syrdal-Lasky, A. K., Millay, K. K., & Knox, C. M. (1981). Performance of dyslexic children on speech perception tests. *Journal of Experimental Child Psychology, 32*, 401–424.

Hulme, C. (1981). The effects of manual tracing on memory in normal and retarded readers: Some implications for multisensory teaching. *Psychological Research, 41*, 179–191.

Ingram, T. T. S. (1962). Delayed development of speech with special reference to dyslexia. *Proceedings of the Royal Society of Medicine, 56*, 199–203.

Ingram, T. T. S. (1969). Developmental disorders of speech. In P. J. Vinken, & G. W. Bruyn (eds.), *Handbook of Clinical Neurology*. Amsterdam: North Holland Publishing Company.

Ingram, T. T. S., Mason, A. W., & Blackburn, I. (1970). A retrospective study of 82 children with reading disability. *Developmental Medicine and Child Neurology, 12*, 271–281.

Karmiloff-Smith, A. (1979). Micro- and macrodevelopmental changes in language acquisition and other representational systems. *Cognitive Science, 3*, 91–118.

Karmiloff-Smith, A. (1984). Children's problem solving. In M. E. Lamb, A. L. Brown, & B. Rogoff (eds.), *Advances in Developmental Psychology, Vol. III*. Hillsdale, NJ: Lawrence Erlbaum Associates Inc.

Liberman, I. Y., Shankweiler, D., Liberman, A. M., Fowler, C., & Fischer, F. W. (1977). Phonetic segmentation and recoding in the beginning reader. In A. S. Reber, & D. Scarborough (eds.), *Towards a Psychology of Reading*. Hillsdale, NJ: Lawrence Erlbaum Associates Inc.

Makita, K. (1968). The rarity of reading disability in Japanese children. *American Journal of Orthopsychiatry, 38*, 599–614.

Marsh, G., & Desberg, P. (1983). Development of strategies in the acquisition of symbolic skills. In D. R. Rogers, & J. A. Sloboda (eds.), *The Acquisition of Symbolic Skills*. New York: Plenum.

Marsh, G. Desberg, P., & Cooper, J. (1977). Developmental changes in strategies of reading. *Journal of Reading Behaviour, 9*, 391–394.

Marsh, G., Friedman, M. P., Desberg, P., & Welch, V. (1980). Development of strategies in learning to spell. In U. Frith (ed.), *Cognitive Processes in Spelling*. London: Academic Press.

Marsh, G., Friedman, M. P., Welch, V., & Desberg, P. (1981). A cognitive-developmental theory of reading acquisition. In T. G. Waller, & G. E. Mackinnon (eds.), *Reading Research: Advances in Theory and Practice*, Vol. 3. New York: Academic Press.

Mason, A. W. (1967). Specific (developmental) dyslexia. *Developmental Medicine and Child Neurology, 9*, 183–190.

McCaughey, M. W., Juola, J. F., Schadler, M., & Ward, N. J. (1980). Whole word units are used before orthographic knowledge in perceptual development. *Journal of Experimental Child Psychology, 30*, 411–421.

Miles, T. R. (1974). *The Dyslexic Child*. Hove, Sussex: Priory Press.

Miles, T. R. (1982). *Dyslexia: The Pattern of Difficulties*. London: Granada.

Miles, T. R., & Ellis, N. C. (1981). A lexical encoding deficiency II: Clinical observations. In G. T. Pavlidis, & T. R. Miles (eds.), *Dyslexia Research and its Applications to Education*. New York: Wiley.

Montgomery, D. (1981). Do dyslexics have difficulty accessing articulatory information? *Psychological Research, 43*, 235–243.

Morton, J. (1980). The logogen model and orthographic structure. In U. Frith (ed.), *Cognitive Processes in Spelling*. London: Academic Press.

Morton, J., & Patterson, K. (1980). A new attempt at an interpretation, or, an attempt at a new interpretation. In M. Coltheart, K. Patterson, & J. C. Marshall, (eds.), *Deep Dyslexia*. London: Routledge & Kegan Paul.

Naidoo, S. (1972). *Specific Dyslexia*. London: Pitman.

Nelson, H. E., & Warrington, E. K. (1974). Developmental spelling retardation and its relations to other cognitive abilities. *British Journal of Psychology, 65,* 265–274.

O'Connor, N., & Hermelin, B. (1963). *Speech and Thought in Severe Subnormality*. Oxford: Pergamon.

Patterson, K. E. (1981). Neuropsychological approaches to the study of reading. *British Journal of Psychology, 72,* 151–174.

Pick, A. D., Unze, M., Brownell, C. A., Drozdal, J. G., & Hopmann, M. K. (1978). Young children's knowledge of word structure. *Child Development, 49,* 669–680.

Read, C. (1971). Pre-school children's knowledge of English phonology. *Harvard Educational Review, 41,* 1–34.

Read, C. (1980). Writing is not the inverse of reading for young children. In C. H. Frederiksen, M. F. Whiteman, & J. G. Dominic (eds.), *Writing: The nature, development and teaching of written communication*. Hillsdale, NJ: Lawrence Erlbaum Associates Inc.

Rozin, P., Poritsky, S., & Sotsky, R. (1971). American children with reading problems can easily learn to read English represented by Chinese characters. *Science, 171,* 1264–1267.

Rutter, M. (1976). Speech delay. In M. Rutter (ed.), *Child Psychiatry, Modern Approaches*. Oxford: Blackwell.

Rutter, M. (1978). Prevalence and types of dyslexia. In A. L. Benton, & D. Pearl (eds.), *Dyslexia: An appraisal of current knowledge*. New York: Oxford University Press.

Rutter, M., & Yule, W. (1975). The concept of specific reading retardation. *Journal of Child Psychology and Psychiatry, 16,* 181–197.

Rutter, M., Tizard, J., & Whitmore, K. (eds.) (1970). *Education, Health and Behaviour*. London: Longman.

Scheerer-Neumann, G. (1981). The utilization of intraword structure in poor readers: Experimental evidence and a training program. *Psychological Research, 43,* 155–178.

Schonell, F. (1942). *Backwardness in the Basic Subjects*. London: Oliver & Boyd.

Seitz, V. (1977). *Social Class and Ethnic Group Differences in Learning to Read*. Newark, Del.: International Reading Association.

Seymour, P. H. K., & MacGregor, C. J. (1984). Developmental dyslexia: A cognitive experimental analysis of phonological, morphemic and visual impairments. *Cognitive Neuropsychology, 1,* 43–82.

Shallice, T., Warrington, E. K., & McCarthy R. (1983). Reading without semantics. *Quarterly Journal of Experimental Psychology, 35A,* 111–138.

Simpson, E. (1980). *Reversals: A Personal Account of Victory over Dyslexia*. London: Gollancz.

Smith, F. (1971). *Understanding Reading: A Psycholinguistic Analysis of Reading and Learning to Read*. New York: Holt, Rinehart & Winston.

Smith, P. T. (1983). Patterns of writing errors in the framework of an information processing model of writing. In D. R. Rogers, & A. J. Sloboda (eds.), *The Acquisition of Symbolic Skills*. New York: Plenum.

Snowling, M. J. (1981). Phonemic deficits in developmental dyslexia. *Psychological Research, 43,* 219–234.

Snowling, M. J. (1983). The comparison of acquired and developmental disorders of reading—A discussion. *Cognition, 14,* 105–118.

Snowling, M. J., & Frith, U. (1981). The role of sound, shape and orthographic cues in early reading. *British Journal of Psychology, 72,* 83–87.

Snowling, M. J., & Stackhouse, J. (1983). Spelling performance of children with developmental verbal dyspraxia. *Developmental Medicine and Child Neurology, 25,* 430–437.

Soderbergh, R. (1971). *Reading in Early Childhood: A linguistic study of a preschool child's gradual acquisition of reading ability*. Stockholm: Almqvist & Wiksell.

Sterling, C. M. (1983). The psychological productivity of inflectional and derivational morphemes. In D. R. Rogers, & J. A. Sloboba (eds.), *The Acquisition of Symbolic Skills*, New York: Plenum.

Stern, C., & Gould, T. S. (1965). *Children Discover Reading. An introduction to structural reading*. New York: Random House.

Strauss, S. (ed.) (1982). *U-Shaped Behavioural Growth*. New York: Academic Press.

Tallal, P. (1980). Auditory temporal perception, phonics, and reading disabilities in children. *Brain and Language*, 9, 182–198.

Tallal, P., & Stark, R. (1981). Speech acoustic-cue discrimination abilities of normally developing and language impaired children. *Journal of Acoustical Society of America*, 69, 568–579.

Tansley, P., & Panckhurst, J. (1981). *Children with Specific Learning Difficulties*. Windsor: NFER–Nelson.

Torrey, J. W. (1979). Reading that comes naturally: The early reader. In T. G. Waller, & G. E. Mackinnon (eds.), *Reading Research: Advances in theory and practice, Vol. 1*. New York: Academic Press.

Vellutino, F. R. (1979). *Dyslexia: Theory and Research*. Cambridge, Mass.: MIT Press.

Weber, R. M. (1970). A linguistic analysis of first-grade reading errors. *Reading Research Quarterly*, 5, 427–451.

V MODELLING THE PRONUNCIATION OF PRINT

V Introduction

Functional accounts of normal skilled reading are of interest to, and relevance to, far more people than are accounts of disordered reading. Moreover, the study of disordered reading is, for many neuropsychologists, only an anticipatory goal response on the path to the ultimate reward sought: an understanding of normal reading. Although there are, of course, specifically clinical motivations (concerned with diagnosis and treatment) for a careful analysis of reading impairments, one major reason for studying patients with acquired reading disorders is that they (should) provide a source of evidence to converge with evidence from normal readers.

Different patterns of disordered reading will of course address different aspects of or issues in normal reading. Furthermore, there are in a sense two different perspectives from which neuropsychological data can address general theory. These two might be called the perspectives of (1) the "privileged view" and (2) the analysis of breakdown. To take a specific and pertinent example, suppose that one wants to understand the procedures involved in pronunciation of a printed word and perhaps especially of a nonword (or an unfamiliar word). In terms of the model on the jacket of this book, this goal can be equated with a study of the routine for subword conversion from orthography to phonology. A neuropsychological foray into this problem may investigate patients with a deficit in the routine(s) for oral reading *other than* this subword translation system. On the twin assumptions that in the normal reader *all* available routines tend to act and interact, and that in a particular impaired reader (ideally) *only* the subword translation routine is available, a study of reading performance by that patient may be thought to afford a privileged view of the operation of this component of reading. This is a common approach in neuropsychology, though of course it is not without its problems or its critics (see Henderson, 1981, for some discussion). The chapter in this section by Shallice and McCarthy can be described as using observations on surface dyslexic patients in an attempt to obtain a privileged view of subword conversion from orthography to phonology.

From the perspective of analysing breakdown, exemplified here by the chapter from Derouesné and Beauvois, one specifically selects a patient with a *deficit* in the routine or procedures of interest. Experimental tasks are cunningly devised so as to fractionate hypothesised subcomponents of this routine; with luck, the patient's pattern of successes and failures on these tasks helps us to assess the appropriateness of our hypotheses about these subcomponents. For the case in point, Derouesné and Beauvois have studied not a surface dyslexic patient who would *rely* on subword phonological reading but rather a phonological dyslexic patient who has a *deficit* in this routine. Such phonological reading must involve a set of different component skills including orthographic segmentation, knowledge of spelling–sound correspondences and assembly or blending of phonological segments. Thus a patient might fail in tasks requiring this routine, such as non-word pronunciation, because of a breakdown in only one of these component skills. If the patient's failure *can* be attributed to a single subcomponent, then our understanding of that subcomponent, and of the structure of that routine as a whole, is advanced.

Evidence from these two neuropsychological perspectives will, one hopes, converge in their implications, both with each other and with data from normal performance. The remaining two chapters in Part V concentrate almost exclusively on the implications of normal data for theories about the procedures involved in the pronunciation of print.

REFERENCE

Henderson, L. (1981). Critical notice: Information-processing approaches to acquired dyslexia. *Quarterly Journal of Experimental Psychology*, *33A*, 507–552.

14 From Orthography to Phonology: An Attempt at an Old Interpretation

K. E. Patterson and J. Morton

INTRODUCTION

Deep dyslexic patients, when confronted with a printed non-word to pronounce, will generally choose to make no response. It is not that they cannot say anything (though of course they cannot say the "correct" thing), and if pressed they often will say something (a visually similar real word); but by preference their response will be "sorry, pass!"

The logogen model, when confronted with the question of how readers assign pronunciation to unfamiliar words or non-words, has generally chosen to make no response. It is not that the model could not say anything, and if pressed it did mumble something ("grapheme–phoneme conversion"); but by preference its response was "sorry, pass."

This disinclination to deal with a particular dimension of reading skill is not necessarily a failing. Every model, after all, has a differential emphasis or focus on components within its domain. The logogen model's primary focus (as regards reading) was on recognition of familiar written words by fluent readers; and precious little unambiguous evidence suggested that the procedures used to assemble a pronunciation for a non-word might be significantly implicated in skilled word recognition. If one were to criticise the logogen model for its hand-waving on the topic of non-word pronunciation, one might as well criticise it for ignoring the question of how visual input logogens are established in the process of reading acquisition. These are simply not questions to which the model specifically addressed itself.

But times moves on. Events of the past few years—both theoretical trends and empirical results—could be said to press any model of word recognition to say something about procedures for assembling pronunciation from print. This chapter represents the first stage of our reluctant compliance with such a demand, reluctant because satisfactory modelling must be based on satisfactory data and we are not convinced that this latter condition obtains at present.

There are many questions or facets in this general topic, but we shall limit ourselves to two: (1) What procedures are involved in the pronunciation of a written non-word like *pove*? (2) Are the same procedures involved (either obligatorily or optionally) in the pronunciation of a familiar written word like *love*? Note that we restrict our questions (and shall accordingly restrict the evidence to be considered) to the issue of pronunciation of words and non-words, including data on both the actual pronunciation given and the latency of the response. Like Henderson (Chapter 17 in this book), and for some of the same reasons, we do not deal here with data from the other major paradigm used in this area, namely lexical decision.

The "standard" hypothesis (e.g. Coltheart, 1978) in response to the first question is that, quite separate or at least separable from the routine whereby a person can "look up" or "address" the pronunciation of a known word, there is a *non-lexical* routine for assembling the pronunciation of any letter string, familiar or otherwise. By non-lexical, we mean that no reference would be made, at the time of assembling the phonological code, to correspondences between orthography and phonology in *specific known* words. To make this quite explicit (and perhaps to reveal straightaway the difficulty confronting such a hypothesis): suppose a person pronounces the non-word *pove*→/pʌv/ (to rhyme with *love*), as indeed occasionally happens (Glushko, 1979; Kay, 1982). The strong hypothesis of a non-lexical phonological routine must deny that such an event demonstrates consultation of the lexically stored pronunciation for *love*. All pronunciations must be capable of being generated by a set of subword-sized correspondences (however complex, context-sensitive, and/or vulnerable to influence by recent experience), without taking advice from lexical advocates.

Note that, in our view, a hypothesis of separable routines (any separable routines; in this case lexical and non-lexical phonology) does not require that the routines operate with complete independence in the normal system. Various aspects of this issue have been discussed by Henderson (1982), also briefly by Patterson (1981). From the point of view of a researcher interested only in the normal operation of cognitive processes, it might seem that, if two routines are not independent, then the question of their separability is without consequence or interest. We would, however, argue against this view. Even if two routines are not independent, variables may act on them independently; in this case, the interaction between these variables would be unintelligible if the two routines were treated as one. From a neuropsychological point of view, of course, the distinction is vital for other reasons. If two routines are separable, then even if they do not normally operate in complete isolation, it will be possible for only one of them to be impaired or lost as a result of neurological insult.

If a model includes a non-lexical routine for assembling phonology, then of course its procedures must ultimately be specified. In particular, it must be determined whether these procedures operate only on a single level such as translation of individual graphemes to phonemes (as in Coltheart, 1978) or on various levels including higher-order units (as in Parkin, 1983, 1984 or Shallice, Warrington, & McCarthy, 1983). The question of the *existence* of a non-lexical routine must, however, be kept separate from the specification of its procedures if it does exist. The two issues tend to be discussed together; as a result, data that may speak only to one of the issues are vulnerable to interpretation with regard to the other. In particular, if there is evidence that a system based solely on grapheme-to-phoneme translation will not suffice, this does not automatically invalidate the hypothesis of a separable non-lexical system.

The major alternative to a non-lexical routine for assembling phonology is, of course, the theory that pronunciations are assigned by analogy with and by specific reference to known lexical items (Baker & Smith, 1976; Baron, 1977; Glushko, 1979; Henderson, 1982; Kay & Marcel, 1981; Marcel, 1980). According to analogy theory, there are no abstract rules by which phonology can be assigned to orthographic segments (of whatever size); there are only orthographic and phonological representations of known words. As both kinds of representations are segmentable, phonology can be assembled for any novel combination of letters by: (1) finding words that contain the appropriate orthographic segments; (2) obtaining the phonology corresponding to those segments; and (3) cobbling together a pronunciation. Precisely the same procedure operates for a letter string that happens to be a real word; but in addition to information about pronunciation of its segments in *other* words, a real word of course also has its *own* whole-string orthographic and phonological specifications.

A non-lexical rule-governed routine and a lexical analogy-based routine do not, presumably, exhaust the theoretical possibilities, but these two are the major bids on the table at present. Needless to say, however, deciding between these alternatives (indeed, at some levels, even discriminating between them) is far from straightforward. As we have already indicated, the most serious current obstacle is not so much the rudimentary state of the theories as the inadequacy of the available data upon which the theories are to be based and evaluated. This complaint is not (or at least nor primarily) directed against the researchers who have collected these data. The degree of complexity of the system and the range of relevant variables are only gradually dawning on us all. Experimenters who have previously failed to consider all of this complexity are therefore scarcely to be condemned. Their *data*, on the other hand, if derived from designs now shown to be inadequate, do not escape this fate. Lest all of this sound arrogant, we hasten to add that even a full awareness of the crucial variables to be manipulated and controlled may not solve the problem. We echo the apt but depressing assessment of Cutler's (1981) title: "Making up materials is a confounded nuisance, or: Will we be able to run any psycholinguistic experiments at all in 1990?"

The confoundings in the existing data base seem sufficiently worrying to warrant description. Accordingly, before selecting a subset of data with which to tweak both non-lexical and lexical theories of assembled phonology, we shall digress to identify some of these problems.

In the 1970s, the only major variables that seemed germane to research on assembling phonology from print were the distinction between words and non-words and, for words, the distinction between regular and irregular (or "exceptional") spelling-to-sound correspondences. There was also the suggestion that a subject's strategy (for example, the extent to which he or she might use or rely on assembled phonology in processing words) could be altered by experimental manipulations like instructions (Stanovich & Bauer, 1978) or the nature of the non-words in a lexical decision task (Davelaar, Coltheart, Besner, & Jonasson, 1978). That, however, was all. In the mid-1980s, we are sadder but wiser, having discovered the following pertinent things:

1. Regularity of spelling-to-sound correspondence appears to be (or to demonstrate its influence as) a continuum rather than a dichotomy (Parkin, 1982; Shallice, Warrington, & McCarthy, 1983). Effects averaged over irregular words spanning the range of this continuum may therefore be misleading.
2. Regularity of spelling-to-sound correspondence is a separate dimension from regularity of spelling pattern: the words *pint* and *yacht* both have an exceptional relationship between orthography and pronunciation, but *pint* has a "normal" or regular spelling pattern whereas *yacht* is orthographically weird.[1] Orthographic irregularity exerts an influence on pronunciation latency over and above that of spelling-to-sound irregularity (Seidenberg, Waters, Barnes, & Tanenhaus, 1984). Experiments where the set of spelling-to-sound irregular words includes orthographically weird words (i.e. most experiments) may therefore be misleading.
3. Word frequency is a potent variable and, most crucially, appears to interact in its influence on pronunciation latency with other relevant

---

[1] As one of our patients remarked when asked to read the word *yacht*, "I know it must be 'yacht' because that is the only word where you get those three letters together," pointing to *cht*.

dimensions such as regularity of orthography or of spelling-to-sound correspondence. Indeed, Seidenberg et al. (1983) conclude that high-frequency words are insensitive to most or all of the other dimensions. Experiments averaging across a range of frequencies within a particular word class, even if frequency was appropriately matched between word classes (again, this will be the majority of experiments), may have to be discounted or reanalysed.

4. As is by now well known, pronunciation may be influenced not only by the word (or non-word's) own spelling-to-sound pattern but by the extent to which other similarly spelled words agree or conflict in pronunciation (Glushko, 1979). This "consistency" effect may be well known, but it is now suffering the same fate (indeed, perhaps an even more distressing version of it) as the regularity effect has done. In Glushko's analysis, consistency was a dichotomy: words and non-words were either consistent (e.g. *wane* or *fane*: all words ending in *ane* are pronounced /eɪn/), or inconsistent (e.g. *save* or *tave*: the word *have* is an unfriendly neighbour). It now seems that all sorts of patterns and degrees of consistency may influence performance (Henderson, Chapter 17, in this book; Kay, 1982; Parkin, 1983). We return to this point later in our chapter. For the moment, suffice it to say that each of the patterns listed in Table 14.1 probably requires separate status in an experimental analysis. Every experiment known to us combines at least several of these patterns into one supposedly homogeneous condition. A further complicating factor is that degree or pattern of consistency may affect words and non-words differently (Parkin, 1983).

5. Finally, the response to a particular word or non-word (its phonology or latency or both) may be influenced by a whole host of variables concerning the nature of other items in the list. This is all very well in (the minority of) studies designed specifically to examine such influences (e.g. the priming studies of Kay & Marcel, 1981, or of Rosson, 1983). In (the majority of) studies that seek only to assess performance on individual items, however, inter-item effects constitute confoundings that are often overlooked. Some of these are relatively simple effects (examples *a* and *b* below), whereas others involve complex interactions (example *c*).

    a. Performance on words (or non-words) in homogeneous lists of words (or non-words) differs from performance on comparable items in mixed lists of words and non-words (Andrews, 1982; Glushko, 1979).

    b. Significant consistency effects like that shown by Glushko may depend upon the (earlier) presence in the list of a conflicting neighbour (Seidenberg et al., 1983). Many experiments repeat spelling patterns with alternative pronunciations (e.g. *cost* and

TABLE 14.1
Fifteen Kinds of Letter String

Word Type	Example	Characteristics
Consistent	*gaze*	All words receive this same *regular* pronunciation of the body.
Consensus	*lint*	All words with one exception receive this same *regular* pronunciation of the body.
Heretic	*pint*	This word is the *irregularly* pronounced exception to the consensus.
Gang	*look*	All words with one exception receive this same *irregular* pronunciation of the body.
Hero	*spook*	This word is the *regularly* pronounced exception to the gang.
Gang without a hero	*cold*	All words receive this same *irregular* pronunciation of the body.
Ambiguous: conformist	*cove*	This is the regular pronunciation; there are many irregular exemplars for this body.
Ambiguous: independent	*love*	This is the (or a) irregular pronunciation; there are many regular exemplars for this body.
Hermit	*yacht*	No other word has this body.

Non-word Type	Example	Characteristics
Consistent	*taze*	Refer to word types above.
Consensus/heretic	*rint*	
Gang/hero	*pook*	
Gang without a hero	*vold*	
Ambiguous	*pove*	
Hermit	*nacht*	

Table 14.1 offers labels for various types of words and non-words reflecting both (1) the agreement (or otherwise) of pronunciation across the set of monosyllabic words sharing the same "body" (vowel plus terminal consonant), and (2) the regularity (or otherwise) of pronunciation with reference to GPC rules. Three of our labels are borrowed from other writers: "consistent" from Glushko (1979), and both "heretic" and "hermit" from Henderson (1982). The remainder, we think, are our own.

post) within one list (Andrews, 1982; Glushko, 1979; Parkin, 1983) and may therefore require caution in interpretation or (once again) reanalysis.

c. A significant effect of word frequency on pronunciation latency for *regular* words apparently obtains only when the list also contains words with an *irregular* spelling-to-sound correspondence (Norris, personal communication). Theoretical interpretation of this observation may have interesting implications. For the moment, this is just another example of the way in which effects are fickle, making generalisation across experiments a nightmare.

There is, in summary, a shortage of sound data available to anyone trying to model the process of assembling phonology from print; it is, however, a shortage rather than a famine, and we do choose to try. As implied by our title, this attempt will take the form of a modified "standard" model, where assembled phonology is produced by a non-lexical system. In the *unmodified* standard model (e.g. as proposed by Coltheart, 1978), the crucial aspects of the system are that it is non-lexical and rule-governed with rules defined only at the level of correspondences between graphemes and phonemes. The modifications that we propose are motivated by the following sets of observations, all of which appear to conflict with the unmodified version:

1. "Inconsistent" non-words are sometimes read aloud with an irregular pronunciation (e.g. *heaf*→/hef/ rather than /hif/). Averaging over a variety of non-word spelling patterns, Glushko (1979) obtained 9% of irregular pronunciations in his experiment 2 (non-words only) and 18% in experiment 1 (mixed words and non-words). Subsequent work establishes that the specific spelling pattern (as in Table 14.1) may substantially alter the obtained percentage of irregular pronunciations (Kay, 1982).

2. Pronunciation latencies may be significantly longer for inconsistent non-words like *heaf* than for consistent ones like *hean*. In Glushko's experiment 2, the mean difference between these two types was 22 msec. Again, subsequent data suggest that a finer-grained analysis of non-word spelling pattern will be required. Parkin (1983), for example, found augmented latencies only for spelling patterns that correspond to several different common pronunciations in words (labelled "ambiguous" in Table 14.1).

3. Pronunciation latencies may be longer for regular inconsistent words like *leaf* than for regular consistent words like *lean* (Andrews, 1982; Glushko, 1979). In Glushko's experiment 3 (words only), the mean difference between these two types was 17 msec. Once again, subsequent research indicates that this effect may require rethinking, given (1) its possible interpretation in terms of bias from other items in the list (Seidenberg et al., 1983); (2) its probable modification in terms of word frequency (Seidenberg et al., 1983); and (3) its uncertain reliability (Parkin, 1983, 1984).

4. Pronunciation of an inconsistent pseudoword can be significantly shifted towards irregularity (e.g. *yead*→/jed/ rather than /jid/) by prior presentation of appropriate irregular words. This was shown by Kay and Marcel (1981), whose experiment included a variety of conditions; for current purposes, the following contrast will suffice: following *head* (the irregular bias condition), *yead*→/jed/ on 39% of occasions; following *shed* (the pronunciation control condition), *yead*→/jed/ on only 10% of occasions.

5. Finally, it appears that the pronunciation assigned to an inconsistent non-word can be shifted towards irregularity by prior presentation of a word

semantically related to a word which would produce the Kay and Marcel bias effect. Rosson (1983) demonstrated that after *sofa, louch*→/lautʃ/ 89% of the time, whereas after *feel, louch*→/lautʃ/ only on 75% of occasions. As far as we can see, Rosson never actually says that the 14% fewer "regular" pronunciations of *louch* preceded by *feel* were /lʌtʃ/ (rhyming with *touch*); but one presumes that they were.

These five sets of observations constitute the data (at least, the most convincing data that we know of) that cause headaches for a standard, non-lexical GPC model. We now try to describe a *modified* standard model to see how it fares in accounting for these awkward observations. Subsequently, we briefly discuss (our understanding of) the procedures of an analogy model for assembling phonology from print. Finally, to share the headaches out equitably, we offer one or two observations awkward for such analogy models.

A MODIFIED STANDARD MODEL

In this model there are effectively three routines for word pronunciation. Two of these are lexical and one is non-lexical. The lexical routines both require that the visual input logogen system is used. In the first, the output from this logogen system accesses the semantics of the item, from which the lexical phonology can be addressed; in the second, the visual input logogen addresses the lexical phonology directly (see Morton & Patterson, 1980).

The central procedure of the non-lexical routine can be described as a set of mapping rules from orthographic strings to phonological strings. Accordingly we label this the orthography-to-phonology correspondence (OPC) system. There are two major senses in which the OPC system differs from and is more complex than Coltheart's (1978) grapheme-to-phoneme correspondence (GPC) system. First, the OPC system deals with two different sizes of orthographic unit: *graphemes* (i.e. the letter or letter combinations that correspond to single phonemes) and bodies (the vowel-plus-terminal-consonant segments of monosyllables that remain when the initial consonants or consonant clusters are removed).[2] Second, although we shall assume for the moment that mappings at the grapheme level are simple one-to-one transla-

---

[2]We have nothing to say at the moment concerning the pronunciation of polysyllabic words. We predict that complex morphophonological processes will exert an influence on the final outcome for polysyllables, and that there will therefore be no simple extension from the account for monosyllables. Data from MacCabe (1984) on the pronunciation of a set of consistent irregular non-words (which, in our terminology, included exemplars from both the gang-without-hero type and the hermit type) indicate that pronunciations corresponding to the irregular word analogy are four to five times more likely for disyllabic than for monosyllabic non-words.

tions, the mapping rules for bodies are more complex and will sometimes require one-to-several translations.

We acknowledge, but have little to say about, the problems entailed by a system operating concurrently with units of more than one size. These problems largely concern the mechanisms whereby, for a given letter string, the "solutions" for the different-length segments are either combined or selected amongst to produce a single response. For some sophisticated theorising on such mechanisms, we commend to you the chapter by Shallice and McCarthy in this volume (Chapter 15).

We have, then, an OPC system forming the centre of the non-lexical routine for assembling a pronunciation of a letter string. It is the centre in that it operates after orthographic parsing and prior to phonological assembly. It has two subsystems, a Coltheartian set of one-to-one mapping rules at the grapheme level and a more complicated set of mapping rules at the body level. To accomplish our goal of accounting for the five awkward sets of data introduced earlier, we shall have to provide considerably more detail regarding the operation of the OPC system and its interaction with the lexical system, and this we shall do almost immediately. It is perhaps worth noting at this stage, however, that the first two of the five observations are already predicted simply by the addition of a body system with one-to-several mapping rules: (1) a non-word with an ambiguous body (e.g. *pove*) may be given an "irregular" pronunciation (/pʌv/) because the OPC mapping rules for this body include *ove*→/ʌv/ as well as *ove*→/oɷv/; (2) whether *pove* is pronounced /poɷv/ or /pʌv/, its latency may be slower than pronunciation of a consistent non-word (like *pote*) because of a time penalty incurred in the choice between alternative pronunciations.

Interaction Between Lexical and Non-lexical Routines

For the pronunciation of a word, there will be two major routines, lexical and non-lexical (the full model of course includes two different lexical routines, but we assume that the fluent adult reader would normally pronounce words utilising direct, that is, non-semantically mediated, input–output connections). As we have already seen, Glushko's (1979) and Andrews' (1982) data indicate that regular but inconsistent words like *rove* take a little longer on average to pronounce than consistent ones (*rote*), though the effect is scarcely robust (Parkin, 1983). We assume that this effect is due to differences in the way that the two kinds of words are processed by the OPC system, because (all other things, e.g. word frequency, being equal) the lexical routine should be equally willing to serve *rote* and *rove*.[3] If pronunciation of a *word* is

---

[3] Note that this is a "strong" version of the visual input lexicon, in which the characteristics of an individual logogen are supposed not to be affected by similarly spelled words (Glushko's "orthographic neighbourhood"), at least under conditions that preclude visual confusions.

affected by the nature of its processing in the non-lexical routine, this suggests that the two routines are interacting. Two different kinds of interaction could be involved, which we label *conflict* and *interference*.

By the *conflict* model, there is a decision process that receives the pronunciations achieved by the two routines. When both pronunciations have been received, they are compared. If they are identical, then that pronunciation is produced. If they are different, then some decision is made which, usually, results in the lexical version being produced. The delay brought about by this extra decision in the case of inconsistent words would account for the latency data. Taken at face value, this model strikes us as silly: if the candidate pronunciations are marked as to their origin, then the lexical candidate might just as well be produced as soon as it arrives. (Note, however, that a model of this sort is considered, and judged not to be silly, by Henderson in this volume.) One rational modification might be that the candidates are not marked as to origin but that in the case of conflict, the two alternatives are checked to see if either corresponds to an entry in the phonological lexicon. This idea yields the following prediction: if the non-lexical routine offers an incorrect word (for example, regularisation of the word *gauge* will give /gɔːdʒ/, which corresponds phonologically to the word *gorge*), then the checking procedure will fail, giving rise either to a major increase in errors (if the process is self-terminating) or to an increase in latency occasioned by the need to carry out more elaborate checks.

We shall opt instead for an *interference* model, in which the phonological codes produced by the two routines both go to a system whose function is to transform the code into a form suitable for production. For the moment, we shall identify this system with the response buffer of Morton's logogen model (e.g. Morton, 1969, 1979; Morton & Patterson, 1980). When the response buffer receives a code from either source, the transformation, which takes time, begins. If nothing else is received before the transformation is complete, then the transformed code is pronounced. If another code is received, it is compared with the first (which may or may not cost time in the transformation). If they agree, then the transformation process continues. If they disagree, then (1) there will be a time penalty due to the interruption and (2) a decision between the alternatives will require a lexical check.

In this modified standard model, the mean time for the lexical routine is faster than that for the non-lexical routine but the distributions have considerable overlap. Indeed, as Henderson (1982) emphasises, the data on pronunciation latencies for most words and non-words indicate such overlap, though the overlap may be negligible in the case of high-frequency words (Seidenberg et al., 1984). The third observation for which we seek an account—the small latency disadvantage suffered by regular inconsistent words (e.g. *rove*) relative to consistent words (*rote*)—can now be seen to arise in the following way. For either word, the lexical code will most often reach the response buffer and indeed begin to be pronounced before any code is received from the non-lexical routine; on some proportion of occasions, however, the code from the OPC system will arrive at the response buffer before processing of the lexical code is complete. Comparison of the two codes for *rote* will always yield a match because (as we shall see shortly) a correctly functioning OPC system can only produce the phonological code /roʊt/ for this string. With *rove*, however, the "body" subsystem of the OPC will sometimes send the code /rʌv/. On those occasions when the non-lexical routine both produces the code /rʌv/ and manages to get it to the response buffer before the lexical code has been pronounced, then whereas the correct pronunciation of *rove* will generally be ensured by a lexical check, the interruption and the lexical check will delay production of the response /roʊv/. Such occasions might be expected to be relatively infrequent; but then it is only a small (if indeed reliable; Parkin, 1983, 1984) average latency difference between *rote* and *rove* that we need to explain.

Regular words like *rove* are very rarely mispronounced, but errors on irregular words (typically regularisations such as *pint*→/pɪnt/) are considerably more common (e.g. 7% regularisation errors in Glushko's (1979) experiment 3 and almost 10% such errors for lower-frequency exception words in Seidenberg et al.'s (1983) experiment 3). In the modified standard model, such errors obviously occur on occasions when the non-lexical routine operates more quickly than the lexical routine; and these occasions, also obviously, derive from the lower end of the latency distribution of the non-lexical routine. Thus, the latency for *pint*→/pɪnt/ (rhyming with *mint*) should be substantially less, on average, than the latency for *nint*→/nɪnt/. We know of no proper data on this *specific* contrast, but some of our own recent data (Evett, Patterson, & Morton, 1985) provide a pertinent observation. One of our experiments, an almost exact repeat of Glushko's (1979) experiment 3, yielded a total of 16 regularisation errors (like *pint*→/pɪnt/), which had a mean latency of 522 msec. The equivalent mean latency for correct pronunciations of regular consistent words (e.g. *pink*) was 515 msec. We did not ask our subjects to pronounce non-words; but both Parkin (1983, using the same subjects in both conditions) and Glushko (1979, using different groups of subjects but from the same population) have shown an 80 msec advantage for consistent words as compared with consistent non-words. This suggests that our subjects' mean latency for pronouncing *nint* would have been at least 595 msec. In other words, there is tentative support for the prediction of the modified standard model that the error response *pint*→/pɪnt/ (measured at 522 msec) ought to be significantly faster than the "correct" response *nint*→/nɪnt/ (estimated at 595 msec). To the best of our understanding (but we postpone this issue until later), an analogy theory of pronunciation would not predict this effect.

The modified standard model as described thus far appears to deal with the first three of the five tasks set for it. The fourth task, an account of Kay and Marcel's (1981) pronunciation bias effect, is more Herculean, and demands a fuller description of how the non-lexical routine operates. A qualitative account is presented here; a quantitative account will be available in Morton, Patterson, Nimmo-Smith, Kay, and Evett (1985).

The OPC System: The "Body" Subsystem

At least four, and possibly five types of bodies require differentiation, and these correspond to the first five body types listed for *non-words* in Table 14.1. For *consistent* bodies like *aze*, the body subsystem offers a single mapping, *aze*→/eɪz/. For *consensus/heretic* bodies like *int*, the overwhelming consensus among words indicates /ɪnt/ (e.g. *mint, lint, hint*, etc.), with the single heretic *pint*. We suggest, along with Parkin (1983), that the OPC system basically treats such letter strings as if they were characterised by *consistency* rather than mere *consensus*. That is, the body subsystem offers a single mapping, *int*→/ɪnt/. Were it to include the alternative pronunciation, *int*→/aɪnt/, we would expect to observe two consequences. First, in "isolation" (that is, uninfluenced by recent exposure to the heretic word), non-words with consensus/heretic bodies such as *rint* or *tave* ought sometimes to be given the heretic pronunciation /raɪnt/ or /tæv/. Data from Kay (1982), however, indicate that under unbiased conditions, 99% of the pronunciations given to such non-words are regular, consensus pronunciations. Second, pronunciation latencies for *rint* and *tave* should be slowed (by the necessity of choosing between alternatives) relative to latencies for consistent non-words. Data from Parkin (1983), however, show no hint of such a latency difference.

Bodies of the *gang* type are, in a sense, the flip side of the coin from consensus and consistent types. A *gang* with a *hero* (e.g. *ook* where every relevant monosyllabic word except *spook*, the hero, is part of the gang: *book, cook, look, hook,* etc.) matches the *consensus/heretic* type precisely in terms of ratio (that is, many: one); but here of course the majority corresponds to the *irregular* pronunciation. A gang without a hero (e.g. *old* where *every* relevant word belongs to the gang: *cold, hold, bold, fold,* etc.) matches the *consistent* type (i.e. no exceptions); but once again the gang pronunciation is irregular rather than regular with respect to GPC rules. Given this parallelism, and because it is our contention that representations in the body subsystem are established on the basis of experience with words (indeed, how could it be otherwise?), then our assumption about *gang* bodies should be that only the majority mapping is represented; thus, from the body subsystem, *ook*→/ʊk/ and *old*→/oʊld/. We do, for the present, make this assumption; and we therefore interpret observations (which we discuss presently) of very frequent pronunciations of *pook*→/puk/ as demonstrating the ascendancy of the GPC subsystem over the body subsystem (which we also discuss presently). Whether gang bodies (especially those with heroes) have only one mapping listed or also include the "regular" pronunciation is, however, an empirical question, not yet resolved but surely resolvable, and so we reserve the right to modify our assumption on the basis of future, better data. After all, although the body subsystem can only learn from words, it may be eclectic in its formative years and be prepared to learn from words with similar but not identical bodies.

Ambiguous bodies are the only type for which it seems clear, at this stage, that at least two OPC mappings must be represented. Thus *ove* will have both /oɔv/ and /ʌv/ listed (and perhaps /uv/ as well, as in *move* and *prove*); *eaf* will have both /if/ and /ɛf/. The evidence forcing this assumption is precisely the evidence that was lacking to suggest OPC mappings for *heretic* pronunciations. First, Parkin (1983) has shown significant slowing of RTs to pronounce ambiguous non-words. Second, Kay (1982) has shown a significant proportion (around .15–.20) of irregular pronunciation assignments (like *pove*→/pʌv/) to ambiguous non-words.[4] In isolation (that is, unbiased by recent pronunciation experience with a word or non-word sharing the same body), we suggest that the body subsystem selects among alternative pronunciations for an ambiguous body at random but incurs a time penalty for this selection relative to bodies with a single candidate pronunciation.

Interaction Between the Two Subsystems of the OPC

We have already noted our current assumption that the GPC subsystem contains only one-to-one mappings (see Temple, Chapter 11 in this book, for a different assumption). Thus the grapheme *ea* will have the single translation /i/; it is only by virtue of the body subsystem that *eaf* can be non-lexically translated as /ɛf/. We expect to be able to account for all non-lexical pronunciation assignments, at least in the absence of factors to prime or bias pronunciation, by normal operation of the two subsystems of the OPC.[5] In the present model, the GPC routine will provide "regular" pronunciations for all letter strings; the body routine will provide: (1) regular pronunciations for both consistent and consensus/heretic bodies; (2) irregular pronunciations for gang bodies; and (3) an equivalent number of each alternative pronunciation for ambiguous bodies. Thus the phonology offered by the two subsystems will match for (1), conflict for (2) and sometimes match,

---

[4]Kay's data do, however, indicate that some ambiguous bodies (e.g. *oll* and *eath*) give rise to *no* exception pronunciations in unbiased non-word reading. This point is discussed further in Morton, et al. (1985).

[5]We acknowledge that at least one (and probably more than one) aspect is missing here, namely some context-sensitive rules like *c* followed by *e*→/s/. At the moment we have not specified how such rules are handled, though we anticipate that it will be by the GPC subsystem.

sometimes conflict for (3). We now need to specify a decision rule between the subsystems. We note (and once again refer to Shallice and McCarthy, Chapter 15) that information from the two levels could in principle be combined; but we shall instead assume for the moment that decisions between the two subsystems of the OPC, like those between the lexical and non-lexical routines, are made on an *or*, not an *and* basis. We have as yet no proposal (and no pertinent data) regarding the relative times required for GPC-level and body-level solutions. Our suggestion for a decision rule is based entirely on an attempt to model the actual proportions of pronunciation assignments to various non-word types obtained by Kay (1982).

Kay's data give us three relevant values for r, that is, the average proportion of unbiased *regular* pronunciations: (1) as already indicated, $r = .99$ for non-words with consensus/heretic bodies like *yint*; (2) for non-words with ambiguous bodies that *in words* have more regular than irregular exemplars, $r = .87$; (3) for non-words with bodies that in words are represented by a majority of *irregular* exemplars, $r = .77$. In Kay's data, this third set includes both gang-with-hero bodies, and ambiguous bodies where the irregular pronunciation in words is the more common.

An assumption that the OPC code produced is controlled by the GPC subsystem on 70% of occasions provides a first-approximation fit for these data: (1) for consensus/heretic non-words, both GPC and body subsystems yield the regular pronunciation, so for these we predict $r = 1.0$ (Kay, 1982, obtained $r = .99$); (2) for ambiguous non-words, the GPC subsystem yields a regular pronunciation on all of its 70% of occasions; random sampling between the regular and irregular pronunciations in the remaining 30% of occasions controlled by the body subsystem means that, overall, predicted $r = .85$ (Kay obtained $r = .87$); (3) for the *ambiguous* non-words in this subset, once again predicted $r = .85$; for the gang non-words (where we have suggested that the body subsystem offers only the irregular pronunciation), predicted $r = .70$. If half of Kay's subset (3) were of each type, then overall predicted $r = .775$ (Kay obtained $r = .77$).

We are now, at long last, ready to attempt an explanation of awkward result number four—Kay and Marcel's (1981) priming or biasing effect. In their experiment, a non-word like *yead* received 39% of irregular pronunciations (/jed/) in the "irregular bias" condition (that is, when it followed the word *head*) but only 10% of irregular pronunciations in the "pronunciation control" condition (i.e. following the word *shed*). The first thing to note is that although Kay and Marcel (1981) label their pronunciation control condition "Rhyming word, different orthography (p. 402)," in fact a minority of the items in this condition *did* rhyme with the irregular bias word (as in *shed* for *head*). The majority of the pronunciation control items only shared vowel phonology with the irregular word (e.g. *wood* for *pull*, *does* for *love*, *aisle* for *pint*, etc.; see Kay & Marcel, 1981, p. 411). Because a proper control condition seemed to us to require rhymes, we (Evett, Patterson, & Morton, 1985) have performed a Kay and Marcel bias experiment with this modification. We replicated their clear and significant bias attributable to shared orthography (after *head*, *yead*→/jed/ on 44% of trials in our experiment). Our more adequate pronunciation control condition did, however, yield a larger value for the bias effect attributable to shared phonology: after *shed*, *yead*→/jed/ on 24% of occasions in our experiment (only 10% in Kay & Marcel), compared with a baseline of about 4%.

Although our replication of Kay and Marcel reduces the *size* of the orthographic bias effect (from about .30 to .20), it does not substantively alter the problem. Why should recent lexical experience affect the operation of a separate non-lexical OPC routine? Such a result of course fits neatly with the idea that all pronunciations, whether addressed directly or assembled by analogy, are obtained from lexical representations.

As Kay and Marcel themselves note, there is a way of explaining their bias result within a framework maintaining separate lexical and non-lexical routines: the lexical event engenders a temporary shift in the probability with which alternative non-lexical pronunciations are selected. We have proposed that, in the absence of a biasing word, the OPC body subsystem selects at random between /jid/ and /jɛd/ as pronunciations for *yead*, producing a body-$r = .50$ (overall r will of course be much higher because of the GPC subsystem). If *head* has just been pronounced, however, this random selection might abruptly shift to favour selection of the /ɛd/ alternative for any *ead* string, and then gradually drift back to its usual lack of preference. For this to work, it would be required that:

1. The stimulus word (*head*) activates the OPC orthographic body *ead*.
2. The phonological response (/hɛd/) activates the OPC phonological code /ɛd/.
3. The OPC system operates in such a way that concurrent activation of the two end elements of a mapping temporarily increments the future likelihood of following the pathway between them. Note that we cannot attribute the facilitation to recent *use* of the appropriate pathway because when *head* is presented, the OPC body subsystem will use the mapping to /hid/ on about 50% of occasions and the OPC system will produce /hid/ on about 85% of occasions.

Kay and Marcel (1981) provide three arguments against the preceding account of their result. The first is that it is a complicated process. We agree, but do not consider this a damning assessment; pronunciation by analogy is also a complex procedure. The second is that "the functional independence of the two processes is almost lost (p. 407)." This might seem a more worrying accusation, but it is not a major snag if one distinguishes, as we do, between separability and independence. Kay and Marcel's results probably rule out the idea of *independent* lexical and non-lexical routines, but not the notion of separable routines. As an example of this, Campbell (1983) has demonstrated an effect similar to Kay and Marcel's biasing result for *spelling* of non-words. When normal subjects have just heard the word "goat," for example, there is a significant shift in the probability with which they will spell the dictated non-word /foɒt/ as *foat* rather than *fote*. Campbell also performed this test on a surface dyslexic patient; his spelling of non-words was adequate (though not error-free), but showed no biasing effect. We interpret this contrast as reflecting the existence of a non-lexical spelling routine, which in the normal system can be influenced by lexical events but whose separability from a lexical spelling system is demonstrated by the neurological patient.[6] Likewise, we might expect certain surface dyslexic patients not to show Kay and Marcel's priming effect in non-word pronunciation. This test does not appear to have been done; however, Shallice, Warrington, and McCarthy (1983) report that their patient H.T.R. showed no significant effect, in pronouncing non-words, of the consistency with which the non-word's orthographic pattern is pronounced in words.

Kay and Marcel's third argument against the dual-routine explanation of priming hinges on the type/token distinction. According to Kay (1982, cited in Kay & Marcel, 1981), it is the number of types rather than the number of of tokens that determines the baseline probability of a particular pronunciation alternative. If this probability shifted with every occurrence of an alternative, then tokens (or frequency) could be expected to provide the dominant influence. To take a specific example, the frequency of *some* (1617 per million; Kucera & Francis, 1967) and that of *come* (630 per million) are both so high as probably to outweigh the combined frequencies of all regularly pronounced *ome* words (e.g. *home, dome, tome*). One's constant encounters with *some* and *come* might therefore be expected, over time, to yield a *permanent* predilection for the /ʌm/ reading of *ome* non-words; but of course the much more likely prouunciation is /oɒm/. Kay and Marcel's interpretation (of the preference for *ome*→oɒm) is, of course, that there are more word tokens with this correspondence (which will therefore weigh heavily in the analogical process) than there are words with the alternative mapping *ome*→/ʌm/. We would argue, however, that whereas Kay (1982) may have convincingly demonstrated that the potent variable is *not* tokens, this does not automatically demonstrate that it *is* types. Indeed, Kay's own data on unbiased non-word pronunciations suggest an effect, but a rather

---

[6] It seems only fair to note that Campbell (1983) offered a somewhat different interpretation of her data. Emphasising the patient's *errors* in non-word spelling (rather than, as we have done, his many correct responses in this task), Campbell concluded that there is no fully competent non-lexical routine for spelling.

surprisingly small one, of the type dimension. Moving from bodies with a majority of regular pronunciations in words to those with a majority of irregular pronunciations only shifted the value of r down by about .10 (from .87 to .77) in Kay's data (an effect that was given a simple account in terms of the OPC system). Even a non-word like *jook*, with an overwhelming gang of *cook, book, look*, etc., was pronounced in a regular way /dʒuk/ by 80% of Kay's subjects. We suggest, therefore, that Kay and Marcel have overemphasised both the power of tokens and the power of the type/token distinction to subvert a dual-routine interpretation of their bias data.

In fact, in the modified standard model, neither types nor tokens are crucial. We need only consider two factors: (1) the effect attributable to shared phonology (i.e. the pronunciation control condition), which produces a bias of about 20% and operates across all body types; (2) the effect attributable to shared orthography, which operates only for ambiguous bodies. The simplest assumption is that, for a brief time after an ambiguous word has been read, the phonological alternative corresponding to that biasing word will always be selected by the body subsystem (instead of its unbiased procedure of selecting at random). After an irregular bias word, ambiguous bodies would then behave like gang bodies, with 30% irregular codes being produced by the OPC system. With a 20% *further* bias attributable to the effect of shared phonology, we are into the range of Kay and Marcel biasing effects without recourse to types, tokens, or the lexicon. The only additional assumption which we have made is that representation of a correspondence in the body subsystem is all-or-none rather than cumulative. This may engender a problem in explaining the mechanism of *acquisition* of body representations; but we hope that theories of reading acquisition will eventually offer solutions to such problems.

In summary, though we acknowledge that lexical biasing of non-lexical pronunciations necessitates a more complex and more interactive model than we might have wished, we do not find anything here which makes the modified standard model unworkable or untenable.

Finally, we face up to what is either the most difficult or the simplest (depending on the solution) observation of all for the modified standard model: Rosson's (1983) demonstration that r (the proportion of regular pronunciations) for an ambiguous non-word can be decreased by a word semantically related to a word that would produce the Kay and Marcel orthographic bias. For example, we know from Kay and Marcel that *louch* preceded by *touch* has a lower value of r than either *louch* in isolation or *louch* preceded by a pronunciation control word like *hutch*. Rosson (1983) has now shown that *louch* preceded by *feel* has a lower value of r than *louch* preceded by *sofa*.

This is a fish from a very different kettle. Trying to explain Kay and Marcel's (1981) bias result in terms of the operation of a non-lexical routine may have given us pause; trying to explain Rosson's (1983) bias result in these terms stops us altogether. The simple but naughty solution is to claim that, until some or all of the following questions are answered, we need not worry ourselves unduly about an account:

1. Rosson's result was certainly statistically reliable and thus should be replicable; but is it? The question may sound mean, but this is not exactly a psychological area noted for replicable phenomena.

2. What are the association values between Rosson's presented bias words and the mediating primed words (i.e. between *feel* and *touch*, *sofa* and *couch*, etc.)? Because these pairs are the only examples from the list given in the article,[7] we cannot answer this question. If the mediating primed words were highly predictable associates of the bias words, then the effect might be attributable to the induction of an association strategy on the subject's part, even though the critical items comprised only 24 pairs randomly interspersed among 82 fillers. Kay and Marcel (1981) went to some lengths to rule out an explanation of *their* bias result in terms of strategy, by demonstrating that the number of biased pronunciations did not increase as the experiment progressed, which one might have expected if the subjects gradually noticed the critical pairs. We are reassured by Kay and Marcel's analysis. None the less, first, it may be that such awareness (and therefore development of the strategy) occurs quickly rather than slowly; and, second, Rosson has provided no comparable reassurance for her result.

3. Rosson's data provide a measure of r for *louch* following either *sofa* (.89) or *feel* (.75), but no baseline measure. A 14% swing in r may seem large; but if average unbiased r for these ambiguous non-words is in fact around .82, then it is only a 7% shift (in each direction) that needs to be explained. The fact that Kay and Marcel (1981) found a major asymmetry, that is, a significantly larger shift from baseline towards irregularity than towards regularity, might make this seem implausible. Recall, however, that Kay and Marcel's critical non-word set contained a number of consensus/heretic bodies like *ave, aid, aste, atch*, etc. For these, according to both our model and Kay's (1982) data, unbiased r is essentially 1.0 and there is thus no room for an effect of a *regular* biasing word. Rosson's (1983) non-word set may have been more homogeneously of the ambiguous body type (again, we cannot tell from the article), permitting more equal (and smaller) effects in the two directions.

4. Finally, it may be critical to measure the duration of Rosson's effect. There are scraps of evidence to suggest that the bias produced by shared orthography, while temporary, may extend over a number of minutes and/or

---

[7]The practice (which is on the increase but obviously not yet universal) of publishing word lists in an appendix to the article seems a very desirable one.

intervening items. First, Kay (1982) found no reduction in the Kay and Marcel bias effect when either one or two items separated the members of a critical pair like *head* and *yead*. Second, and perhaps more dramatically, Seidenberg et al. (1983) have reinterpreted Glushko's (1979) finding of slowed pronunciation for regular inconsistent words (like *cost*) as dependent on the prior occurrence in the list of an irregularly pronounced word with the same body (e.g. *post*). In Seidenberg et al.'s experiment to demonstrate this influence, "prior occurrence" might mean something like 30 items intervening between *post* and *cost*. This effect of shared orthography on pronunciation (shown by Kay & Marcel, 1981; Seidenberg et al., 1983, etc.), which in the modified standard model represents an influence of a lexical event on the operation of the non-lexical routine, thus appears to have a moderate lifespan. Rosson's bias result, if reliable, must be attributable to a very different set of processes and influences, and we predict that one indication of this difference may be a substantially reduced temporal durability relative to the bias from shared orthography.

With all of the foregoing queries unanswered, we still ought to give an indication of how our model might deal with Rosson's (1983) finding. This will require some further assumptions about the operation of the visual input logogen system with non-word stimuli. The simplest would involve the logogen for *touch* being affected by the stimulus *louch*, together with feedback from the cognitive system following prior presentation of *feel*. In the response buffer, the resulting lexical phonological code /tʌtʃ/ would then have to be segmented into /t-/ and /-ʌtʃ/, with the latter combining with /l-/ from the GPC subsystem of the OPC. A more detailed account awaits more detailed data.

Having tweaked the standard model of assembled pronunciation with the data most awkward for it, and having done our best (which is in some cases better than others) to modify the standard model such that it can accommodate these awkward observations, we feel that we have earned the right to subject analogy theory to some of the same treatment (the tweaking part, that is; the modifying we shall obviously leave to others).

ANALOGY THEORY

In order to see what unsolved problems might be lurking in the shadows for analogy theory yet to accommodate, we need to review, at least superficially, how the theory works. Its best specified version is to be found in Marcel (1980). One major question is whether links between orthographic and phonological representations exist only at the word (or morpheme) level, or whether these links also exist from individual letters and letter combinations to their phonological counterparts. At times, Marcel's account suggests the former, and thus seems to warrant its description as a purely lexical system. For example, "Each of the addresses in the visual input lexicon has at least two pointers. One of these leads to a semantic description. . . . The other is to an entry . . . in the output lexicon or speech vocabulary (p. 243)." The implication might be that whole-morpheme orthographic codes access whole-morpheme phonological codes, and all additional necessary operations (to account for non-word reading, specification of orthographic neighbourhood on the basis of similar segments, etc.) are handled by the fact that both types of code are *segmentable*.

In our view, the segmentability of these representations is not the issue and indeed is relatively uncontroversial. If the system truly managed with segmentable word or morpheme representations, we would not challenge the analogy theorists' claim to have an entirely lexical system. Our assessment, however, is that the model contains not just segmentable representations but already *segmented* ones. When discussing assignment of pronunciation to the non-word *kwib*, Marcel (1980) says: ". . . each letter, as it appears in words, will be accessed as a segment in the input lexicon. The most frequent pronunciation of each segment or letter (in the equivalent position in a word) will then be retrieved (p. 247)." In the limit, this system operates *like* a grapheme-to-phoneme converter, but "by recourse to lexical knowledge (p. 247)." It thus appears that a lexical entry in this model effectively includes all possible pairings between an orthographic string (of length from 1 to N letters) and its phonological equivalent that are derivable from the word in question. For a simple word like *mat*, we guess that the entry might look like this:

$$m_1\, a_2\, t_3 \rightarrow /m_1\, \text{æ}_2\, t_3/$$
$$m_1\, a_2\quad \rightarrow /m_1\, \text{æ}_2\quad /$$
$$a_2\, t_3 \rightarrow /\quad \text{æ}_2\, t_3/$$
$$m_1\quad \rightarrow /m_1\quad /$$
$$a_2\quad \rightarrow /\quad \text{æ}_2\quad /$$
$$t_3 \rightarrow /\quad t_3/$$

We thus interpret Marcel as postulating mappings from orthographic segments to phonological segments at submorphemic levels, indeed, at individual grapheme and phoneme levels. This is *our* interpretation, but we do not see an alternative one. Without such mappings, given the two strings *have* and /hæv/, it is by no means clear how one could determine which orthographic segment yields which phonological segment—unless one were to use the kind of rule-based information that is explicitly prohibited from an analogy model. Despite the fact that these multi-level mappings are to be found within lexical entries, their existence leads us to think that the distinction between an analogy theory and our modified standard model is not best captured by the question of whether there is "non-lexical" information concerning pronunciation. Rather, the issue seems to be that information in the analogy model resides only in specific instances whereas, according to our model, the system "knows" about abstractions from the instances.

At least two issues appear to us to require specification in an analogy framework. The first concerns procedures for matching analogous segments. Terminal segments are supposed (by Glushko, 1979; Marcel, 1980) to form the primary source of analogy words. In a non-word like *kwib*, Marcel (1980) acknowledged that *k* and *w* will not constitute a single segment because they do not do so in any lexical entry. The question then arises, will the *ib* in *kwib* activate the entry for, for example, *bib*? With a non-word like *phave*, it is possible that the initial *ph* will be specially bracketed, thus preserving the indexing to give (ph)$_1$ a$_2$ v$_3$ e$_4$. (This would also obviate the need to have some special means of blocking access to the large segment *have*.) In general, however, the procedures for creating the appropriate segments needed to access appropriate analogy words remain as yet underspecified. The second issue that requires attention is the mechanism by which larger (and, in the case of words, whole-string) segments over-ride smaller segments. The postulate that all and only conflicting subsegments are over-ruled, which Marcel used to account for the difference in latencies between consistent and inconsistent words, requires complex processes of comparison. Furthermore, the general over-riding principle reawakens a disquiet similar to that which we expressed in discussing a conflict version of the modified standard model. If the whole-string specification is marked as having some special quality (lexicality, or economical accounting for the input string, or whatever), then why would the system not just accept that specification and output its corresponding phonology? Why attend to the contents of smaller segments, only to militate reliably against them?

Having noted the major issues that seem to us to be underspecified in analogy theory, we turn now to two sets of observations awkward for such a theory, both of which have been mentioned in passing earlier in our chapter.

First, there are certain non-words for which analogy theory must predict a preponderance of "irregular" pronunciations. Examples given by Kay (1982) are *jook* and *nind*. Against the "regular" pronunciation of each (/dʒuk/ and /nɪnd/ respectively), there are what Henderson (1982) calls a maximum of lexical neighbours "... united in a hostile orthodoxy (p. 159)" and what we call simply "the gang." For *jook*, virtually every similar-ending word is pronounced like *book* (*book, cook, hook, look, rook, took*); only the hero *spook* accords with the "regular" pronunciation. For *nind*, virtually every similar-ending word is pronounced like *find* (*bind, find, hind, kind, mind, rind*); only *wind* (and even then only one of *its* versions) is a hero (or half-hero). Are these overwhelming analogies apparent in the assignment of pronunciations to non-words like *jook* and *nind*? We offer two sets of observations. The first comes from Kay (1982): out of 25 pronunciations, *jook*→/dʒuk/ (the "regular" pronunciation) 20 times (.80) and *nind*→/nɪnd/ 18 times (.72).

We also collected some data of our own, using the similar non-words *pook* and *lind*. We have often wondered if experiments that ask subjects to pronounce long lists of non-words, giving elaborate instructions about the task, might not encourage the development of unusual strategies. In our mini-experiment, therefore, we simply asked 60 people to pronounce each of the two items (printed on index cards, in lowercase letters), giving no previous explanation, and no warning that the items would be non-words. The subjects included a wide cross-section of people: secretaries, cleaners, students, psychologists, housewives, technicians. The results were as follows: 55/60 (.93) people produced a regular pronunciation of *pook* /puk/; only 4/60 pronounced it /pɒk/ to rhyme with the overwhelmingly common analogy of *book* and *cook*. For *lind*, all 60 people gave the regular pronunciation /lɪnd/; no one said /laɪnd/ as in *find*.

The results of our mini-experiment appear to conflict with the notion of pronunciation by lexical analogy. Of course one can (*post hoc*) find plenty of analogies to support the regular pronunciations obtained (e.g. *pool* for *pook*, *lint* for *lind*); but if analogy theory is forced to adopt such an open-door admission policy, it would seem to become rather unwieldy. Furthermore, in at least Glushko's version of the theory, choice of analogy is explicitly based on *terminal* orthographic segments. (Otherwise how could Glushko, 1979, define a pseudoword like *hean* as "regular"? It is regular by analogy with *lean* but irregular by analogy with *head*.) Yet it seems that our results *do* force analogy theory to the assumption of analogies based on other than terminal segments and indeed to the unpalatable assumption that more remote and/or smaller segment analogy words can exceed the influence of close analogies. As it seems implausible that the single hero word *spook* could dominate the 11-member gang of *book*, *cook*, *look*, etc., it would surely have to be the influence of words like *pool*, *moon*, and *food* that produces the high *r* for a non-word like *jook*. Most analogy theorists of our acquaintance (e.g. Henderson, 1982) have a proper respect for the palate, and we cannot imagine that they would prefer distant *food* to a nearby *cook*.

Second, as noted earlier, both Glushko (1979) and Parkin (1983) have data showing an average latency difference of 80 msec between pronunciation of consistent words and consistent non-words. In the modified standard model, this difference arises simply from the greater mean time of the non-lexical routine than of the lexical routine. In an analogy model, the slower time for non-words presumably reflects the time needed, in the absence of a whole-string specification, to consult the entire orthographic neighbourhood, obtain the appropriate segments of phonology from these various sources, and assemble a pronunciation. The problem for such an account, we suggest, is our recent observation (Evett, Patterson, & Morton, 1985) that the average latency for a regularisation error like *pint*→/pɪnt/ is scarcely longer than the latency for correctly pronouncing a consistent word and therefore, by implication, is substantially *shorter* than the latency for correctly pronouncing a consistent non-word. For reasons given earlier, our model predicts this result. In an analogy model, errors like *pint*→/pɪnt/ must derive from a failure of the lexical over-riding operation. When this fails, the procedure for producing a pronunciation must be the same as that for pronouncing a non-word, namely assembly of phonology from the neighbours.

Thus, it seems to us that an analogy theorist must predict equal latencies for *pint*→/pɪnt/ and *nint*→/nɪnt/. We suppose that he or she might argue (along similar lines to our argument for lexical and non-lexical distributions) that whole-string addressing and assembly from neighbours are procedures with overlapping time distributions, with the former producing a faster solution on the great majority of but not all of the occasions. Apart from the fact that this would involve abandoning the principle of lexical over-riding, it seems implausible to us. Majority rule (which is how the analogical process is supposed to work) requires one to wait until all of the votes have come in; how could this procedure ever be quicker than direct addressing of the single correct lexical candidate?

CONCLUSION

We have shown how a very simple expansion of the standard dual-routine model can account for a set of observations that seemed, on first glance, to controvert such a model. Our orthography-to-phonology correspondence system maintains an old grapheme-to-phoneme subsystem and postulates a new "body" subsystem. The addition of the latter allows us to account for (indeed, to predict) variable pronunciation *assignments* to ambiguous non-words and augmented pronunciation latencies for both ambiguous words and non-words. Though Kay and Marcel's (1981) observation (biasing of non-word pronunciation by orthographically similar words) has forced us to complicate our model by permitting lexical events to alter the operation of the non-lexical routine, the actual *performance* of our model probably predicts these bias effects more accurately than an analogy theory would do. The detailed, quantified performance of the model in terms of values of *r* for both unbiased and biased pronunciations of non-words will shortly be available in Morton, Patterson, Nimmo-Smith, Kay, and Evett (1985).

We look forward eagerly to reading an account of analogy theory drawn in sufficient detail to enable proper qualitative and quantitative comparisons between the two sorts of models. In closing, however, we reiterate the warning note on which we began, to ourselves and all others who would attempt an evaluation of these theories. Differences between the various body "types" and even between exemplars within one "type" are very large indeed; averaging over exemplars that behave differently can only obscure the issues. This is a depressing conclusion in its implications for the difficulty of constructing appropriate control items and for the necessity, given the inevitably small N for item type, of having a large N for subjects. It is, however, clear that even the atypically restrained generalisation across items in which we have indulged will turn out to be excessive.

REFERENCES

Andrews, S. (1982). Phonological recoding: Is the regularity effect consistent? *Memory & Cognition, 10*, 565–575.

Baker, R. G., & Smith, P. T. (1976). A psycholinguistic study of English stress assignment rules. *Language and Speech, 19*, 9–27.

Baron, J. (1977). Mechanisms for pronouncing printed words: Use and acquisition. In D. LaBerge, & S. Samuels (eds.), *Basic Processes in Reading: Perception and Comprehension.* Hillsdale, NJ: Lawrence Erlbaum Associates Inc.

Campbell, R. (1983). Writing nonwords to dictation. *Brain and Language, 19*, 153–178.

Coltheart, M. (1978). Lexical access in simple reading tasks. In G. Underwood (ed.), *Strategies of Information Processing.* London: Academic Press.

Cutler, A. (1981). Making up materials is a confounded nuisance, or: Will we able to run any psycholinguistic experiments at all in 1990? *Cognition, 10*, 65–70.

Davelaar, E., Coltheart, M., Besner, D., & Jonasson, J. T. (1978). Phonological recoding and lexical access. *Memory and Cognition, 6*, 391–402.

Evett, L. J., Patterson, K., & Morton, J. (1985). Replicable phenomena in the pronunciation of words and nonwords. (In preparation.)

Glushko, R. J. (1979). The organization and activaton of orthographic knowledge in reading aloud. *Journal of Experimental Psychology: Human Perception and Performance, 5*, 674–691.

Henderson, L. (1982). *Orthography and Word Recognition in Reading.* London: Academic Press.

Kay, J. (1982). Psychological Mechanisms of Oral Reading of Single Words. Unpublished PhD. thesis, University of Cambridge.

Kay, J., & Marcel, T. (1981). One process, not two, in reading aloud: Lexical analogies do the work of non-lexical rules. *Quarterly Journal of Experimental Psychology, 33A*, 397–413.

Kucera, H., & Francis, W. N. (1967). *Computational Analysis of Present-Day American English.* Providence, RI: Brown University Press.

MacCabe, I. D. (1984). Phonography: Data and speculations. Paper presented at a meeting of the Experimental Psychology Society, London, January 1984.

Marcel, T. (1980). Surface dyslexia and beginning reading: A revised hypothesis of the pronunciation of print and its impairments. In M. Coltheart, K. Patterson, & J. C. Marshall (eds.), *Deep Dyslexia.* London: Routledge & Kegan Paul.

Morton, J. (1969). The interaction of information in word recognition. *Psychological Review, 76*, 165–178.

Morton, J. (1979). Facilitation in word recognition: Experiments causing change in the logogen model. In P. A. Kolers, M. E. Wrolstad, & H. Bouma (eds.), *Processing of Visible Language,* Vol. 1. New York: Plenum.

Morton, J., & Patterson, K. (1980). A new attempt at an interpretation, or, an attempt at a new interpretation. In M. Coltheart, K. Patterson, & J. C. Marshall (eds.), *Deep Dyslexia*. London: Routledge & Kegan Paul.

Morton, J., Patterson, K., Nimmo-Smith, I., Kay, J. & Evett, L. J. (1985). The modified standard model for the conversion of orthography to phonology. (In preparation.)

Parkin, A. J. (1982). Phonological recoding in lexical decision: Effects of spelling-to-sound regularity depend on how regularity is defined. *Memory and Cognition*, *10*, 43–53.

Parkin, A. J. (1983). Two processes not one in reading aloud. Paper presented at a meeting of the Experimental Psychology Society, Oxford, July, 1983.

Parkin, A. J. (1984). Redefining the regularity effect. *Memory and Cognition 12*, 287–292.

Patterson, K. E. (1981). Neuropsychological approaches to the study of reading. *British Journal of Psychology*, *72*, 151–174.

Rosson, M. B. (1983). From SOFA to LOUCH: Lexical contributions to pseudoword pronunciation. *Memory & Cognition*, *11*, 152–160.

Seidenberg, M. S., Waters, G. S., Barnes, M. A., & Tanenhaus, M. K. (1984). When does irregular spelling or pronunciation influence word recognition? *Journal of Verbal Learning and Verbal Behaviour*, *23*, 383–404.

Shallice, T., Warrington, E. K., & McCarthy, R. (1983). Reading without semantics. *Quarterly Journal of Experimental Psychology*, *35A*, 111–138.

Stanovich, K. E., & Bauer, D. W. (1978). Experiments on the spelling-to-sound regularity effect in word recognition. *Memory & Cognition*, *6*, 410–415.

15 Phonological Reading: From Patterns of Impairment to Possible Procedures

T. Shallice and R. McCarthy

INTRODUCTION

It has been standard to assume that the normal reader can read aloud by transforming the orthographic representation of a letter string into a phonological form without the involvement of semantic processing, and also that certain acquired dyslexic patients read aloud using basically the same procedure (e.g. Coltheart, 1978; Marshall & Newcombe, 1973; Morton & Patterson, 1980; Shallice & Warrington, 1980). A common proviso has been that in at least some of these patients the operation of the "phonological reading" procedure is itself impaired although to a lesser degree than is the process of reading aloud mediated by semantics.

There has, however, been no agreement on how "phonological reading" operates in both normal subjects and patients. Even within the relatively restricted set of theories that have been applied in the acquired dyslexia literature, at least three distinct views may be distinguished.

1. *The Standard Position.* Independent lexical and non-lexical procedures are assumed to exist (in addition to the semantic route) and the patient relies on the non-lexical procedures only if the lexical ones are unavailable (e.g. Coltheart, 1982; Morton & Patterson, 1980). The non-lexical route has typically been assumed to involve grapheme–phoneme conversion rules, and until recently (where the process has been specified) to depend on rules based on functional spelling units (e.g. Coltheart 1978; but see Patterson & Morton, Chapter 14 in this book).

2. *The Multiple-Levels Position.* Spelling-to-sound transformations are

assumed to take place at a number of levels in parallel. The units range from graphemes through subsyllabic units (similar to Fujimura's, 1975, "demisyllable," e.g. the "rhyme"), syllables to morphemes; higher levels can be used more rapidly but are more sensitive to neurological degeneration (Shallice & Warrington, 1980; Shallice, Warrington, & McCarthy, 1983).

3. *The Lexical Analogy Position* (Henderson, 1982; Marcel, 1980). According to Marcel's version, segmentation of the letter string in all possible ways occurs, and each segment then automatically accesses (at the time the letter string is encountered) all words that contain those segments in equivalent positions. (The effect of morphemic segments predominates.) This in turn activates the pronunciations of those segments as they occur in each of those words. From this the pronunciation of the letter string is achieved (see Kay & Marcel, 1981). It is presupposed that in surface dyslexia some of the orthographic specifications have been lost in the input lexicon so that the pool of words on which the analogy process can operate has shrunk.

These three theories are not sharply conceptually distinct. Thus by complicating the nature of the non-lexical process the first theory becomes quite similar to the second, except for the assumption of a differential sensitivity to neurological degeneration (see, for example, Patterson & Morton, Chapter 14 in this book). In addition the second and third theories can make many similar predictions. However, they differ on whether lexical activation of similar words is crucially involved in phonological reading. Also the second theory, but not the third, predicts that lexical and non-lexical processing could be dissociated, so that a patient could exist who could read no irregular morphemes and yet could read non-words. Moreover, all the assumptions of any particular theory are not central to the theory. Thus the specific assumptions made by Marcel (1980) about the parsing process could be replaced within the general lexical analogy theory. However, for convenience of analysis three core theories will be contrasted.

The primary purpose of this Chapter is to assess which of these theories best explains the evidence from phonological reading in acquired dyslexia. However, a wide range of reading patterns are subsumed by the term "phonological reading." The reading of patients already reported in the literature differs very considerably. We therefore first describe briefly the characteristics of the reading of three possible subgroups of patients before assessing their theoretical significance. The subdivision we use was introduced by us in collaboration with Elizabeth Warrington (Shallice, Warrington, & McCarthy, 1983).

In all the patients being considered there is evidence that reading aloud by means of the semantic system is grossly impaired. The patient reported whose phonological reading was most intact is W.L.P. (Schwartz, Saffran, &

Marin, 1980). She was able to read nearly all words (with the exception of a few irregular words) at a nearly normal speed. At a later stage of her illness W.L.P. showed characteristics observed in a second group of patients, namely E.M. (Warrington, 1975), H.T.R. (Shallice, Warrington, & McCarthy, 1983), and probably also M.P. (Bub, Cancellière, & Kertesz, Chapter 1 in this book). The four major characteristics of this subtype are:

1. A strong effect of the regularity of the word's grapheme–phoneme correspondences on reading; regular words being read more easily than irregular ones.
2. Nonsense syllables are read as well as regular monosyllabic words (when matched in their non-semantic characteristics).
3. Errors are prototypically (non-lexical) regularisations.
4. Reading speed is relatively normal.

We have previously referred to this subtype as "semantic dyslexia" and for convenience we will continue to use this label in this Chapter.

A third subtype of acquired dyslexia held to be relevant to theories of phonological reading is, of course, "surface dyslexia" as originally described by Marshall & Newcombe (1973) in their patients J.C. and S.T. These patients differed from the previous subtype in at least three respects, namely:

1. Basic grapheme–phoneme correspondences are much less reliable. For instance, markers (e.g. rule of *e*) are frequently ignored and vowel digraphs give trouble.
2. Errors seem to represent the operation of a spelling-to-sound translation process but errors of perfect regularisation are atypical. Lexicalisations frequently occur.
3. Phonological reading is often slow with frequent corrections.

In Shallice, Warrington, and McCarthy (1983) we previously argued that these three subtypes are on a continuum. Authors who support the standard model would, however, make a qualitative distinction between the first two. In this Chapter we argue that a qualitative distinction should indeed be drawn, but between semantic dyslexia and surface dyslexia; semantic dyslexia is not, in our view, simply a purer form of surface dyslexia. In the next section we discuss surface dyslexia in somewhat more detail, basically relying on the descriptions of J.C. and S.T. given by Holmes (1973). The conclusion of this section is that it would be dangerous to make inferences from the properties of surface dyslexia to the operation of the phonological route in normal subjects.

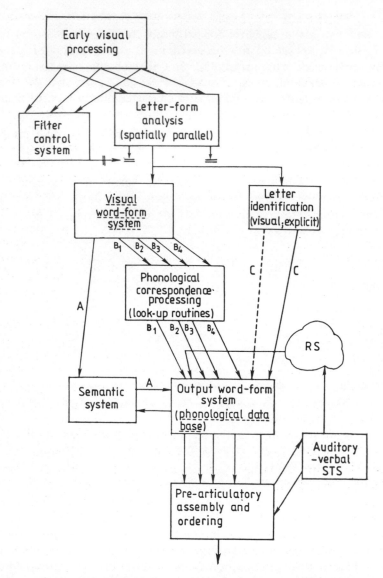

FIG. 15.1. Model of the word-form multiple-levels approach to the reading process. A = the semantic "route," B = the phonological "route," and C = the compensatory strategy "route." B_1–B_4 represent different levels of operation of the multiple-level system, and the divisions within subsystems. For the compensatory strategy, the continuous line C represents the use of letter names as the unit transmitted; the dotted line C is one possibility for the use of conventional letter sounds (the other is B_4). The "cloud"-shape (RS) represents the operation of the hypothetical reversed spelling procedure. (The earlier parts of the system are discussed in the paper from which this model is derived, namely Shallice, 1981.)

SURFACE DYSLEXIA AND LETTER-SOUND BY LETTER-SOUND READING

In their initial account of surface dyslexia–in conjunction with deep dyslexia and visual dyslexia–Marshall and Newcombe (1973) wrote: "We wish to emphasise the essential 'normality' of the errors characteristic of acquired dyslexia. That is we shall interpret dyslexic mistakes in terms of a functional analysis of normal processes (p. 188)." It has since been standard to conceive of surface dyslexia within such a framework (e.g. Coltheart, 1978; Marcel, 1980; Patterson, 1981; Shallice, 1981), although there has been at least one major exception (Henderson, 1981, 1982).

Not all acquired dyslexic syndromes have been treated in this way. In particular the letter-by-letter reading observed most commonly in the syndrome known variously as "word-form dyslexia," "pure alexia," and "alexia without agraphia" is normally viewed as the result of a compensatory procedure to bypass a specific impairment in the normal reading process, but itself (the compensatory procedure) having no relevance for normal reading (see, for instance, Patterson & Kay, 1982; and for a related, more extreme example Beauvois and Derouesné, 1982).

In the present section we argue that surface dyslexia as originally described is best understood as the result of an analogous compensatory procedure. Its properties therefore become less relevant for understanding the normal reading process. An issue of this sort cannot be tackled atheoretically. We will address it from the standpoint of the multiple-levels position, adopting an extension of the flow diagram used previously by one of us (Shallice, 1981) (see Fig. 15.1).

On this position, intact phonological reading involves at least three different stages of processing: (1) orthographically categorising and parsing the letter string (in the visual word-form system); (2) the use of "look-up" routines for accessing the appropriate phonological correspondences; (3) the assembling of pre-articulatory phonological instructions (and then articulatory production).

Theoretically on our approach entry to both the semantic and phonological routes requires the integrity of the visual word-form system (see Shallice & Warrington, 1980; Warrington & Shallice, 1980). Following a severe impairment of that system "reading" may still be possible if, as in one of the classic forms of dyslexia without dysgraphia, information about the identity of individual letters can still be obtained. Whether such identification involves direct transmission by the faulty visual word-form system or a process analogous to object naming is uncertain—and indeed both options are possible. Information about the individual letters that make up a written word can subsequently be transmitted sequentially to the phonological system and held there in a similar fashion to a heard sequence of letter names, as has repeatedly been shown in standard short-term memory experiments with visual input (e.g. Conrad, 1964; Sperling & Speelman, 1970).

After a sequence of letters has been presented auditorily it is possible to use a "reverse spelling" procedure and deduce what word they comprise. Although it is unclear how such a process operates in the successful identification of a word that has been spelled aloud, we would assume that it is parasitic upon operations involved in spelling. Combining these two procedures we would suggest that letter-by-letter reading utilises "reverse spelling" on information about individual letter identities transmitted to auditory verbal short-term memory. Warrington and Shallice (1980) showed that a number of the properties of letter-by-letter reading are consistent with this interpretation and indeed it is a reformulation of the classic account of this syndrome (see Hécaen & Kremin, 1976).

More recently Patterson and Kay (1982) have presented an alternative interpretation of the syndrome. They consider the possibility that in word-form dyslexia, it is not the visual word-form system itself that is damaged, but the input to it; this is, of course, a position that is more consistent with the traditional disconnection explanation for the syndrome (e.g. Dejerine, 1892). They assume that in letter-by-letter reading information about letters enters the visual word-form system serially rather than in parallel.

In the same paper Patterson and Kay showed that letter-by-letter readers can be subdivided into two types. One of these (type I) is similar to the patients studied by Warrington and Shallice (1980) and earlier by Staller et al. (1978), who generally produce the word correctly if they identify all its letters. For the others (type II), however (patients T.P. and K.C. of Patterson & Kay), correct identification of letters does not eliminate errors, but in the majority of the errors the response "represents a pronunciation of the graphemic string which, though lexically incorrect, is either phonologically plausible or nearly so."

Patterson and Kay (1982) considered two alternative explanations for this difference. The first, based on the classic account of the letter-by-letter reading process, they describe thus: "letter-by-letter reading arises from impairment of the visual word-form system which (in the normal reader) recognises or categorises written letter strings. A sequence of explicit letter names or identities permits word recognition via processes which belong to the spelling system. The reason that we have two types of letter-by-letter reader is that in fact we have two types of speller. C.H. and M.W. have reasonably normal lexical knowledge of spelling, and so they can correctly identify and assign lexical pronunciations to words once they have identified the component letters. T.P. and K.C., on the other hand, have a neurologically acquired impairment of lexical spelling. When they try to use this deficient spelling system in reverse for word identification, not surprisingly it produces errors (pp. 432-433)."

In fact T.P. and K.C. spelled with an over-reliance on the typical sound-to-spelling correspondences of English (as in the syndrome of lexical agraphia–Beauvois & Derouesné, 1981; Hatfield & Patterson, 1983). If this spelling process were "reversed" then one would indeed expect that patients with the appropriate "double deficit" would try out "pronunciations" rather than words per se.

The second type of explanation offered by Patterson and Kay (1982) is related to the disconnection explanations often given for word-form dyslexia, namely "letter-by-letter reading arises because of a disconnection between the letter-form analysis system and the visual word-form system. Although the word-form system is primarily suited to operating on abstract letter identities in parallel, it can also accept a sequence of letter identities. If this disconnection is the only deficit, one will find the pattern shown by classical letter-by-letter readers such as C.H. and M.W. However, in some cases there is a further impairment in the recognition system itself; in models like those proposed by Marcel (1980) and Shallice (1981) (and the one presented in Fig. 15.1), this impairment would correspond to whole-word or whole-morpheme specifications in the visual word-form system. The patient with this additional deficit would be forced to assign phonology to sub-word-sized graphemic segments and then cobble together a pronunciation. The result would be many eading errors characteristic of surface dyslexic patients (p. 433)."

Patterson and Kay (1982) point out that the first account is the more parsimonious as it explains the relation between reading and spelling characteristics, which the second account does not. In addition, on the second account if the type-II patients are reading by sounding out "subword-sized graphemic units" their strategy of producing letter *names* (e.g. T.P.: *head*→"h, e, a, d, heed") would be epiphenomenal. We will therefore adopt the first of these two explanations.

On this explanation a type-II word-form dyslexic reads by transferring information about letter names to the phonological system, and then reversing "lexical agraphic" spelling. This process could also operate on characteristic letter sounds derived directly from visual letter forms (see Fig. 15.1). Such an independent option presumably exists because there are patients who can give the characteristic sound of an individual letter (e.g. b→/bə/, c→/kə/, or u→/ʌ/) but not its name (e.g. R.O.G., Shallice & Warrington, 1980). Hypothetical word-form dyslexic patients who read in this fashion we will term "letter-sound by letter-sound readers," or "word-form dyslexics type IIB." (The term "letter-sound by letter-sound reader" has also been used by Newcombe and Marshall, Chapter 2 in this book; the two types of usage appear compatible.)

On this revised form of the word-form dyslexia theory, a word-form dyslexic with intact spelling and preserved letter naming (type I) would use the letter-by-letter procedure as it is more reliable (given English orthography) and also because the oral spelling process it reverses is the more familiar. A word-form dyslexic with lexical agraphia would use one or other form of letter-sound by letter-sound reading as the best procedure available.

The errors of these word-form type-II patients are, as Patterson and Kay (1982) demonstrated, very similar to those of classic surface dyslexia. The following types of errors are made by both: exact regularisation, violation of final e rule, pronunciation of silent letters, confusion of hard/soft consonants, and vowel digraphs give problems. Yet, in our view quite correctly, Patterson and Kay (1982) consider these patients as word-form dyslexics, because of the many features they have in common with the type-I patient. Reading in these patients clearly depends upon sequential conscious identification of individual letters.

Moreover, the characteristics of the reading of these word-form type-II patients, like those of the type-I patients, depend heavily on abnormal compensatory procedures. The whole process is under effortful conscious control, letters have to be explicitly identified one at a time, phonological information has to be moved into and out of auditory-verbal short-term store and there is ample opportunity for guessing strategies to be used.

As certain aspects of the reading of classic surface dyslexia are reminiscent of the properties of word-form dyslexia type II, could it be that surface dyslexia, as originally described by Marshall and Newcombe (1973), should be considered from within the framework of letter-sound by letter-sound reading and word-form dyslexia (a position related to that suggested by Henderson, 1982, for patient S.T.) rather than in terms of reading by an impaired phonological route? One characteristic of "phonological reading" considered critical by Shallice and Warrington (1980) and Coltheart (1982), namely the existence of "regularisation" errors (called, by Shallice and Warrington, "misapplications of valid correspondence rules"), does not appear to be a major aspect of the reading of J.C. and S.T., to judge from the Holmes (1973) corpus. Thus, as Henderson (1982) has pointed out, the characteristics that one would expect of phonological reading are not all necessary characteristics of surface dyslexia. In addition, although errors of the "partial failure of grapheme–phoneme correspondence rules" could be arising from the use of an impaired phonological route, they could also be an epiphenomenon of letter-sound by letter-sound reading.

The detailed account given by Holmes (1973) of patients J.C. and S.T. is consistent with this interpretation. According to Holmes, both patients have impaired spelling. Therefore, on the argument presented earlier, a word-form dyslexia could (at best) manifest itself as a type II, namely letter-sound by letter-sound reading. Moreover Holmes, herself, argues: "... to be able to read English (and many other languages) one has to be able to take in information in chunks, to process it in parallel, since information about the actual vowel represented by a particular vowel grapheme is given by the following consonantal environment represented by the appropriate consonant grapheme or group thereof. But this is coding and coding is what the subjects should be doing in order to read. When these subjects give an erroneous response, however, a failure of coding occurs; they operate at the level of the cipher. Descriptively it is as though cerebral injury in the case of J.C. and S.T., ... has resulted in their being unable to 'hold in mind' and process the sequence of graphemic items over which context-sensitive rules operate (p. 104)." Her view appears to be similar to ours, namely that these two patients base their responses on the information they can extract from the stimulus as a set of letters rather than as a sequence of graphemes. With their impaired spelling, on the argument presented earlier, they would be reduced to letter-sound by letter-sound reading.

Letter-sound by letter-sound reading is a procedure that patients apply as a clear strategy of which they are normally explicitly aware. The surface dyslexic patients J.C. and S.T. appear to have used such strategies. Thus Holmes (1973) says of J.C.: "J.C. makes great use of 'practice'; his approach is to realize a consonant 'frame' (by means of grapheme to phoneme match?) and to try out different possible vowel sequences until he *hears* one that has a match in his lexicon (p. 111)." Of S.T. she says: "S.T. also has a strategy to be employed when he has difficulty in reading a word. ... He attempts to spell out the presented words. This kind of spelling, that is, by the names of the letters, is in fact object-naming, and gives S.T. little or no help as to the pronunciation (p. 114)." (In addition S.T. makes letter-naming errors, a characteristic frequently associated with word-form dyslexia.) In both cases, though, other words are "recognised" more rapidly, apparently without the use of this conscious strategy. However, the errors that arise through this rapid process appear to be those classified by Holmes (1973) as visual—this point is explicitly made about 57 such errors of J.C. (p. 117); they would therefore seem to arise from a process different from the ones traditionally classified as "surface dyslexic." Thus the surface dyslexic type of errors appear, from the corpus, to be those in which the aforementioned conscious strategy is coming into play.

It might be argued that the existence of these rapid "recognition" responses is in conflict with the suggestion of a word-form dyslexia type II. Indeed severe word-form dyslexics *recognise* very few words rapidly, but they may make educated guesses that would operationally be classified as "visual errors," although arising by a different process from errors categorised in this way in deep dyslexia. If they do make rapid error responses these are visual in nature. Moreover, in a milder deficit of the visual word-form system one might well expect some words to be read relatively normally. Thus the patient B.Y. of Staller et al. (1978), who was said to decode words in a letter-by-letter fashion, had a mean naming time per word of 3.16 sec and an SD of 3.47 sec. Thus some words must have been read rapidly.

Other aspects of J.C. and S.T.'s surface dyslexia are what one expects from letter-sound by letter-sound reading. Reading speed on the critical errors is typically very slow, repeated attempts are made to read the word, and often these attempts are to read segments shorter than the whole word. Thus Holmes says of J.C. : "the words he has difficulty with are all characterised by repeated attempts to find a pronunciation that sounds like a genuine lexical item of English (p. 78)." Moreover, the characteristic inability to cope with rule of *e*, hardening or softening of *g* or *c*, and difficulty with vowel digraphs would all follow from a strategy of sounding each letter in a sequential left-to-right pass.

The account we have presented is related in spirit to that of Henderson (1981), who argues that surface dyslexia arises from a deficit of the graphemic buffer. However, given that some word-form dyslexics can perform well on visual short-term store tasks (e.g. R.A.V. of Warrington & Shallice, 1980), we prefer the present interpretation. With respect to the functional locus of the impairment, the account is closely similar to that of Marcel (1980)—loss of orthographic specification for some words—and is quite close to that of Coltheart (1981)—"failure of access to the word recognition component." However, our position, as a whole, differs from these two in certain important respects.

First, it differs from Coltheart's in providing a motivated account of why difficulties at the level of the visual word form produce a problem in non-lexical as well as lexical spelling-to-sound translation—this follows from the difference between the word-form conceptual framework and the logogen one that he adopts. On the logogen approach there is no principled reason why patients who have a visual logogen deficit should have a deficit in reading by the GPC route (see Coltheart, Masterson, Byng, Prior & Riddoch, 1983, for a discussion of this point). The difficulties that surface dyslexic patients have (failure to use the "rule of *e*" etc.) must be attributed to an additional deficit in that route. On our account a word-form type-II dyslexic patient whose word-form deficit is severe must show surface dyslexic characteristics if attempting to read as this involves sounding out words.

More fundamentally the present approach differs from those of both Marcel (1980) and Coltheart (1981) in suggesting a *qualitative* not a *quantitative* distinction between the reading of surface dyslexic patients J.C.

and S.T., on the one hand, and of semantic dyslexic patients such as E.M., H.T.R., and M.P. on the other. (In which category patients classified by other authors as "surface dyslexic" should be placed is unclear.)

In semantic dyslexia the phonological route would be used to read, but its operation would be impaired through loss of or inability to access morphemic representations at any of three stages of processing—orthographic (in the visual word-form system), orthographic-to-phonological correspondences (in the look-up routine system), or phonological (in the phonological assembly and production system). However, J.C. and S.T.'s reading, far from being comprehensible just in terms of a selective preservation of a component of the reading process, would be better understood as the consequence of a special type of compensatory process.

The possibility that a compensatory process using associations between visually identified letters and their characteristic sounds might be functionally independent of the operation of the phonological route, receives some support from the reading of a patient, F.L., briefly described by Funnell (1983). F.L. performed fairly well on reading single-syllable nonwords (74%) but was quite unable to give the characteristic sound of a visually presented letter (0/15), even though she could nearly always give the name of the letter, could always repeat the characteristic sound, and could always write the letter given the characteristic sound!

This distinction between the compensatory process and the operation of a somewhat impaired phonological route is of relevance for the issue of extrapolation to normal reading, as can be seen by considering some of the arguments of Marcel (1980). He argues that parsing of letter strings in normal subjects involves two processes: a left-to-right procedure in which every possible continuous sequence of letters is bracketed and a morphemic "marking," which specifies certain of these letter sequences as potentally critical. In his article Marcel uses characteristics of surface dyslexia to support his position. The apparent support that the evidence from surface dyslexia provides for this theory is, we would claim, illusory because the characteristics correspond to properties of the compensatory procedure rather than those of the reading process itself.

Although we have argued that the reading characteristics of J.C. and S.T. would be compatible with a deficit at the level of the visual word form, it would be premature to suggest that such patterns of reading aloud are *diagnostic* of deficits at this level or that all surface dyslexics are word-form dyslexics. In Appendix I we discuss the patient described by Deloche et al. (1982) who also appears to have used a compensatory strategy, and for whom an explanation in terms of visual word-form impairment may well be appropriate. Patients may also attempt to use a sounding-out (or letter-naming) strategy in order to circumvent other types of dyslexic (or even nominal) difficulties. Thus sounding-out may be used in order to circumvent impaired semantic processing of the written word when auditory semantic processing is intact, or when output phonology cannot be efficiently accessed in "nominal" dyslexic patients. Whether such patients are attempting to make use of a very degraded phonological route or of explicit associations between letters and their characteristic sounds (e.g. $b \rightarrow /b\partial/$) will probably prove difficult to determine. However, even in the former case their reading is likely to reflect the nature of the compensatory procedure rather than the properties of the phonological route itself. From clinical experience this seems especially likely if the patients have intact auditory comprehension. In such a situation the attempt to apply conscious guessing strategies to the inadequate products of the spelling-to-sound translation process could be entirely natural and may be impossible to avoid. Therefore, even such forms of surface dyslexia need to be qualitatively distinguished from semantic dyslexia.

THE IMPLICATIONS OF SEMANTIC DYSLEXIA

We argued in an earlier section that three acquired dyslexic syndromes have been described in which phonological reading is the most prominent aspect. The second of these, semantic dyslexia, was, to our knowledge, first observed by Warrington (1975) in two patients, A.B. and E.M., whose severe semantic memory deficits were the primary object of study. It was observed that these patients had only a mild deficit on the Schonell (1942) graded reading test— which involves mainly regular words—but that "words departing from the standard phonetic rules of English presented most difficulty." Indeed on an early version of the National Adult Reading Test (Nelson, 1983), which uses only irregular words, both patients showed a clearcut deficit. Unlike J.C. and S.T. these patients read at a roughly normal speed. Warrington (1975) concluded: "That words which are spelt in a bizarre manner (i.e. very irregular words) presented difficulty for these patients is consistent with the notion that the direct graphemic route (i.e. the semantic route) was inoperative. That phonetically (i.e. regularly) spelt words could be read with relatively little difficulty indicates that reading by the phonetic (i.e. phonological) route can be quite effective (p.654)." The reading of one of these patients, E.M., was analysed in somewhat more detail later (Shallice & Warrington, 1980). At a time when her dementing illness had reached a very advanced stage, she showed a very pronounced effect of regularity on reading; on the Coltheart et al. (1979) list she read 28/39 of the regular words correctly but only 5/39 of the irregular ones.

The patient of this type who has been investigated in most detail is H.T.R.

(Shallice, Warrington, & McCarthy, 1983). H.T.R. read 79% of regular words correctly but only 48% of matched irregular words. Her performance on words classed as "very irregular" was even worse (29%). By contrast nonsense syllables were read as well as regular words (84%). Semantic dyslexia cannot be attributed to any compensatory procedure of the type found in letter-by-letter or letter-sound by letter-sound reading. Reading is rapid, repeated attempts to read a word are rare, the prototypic error is a perfect regularisation, and lexicalisation is not a prominent aspect. It therefore seems appropriate to consider the relation of semantic dyslexia to theories of the operation of the phonological route in normal reading.

Most of the characteristics of semantic dyslexia, and in particular of H.T.R.'s reading, described in the introduction to this chapter are compatible with each of the three positions described there. However, certain aspects of the reading of H.T.R. present problems for the first and third positions.

Two aspects of H.T.R.'s reading present difficulties for the strong version of the standard position. "Mildly irregular" words—words that contained a single GPC that was not the most common one in English (e.g. *crow*, *remind*)—were read significantly better than "very irregular" words that contained either multiple irregularities (e.g. *colonel*, *yacht*, *area*) or an exceptional correspondence (e.g. *gauge*, *busy*). Yet on the strong form of the independence position neither type of word can be read correctly by means of the non-lexical phonological route and therefore requires the use of the lexical phonological route. There should therefore be no difference in how well these two types of word are read, as the degree of irregularity of their GPCs should be irrelevant to whether information about them can be transmitted by lexical routes.

It has been suggested that the superiority of H.T.R.'s reading of "mildly irregular" words compared with "very irregular" words may arise due to the variability with which a phoneme is produced for a given grapheme; for instance, that a word like *dread* is read relatively easily because *ea* is occasionally pronounced /ɛ/ independently of its context. There is no evidence for this position in the H.T.R. corpus. It is very rare for a vowel in a regular word to be pronounced by her as a minor (but not exceptional) correspondence. Thus in over 30 occurrences of *ea* in regular words it was never pronounced /ɛ/ although this frequently happened in words containing *ead*; in over 70 occurrences of *a* in regular words, the pronunciation /ɔ/ never occurred (although it was frequent for words containing *all*).

A second finding we made with H.T.R. is that when words in which a single GPC is irregular but not exceptional are analysed, the context of the vowel critically affects the chance of the word being read. To slightly simplify the analysis, if the word is *typically divergent* in that the vowel correspondence is not the most frequent in English but the V + CC correspondence is the most frequent (e.g. *head*), then the word is read nearly as well as comparable regular words (75% vs. 78%) and much better than *atypically divergent* words where both the vowel correspondence and V + CC are not the most frequent (e.g. *bowl*) (42%). These analyses suggest that for H.T.R. a critical unit for spelling-to-sound correspondences is that of what we call the subsyllabic unit, namely V + CC (the "rhyme") or in certain cases its complement CC + V. This means that non-lexical correspondences other than standard GPCs based on functional spelling units can be used by the phonological route, in conflict with the strong form of the standard theory. Parkin (1982) makes a similar deduction from his results on normal subjects, which we discuss later. He too argues that correspondence rules could apply to units larger than graphemes but smaller than morphemes.

Certain other aspects of H.T.R.'s reading present difficulties for the lexical analogy theory. Thus Marcel (1980), who sees surface dyslexia as arising from a lack of orthographic lexical addresses, in other words the loss of visual logogens, argues that this results in five effects: (1) removal of the effect of *e* and *i* on *c* and *g*; (2) removal of the effect of final *e* on vowels preceding the consonant before the *e*; (3) removal of the effects of digraphs for synthesis or diphthongisation; (4) silent letters are given a phonetic value; (5) morphemic segments are not over-ridden (e.g. island→*is* + *land*).

In general for H.T.R. these phenomena are very rare, except for (4). She makes only one error where the rule of *e* is not applied (*done*→"don") as opposed to many regularisations where it is applied (e.g. *some*→"soam"). On only two occasions did she pronounce *g* or *c* in the inappropriate hard or soft form: *circuit*→/koʊkʌt/ and *tragic*→/trægɪt/; on many occasions appropriate softening/hardening occurs as in the regularisation error of *mortgage*. Many, but not all, digraphs are appropriately pronounced as in the regularisations of *measure, bowl, shoulder, leather, steady, wear, plaid, gauge*, etc. Finally, lexicalisation is a much less strong tendency in H.T.R.'s reading than regularisation; errors of the non-over-riding of morphemic segments (e.g. *myth*→/maɪθ/) that were not regularisations were rare—only six errors of this type were noted. According to Marcel's (1980) theory all these effects should be major characteristics of phonological reading. Thus the predictions from Marcel's theory, whose success in accounting for surface dyslexia we explained in terms of compensatory strategies, do not fit H.T.R.'s reading.

CAN THESE THEORIES BE IMPLEMENTED?

These three theories can, however, be approached from an entirely different viewpoint. It is easy to see how a system based on the strong version of the standard theory might operate (see Coltheart, 1978). Indeed Coltheart (1982) reports that a computer simulation related to it exists. By contrast it is much less clear how a system functioning on one of the other two theories might work. Thus, of their version of the lexical analogy theory Kay and Marcel (1981) say: "A printed letter string is segmented in all possible ways....Each segment automatically accesses matching segments in the orthographic lexical input addresses of all words which contain those segments in equivalent positions (p. 401)." Leaving aside what counts as an "equivalent position," this requires that for any word the pronunciation of all possible segments must be stored. For a seven-letter word there are 28 of these (seven of length one, six of length two, and so on) and even if ones that disrupt functional spelling units are excluded, this approach to phonological reading requires that far more information be stored and accessed than does simple morphemic reading. This makes it a priori implausible. In addition how the mêlée of information accessed is recombined is unclear.

Henderson's (1982) development of Glushko's (1979) lexical pooling model avoids the computational largesse of Kay and Marcel's (1981) approach. Henderson assumes that each letter string activates all visually similar words by an amount proportional to the degree of relatedness and that each entry in a visual lexicon in turn activates its phonological counterpart proportionately. The "most heavily weighted" candidate is chosen. It is unclear to us how this process would work without considerably more assumptions. Consider attempting to pronounce *ehelf*; *h* almost never occurs in the second position in English words other than as part of the graphemes *ch*, *ph*, *sh*, and *th*. How are these pronunciations over-ridden when one produces say /əhɛlf/ or alternatively, why is *shelf* not a visually similar word? If position in the word is irrelevant, then making sense of the chaos of information activated would seem even more difficult. Maybe a lexical analogy process could work, but this definitely remains to be demonstrated. (For other criticisms of lexical analogy theory see Saffran, 1983.)

Is the multiple-levels position any better in this respect? There appear to be two different problems. First, for some of the levels (e.g. the subsyllabic one), can one be sure that an appropriate phonological correspondence could be produced for the letter string as a whole? This problem may remind the reader of Coltheart's (1978) discussion of whether a process based purely on syllabic correspondences could lead to the correct pronunciation of all English words and in particular the difficulties his analysis produces for the Hansen and Rogers (1973) Vocalic Centre Group theory. In fact this is not the issue here. As far as any one level is concerned (e.g. the subsyllabic), the relevant question is whether a process using units of this type can produce one or more phonological candidates for all orthographically regular letter strings. We are not concerned, as Coltheart was, about whether the process would lead to the correct pronunciation of specific English words not covered by rules, such as whether a CVCVC word should be parsed as CV + CVC or CVC + VC; much information of this type is likely to be carried by the morphemic level rather than the subsyllabic.

Intuitively a much more difficult problem is the second one of how the different levels of processing are integrated. How does one ensure that contradictory parsing does not occur at the different levels? How are they kept in step in the time domain while allowing the morphemic level to dominate or be fastest, as it must in the reading of irregular words? In the next section, a hypothetical scheme is developed to show that these problems may be resolvable.

THE MULTIPLE-LEVELS APPROACH

The Analogy from Scene Recognition

The multiple-levels approach differs from the standard position on phonological reading in two ways. First, it is claimed that differenty levels of unit are used, particularly subsyllabic units and also syllables. The assumption that levels between the grapheme and the morpheme are relevant has, of course, been held by theories of the norla reading process; for instance Spoehr and Smith (1973) argue that phological translation operates at the syllabic level and Laberge (1979) considers that letter clusters are important. In the present discussion we pay particular attention to the subsyllabic unit (which corresponds closely to Fujimura's (1975) concept of a demisyllable in the speech production literature) as it has rarely been considered by theoriests of the reading process.

The second difference is that on the multiple-levels position it is held that different levels of the process operate in an integrated way in parallel. Consider the following subcomponents of a spoken word: vowels, initial and terminal consonant clusters of one element or more, syllable onsets (SO) (i.e. initial consonant cluster plus vowel nucleus), rhymes (i.e. vowel nucleus plus terminal consonant cluster), syllables, and morphemes. Any particular phonological representation of one of these types will have one or more corresponding orthographic units. (In some cases an orthographic unit will have two or more phonological representations, for example *ead* can be /id/ (as in *bead*) or /ɛd/ (as in *head*).) We will assume that for each orthographic unit on every one of these levels there exists a specific detector within the visual word-form system. Table 15.1 illustrates the detectors assumed to be activated in orthographic analysis of the word *prostrate*.

To show that the multiple-levels theory could work one needs to indicate for each level how a set of these visual word-form units could be selected that

TABLE 15.1
Detectors Activated (Example— *Prostrate*)

Initial consonant cluster: *p, pr, r, s, st, str, t, tr, r.*
Terminal consonant cluster: *p, r, s, st, t.*
Vowel: *o, a, e.*
Syllable onset: *pro, ro, o, stra, tra, ra, a, te, e.*
"Rhyme": *o, os, ost, a, at, ate, e.*
Syllable:[a] *pro, pros, prost, ro, ros, rost, o, os, ost, stra, tra, ra, a, strat, trat, rat, at, strate, rate, ate, te, e.*
Morpheme: *pro, prostrate, rat, rate, ate, at.*

Possible parsing in subsyllabic units

1	*pro*	2,3 *o, stra*	4,5 *ate, –*
		os, tra	*at, e*
		ost, ra	*a, te*

Select any one of the (2,3) pairs and any one of the (4,5) pairs.

---

[a] These detectors would only be presumed to exist if they correspond to syllables within words in the language.

do not overlap and yet "cover" the word completely, and also how this selection process is ensured to be compatible between levels (for instance, to select *-ate* as a rhyme and *-e* as a syllable would be contradictory). The process of obtaining a complete but non-overlapping set of units to cover a word—part of the parsing process—would involve sensitivity to the logical constraints between different potential parsings.

These constraints can be divided into three types. First, there are incompatibilities for individual letters. Thus if one considers the first letter *t* there are six mutually exclusive initial and terminal consonant clusters of which it can be a part—*t-, st-, str-, tr-, -t, -st*, and each of these has entailments and incompatibilities with other levels of unit. Second, there are entailments between neighbouring letters, in particular the end of a terminal consonant cluster, rhyme, and syllable must be followed by the start of an initial consonant cluster, syllable onset, and syllable if the letter string does not end. (For the present we are ignoring the complications introduced by ambisyllabic parsing, for example, McCawley, 1978.) Combining these entailments produces more complex ones. Thus in the foregoing example if the first syllable ends with *-o* then *-tr* cannot be a syllable onset. Indeed, just considering syllable onset and rhymes there are nine permissible parsings of this letter string (see Table 15.1).

These sorts of constraints resemble those used in automatic scene recognition. Early approaches to computer vision attempted to parse scenes using, as basic data, noisy information about lines in the visual field. (For introduction see Boden, 1977, Part IV.) Two sorts of constraints were sufficient to allow overall interpretations to be obtained for these scenes that were consistent. One type of constraint is that the sets of lines meeting in a point (a vertex) fall into a number of types, for each of which there is a different small set of mutually exclusive alternative interpretations. For instance, an "arrow-head" of three lines meeting at a point has three possible interpretations: an open corner, its reverse, or a vertex of a solid viewed against a background plane. The second type of constraint is that the interpretations given to different vertices must be consistent; for instance, if an edge is interpreted as concave at one end it must be concave at the other too.

In Appendix II we attempt to show that the constraints in the domain of orthographically parsing a letter string are analogous to those which proved sufficient to allow satisfactory parsing in the scene recognition domain. From this similarity in constraints we infer that parsing procedures that have been shown to work in the scene recognition domain are likely also to work in the present domain too.

Early scene recognition programmes use an essentially serial approach. They first try to interpret one vertex then another and so on, backtracking where necessary. However, later programmes that were simulating human vision have attempted to use a more parallel approach, which is more plausible both psychologically and physiologically. In so-called "relaxation" procedures each possible hypothesis about how a particular part of the whole scene is to be interpreted is given a "degree of belief" parameter whose value interacts with the value of parameters corresponding to neighbouring parts of the scene (see, for example, Hinton, 1977; Hinton & Anderson, 1981). The form of the interaction depends on the nature of the constraint. For instance, if a local hypothesis about what happens at one end of a line provides the same interpretation of the line as a local hypothesis about what happens at the other end, then the two degrees-of-belief parameters are strongly mutually excitatory. In other words, if both hypotheses assume that the line is a concave edge, say, or both consider it the border of a shadow they "support" each other. If, by contrast, the two hypotheses provide different interpretations they are strongly mutually inhibitory. It has been shown in a number of cases that given reasonable starting points for the degree-of-belief parameters, the excitatory and inhibitory constraints will over time tend to result in stable maximum or minimum values of the parameters (i.e. produce a fixed interpretation of the scene).

That relaxation is the most plausible approach for the simulation of human scene recognition suggests that it should be considered for the orthographic parsing preceding spelling-to-sound translation. Applying relaxation to the spelling-to-sound domain one would require a set of detectors such that for each visual unit defined earlier (such as a particular subsyllabic unit, e.g. -*ost* as rhyme) there would be a detector (or better, more than one—see later). The detector would be activated by the appropriate visual input such that, in the absence of interactions with other detectors, its activation level would rise towards maximum. The two sorts of constraint would be provided by strongly inhibitory links for different incompatible hypotheses for the role of the individual letters and by both strongly facilitatory and strongly inhibitory links for the "neighbour" constraints. The most plausible consistent interpretation could be achieved by allowing the parameter controlling the rate of increase in activation of individual isolated detectors (the gain parameter) to vary such that the more frequently the unit occurred in the language the higher its gain parameter would be. For instance, the rhyme unit -*ate* would have a higher gain parameter than terminal syllable unit *e*. This would mean that parsings based on frequently occurring units would inhibit those based on infrequently occurring units. (For related formalisations see Hinton, 1977, p. 90; Shallice, 1972, Appendix 1.)

How would the relation between different levels operate on this system? If compatible units on different levels are made mutually facilitatory and possibly also incompatible ones on different levels mutually inhibitory, then because of their simple hierarchical relation it would seem possible for all levels of unit to be activated together and for the different levels of parsing to reinforce each other in the overall relaxation process (see Appendix II).

To summarise, three important characteristics of this procedure should be noted. First, the parsing constraints occur between all levels of orthographic units with the exception of the morphemic level. Therefore, in the orthographic "part" of the spelling-to-sound translation process parsings can take place on all orthographic levels at the same time, and incompatible parsings on different levels will not occur (with the possible exception of the morphemic level). Second, the units that are detected are ones with immediate phonological correspondences. Thus the orthographic parsing minimises any supplementary reading-specific spelling-to-sound parsing process. Individual orthographic units, when activated, can in turn activate a corresponding phonological unit (or possibly more than one, to different extents; see the discussion by Patterson and Morton, Chapter 14 in this book). Third and most basic of all, it seems likely that the multiple-level approach would be computationally tractable as the constraints in the present domain are so analogous to those in the scene recognition domain.

This account is, though, only a mere sketch of how the theory might be implemented. There are a number of obvious problems with it that need to be discussed. However, before they are considered a theoretical comparison is made between the multiple-level and rival approaches.

Costs and Benefits of This Approach

A procedure has been described that parses a letter string orthographically in terms of a set of units of different size. Computationally, what are the advantages and disadvantages of such a procedure by comparison with relying on just two sizes of unit—functional spelling units and morphemes— or just one, morphemes, but also allowing partial mappings (lexical analogy)?

The most obvious cost incurred by the present approach, which allows for visual analysis at the level of grapheme, consonant cluster, subsyllablic unit, syllable, and morpheme, lies in the increased number of orthographic processing units and spelling-to-sound correspondences that are required. Such an increase produces greater loads in acquisition, discrimination, and transmission.

We have seen that for the Kay and Marcel version of the lexical analogy model, the problem of the number of units required is severe. However, the number of additional units required by the multiple-levels model may be relatively small. Fujimura (1976) estimated that syllable level processing would require an additional 10,000 units whereas demisyllable-level processing (comparable to our subsyllabic units) would only require an additional 1000. Therefore the increased load would not be all that great and certainly the units involved would be fewer in number than those at the morpheme level, which are allowed on all three theoretical positions. The present approach also has the possible benefit of facilitating the learning processes required in the establishment of new morphemic-level correspondences; the use of orthographic subsyllabic units in expanding a reading vocabulary would be likely to be quite efficient.

Moreover, there are problems with the standard GPC approach. On the standard model the analysis of a letter string is considered to operate in a sequential left-to-right manner with backtracking when contextual factors modify the initial analysis (thus allowing for the rule of *e*, and softening of *g* or *c*). Current accounts are somewhat unclear as to whether these contextual effects operate at the level of graphemic parsing or at a subsequent processing stage. In either case in the reassignment of phonological correspondences, the GPC approach will be more costly in its processing requirements than the multiple-levels one.

The basic advantage of the multiple-levels approach is that at little extra cost in terms of the number of orthographic processing units, considerable power has been added to the procedures available for converting print to sound. The orthographic processing units that enter into the conversion process correspond closely to those that have been postulated empirically and theoretically as relevant for pre-articulatory phonological processing in speech production. Behavioural evidence from "slips of the tongue," for example, strongly suggests that there is a level of phonological processing intermediate between the segment (phoneme) and the morpheme (Crompton, 1982; Fromkin, 1973; MacKay, 1972; Shattuck-Hufnagel, 1979). Similarly there has recently been some recognition within generative phonology that considerable economy can be achieved with respect to derivation of some varieties of allophonic variation if units of syllable size are considered (Anderson & Jones, 1977; Kahn, 1980). Simulations of the speech production process have also used the elements of syllable or demisyllabic size (Fujimura, 1976; Perkell, 1980).

If one considers the non-lexical spelling-to-sound translation process in detail, two conceptually distinct types of operation following any orthographically based analysis of the letter string may be implicated: (1) Access to the appropriate phonological correspondences; and (2) the ordering and structuring of phonological output. We argue that the present approach has advantages for both of these types of operation.

Phonological Access

If in speech production the phonological information required is retrieved from a system containing an organised set of phonological data, then questions about the level at which it is represented become relevant. Opinion varies on this particular issue (see, for example, Crompton, 1982) but there is some consensus that units of approximately phoneme segment size or greater are involved in storage, although as Cutler and Isard (1980) and Fromkin (1973) have argued, such information is likely to be represented at a more abstract level than appears on the surface of speech production (given the existence of phenomena such as voicing agreement in consonant + s constructions in certain speech errors).

Whereas a phonological access procedure based upon the sequential retrieval of grapheme–phoneme correspondences is possible, the computational requirements of such a system would appear likely to be large and cumbersome. The GPC model is rarely spelled out in detail, but this criticism would be particularly apposite if one adopted a variant in which the bulk of computation occurs at phonological retrieval. The input from a graphemic parser would be constantly varying as a result of backtracking "error correcting processes" and an activation-based model of phonological retrieval (e.g. Crompton, 1980; MacKay, 1982) would presumably have considerable difficulties in coping with such input. On the approach we have adopted, sublexical phonological access would operate through "windows" of approximately syllable size and could be based on parallel access from units of syllable size or less. For instance, detectors would exist for units such as -obe and sci-, thus reducing the need for backtracking.

Ordering and Structuring of Phonology for Output Processing

We have already pointed out that it is now widely believed that units of the order of a syllable are involved at one level of the speech production process. If information were transmitted to the phonological system on a phoneme-by-phoneme basis (as in the GPC framework), subsequent concatenation into larger (possibly syllabic) units would be required for further pre-articulatory processing. The output from a system based upon the types of unit that we have described would not require such complex routines and could therefore be more efficient.

Problems With the Multiple-levels Approach

There are, however, a number of problems with this approach that have been glossed over so far. They are discussed separately.

Letter Order and Multiple Representations

A classic problem for systems of this sort is that there can be multiple representations of the same element in a letter string. For instance, in parsing the letter string *prorogue*, for the first syllable the unit detecting syllable onset *ro-* needs to be inhibited by that detecting *pro-* through the operation of the neighbour constraint, but for the second syllable the *ro-* unit should not be inhibited. A related issue is that the ordering of units needs to be transmitted.

There are a number of possible ways by which this problem could be overcome:

1. Instead of a single detector for a particular unit, it would be possible to have a number of them—neither mutually facilitatory nor mutually inhibitory—sensitive to different parts of the word, where this is roughly defined. Such intra-word position-specific units have already been suggested by the properties of segmentation errors (see Allport, 1977; Shallice & McGill, 1978; Shallice & Warrington, 1977). For the rhyme unit level, four detectors most sensitive to different quarters of a word would probably be sufficient.

2. An activation gradient (e.g. MacKay, 1970, related to Rumelhart & Norman, 1981). In this sort of approach the beginnings of letter strings would initially activate the detectors more than the ends; but once the initial letters are parsed, the subsequent ones provide more activation. The problem with such a procedure is that the same variable has to control both order and optimality.

3. A Wickelgren (1969) overlap model, in which the basic unit used in the correspondence process would be the triad of a letter and the immediately preceding and following letters (e.g. the two *ts* in *prostrate* would be coded as

$_st_r$ and $_at_e$). Activation of the preceding letter triad in the correspondence process primes the present one (e.g. detection of $_os_t$ primes $_st_r$ and not $_at_e$). Some aspects of this approach are present, in, say, the relation between syllable onsets and rhyme. However, a proper Wickelgren approach would require qualitatively different sorts of unit to be postulated.

The most likely possibility seems the first, with some possible contribution from the second and third, as the three procedures are not mutually exclusive.

The Morphemic Level

How does the morphemic level interact with the others? Morphemic boundaries mainly occur within letter strings between stems and affixes. With the exception of the two suffixes *s* and *ed*, affixes are syllables, and the latter is still orthographically a syllable even when it is not one phonologically. Therefore if affix stripping were to occur by relaxation processes operating in parallel on the stem and the affix, then in general the morphemic boundaries produced would be reinforcing with boundaries produced in lower-level relaxation processes (e.g. syllabic ones). Therefore the different levels of relaxation process would fit naturally together.

There are some complications in assuming that affix stripping occurs through two relaxation processes operating in parallel. For most stem-affix boundaries the standard neighbour relation assumed earlier would work; this would follow if stripping the affix left the stem itself (e.g. *lightly*). However, there would be complications in cases where adding an affix to a stem required the doubling of a terminal consonant (e.g. *fitted*) or removal of an *e* (e.g. *timing*). In these cases, the extra complication produced at the morphemic level has the effect of maintaining spelling-to-sound correspondences. Therefore the assumption that all levels of parsing operate together helps to reduce any anomalies on the purely morphemic level.

Why should the morphemic level operate the most rapidly or strongly (as it needs to, given the fact that irregular words are on the whole read correctly)? Information is sent to the phonological system about the whole morpheme simultaneously so that if there is any non-simultaneity in the parsing—either orthographic or post-orthographic—of lower levels (e.g. in the use of an activation gradient), the later parts of the letter string would be processed more rapidly morphemically. In addition the gain of morpheme detectors could be greater than those corresponding to lower levels.

The Neighbour Constraint

The main difficulty in attempting to parse a letter string in a parallel fashion is how constraints can be made to operate on the particular letters they are supposed to affect. In particular, how can the neighbour constraint operate, given that the detectors are not sensitive to a specific position in the letter string alone? Thus in Table 15.1, the potential syllabification *pro, trate* of *prostrate* is not supported as the *o* and *t* are not neighbours, whereas *pros, trate* is supported because the two syllables have a common boundary between the *s* and the *t*.

There appear to be two ways in which this neighbour relation could be established. One is through the use of the integer position of neighbours within the letter string, for instance, in the example position (*t*), position $(s) = 5 - 4 = 1$. This, though, has the disadvantage that the exact position of letters in words must be coded and subtraction operations performed.

A second possibility is to use the relative position of the letters in the visual field. An earlier level of processing than that of letter-form identification could well signal that the *s*-shape and the *t*-shape were neighbouring figures in the visual field. This level of processing would presumably be related to that of figure-ground separation. (It would, though, in addition need to distinguish pairs of neighbouring characters within letter strings from pairs of characters separated by an inter-word space.) In this approach the neighbour property is deduced from a property of the letters as elements in the visual field (i.e. from general visual perceptual processes) and not from their positions in a letter string (i.e. orthographic processes). Computationally it seems preferable to the first approach as it could be performed in parallel for different pairs of letters in the visual field much more easily. However, there is at present little evidence available on the point, and it remains an unsupported assumption for the theory.

It does, however, make it easy to understand how the reading system can cope with spatial distortion of the letter string provided that the letters still form a line, which on the whole goes or can be translated into a form that goes from left (top) to right (bottom) (see, for example, Seymour & May, 1981). The visual system is generally capable of processing stimuli satisfactorily if they do not deviate too grossly from their standard orientation, and the word-form system would be parasitic on general visual-perceptual processes for the determination of *which* characters were left and right neighbours of any given one.

A drastic way of avoiding the computational problems produced by the determination of which characters are and are not neighbours might be possible if the maximalist position on syllabic boundaries (e.g. Anderson & Jones, 1977) were accepted. On the maximalist position each syllable is assumed to have the maximum possible extent subject to Venneman's (1972) laws on legitimate initial and terminal consonant clusters. Syllables are allowed to overlap. The theoretical motivation for this position within modern phonology has been that it allows the retention of the syllable as a valuable theoretical construct while eliminating the thorny issue of where syllables begin and end.

The relaxation model could then operate with no inhibition between rhyme and syllable onset units containing the same elements. In Table 15.1 -*ost* would not compete with *stra*-. Within the set of subsyllabic units that still compete with each other (e.g. *ra*-, *tra*-, *stra*- in Table 15.1) it would be assumed that the activation gain was in general greater for the longest unit, so that this would tend to inhibit the others. "Neighbour" facilitation would then not be required. The theoretical consequences of these assumptions have not been considered in detail.

The Relation of the Model to Normal Reading

A variety of theorists on normal reading have suggested the existence of orthographic units intermediate between the letter and the word, having been influenced particularly by the ideas of Gibson et al. (1962). Attempts to demonstrate the existence of these units using normal experimentation have not provided clear support for them (see Henderson, 1982). Two recent groups of experiments seem, however, to provide more powerful support.

Mewhort and Beal (1977) have shown that presenting a word tachistoscopically as a sequence of syllables makes little difference to the ease with which it can be identified, provided that the syllables are displayed in a left-to-right sequence. If, however, the words were segmented non-syllabically (e.g. *ho-sp-ital* or *sp-eci-fic* instead of *hos-pi-tal* or *spe-cif-ic*) the error rate went up by a few hundred percent. It might be argued that the use of stimuli segmented in this way encourages the use of phonological recoding and the effect arises because the syllabic stimuli are more easily held in auditory-verbal short-term store. Such an explanation is, in fact, very implausible. When the *groups* of letters were presented at a 125-msec rate there was much greater difficulty in identifying the non-syllabic stimuli (over 30% of errors by comparison with about 10% in the syllable case). Such a rate is far too fast to allow effective coding into auditory-verbal short-term store (see Mewhort & Campbell, 1980, for further problems for this explanation). The most plausible explanation is that the syllable or the subsyllable—the non-syllabic condition affected that level of unit too—is an orthographic processing unit.

Another demonstration comes from the experiments of Santa, Santa, and Smith (1977) and Santa and Santa (1979). In these experiments a subject is simultaneously presented with a word and a letter group (e.g. *blast:las*) and must decide whether the letter group is contained in the word. In their main experiment some responses to initial consonant clusters (*bl*) and subsyllabic units (*bla, ast*) were as fast as to individual letters and faster than to the other doublets and the middle triplet (*las*). A serial position explanation was refuted in Santa and Santa (1979) where it was shown that if the same letter positions are compared across different words, then those that fit with the orthographic structure are detected more rapidly (e.g. *ea* in *treat* by comparison with *in* in *paint*). The most plausible explanation, again, appears to be that consonant clusters, vowel digraphs, and subsyllabic units exist as orthographic-processing units in the reading process. However, in this case it is not so easy to dismiss an explanation in terms of the differential ease in the use of phonological mediation.

Turning to spelling-to-sound correspondences there were two findings with H.T.R. that were easier to explain on the multiple-levels position than on standard three-route theory. To each there exists a related finding on normal subjects. One such finding, related to the greater ease H.T.R. had in reading mildly irregular than very irregular words, has been obtained by Parkin (1982). Parkin found that lexical decision responses to words considered sufficiently irregular to have their pronunciation listed in the *Oxford Paperback Dictionary* (OPD words) took significantly longer than regular control words matched for frequency and length (R words). By contrast, words which are technically irregular by Venezky's (1970) criteria in that they use minor correspondences (MC words) (e.g. *steak*) took no longer than control words. Thus in one experiment lexical decision times were: MC words, 688 msec; R words, 709 msec; OPD words, 741 msec. Pronunciation time showed similar effects. For instance, for lists of 16 words R words took 9.33 sec, MC words 9.56 sec (not significantly longer), and OPD words 10.85 sec (significantly slower). Parkin (1982) also showed by a *post-hoc* analysis of the lexical decision results of Bauer and Stanovich (1980) that a similar pattern is found there too. In a later paper Parkin and Underwood (1983) showed that the "OPD effect" was a spelling-to-sound correspondence phenomenon not due to unusual orthographic characteristics of the stimuli.

The second finding relates to the greater chance H.T.R. had of reading a typically irregular word—one where the rhyme is more frequently given the irregular pronunciation (e.g. *head*)—than an atypically irregular word (e.g. *bowl*). Seymour and McCabe (personal communication) found that normal subjects presented with nonsense syllables derived from the first sort of irregular word produced the irregular pronunciation of the vowel far more often than when the non-word was derived from an atypically irregular word. (However, see Patterson and Morton, Chapter 14 in this book, for apparently conflicting evidence.)

Relation of the Model to Semantic Dyslexia

The theoretical analysis of the previous sections has moved rather far from the acquired dyslexias. Can the model account for the characteristics of the reading of patients who read by an impaired phonological route?

According to the model, phonological reading involves three processing stages specific to language: orthographic analysis in the visual word-form system, the attaining of the appropriate phonological correspondences for the orthographic units detected, and the structuring and organising of the phonological output. The computational aim of the present model has been to reduce the processing load required in the second and third stages.

In patients with an inability to read by the semantic route, any impairment in phonological reading could theoretically arise at one of three sources—the visual word-form stage, the stage of attaining phonological correspondences, and the phonological organisation stage (a related point is made by Coltheart et al., 1983). For the purpose of the present discussion we will ignore disorders arising from impairments to the third of these, or access to it, as this would require extensive analysis of speech production and of corresponding aphasic disorders (but see Derouesné & Beauvois, 1979, and McCarthy & Warrington, 1984, for relevant discussion). The other two stages have, however, both been assumed to be the locus of the deficits in impaired phonological reading (e.g. Coltheart, 1981; Marcel, 1980; Marshall & Newcombe, 1973; Shallice & Warrington, 1980).

Determining which of these two stages is the locus of the impairment in any particular patient can prove difficult. However, an equivalent problem arises for either possible locus: how to explain an impairment that results in relatively preserved phonological reading using correspondences smaller in size than the morpheme, as in H.T.R. Does the contrast between a relatively intact submorphemic level and an impaired morphemic one require that a functional subdivision within the relevant subsystems be postulated? In this case the theory would become quite similar to the elaboration of the standard position, held by Patterson and Morton (chapter 14 in this book), in which separate morphemic and submorphemic systems are postulated.

As an alternative can a principled argument be produced as to why morphemic correspondences might be expected to be more vulnerable to neurological disease than smaller-size ones? In Shallice, Warrington, and McCarthy (1983), we argued that such a principle would enable one to explain the clinical course of the increasing impairment to phonological reading observed in two patients, E.M. (see Shallice & Warrington, 1980) and W.L.P. (Schwartz, Saffran, & Marin, 1980).

We considered three types of principle, including differential frequency of spelling-to-sound correspondences in the language and age of acquisition. However, the one we most favoured relies on the fact that a smaller amount of information needs to be transmitted to differentiate one subsyllabic unit from the set of all competing subsyllabic units compared with the amount required to differentiate one morpheme from the set of all other morphemes. In the former case one needs to differentiate between, say, 1000 possibilities as compared with over 20,000 in the latter. If the transmitted signal became increasingly weak or noisy, then one would expect that the size of the set of units between which discrimination could occur would decline, and this could produce qualitative changes in the reading given that the different levels of orthographic unit were in different discrimination sets. In particular, three qualitative levels can be distinguished depending on whether the highest level of reliable reading is based on morphemes, subsyllabic units, or functional spelling units.

On this approach, preservation of the whole system in the absence of semantic processing is clearly compatible with the reading of a patient like W.L.P. In some respects phonological reading in which even the middle level of correspondences have become unreliable would appear to relate to some forms of surface dyslexia. However, until some patients who read with surface dyslexic characteristics can be shown not to be better described as utilising compensatory strategies (such as word-form dyslexia type II), discussion of this relation seems premature.

How about the syndrome we termed "semantic dyslexia"? Semantic dyslexia would correspond to phonological reading when a phonological route is being used in which the amount of information transmitted is sufficient in general to allow effective discrimination between subsyllabic units but not between morphemes. Such an account predicts the effects of regularity, the effects of typicality of divergence, the prototypic regularisation error, and the relatively good performance with nonsense syllables. However, the effects of morphemic correspondences would not be expected to be eliminated completely; they would be weakened and slowed by comparison with normal. There is good evidence for this in the 10 errors made by H.T.R., in which one part of a very irregular word was regularised but another was not, for example, *yacht*→/jæt/, *castle*→kæsəl/, *suede*→/swid/. In such errors one part of the word seems to be pronounced under the influence of a morphemic correspondence (e.g. the *ch* in *yacht*) but another part under the influence of a subsyllabic correspondence or GPC (e.g. the *a* in *yacht*). Such weak parallel effects of the morphemic correspondences may well contribute to H.T.R.'s relatively good performance on mildly irregular words by contrast with very irregular words. It also fits with the fact that she can still read some very irregular words.

Another syndrome that seems to offer the possibility of a clear choice between the separable morphemic and submorphemic routes position and the differential sensitivity to disease is phonological alexia (Beauvois & Derouesné, 1979; Patterson, 1982; Shallice & Warrington, 1980). If the phonological alexic patient is reading words by a non-semantic process then this suggests that there are functionally distinct morphemic and submorphemic phonological routes (see Saffran, 1983, for discussion).

A patient that appears to offer evidence for this form of alexia is W.B., described by Funnell (1983). W.B. was able to read all types of word aloud at better than 85% accuracy and yet could read hardly any non-words correctly. In addition he made errors on tests of comprehending written words. It was therefore argued by Funnell that W.B. provides evidence for a functional separation between morphemic and submorphemic phonological routes.

In fact the evidence presented by W.B. is far from compelling. It is clear that the patient was severely aphasic and had considerable expressive speech difficulties. He made 50% errors on the repetition of nonsense syllables. Therefore it remains possible that the patient's difficulty in reading non-words could arise at a phonological organisation stage or access to it following translation from orthography. Funnell's main argument against this is that W.B. could not sound out single letters as syllabic sounds, although syllabic sounds could be repeated perfectly. However in the same paper she describes a second patient, F.L., who could read non-words fairly well but not sound out letters at all as we described in an earlier section. This suggests that sounding out single letters in a conventional fashion may be a process distinct from the operation of the phonological route, as discussed earlier. Therefore the existence of an impairment in the sounding-out of individual visually presented letters prior to the phonological organisation stage does not necessitate that the reading of nonsense syllables will be impaired at those stages too.

In addition the evidence that W.B. was not using the semantic route to read words is also debatable. The best evidence comes from a task in which W.B. had to choose which of the two written words (e.g. *lemon/orange*) was the more similar to a spoken word (e.g. "tangerine"). Performance was poorer than if unrelated written words were used (e.g. *comb/orange*). However, the coordinate relation is known to be an operation that aphasics find difficult (see Goodglass & Baker, 1976). Decisions about the relative closeness of two coordinate relations may well present especial difficulty for a severe aphasic like W.B., even if the semantic access process is intact (consider, for example, *motorway: road* or *lane*; and *linen: cotton* or *nylon*).

The evidence from Funnell's patient W.B. is not, therefore, at all clearcut. At present it remains unclear to what extent the different levels of operation of the phonological route are dissociable. However, even if "subroutes" can be dissociated, it seems unlikely that they involve a set of completely distinct processes.

The primary emphasis of this Chapter has been on the multiple-levels theory of phonological reading. We first argued that the characteristics of surface dyslexia as originally described are probably irrelevant for the understanding of the way phonological reading operates. The multiple-levels position gives a satisfactory explanation of the properties of the phonological reading of other acquired dyslexic patients and also seems well supported by the evidence from normal subjects. Moreover, the theory seems computationally tractable. Whether the different levels of the spelling-to-sound translation process are themselves functionally distinct appears to be still an open question.

REFERENCES

Allport, D. A. (1977). On knowing the meaning of words we are unable to report: The effects of visual masking. In S. Dornic (ed), *Attention and Peformance VI*. Hillsdale, NJ: Lawrence Erlbaum Associates Inc.

Anderson, J. M., & Jones, C. (1977). *Phonological Structure and the History of English*. North-Holland Linguistic Series. Amsterdam: North-Holland.

Bauer, D. W., & Stanovich, K. E. (1980). Lexical access and the spelling-to-sound regularity effect. *Memory and Cognition*, *8*, 424–432.

Beauvois, M. F., & Derouesné, J. (1979). Phonological alexia: Three dissociations. *Journal of Neurology, Neurosurgery and Psychiatry*, *42*, 1115–1124.

Beauvois, M. F., & Derouesné, J. (1981). Lexical or orthographic agraphia. *Brain*, *104*, 21–49.

Beauvois, M. F., & Derouesné, J. (1982). Recherche en neuropsychologie et rééducation: Quels rapports? In X. Seron, & C. Laterre (eds.), *Rééduquer le Cerveau*. Bruxelles: Pierre Mardaga, pp. 163–189.

Boden, M. (1977). *Artificial Intelligence and Natural Man*. Hassocks, Sussex: Harvester.

Coltheart, M. (1978). Lexical access in simple reading tasks. In G. Underwood (ed.), *Strategies of Information Processing*. London: Academic Press.

Coltheart, M. (1981). Disorders of reading and their implications for models of normal reading. *Visible Language*, *15*, 245–286.

Coltheart, M. (1982). The psycholinguistic analysis of acquired dyslexias: Some illustrations. *Philosophical Transactions of the Royal Society, London, B298*, 151–164.

Coltheart, M., Besner, D., Jonasson, J. T., & Davelaar, E. (1979). Phonological recoding in the lexical decision task. *Quarterly Journal of Experimental Psychology*, *31*, 489–508.

Coltheart, M., Masterson, J., Byng, S., Prior, M., & Riddoch, J. (1983). Surface dyslexia. *Quarterly Journal of Experimental Psychology*, *35A*, 469–495.

Conrad, R. (1964). Acoustic confusions in immediate memory. *British Journal of Psychology*, *55*, 75–84.

Crompton, A. (1982). Syllables and segments in speech production. In A. Cutler (ed.), *Slips of the Tongue and Language Production*. Berlin: Mouton.

Cutler, A., & Isard, S. (1980). The production of prosody. In B. L. Butterworth (ed.), *Language Production Vol. 1, Speech and Talk*. London: Academic Press.

Dejerine, J. (1892). Contribution à l'étude anatomoclinique et clinique des différentes varietiés de cécité verbale. *Compte Rendu Hebdomadaire des Scéances et Memoires de la Société de Biologie*, *4*, 61–90.

Deloche, G., Andreewsky, E., & Desi, M. (1982) Surface dyslexia: A case report and some theoretical implications to reading models. *Brain and Language*, *15*, 12–31.

Derouesné, J., & Beauvois, M. F. (1979). Phonological processing in reading: Data from alexia. *Journal of Neurology, Neurosurgery and Psychiatry*, *42*, 1125–1132.

Fromkin, V. A. (1973). *Speech Errors as Linguistic Evidence*. Mouton: The Hague.

Fujimura, O. (1975). Syllable as a unit of speech recognition. *IEEE Transactions on Acoustics, Speech and Signal Processing*, *23*, 82–87.

Fujimura, O. (1976). Syllables as concatenated demisyllables and affixes. Paper presented to the Acoustical Society of America, Washington, DC.

Fujimura, O., & Lovins, J. B. (1978). Syllables as concatenative phonetic units. In A. Bell, & J. B. Hooper (eds.), *Syllables and Segments*. Amsterdam: North-Holland.

Funnell, E. (1983). Phonological processes in reading: New evidence from acquired dyslexia. *British Journal of Psychology*, *74*, 159–180.

Gibson, E. J., Pick, A. D., Osser, H., & Hammond, M. (1962). The role of grapheme–phoneme correspondence in the perception of words. *American Journal of Psychology*, *75*, 554–570.

Glushko, R. J. (1979). The organisation and activation of lexical knowledge in reading aloud. *Journal of Experimental Psychology: Human Perception and Performance*, *5*, 674–691.

Goodglass, H., & Baker, E. (1976). Semantic field, naming and auditory comprehension in aphasia. *Brain and Language*, *3*, 359–374.

Hansen, D., & Rodgers, T. S. (1973). An exploration of psycholinguistic units in beginning reading. In K. S. Goodman (ed.), *The Psycholinguistic Nature of the Reading Process*. Detroit: Wayne State Press.

Hatfield, F. M., & Patterson, K. E. (1983). Phonological spelling. *Quarterly Journal of Experimental Psychology*, *35*, 451–468.

Hécaen, H., & Kremin, H. (1976). Neurolinguistic research on reading disorders resulting from left hemisphere lesions: Aphasic and "pure" alexia. In H. Whitaker, & H. A. Whitaker (eds.), *Studies in Neurolinguistics, Vol. 2*. New York: Academic Press.

Henderson, L. (1981). Information processing approaches to acquired dyslexia. *Quarterly Journal of Experimental Psychology*, *33A*, 507–522.

Henderson, L. (1982). *Orthography and Word Recognition in Reading*. London: Academic Press.

Hinton, G. E. (1977). Relaxation and its role in vision. PhD. thesis, University of Edinburgh.

Hinton, G. E., & Anderson, J. A. (1981). *Parallel Models of Associative Memory*. Hillsdale, NJ: Lawrence Erlbaum Associates Inc.

Holmes, J. M. (1973). Dyslexia: A neurolinguistic study of traumatic and developmental disorders of reading. PhD thesis, University of Edinburgh.

Huffman, D. A. (1971). Impossible objects as nonsense sentences. *Machine Intelligence*, *6*, 295–305.

Kahn, D. (1980). Syllable-structure specification in phonological rules. In M. Aronoff, and M. L. Kean (eds.), *On Juncture*. San Francisco: AMNI LIBRI.

Kay, J., & Marcel, A. J. (1981). One process, not two, in reading aloud: Lexical analogies do the work of non-lexical rules. *Quarterly Journal of Experimental Psychology*, *33*, 397–413.

Laberge, D. (1979). The perception of units in beginning reading. In L. B. Resnick, & P. A. Weaver (eds.), *Theory and Practice of Early Reading, Vol. 3*. Hillsdale, NJ: Lawrence Erlbaum Associates Inc.

McCarthy, R., & Warrington, E. K. (1984). A two-route model of speech production: Evidence from aphasia. *Brain*, *107*, 463–485.

McCawley, J. D. (1978). Where you can shove infixes. In A. Bell, and J. B. Hooper (eds.), *Syllables and Segments*. Amsterdam: North-Holland.

MacKay, D. G. (1970). Spoonerisms: The structure of errors in the serial order of speech. *Neuropsychologia*, *8*, 323–350.

MacKay, D. G. (1972). The structure of words and syllables: Evidence from errors in speech. *Cognitive Psychology*, *3*, 210–227.

MacKay, D. G. (1982). The problems of flexibility, fluency, and speed-accuracy trade-off in skilled behaviour. *Psychological Review*, *89*, 483–506.

Marcel, A. J. (1980). Surface dyslexia and beginning reading: A revised version of the pronunciation of print and its impairments. In M. Coltheart, K. E. Patterson, & J. C. Marshall (eds.), *Deep Dyslexia*. London: Routledge & Kegan Paul.

Marshall, J. C., & Newcombe, F. (1973). Patterns of paralexia: A psycholinguistic approach. *Journal of Psycholinguistic Research*, *2*, 175–199.

Mewhort, D. J. K., & Beal, A. L. (1977). Mechanisms of word identification. *Journal of Experimental Psychology: Human Perception and Performance*, *3*, 629–640.

Mewhort, D. J. K., & Campbell, A. J. (1980). The rate of word integration and the overprinting paradigm. *Memory and Cognition*, *8*, 15–25.

Morton, J., & Patterson, K. E. (1980). A new attempt at an interpretation, or an attempt at a new interpretation. In M. Coltheart, K. E. Patterson, & J. C. Marshall (eds.), *Deep Dyslexia*, London: Routledge & Kegan Paul.

Nelson, H. (1983). *The National Adult Reading Test*. Windsor, England: NFER Publishing Co.

Nilsson, N. J. (1971). *Problem-solving Methods in Artificial Intelligence*. New York: McGraw-Hill.

Parkin, A. J. (1982). Phonological recoding in lexical decision: Effects of spelling-to-sound regularity depend on how regularity is defined. *Memory and Cognition, 10*, 43–53.

Parkin, A. J., & Underwood, G. (1983). Orthographic versus phonological irregularity in lexical decision. *Memory and Cognition, 11*, 351–355.

Patterson, K. E. (1981). Neuropsychological approaches to the study of reading. *British Journal of Psychology, 72*, 151–174.

Patterson, K. E. (1982). The relation between reading and phonological coding: Further neuropsychological observations. In A. W. Ellis (ed.), *Normality and Pathology in Cognitive Functions*. London: Academic Press.

Patterson, K. E., & Kay, J. (1982). Letter-by-letter reading: Psychological descriptions of a neurological syndrome. *Quarterly Journal of Experimental Psychology, 34A*, 411–441.

Perkell, J. S. (1980). Phonetic features and the physiology of speech production. In B. Butterworth (ed.), *Language Production, Vol. 1*. London: Academic Press.

Rumelhart, D. E., & Norman, D. A. (1981). Simulating a skilled typist: A study of skilled cognitive-motor performance. *Center for Human Information Processing Technical Report No. 102*.

Saffran, E. M. (1983). Acquired dyslexia: Implications for models of reading. In G. Mackinnon, & T. C. Waller (eds.), *Reading Research: Advances in Theory and Practice, Vol. 4*. New York: Academic Press.

Santa, J. L., & Santa, C. (1979). Vowel and consonant clusters in word recognition. *Perception and Motor Skills, 48*, 951–954.

Santa, J. L., Santa, C., & Smith, E. E. (1977). Units of word recognition: Evidence for the use of multiple units. *Perception and Psychophysics, 22*, 585–591.

Schonell, F. J. (1942). *Backwardness in Basic Subjects*. Edinburgh: Oliver & Boyd.

Schwartz, M. F., Saffran, E. M., & Marin, O. S. M. (1980). Fractionating the reading process in dementia: Evidence for word specific print-to-sound associations. In M. Coltheart, K. E. Patterson, & J. C. Marshall (eds.), *Deep Dyslexia*. London: Routledge & Kegan Paul.

Seymour, P. H. K., & May, G. P. (1981). Locus of format effects in word recognition. Paper presented to the Experimental Psychology Society, Oxford.

Shallice, T. (1972). Dual functions of consciousness. *Psychological Review, 79*, 383–393.

Shallice, T. (1981). Neurological impairments of cognitive processes. *British Medical Bulletin, 37*, 187–192.

Shallice, T., & McGill, J. (1978). The origins of mixed errors. In J. Requin (ed.), *Attention and Performance, Vol. 7*. Hillsdale, NJ: Lawrence Erlbaum Associates Inc.

Shallice, T., & Warrington, E. K. (1977). The probable role of selective attention in acquired dyslexia. *Neuropsychologia, 15*, 31–41.

Shallice, T., & Warrington, E. K. (1980). Single and multiple component central dyslexic syndromes. In M. Coltheart, K. E. Patterson, & J. C. Marshall (eds.), *Deep Dyslexia*. London: Routledge & Kegan Paul.

Shallice, T., Warrington, E. K., & McCarthy, R. (1983). Reading without semantics. *Quarterly Journal of Experimental Psychology, 35A*, 111–138.

Shattuck-Hufnagel, S. (1979). Speech errors as evidence for a serial ordering mechanism in sentence production. In W. E. Cooper, & E. C. T. Walker (eds.), *Sentence Processing: Psycholinguistic Studies Presented to Merrill Garrett*. Hillsdale, NJ: Lawrence Erlbaum Associates Inc.

Sperling, G., & Speelman, R. G. (1970). Acoustic similarity and auditory short-term memory: Experiments and a model. In D. A. Norman (ed.), *Models of Human Memory*. New York: Academic Press.

Spoehr, K. T., & Smith, E. E. (1973). The role of syllables in perceptual processing. *Cognitive Psychology*, 5, 71–89.

Staller, J., Buchanan, D., Singer, M., Lappin, J., & Webb, W. (1978). Alexia without agraphia: An experimental case study. *Brain and Language*, 5, 378–387.

Venezky, R. L. (1970). *The Structure of English Orthography*. The Hague: Mouton.

Venneman, T. (1972). On the theory of syllabic phonology. *Linguistische Berichte*, 18 (1), 1–18.

Warrington, E. K. (1975). The selective impairment of semantic memory. *Quarterly Journal of Experimental Psychology*, 27, 635–657.

Warrington, E. K., & Shallice, T. (1980). Word form dyslexia. *Brain*, 102, 43–63.

Wickelgren, W. (1969). Context sensitive coding, associative memory and serial order in (speech) behavior. *Psychological Review*, 76, 1–15.

APPENDIX I

That "letter-sound by letter-sound" reading may be the appropriate analysis of the reading of patients other than J.C. and S.T. who have been labelled as "surface dyslexic," can be shown by considering one of the first detailed reports on another patient, namely that of Deloche, Andreewsky, and Desi (1982). They reported a patient (A.D.) whom they described as "surface dyslexic"; he was, however, comparatively mildly affected. His success at reading individual words was initially 74% correct. Spontaneous self-corrections raised his performance to 92%.

His reading is described as slow with phonemic paraphasias. He showed a significant effect of letter-string length (but not syllabic structure). The patient's errors on 50 words (including those subsequently read correctly) are presented as a corpus in phonemic transcription. The majority of such errors are described as the result of "inappropriate assigning (as regards the particular item to be read aloud) of some phonemic value to a letter substring in the item ... from a set of legal candidates (p.19)." Errors appeared to involve both individual letter-sound misapplications of correspondence rules and multiple letter-sound parsing errors. Deloche et al. (1982) hypothesise that the reading process "might be described as a parser operating from left to right extracting letter substrings which might be grapheme candidates, assigning phonemic values to these graphemes and building up the response by phoneme concatenations." This interpretation bears a strong resemblance to that provided by Holmes (1973) for the reading strategies adopted by J.C. and S.T.

A.D., like J.C. and S.T., had impaired spelling as required on the letter-sound by letter-sound theory. Data on his spelling errors are provided and these too fit, being comparable to the type-II patients of Patterson and Kay (1982), namely replacement of the appropriate graphemes with phonologically plausible alternatives (87%), in other words lexical agraphia (see Beauvois & Derouesné, 1981).

Two experiments are reported that bear directly on the issue of whether A.D. can be considered as a letter-sound by letter-sound reader, that is, a patient with word-form dyslexia and impaired spelling. A.D. was required to make rapid lexical decisions to words presented for a brief but unspecified duration with and without pattern masking. Under pattern masking d' was very low (.62) as it typically is in word-form dyslexia even without pattern masking (see Patterson & Kay, 1982). There was, however, a regularity effect with nouns for A.D., significantly poorer performance being obtained on irregular items. However, a subset of the non-words were homophonic with irregular words on the stimulus list: if A.D. was employing a phonological reading strategy, then a high proportion of false positives to homophone distractors would be expected. The difference between these two sets of non-words was not significant ($\chi^2 = .7$), which suggests that the regularity effect may be attributable to orthographic factors alone.

When stimuli were presented without a pattern mask d' was larger overall (2.17). In addition homophonic non-words were more likely to be accepted as words ($\chi^2 = 9.2$) than were non-homophones. This latter effect suggests that the patient was employing a phonological-processing strategy, but paradoxically, no effect of stimulus regularity occurred for the noun stimuli. As quite high d' values can occur in letter-by-letter readers (Shallice & Saffran, in preparation) the explanation of this final set of results is obscure. Insufficient evidence is presented on the patient's visual short-term store abilities and on characteristics of the stimuli (e.g. word length) for it to be possible to refute a letter-sound by letter-sound explanation. As A.D. had very impaired performance with pattern masking, was only able to read slowly, and had impaired spelling, the possibility remains that he too should be considered as a letter-sound by letter-sound reader.

APPENDIX II

In standard scene recognition programs using so-called Huffman-Clowes labelling the two types of constraint operate at one basic level. In the present domain the parsing is occurring at a number of different levels. For simplicity we will first take one level—the syllable level—and illustrate the analogy on that level.

Table 15.2 shows the analogy between the constraints operating in the two domains. The first type of constraint is that each basic input element on which the parsing operates can be interpreted in one of a number of mutually exclusive ways. The second type of constraint concerns the relation between the ways that neighbouring elements are interpreted; these must be compatible.

In the scene recognition domain the elements are the vertices where sets of straight lines meet. The first constraint is that for each configuration of lines forming a vertex only a small number of interpretations is possible (see Fig. 15.2). The second type of constraint is that if at one point on a line the line is interpreted as, say, a concave edge then at any point on the same (straight) line the interpretation must be the same. A line cannot change from being interpreted as, say, a convex edge at one vertex and become, say, a concave one at another.

In scene recognition programmes many different types of parsing procedure use these two types of constraint to produce consistent interpretations of scenes based on blocks. Some are very simple as in so-called Waltz filtering, where a simple sequential procedure of exhaustive logical inferences works because there are sufficient con-

TABLE 15.2
Analogy Between Scene Recognition and Orthographic Parsing

	Element	*Constraint 1*	*Constraint 2*
Scene recognition	Vertex	Has a limited number of interpretations.	Lines joining vertices must have a consistent interpretation.
Orthographic parsing	Letter	Is contained in a limited number of potential syllables.	Neighbouring letters must have a consistent boundary relation (see Table 15.3).

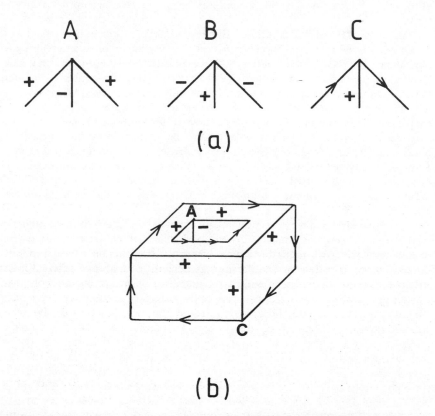

FIG. 15.2.   An example of the first type of scene recognition constraint (a). An "arrow" configuration is when three lines meet at a point, with one of the angles greater than 180°. It can have only three possible interpretations. + = a convex edge, − = a concave edge, < = an "occluding" edge, in which one side is a surface that obscures the extension of the other surface (or background). Two examples of interpreted arrows are illustrated in the very simple scene (b). One is a type A, the other a type C. (Adapted from Huffman, 1971.)

straints to prevent combinatorial explosions. Some require the *sequential* interleaving of the construction and development of a number of competing parsings, as in the popular branch-and-bound search procedure (e.g. Nilsson, 1971). This sort of approach is appropriate for a computer program, but not for a brain. Finally some, as discussed in the main text, operate with the much more psychologically and physiologically plausible procedure of parallel computation.

If we turn, now, to the present domain the interpretation we are seeking concerns the set of possible syllabic parsings of a given letter string. Again we may distinguish two types of constraint. If one considers only the syllables in the language that are physically present in the string, then there are only a small number of them that contain any particular letter in the string. Thus from Table 15.1 it can be seen that the letter *o* is part of nine potential syllables. The purpose of the overall parsing procedure is to select, from those nine, the ones that are possible given the constraints of the other choices. (In relaxation procedures the system selects a plausible candidate set.)

The parsing process also utilises the second type of constraint—the lateral constraint. A syllable must begin either at the beginning of a letter string or immediately another syllable finishes. So if we consider any letter in the string it can have a syllabic boundary on its left side (L), its right side (R), neither (-), or both (LR), and a simple general rule applies. If and only if a letter has a boundary to its left, its left-hand neighbour must have a boundary to its right. Application of this simple principle reduces the set of possible parsings, for *prostrate*, to nine alternatives. For instance, *ro* can be rejected as a syllable because the boundary preceding *r* requires a left-hand neighbour letter that terminates a syllable; no such unit exists among the activated syllable set for *p*. As a slightly more complex example, *pro* and *ate* cannot both be selected; the former requires a syllable beginning *s* and all such syllables contain no boundary following *r* and therefore conflict with the requirements for *ate*.

As the present domain has very analogous types of constraints to those occurring in the scene recognition domain, it seems plausible that similar types of parsing procedures would work in this domain too, in particular relaxation. In one respect the present domain is more complex. Parsing can occur at a number of different levels. Syllables contain syllable onset and rhyme units, which in turn contain consonant clusters and vowels. Moreover, the nature of the boundary relations are different for the different levels. This is illustrated in Table 15.3, which shows the boundary condition constraints between all levels of unit. To indicate how Table 15.3 should be interpreted consider the syllable onset, vowel cell. This says that only one type of situation can be ruled out, where the syllable onset unit finishes with the left-hand letter but the vowel unit does not start with the right-hand one. To illustrate the other three possibilities consider the possible boundaries between letters 1 and 2: (1) fa$_1$i$_2$nt with no boundary for either *fai* (syllable onset) or *ai* (vowel) between *a* and *i*; (2) f$_1$a$_2$int with a boundary for *ai* (vowel) but not for *fai* (syllable onset); (3) cha$_1$o$_2$s with a boundary for both *cha* (syllable onset) and *o* (vowel).

However, because the units are hierarchically related, it seems possible for the parsings to operate in parallel. Thus on a relaxation process the syllable unit *rost* would be strongly linked to the syllable onset unit *ro-* and the rhyme *-ost* and then in turn to the appropriate vowel and consonant cluster units. To reduce the complexities

TABLE 15.3
Boundary Condition Constraints Between Orthographic Processing
Units

	Type of Detector	Second Letter of Pair					
		Vowel	*ICC*	*TCC*	*SO*	*Rhyme*	*Syllable*
First Letter of Pair	Vowel	S	B	B	S	not N_1B_2	not N_1B_2
	Initial consonant cluster (ICC)	B	N	I	N_2	B	N_2
	Terminal consonant cluster (TCC)	B	B	N	B_2	S	S_2
	Syllable onset (SO)	not B_1N_2	S	B	S	–	not N_1B_2
	Rhyme	S	B	N_1	S	S	S
	Syllable	not B_1N_2	S	not B_1N_2	S	not B_1N_2	S

This table shows the boundary relations that exist between one type of unit detecting the first of two neighbouring letters and another type of unit detecting the second of them. The relation concerns the right-hand potential boundary of the first unit (1) and the left-hand one of the second (2).

Key: B = There must be a boundary (applies to both units unless 1/2 specified). N = There must be no boundary (applies to both units unless 1/2 specified). S = Boundary conditions must be the same for both. I = Impossible for the two units to be neighbours. – = All alternatives are possible.

of boundary relations between different types of unit, one level could be taken (say the syllable onset/rhyme one) and made the primary determinant for establishing neighbour relations.

It is thus quite possible in a relaxation process for all levels of detection, or at least from vowel/consonant cluster through to syllable, to operate together with the parsings on the different levels acting to reinforce each other.

16

The "Phonemic" Stage in the Non-lexical Reading Process: Evidence From a Case of Phonological Alexia

J. Derouesné and M.-F. Beauvois

INTRODUCTION

The purpose of the first cognitive studies on dyslexia that were concerned with phonological reading was to try to establish whether there did exist a reading process that would be functionally distinct from a lexical and/or semantic reading process. This was discussed mainly by contrasting surface dyslexic patients (Marshall & Newcombe, 1973), in whom lexical reading would have been impaired while phonological reading would have been rather good, with first deep dyslexic (Marshall & Newcombe, 1973; Patterson & Marcel, 1977; Saffran & Marin, 1977; Shallice & Warrington, 1975) and then phonological alexic patients (Beauvois & Derouesné, 1979; Patterson, 1982; Shallice & Warrington, 1980) in whom phonological reading would have been impaired while lexical reading would have been rather good. However, until 1978–79, little neuropsychological investigation was devoted to the question of how such a hypothetical phonological process could operate; it was only assumed that it involved grapheme-to-phoneme conversion (GPC) rules.

In 1979 Derouesné and Beauvois postulated functional distinction between two stages in the phonological reading process: a graphemic and a phonemic one. We obtained evidence that they could be impaired separately in two different forms of phonological alexia. Later (Beauvois, Derouesné, & Saillant, 1980), we came to the conclusion that both stages may be distinct from grapheme–phoneme conversion. Since then, a number of neuropsychologists have become interested in the operation of the phonological reading process and made certain proposals on this topic. It is therefore necessary now to define more precisely the way we conceive these two stages and to compare it with other conceptions of how phonological reading can operate.

By our definition, both stages are non-lexical. In other words, the kinds of processing involved in these two stages can be carried out without reference to the lexicon, unlike what is postulated in analogy theories (Henderson, 1982; Marcel, 1980) or multiple-level theory (Shallice, Warrington, & McCarthy, 1983).

The graphemic stage is conceived as distinct both from visual analysis (phonological alexic patients suffering from an impairment of the graphemic stage can analyse sequences of letters when reading words) and from print-to-sound conversion. It is assumed to bring into play the use of rules specific to written language, which are the basis of its translation into sounds. It involves a store of graphemic information that can be used for the parsing of a sequence of letters. Depending on the theory, the kind of unit that is stored and has to be converted into sound varies to a considerable extent. In the best known version of the way the non-lexical process could operate (Coltheart, 1978), the units that are stored are single graphemes (i.e. letters or letter strings that should be converted into one phoneme). In the multiple-level theory (Shallice, Warrington, & McCarthy, 1983; Shallice & McCarthy, Chapter 15 in this book) the units go from graphemes up to lexical units. In the analogy theory only lexical units are stored. According to our view, the information that is stored concerns not only the identification of graphemes but also of certain sequences of graphemes such as subsyllables and maybe syllabic units (see also Patterson & Morton, Chapter 14 in this book). This implies that syllabic or at least subsyllabic units, or alternatively orthographic rules concerning them (e.g. *c* should be converted into /k/ when followed by *a*, *o*, and *u* and into /s/ when followed by *i* or *e*) are stored at the graphemic stage.

On a flow diagram, the phonemic stage: (1) follows print-to-sound conversion; (2) precedes explicit articulation of non-words as well as their phonetic planning; (3) is specific to reading. In other words, it would be located between the stage resulting in the retrieval of phonemes and clusters of phonemes from print, and the one making their utterance possible. It would consist in the building of the whole phonological form. From (1) it follows that the kind of unit processed at this stage corresponds to the one resulting from the graphemic stage once the unit has been converted into sound. A consequence of (2) is that, unlike what was assumed by certain authors (Marcel, 1980; Newcombe & Marshall, Chapter 2 in this book), the phonemic processing does not obey phonetic rules but only phonological ones. Finally, (3) means that it is clearly located before the response buffer; therefore an impairment of phonemic processing is clearly different from the impairment assumed by Bub (1983) to account for the impairment of his phonological alexic patient.

Since 1979 certain authors have been concerned by what could occur between grapheme–phoneme conversion and speech output. Morton and Patterson (1980) first considered the idea of "a transmission of phonological information adequately obtained by application of grapheme–phoneme rules to the response buffer (p.110)." However, it is in the present book mainly that the idea of a particular phonological assembly processing appears: Patterson and Morton no longer speak of simple transmission but rather of the "transformation of the phonological code into a form suitable for production"; Temple and Marshall include a phonological assembler in their model; Shallice and McCarthy, too, assume a "phonological organisation stage" located after the stage of attaining phonological correspondences.

Despite this increasing interest, there are still few experimental data concerning the possible existence of such a phonemic stage. In a previous study (Derouesné & Beauvois, 1979), the existence of what we called the phonemic stage in non-lexical reading was inferred from the experimental evidence that certain phonological alexic patients could more successfully read aloud non-words pseudohomophonic to a word than non-words not homophonic to a word. We assumed that, after print-to-sound conversion has been done, the use of an alternative strategy, that is the evocation of the sound form of the word, allows the patients to get over their impairment of the phonemic processing. For instance, when presented with the non-word *tono*, the patients would be able to read it only because they have recourse to the phonology of the word that sounds like it (*tonneau*, pronounced /tɔno/). They would not be able to produce directly the phonology of a non-word from print, even though they are able to carry out properly the print-to-sound conversion.

However, one might wonder how these patients could find the lexical phonology corresponding to the one of a pseudohomophone if they had not yet assembled the bits of phonology for this pseudohomophone. This has now to be specified. Assume that the information resulting from print-to-sound conversion is of two sorts: phonemes and subsyllabic units on the one hand, some index concerning their serial order on the other. This does not automatically produce a phonological whole form, which has to be constructed (in the case of a non-word) or retrieved (in the case of a word). However, it is very likely that the amount of information obtained from print-to-sound conversion is sufficient to allow the patient to retrieve the phonology of a word that sounds like the non-word, as it should be sufficient to allow a normal subject to build the whole phonological form of the non-word.

More recently, Patterson (1982) did in fact find that a phonological alexic patient, A.M., could read pseudohomophones better than ordinary non-words. However, she thought that this effect was "attributable to the use at least in part of a particular strategy for reading non-words." She assumed that for non-words A.M. would avoid the phonological route and use the visual/lexical route. From her account, therefore, it would not be possible to use the observation of a pseudohomophonic effect in certain phonological alexic patients as evidence supporting the existence of a phonemic stage in reading. Although most of the authors who tested a possible pseudohomophone effect in phonological alexic patients (Bub, 1983; Funnell, 1983; Temple & Marshall, 1983) used it as a way of establishing whether grapheme–phoneme conversion has been carried out, the question still remains. It is obviously possible that certain phonological alexic patients use a complete visual/lexical strategy (this is very likely for A.M. who makes a lot of errors that are lexicalisations) whereas others, at least under certain circumstances (depending, for instance, on the instructions which they receive, as suggested by Patterson, 1982) are able to carry out phonological reading including print-to-sound conversion, and then have recourse to the pseudohomophony with a word. Fortunately, it is possible to test experimentally the validity of each of these accounts in a particular patient, as they lead to different kinds of predictions. Consider the following four experimental conditions: (1) non-homophonic non-words visually similar to a word; (2) non-homophonic non-words visually distant from a word; (3) pseudohomophonic non-words visually similar to a word; (4) pseudohomophonic non-words visually distant from a word. The "visual/lexical strategy" theory would predict that only (3) non-words will be better read than the others (in particular there is no reason to assume that (4) non-words will be better read). The "phonemic" theory would predict that both (3) and (4) non-words will be better read than (1) and (2) non-words. Among the authors who found a pseudohomophone effect in cases of phonological alexia (Derouesné & Beauvois, 1979; Bub, 1983; Patterson, 1982; Temple & Marshall, 1983) only Temple and Marshall's data allow us to make a distinction between the two theories and seem to support the "phonemic" theory. However, unlike the other cases, their patient is a developmental dyslexic who may behave in a slightly different way from cases of acquired dyslexia. In addition, unfortunately their study does not include a large number of items in each experimental condition.

In the present study we show with a new case of acquired phonological alexia, L.B., that whether non-words are pseudohomophonic to a word does affect his performance and that this effect is not confined to the condition of visual similarity with real words. Second we would like to specify the level of the phonemic processing involved in phonological reading.

CASE REPORT

History

L.B., a right-handed man, was born in 1926. After four years of secondary school and doing a number of different kinds of job, he became a draughts-man. In 1971, aged 45, he suddenly suffered from left hemiplegia, sensory disturbances of the left part of his body, finger agnosia, alexia, and agraphia. He never showed any evidence of aphasia in French, although he complained of having forgotten English and Russian that he would have learned previously. On the basis of right carotid angiography, it was inferred that he had had a stroke involving the territory of the right middle cerebral artery; this was confirmed later by CT scans (see Chapter 18).

The experimental investigation of L.B.'s reading impairment was carried out between 1981 and 1983, in other words 10 years after the stroke. At that time, the neurological picture remained roughly the same, apart from an improvement in his motor difficulties, such that the patient was able to perform activities in everyday life almost normally. Indeed, although his wife died suddenly at the beginning of 1982, the patient was able to stay at home and managed to take care of himself without any assistance. He did not complain of any serious problems apart from left motor awkwardness and difficulties in reading, writing, and counting.

Neuropsychological Examination

Handedness

Because L.B.'s alexia and agraphia were apparently due to damage in the right hemisphere, special care was devoted to the examination of his handedness. However, no evidence of left-handedness could be found: his LQ on the Edinburgh Handedness Inventory (Oldfield, 1971), was +90, Decile R.8; as far as the patient could remember he had always used his right hand to write, draw, etc.; after the stroke, he was not particularly impeded by the impairment of his left hand, except for a slight awkwardness in the simultaneous use of both hands; no evidence of sinistrality or ambidexterity could be found in his family, with the possible exception of one of his mother's brothers whom the patient had not known.

Perceptual Processes

Clinically, there was no sign of visual neglect; L.B. was able to cross out correctly all the examples of a particular sign on a page (22/22 A, 20/20 circles) and he performed a test of bisection of lines correctly. There was no evidence of visual agnosia: he named 49/50 perceptually difficult pictures of objects, 20/20 colours, and 19/20 famous faces.

Praxis

There was no evidence of gestural apraxia. L.B. could mime the use of objects upon spoken request with either hand (13/13 with his left hand; 13/13 with his right hand), even if they involved a complex programme of action (8/8); he could perform symbolic gestures upon spoken request (14/15); imitation of single meaningless gestures was also carried out correctly with his right hand (13/13), his left hand (13/13), and both hands (15/15). In contrast, signs of constructional apraxia were observed, which were of particular significance as the patient had been a draughtsman, whereas his copying of rather simple drawings like the test of Bender (1967) was almost normal. The copy of the Rey figure was drastically impaired (score 24, far below the 10th percentile and exhibiting a total lack of organisation); when asked to draw a house from two different perspectives (front and side) he was unable to do it and also could not draw a bicycle properly. This impairment of constructional abilities when drawing contrasted strongly with excellent ability to copy figurative images, which was one of his favourite hobbies. For instance, he made a copy of the face of the singer G. Brassens that really looked like a photograph.

Body Image and Finger Agnosia

Tests concerned with the body image and left–right orientation were performed normally. In contrast, signs of finger agnosia were observed. Mistakes were recorded on tests involving naming fingers and pointing to fingers upon spoken request, as well as when the patient was asked to point to the finger of his that corresponded to one of the examiner's.

Calculation

Evidence of dyscalculia was observed: L.B. made mistakes in oral performance of simple additions (4/8 correct), subtractions (2/8), divisions (6/7), and multiplications (2/8); he had trouble in counting backwards in threes as required in a subtest of the Wechsler Memory Scale. He also had difficulty with written arithmetic operations; possibly, this was partially due to his problem in reading numbers, but not to visual neglect of which no evidence was ever observed. However, he quite often managed to correct himself when necessary in everyday life and his standard score (7) on the arithmetic subtest of the Wechsler Adult Intelligence Scale (WAIS) was in the dull normal range.

Memory

Clinically L.B. did not have obvious memory impairment: he was well oriented for time and space; he used to take long walks in Paris and the suburbs and to make complicated journeys by Underground; living by himself, he did not seem to forget anything and was able to have a normal everyday life, taking part in a lot of social activities. However, memory tests revealed impairments both for the short-term component and for the long-term one. His auditory verbal span was poor (four digits, five letter names, four phonemes), as was his span for written letters (five). His MQ was 76 on the Wechsler Memory Scale and his score (35/50) was very low on the Forced Choice Recognition Test of Warrington (1984).

Intellectual Efficiency

L.B. was in the normal range: on the WAIS his verbal IQ was 99 and his performance IQ was 87; on Raven's Progressive Matrices he scored between the 25th and the 50th percentile.

Speech

L.B. had never shown any sign of aphasia. His speech examination was entirely normal. Repetition was perfect for 50 words, 40 long and complex non-words (e.g. /birystek/), and for all the sentences of the Terman–Merrill Intelligence Scale, up to the highest level. Production of words was fast and accurate. L.B. could name pictures of objects (50/50) easily and could produce the opposite of a given word (50/50) quickly. Word definitions were good (his standard score was 12 on the WAIS vocabulary subtest). L.B. could construct sentences easily from two or three given words (score 6/7 on the sentence constructing test of the *Examen de l'Aphasie*, Ducarne, 1976).

Understanding of Spoken Language

L.B.'s understanding of spoken language was fairly good. He was able to carry out correctly all the tests of oral understanding of the *Examen de l'Aphasie*: pointing to an object named by the examiner (35/35), performing orders (10/10), and the Three-Paper Test of Pierre Marie. The critique of irrational stories of the Terman–Merrill Intelligence Scale was correctly performed up to the highest level. L.B. did have some troubles only at the fifth level of the Token Test (de Renzi & Vignolo, 1962) where he scored 11/20. This abnormal performance was due very probably to his verbal short-term memory impairment.

Writing

Spontaneous writing was very disturbed. It was slow, severely paragraphic (e.g. *kilo→kiolo; prendre→predente*) with, in addition, substitutions of function words (e.g. *pour→sous*). In contrast, copying was perfect, without being slavish, for letters, non-words, words, and sentences. Writing to dictation was very impaired. Because this writing impairment raises the question of the relationship between reading and writing, it is described more formally in the experimental section.

Reading

L.B. had been a good reader: before his illness he used to read a newspaper every day and quite often novels and books on history. After the stroke, his reading abilities became very impaired and remained abnormal, in spite of a 4-year rehabilitation attempt. In 1983, he was still very impaired: he did not read newspapers any more, and had tried to read two novels without success and complained that he did not understand them; in addition, he could not follow subtitled films, and had trouble in understanding administrative forms that he had to fill in by himself after his wife died. On the whole, he read mainly TV programme listings and comics. However, he managed to do essential tasks involving reading in everyday life, by taking time to understand and by checking everything. The Alouette Reading Test (Lefavrais, 1963), which consists of a text that is particularly difficult to read because its meaningfulness is low or unexpected, confirmed his serious reading impairment. L.B.'s reading level corresponded to the level of the beginning of the second year of elementary school (he could read only 183 words in 180 sec, making 35 errors, mainly on function words and verb inflexions).

Reading Aloud and Pointing

Letters were named correctly (40/40) and quickly and could also be sounded virtually without any mistake (38/40). L.B. could point out from among a set of 20 letters the printed letter corresponding to a letter name (39/40) or to a letter sound (37/40) pronounced by the examiner. *Non-word reading* was impaired: L.B. made mistakes in reading aloud simple two-letter syllables (34/40 correct responses) and he could read only 19/40 (48%) simple non-words of four or five letters. His ability to point to the printed syllable or non-word corresponding to the one pronounced by the examiner from among a set of 20 was also impaired (35/40 for syllables; 31/40 for four- or five-letter non-words). *Reading aloud of numbers* was impaired in the same way (L.B.'s performance was as follows: one-digit numbers, 20/20; two-digit numbers, 8/10; three-digit numbers, 6/10; four-digit numbers, 4/10; five-digit numbers, 1/10). *Word reading* is described in detail elsewhere; therefore it is only briefly summarised here. Two tests are of interest. First L.B. correctly read 59/60 irregular words. Second, the word reading test that had been constructed for the first reported case of phonological alexia, R.G. (see Beauvois & Derouesné, 1979b; Beauvois, Derouesné, & Saillant, 1980) was administered to L.B. The test consisted of 1080 words, which had been selected in order to allow us to manipulate five variables, combined in a systematic experimental design: length, frequency, part of speech, concreteness, and word meaningfulness. Overall, L.B. read 87% of the words correctly. All the variables affected his reading performances; in particular, the effect of part of speech was important (nouns, 95%; adjectives, 93%;

function words, 82%; inflected verbs, 74%). Incorrect reading consisted mainly in derivational and so-called visual errors, substitution of function words and of verb inflexions, whereas no semantic error occurred and neologisms and omissions were very rarely recorded. *Reading aloud of sentences* of varying grammatical complexity and length was slightly impaired. L.B. read 30/40 sentences correctly, making 15 errors out of 312 words (95% correct). The errors occurred only on function words and inflected verbs.

Understanding of written language paralleled reading aloud, both for single words and for sentences. L.B. understood single content words normally (his IQ was 104 on the Synonym Test of Binois and Pichot (1958); he scored 101/103 on the French form of the Picture Vocabulary Test (Légé & Dague, 1976). By contrast, verb inflexions were rarely understood: in a test that is easy for normal subjects, namely where L.B. had to select from among three pronouns or among three adverbs (e.g. *now, yesterday, tomorrow*) the one corresponding to a given inflected verb, he scored only 65/120 (chance level = 40). Written sentences whose meaning depended upon function words were poorly understood. For instance, his score on the written form of the fifth part of the Token Test was only 15/22. This, unlike what happened with oral presentation, could not be entirely due to a verbal short-term memory impairment because the written sentence was left in front of the patient as long as necessary for him to perform his action. Most of the errors were apparently due to substitutions of function words (*behind→on*; *I→him*; *in front of→under*; *under→on*).

Lexical decision

Two tests of lexical decision were administered to L.B. The first one was made up from four sets of stimuli: set 1 included 50 words (e.g. *pièce*); set 2 included 50 non-words pseudohomophonic to the ones in set 1 and most often visually distant from it (e.g. *piaisse*); set 3 included 50 non-words that were not homophonic but visually similar (i.e. differing by one letter only) to words of set 1 (e.g. *pièle*); set 4 included 50 non-words very different from a real word but orthographically legal (e.g. *banfi*). The second test was made up from two sets: set 5 included 50 words; set 6 included 50 non-words that were both pseudohomophonic and visually close to the words of set 5 (e.g. *musicien* in set 5 became *muzicien* in set 6).

L.B.'s performance was fairly good (see Table 16·1). His false-positive rate can be considered as similar to or lower than that of Martin's (1982) normal subjects, although the measure of visual similarity was somewhat different in the two experiments, and of course Martin's subjects were instructed to respond as fast as possible. L.B. made errors only when non-words were both pseudohomophonic and visually close to a real word; in this condition (set 6), he obtained the same rate of errors as the mean of Martin's normal subjects.

TABLE 16.1
Errors in Lexical Decision

	Errors	
First test		
Set 1: Words (50)	2	4%
Set 2: Pseudohomophones visually dissimilar to words (50)	0	
Set 3: Non-words visually similar to words (50)	0	
Set 4: Non-words visually dissimilar to words (50)	0	
Second test		
Set 5: Words (50)	6	12%
Set 6: Pseudohomophones visually similar to words (50)	3	6%

Unlike Martin's normal subjects, he did not make errors when non-words were only visually close to a real word (the mean of Martin's normal subjects was 7.6%). As far as his false-negative rate is concerned, it tended to be slightly higher than his false-positive rate, especially on a test involving only non-words that were both pseudohomophonic and visually close to a real word.

In a control test, L.B. was presented simultaneously with a stimulus of set 5 and the one of set 6 derived from it (*musicien–muzicien*) and was asked to underline the correct spelling. He was 100% correct (50/50). His mistakes on the lexical decision task might therefore result from the use of a particular strategy rather than from lack of knowledge.

How does one explain the difference (if it was significant) between the performance of L.B. and that of normal subjects? If, unlike Martin's normal subjects, L.B. sometimes had used a phonological coding strategy, this would have led to his not making mistakes with non-words that were close to a real word but not pseudohomophonic with it. As it would presumably also have led to less use of direct visual lexical access, the strategy would have been less efficient for word stimuli; his attention being less strongly focused on the specific spelling of the word, he would have been less able to distinguish a word from its pseudohomophone. An additional item of clinical evidence that L.B. sometimes used a phonological strategy is that he noticed spontaneously, while doing the test, that certain stimuli were not words but sounded like words. It is noticeable that one of Martin's (1982) deep dyslexic patients, B.L., showed the same tendency to use phonological coding in lexical decision, because he made significantly more errors with non-words that were pseudohomophonic with a real word than with non-words visually similar to a word.

Why would L.B. have made more use of phonological coding than Martin's normal subjects? Several alternatives seem plausible. First, L.B. had had four years of rehabilitation based on attempting to train phonological reading, as is still generally done by French speech therapists with patients suffering from phonological or deep dyslexia. Second, he was trained to use phonological coding in certain experiments (i.e. reading aloud pseudohomophonic non-words) and may have applied the same strategy in the lexical decision task. However, the use of phonological coding could be due to certain differences between the two kinds of lexical decision task. First, as was first argued by Coltheart, Besner, Jonasson, and Davelaar (1979) and recently supported by Parkin and Underwood's (1983) results, if phonological coding occurs in normal reading but is slower than direct visual access, it would occur when there is no pressure of time (which was the case with L.B. and B.L.), whereas it would be less important when the subject is asked to answer as fast as possible (which is generally the case in experiments with normal subjects). Second, when non-words are both pseudohomophonic and visually similar to a real word, the subjects might understand or guess that their decision depends only on one letter; their attention might therefore be sometimes drawn to particular letters rather than spread over the whole word, which, when there is no pressure of time, could favour phonological coding.

To summarise, L.B.'s performance in lexical decision tasks was at least as good as that of normal subjects. It is noticeable that even in lexical decision there is some suggestion that phonological coding occurred.

Awareness of the Impairment of Non-Word Reading

Clinically, L.B. seemed to be very aware that he had trouble in reading non-words. His awareness was tested more formally. In a test involving 150 non-words, he was asked, after having read each non-word, to specify if he thought that his response was correct, incorrect, or if he was unsure about it. He read 49% of the non-words correctly. When his responses were correct he never thought that he had been wrong, but sometimes (17%) he was not certain that he had been right. When the responses were incorrect, he thought he had been correct for 66% of them and thought that he had been wrong for only 17% of these items. On the whole, L.B. tended therefore to underestimate his impairment.

Summary

L.B., a right-handed man, who had had a right hemisphere stroke 10 years before, still suffered from left motor and sensory disturbances, finger agnosia, constructional apraxia, dyscalculia, memory impairments, and alexia with agraphia.

L.B.'s reading impairment was characteristic of phonological alexia: whereas he could read words fairly well, including irregular ones, his reading of non-words was impaired. This pattern of results may be understood in the theoretical framework that was used in the original definition of the syndrome (Beauvois & Derouesné, 1979a): in our view, it reflects good operation of the lexical reading process, whereas the non-lexical reading process was not functioning properly.

Unlike most of the phonological alexic patients described in the literature, L.B. was able to sound letters. This is compatible with the conceptual definition of the syndrome. Indeed, when non-lexical reading is not operating properly, this does not mean that every kind of processing it entails should be inoperative. In theory, it is obviously conceivable that sounding letters may involve a different kind of phonological processing from those involved in the reading of non-words, even though they are both non-lexical; in particular, it is probably not necessary to sound letters to read non-words. And indeed, a patient has been reported who could not sound letters whereas she could sound non-words (F.L. reported by Funnell, 1983).

Other results, often described in cases of phonological alexia, are more difficult to understand in the theoretical framework in which the syndrome was originally described. They are the impairments observed in the reading of certain categories of single words and of sentences. The question still remains of whether at least some of these problems result from the impairment of non-lexical reading or whether they are additional deficits.

EFFECT OF HOMOPHONY ON NON-WORD READING

In order to decide whether L.B. could read pseudohomophones more successfully than ordinary non-words the simple manipulation of homophony (present↔absent) would be insufficient. Other points should be considered.

The first one is that other variables have to be taken into account, as they may interfere with the specific manipulation of homophony. For example, it has been suggested that the apparent effect of homophony, which was found with certain phonological alexic patients (Patterson, 1982) as well as with normals (Martin, 1982), could be due to an artefact, that is, to the fact that in these experiments homophony was overlapping with visual similarity. It is therefore obvious that a *distinct* manipulation of visual similarity has also to be included in the experimental design. Furthermore, as we have already emphasised (Derouesné & Beauvois, 1979), even though there do exist certain phonological alexic patients who specifically suffer from a disturbance of phonemic processing without impairment of graphemic processing, a large majority of patients have both kinds of impairment. In those cases the effect of homophony may vary with the graphemic complexity of the stimuli. This last variable has therefore to be included, too, in the experimental design.

The second point to consider is the kind of strategy (i.e. approximate visual access or homophony) that is used by the patient, either spontaneously, or according to special instructions given by the examiner. If not controlled, the strategy can therefore interfere with or prevent the effect of the variables under consideration. Thus we found a significant effect of homophony in certain phonological alexic patients by suggesting that they use a homophonic strategy, whereas Temple and Marshall (1983) obtained the same effect without using such a suggestion. It was therefore decided to include in the present experiment the manipulation of the kind of strategy suggested to the patient.

Consequently, the investigation of L.B.'s reading aloud of non-words was divided into two parts. In the main experiment the effect of the three following variables, combined in a factorial design, was studied simultaneously: homophony, visual similarity with a word, and graphemic complexity. In this experiment L.B. was instructed to use a homophonic strategy, because it was assumed that the effect of homophony depended on the fact that he intentionally decided to use it. Then two control tests were carried out to allow us to decide whether the suggestion of using a particular strategy (homophonic or visual) affected the patient's performance.

Main Experiment

Experimental Design

An experimental design involving the reading aloud of 240 four- or five-letter non-words was constructed in order to allow us to manipulate three distinct variables (Table 16·2). The first variable was whether or not a non-word was homophonic to a real word. This was done by contrasting pseudohomophones (e.g. *kacé*, pronounced /kɑse/ like the word *cassé*) with non-words that were not homophonic to a real word (e.g. *zida*, pronounced /zida/). In this experiment when the patient had to read pseudohomophones, he was instructed to try to use a homophonic strategy (i.e. he was told that he should try to find a word that sounded like the non-word). For this reason the 120 pseudohomophones were presented separately. The second variable, graphemic complexity was manipulated by contrasting non-words in which every letter corresponded to one phoneme (e.g. *pami*, pronounced /pami/) with non-words in which two letters had to be processed together to be converted into one phoneme (e.g. *aufo*, pronounced /ofo/). Finally, the effect of visual similarity between a word and a non-word was tested by contrasting non-words considered to be visually dissimilar to any word with non-words

TABLE 16.2
Factorial Design

Homophony	Graphemic Complexity	Visual Similarity	Examples	
			Non-words	Corresponding Words
Pseudo-homophonic non-words	1 letter→1 phoneme	low	kacé /kase/	cassé
		high	galo /galo/	galop
	2 letters→1 phoneme	low	ylau /ilo/	îlot
		high	aizé /eze/	aisé
Non-homophonic non-words	1 letter→1 phoneme	low	tiko /tiko/	
		high	pami /pami/	pari
	2 letters→1 phoneme	low	eulo /ølo/	
		high	aufo /ofo/	auto

considered to be visually similar to a real word. A non-word was considered visually dissimilar to a word when it did not have more than 42% of its letters in common with a word. These non-words were constructed by changing certain letters of four- to eight-letter words: when they were constructed from short words (four to six letters) they did not have more than one letter (for four-letter words) or two letters (for five- and six-letter words) in common with the word (e.g. the word *îlot* was changed into the non-word *ylau*); when they were constructed from long words (seven or eight letters) they did not have more than three letters in common with the word (e.g. *tonneau* was changed into *tono*). A non-word was considered as being visually similar to a word when it had more than 75% of its letters in common with it. These non-words were constructed from four- to six-letter words in which only one letter was changed or deleted (e.g. the word *aisé* was changed into *aizé*; *galop* was changed into *galo*; *auto* into *aufo*).

The three variables were combined into a factorial design, giving rise to eight experimental conditions (see Table 16·2). Each condition included 30 non-words. Three other variables were balanced in each condition: the syllabic structure of the non-words was kept constant (i.e. every non-word had two syllables); length was matched (10 non-words had four letters and 20 had five letters); the frequency of the words from which the non-words had been constructed was also balanced whenever it was possible, in other words when non-words were not too different from a word either visually or phonologically (which was the case for the 120 pseudohomophones and the 60 non-words that were not homophonic but visually similar to a real word). In each of these conditions the frequency was $\geqslant 30$ for 1–5 words, 1–29 for 16–20 words, and < 1 for 7–10 words (Juilland et al., 1970). The non-words were printed in lower case and presented to the patient one at a time.

Two comments have to be made concerning the construction of the non-words:

1. *Vowel aperture in grapheme-phoneme correspondence.* Even though, in principle, certain graphemes should correspond to a given vowel, there is a degree of uncertainty in French grapheme–vowel correspondence, which is related to the variability in the aperture of certain vowels. Consider a simple example involving a single letter, independently of the context: *è* and *ê* should, in principle, be pronounced /ɛ/, whereas *é* should be pronounced /e/. However, a number of French speakers make no distinction between /ɛ/ and /e/ and consequently pronounce in the same way *é*, *è*, and *ê*. In the construction of pseudohomophones we therefore sometimes took the liberty of considering as equivalent /ɛ/ and /e/. For the same reason, the same approximation was sometimes made with /o/ and /ɔ/, with /ə/, /œ/, and /ø/, with /y/ and /ɥ/, with /ɛ̃/ and /œ̃/, with /u/ and /w/, with /a/ and /ɑ/. Conversely, the relative aperture of such vowels was not taken into account in the analysis of the errors.

2. *Orthographic legality versus visual familiarity.* In the studies involving reading of non-words it is customary to use non-words that are orthographically legal. Roughly speaking, this means that non-words are made of sequences of letters that exist in the corresponding position in certain words of the language under consideration. This, to our mind, imposes unnecessary constraints on the experiments. Indeed, when testing the operation of the grapheme–phoneme conversion process, what matters is not whether a particular sequence of letters exists in a word of this particular language (which would be only a linguistic but not necessarily a psychological question); it is whether the reader can be expected to have ever carried out such a conversion in reading. This does not necessarily coincide with orthographic legality. There are circumstances in everyday life, under which a reader has to read written material that is not orthographically legal. Here are two examples related to some of the stimuli that we used. When you read comics that imitate spoken language you are quite often faced with orthographically illegal sequences. However, you can read them. Also, there are certain sequences that do not exist in a particular language but which look familiar, and which you can pronounce because they often appear in a newspaper as foreign names and they are pronounceable by using French rules. For instance, the non-word *kubov* for French readers looks like a Russian name and is easily pronounceable. It is therefore familiar and can be used in certain experiments even though *ov* is not a legal final sequence in French. This is obviously not the case for every kind of sequence in foreign words. In our experiments we used non-words that were sometimes illegal but were both easily pronounceable and familiar from the point of view of grapheme-phoneme conversion.

TABLE 16.3
Main Experiment: Correct Responses in Reading

Homophony	Graphemic Complexity	Visual Similarity	Correct Responses
Pseudohomophonic non-words	1 letter→1 phoneme	low	20/30
		high	26/30
	2 letters→1 phoneme	low	11/30
		high	25/30
Non-homophonic non-words	1 letter→1 phoneme	low	10/30
		high	11/30
	2 letters→1 phoneme	low	5/30
		high	10/30

Results (see Table 16·3)

A multi-variate analysis of the $2 \times 2 \times 2 \times 2$ contingency table was performed following a logistic transformation (Cox, 1970). There were highly significant effects of both homophony ($z = 5.77$, $P < .001$) and visual similarity ($z = 3.51$, $P < .001$). The effect of graphemic complexity was also significant ($z = 2.06$, $P = .02$). On a one-tailed test there was also a significant interaction between homophony and visual similarity ($z = 1.82$, $P = .03$). However, it should be noted that, combining over the two levels of graphemic complexity, the effect of homophony was significant for both high visual similarity stimuli and low visual similarity stimuli ($\chi^2 = 31.24$, $P < .001$; $\chi^2 = 20.3$, $P < .001$). In contrast, the effect of visual similarity was significant only for pseudohomophones ($\chi^2 = 15.38$, $P < .001$) but not for ordinary non-words ($\chi^2 = 1.42$, NS).

A control test was carried out to analyse whether the frequency of the words from which the non-words had been constructed affected the patient's performance. The words having been classified in three categories of frequency, the percentages of errors were, respectively, 43% when F < 1; 45% when 1 < F < 15; 38% when F ≥ 16. None of these differences was statistically significant.

Error Analysis

Were Error Responses Mainly Words or Non-words? (see Table 16·4). We recorded 122 incorrect responses out of 240 stimuli (51%). About two-thirds were non-words and one-third were words; very few omissions were observed (3% of the incorrect responses).

On the whole, the number of errors that were words or non-words was not significantly affected either by visual similarity ($\chi^2 = .002$, NS; $\chi^2 = .53$, NS) or by graphemic complexity ($\chi^2 = .57$, NS; $\chi^2 = .19$, NS). In contrast, there were significantly more errors that were words ($\chi^2 = 23.37$, $P < .001$) when the non-

TABLE 16.4

Main Experiment: Number of Incorrect Words and Incorrect Non-words (Each Condition Included 30 Stimuli) — Reading Errors

Homophony	Graphemic Complexity	Visual Similarity	Errors			Total
			Words	Non-words	No Response	
Pseudohomophonic non-words	1 letter→1 phoneme	low	9	1	0	10
		high	3	1	0	4
	2 letters→1 phoneme	low	10	9	0	19
		high	2	2	1	5
Non-homophonic non-words	1 letter→1 phoneme	low	0	20	0	20
		high	6	12	1	19
	2 letters→1 phoneme	low	2	21	2	25
		high	5	15	0	20
Total			37 (30%)	81 (67%)	4 (3%)	122

words were pseudohomophonic (and the patient was instructed to apply a homophonic strategy) than when they were not homophonic to a word; the opposite effect was observed with errors that were non-words ($\chi^2 = 25.56$, $P < .001$). If we analyse the relationship between the effect of visual similarity and the one of homophony two results should be underlined: (1) the effect of homophony on the production of errors that were words was significant even for non-words that were visually dissimilar to a word ($\chi^2 = 42.05$, $P < .001$); (2) the effect of visual similarity was significant even for non-words that were not homophonic to a word ($\chi^2 = 8.98$, $P < .01$).

The frequency of the words that L.B. produced as erroneous responses, compared with that of the words from which the non-words were constructed, was lower for 48% of the examples, higher for 26% of the examples, and roughly similar for 26% of the examples.

Were the Errors "Visually" Similar to the Stimulus?   It has now become standard in the literature to consider whether an error bears a so-called "visual" similarity with the stimulus. According to Morton and Patterson (1980), an error is considered as being "visual" when at least 50% of the letters of the stimulus are present in the same order in the erroneous response. This criterion was adopted in our analysis. Previously, a number of authors (Coltheart, 1980; Shallice & Warrington, 1975) considered only the requirement of 50% of the letters in common, without taking into account their serial order.

As the non-words used in our experiment were composed of four or five letters, the number of letters that had to be shared between stimulus and response to determine a "visual" error was two for four-letter non-words and three for five-letter non-words. Four types of errors were distinguished: (1) substitutions (one of the letters of the stimulus had been converted into a phoneme that could not correspond to a letter of the stimulus); (2) deletions (one of the letters of the stimulus had not been taken into account in the erroneous response); (3) additions (one of the phonemes produced in the erroneous response did not correspond to a real letter of the stimulus, or to a letter that could have been wrongly converted); (4) serial order (a phoneme corresponding to a letter of the stimulus was produced at a wrong place in the response). Obviously, combinations of different types of errors were recorded (see Tables 16·5 and 16·6).

On the whole a majority of errors (86/122, 73%) could be considered as visual. Moreover, most of the errors (92%) had a strong similarity with the stimuli, because at least 50% of the letters of the stimuli were present in these erroneous responses. As it is more frequent in the literature to analyse visual errors when they are words than when they are non-words (given the assumption that visual errors that are words result from the use of approximate visual access to the lexical route), a distinction was made between errors

TABLE 16.5

Main Experiment: Analysis of the "Visual" Similarity Between the Stimulus and the Error When Errors Were Non-words (81 Examples)[a]

Substitutions and/or deletions of letters	Other Letter Errors			
	No Error	Addition (1 Letter)	Position Change	Addition (1 Letter) and Position Change
No error		14 solé /sole/→ solré /solʀe/	3 ilogu /ilogy/→ igolu /igoly/	3 spour /spuʀ/→ sproud /spʀud/
1 letter	35 guzé /gyze/→ duzé /dyse/	5 kubol /kybol/→ trubol /tʀybol/	5 kurpa /kyʀpa/→ purda /pyʀda/	0
2 letters	8 fisaf /fisaf/→ fita /fita/	1 jofʃé /ʒofʃe/→ éjoksé /eʒokse/	3 baklé /bakle/→ kavé /kave/	0
3 letters	3 ukobi /ykobi/→ urudi /yʀydi/		1 ozajo /ozaʒo/→ zamak /zamak/	

[a] "Visual" errors are on the left upper part of the table.

TABLE 16.6

Main Experiment: Analysis of the "Visual" Similarity Between the Stimulus and the Error When Errors Were Words (37 Examples)[a]

Substitutions and/or deletions of letters	Other Letter Errors			
	No Error	Addition	Position Change	Addition and Position Change
No error		4 toué /twe/→ troué /tRue/	1 aigo /ego/→ agio /aʒjo/	3 afecé /afese/→ éffacé /efase/
1 letter	5 abovi /abovi/→ aboli /aboli/	3 angré /ɑ̃gRe/→ agrès /agRɛ/	1 pholy /fɔli/→ philo /filɔ/	4 augur /ɔgyR/→ agrume /agRym/
2 letters	5 rauzé /Roze/→ rasé /Raze/	6 préry /pReRi/→ précis /pResi/	0	0
3 letters	2 kasyé /kazje/→ café /kafe/	1 serso /seRso/→ cerveau /seRvo/	1 dazon /dazɔ̃/→ drap /dRa/	1 kozé /koze/→ écho /eko/

[a]"Visual" errors are on the left upper part of the table.

that were non-words (see Table 16·5) and errors that were words (see Table 16·6). If visual errors resulted from approximate visual/lexical access, one should expect them to be more frequent when errors were words than when they were non-words. However, this was not at all the case. There was a tendency ($\chi^2 = 3.19$, $P < .10$) to produce more visual errors when errors were non-words than when errors were words. In the same way, the percentage of errors that had a strong visual similarity with the stimuli (i.e. in which at least 50% of the letters of the stimuli were present) was slightly greater when errors were non-words (95%) than when they were words (86%). It is also noticeable (see Table 16·7) that visual errors that were words were more frequent ($\chi^2 = 6.9$, $P < .01$) when the stimuli were not homophonic but visually similar to a real word than when the stimuli were pseudohomophonic but visually dissimilar to a word.

Was the Similarity Between the Stimulus and the Error Orthographic or Phonological?   In a previous paper (Beauvois, Derouesné, & Saillant, 1980) it was suggested, concerning a case of phonological alexia, that certain errors on words generally considered as visual on the basis of the above criterion, might be in fact phonological errors. (See also Chapter 7 by Goldblum, in this book, for a discussion of this issue.) What we meant was that they might not be due to a dysfunctioning of the visual/lexical process of reading as it is generally assumed, but to the inappropriate use of the impaired non-lexical reading process. In the following analysis, we tried to make a distinction between errors on non-words that would be rather orthographic and errors that would be rather phonological. This was done in the following way. When, for instance, /seʀvo/ is produced as an erroneous response to the stimulus *serso*, the error can be, in principle, transcribed either *phonologically* (*servo*) or lexically, namely like the word it sounds like (*cerveau*). Two calculations were therefore made for each of the 37 words (the lexical translation being impossible for non-words) that was produced as an

TABLE 16.7
Number of Incorrect Words Visually Similar to the Stimuli in Relation With
the Number of Incorrect Words

Stimuli	Pseudohomophonic Non-words	Non-homophonic Non-words	Total
Low visual similarity	8/19	1/2	9/21 (43%)
High visual similarity	4/5	10/11	14/16 (87%)
Total	12/24 (50%)	11/13 (85%)	23/37 (62%)

erroneous response: (1) the percentage of letters belonging to the word's correct spelling that were also present in the stimulus (e.g. the erroneous word *cerveau* had two letters out of seven that were the same as certain letters of the stimulus *serso*, which gave 29%); (2) the percentage of phonemes of its phonological form that were present in the phonological form of the stimulus (e.g. in /sɛʀvo/ there were four phonemes out of five that belonged also to the stimulus *serso*, of which the correct pronunciation is /sɛʀso/, which gave 80%). When the difference between the two percentages was greater than 25%, the error was considered as being rather phonological or rather visual (in the foregoing example the error was counted as rather phonological).

Errors for which it was not possible to decide whether they were phonological or orthographic were the most frequent (see Table 16·8). However, phonological errors were statistically more frequent than orthographic errors (binomial test, $P < 0.05$). It is also of interest that phonological errors tended (even though this was not significant) to be more frequent when the stimuli were pseudohomoponic but visually not similar to a word (8/19, 42%) than when the stimuli were not homophonic but were visually similar to a word (2/11, 18%). The reverse pattern was observed with errors that were phonological and orthographic (10/19↔8/11). Orthographic errors were virtually nil in both conditions.

Graphemic Errors.   It had been presupposed (Derouesné & Beauvois, 1979) that a significant effect of graphemic complexity would reflect an impairment of the graphemic processing stage. If so, certain errors on graphemically complex stimuli should be "graphemic" errors, in other words they should correspond to the ones that would be expected when the graphemic stage is dysfunctioning. In particular, if one considers errors in digraphs, one should expect to find some evidence that the two letters have not been processed together before being converted into a single phoneme, but that they have been processed separately. For instance, a single letter of the digraph would have been converted into a phoneme, the other letter being deleted (Coltheart, 1978), or the two letters would have been converted into two different phonemes.

The 69 errors made on the 120 stimuli that were graphemically complex (i.e. in which two letters had to be converted into a single phoneme) were analysed. In about half of them (36/69) the erroneous response included an error on the digraph (often together with an error on other letters of the non-word). It was found (see Table 16·9) that often (13/36) the two letters of the digraph seemed to have been processed separately, in other words they had been converted into two different phonemes, either correctly or incorrectly. (The patient described by Newcombe and Marshall in Chapter 2 in this book also frequently made just this kind of graphemic parsing error.) Very often too (16/36), a single letter was processed, the other being deleted. There were

TABLE 16.8

Main Experiment: Orthographic and Phonological Similarity Between the Stimuli and the Erroneous Word Responses

Stimuli		Responses			
		Similarity With Stimuli			
Homophony	Visual Similarity	More Phonological	Phonological= Orthographic	More Orthographic	Total
Pseudohomophonic non-words	low	8 kozé /koze/→ écho /eko/	10 fisik /fisik/→ finish /finiʃ/	1 aigo /egɔ/→ agio /aʒio/	19
	high	2 sakré /sakʀe/→ saqué /sake/	2 ésité /ezite/→ obésité /ɔbezite/	1 augur /ɔgyʀ/→ agrume /agʀym/	5
Non-homophonic non-words	low	0	2 phiko /fiko/→ picot /piko/	0	2
	high	2 paidi /pedi/→ prédit /pʀedi/	8 blisé /blize/→ brisé /bʀize/	1 ilan /ilɑ̃/→ alain /alɛ̃/	11
Total		12 (32%)	22 (59%)	3 (8%)	37

421

TABLE 16.9
Main Experiment: Errors in Reading the Groups of 2 Letters→1 Phoneme

		Number of Groups	Examples
No deleted letter	2 letters→		
	2 "correct" phonemes	8	an /ɑ̃/→an(e) /an/
	2 letters→		
	1 "correct" phoneme and		
	1 "incorrect" phoneme	4	en /ɑ̃/→on(e) /on/
	2 letters→		
	2 "incorrect" phonemes	1	ch /ʃ/→sv /sv/
	2 letters→		
	1 "incorrect" phoneme	3	on /ɔ̃/→ou /u/
1 Deleted letter	1 letter→		
	1 "correct" phoneme	14	ei /ɛ/→i /i/
	1 letter→		
	1 "incorrect" phoneme	2	in /ɛ̃/→u /y/
No response		4	an /ɑ̃/→ ...

few omissions of both letters and, most important, very few cases (3/36) in which both letters had been converted together into a single wrong phoneme. On the whole, therefore, most (81%) of the errors made on the digraphs of graphemically complex non-words were graphemic errors.

Control Experiments

These were carried out several months after the main experiment.

Effect of the Suggestion of Using a Homophonic Strategy

Experiment.   Sixty pseudohomophones and 60 ordinary non-words were mixed in a list (these 120 stimuli were those of the previous experiment that were graphemically simple). The patient was asked to read them one at a time, without having received any particular instruction.

Results (see Table 16·10).   There was a tendency, which was not significant ($\chi^2 = 3.42$, $P < .10$), for pseudohomophones to be read better than ordinary non-words. L.B.'s performance for pseudohomophones was significantly worse ($\chi^2 = 9.16$, $P < .01$) when he did not receive the instruction of using a homophonic strategy than when he received this instruction; this was not the case for ordinary non-words ($\chi^2 = 0.3$, NS). The kind of errors (see Table 16·11) was significantly affected by the instruction of using a homophonic strategy, but only for pseudohomophones: L.B. produced more

TABLE 16.10
Suggested and Non-suggested Homophonic Strategy—Correct
Responses in Reading

| | Homophonic Strategy | | |
	Suggested	Non-suggested	Comparisons
Pseudohomophonic non-words	44/60 (77%)	30/60 (50%)	$\chi_i^2 = 9.16$, $P < .01$
Non-homophonic non-words	21/60 (35%)	20/60 (33%)	$\chi_i^2 = 0.03$, NS
Total	67/120 (56%)	50/120 (42%)	$\chi_i^2 = 8.82$, $P < .01$

words ($\chi^2 = 7.73$, $P < .01$) and fewer non-words ($\chi^2 = 5.51$, $P < .05$) when he received the instruction of using a homophonic strategy than when he did not receive it.

Effect of the Suggestion of Using a Strategy of Approximate Visual Access to the Lexicon

Experiment. In this experiment the patient was told that the non-words looked like words although they were not words and that if, for each of them, he could find a word that looked like the non-word, this could help him to read aloud the non-word. The test included the 30 non-words of the main experiment that were non-homophonic, graphemically simple, and visually similar to words.

Result (see Table 16·12). The suggestion of using a strategy of approximate visual access to the lexicon did not significantly improve L.B.'s performance ($\chi^2 = 1.08$, NS); neither did it affect the relative number of errors that were words and non-words.

Control Experiment. In theory, this lack of effect could have been due to the fact that the patient, for whatever reason, had been unable to find a word that looked like the non-word. This was checked by presenting him with the same stimuli again and asking him to produce a word that looked like the non-word. He performed fairly well: in 27/30 examples he found a word that, most often (23/27), did have a visual similarity with the non-word. Even though, therefore, the patient was able to find a word that looked like a non-word when it was possible (i.e. when non-words were visually similar to a word), the deliberate use of approximate visual access to the lexicon did not help him to read non-words.

TABLE 16.11
Suggested and Non-suggested Homophonic Strategy—Reading Errors

	Suggested				Non-suggested			
	Errors				Errors			
	Words	Non-words	No Response	Total	Words	Non-words	No Response	Total
Pseudohomophonic non-words	12 (86%)	2 (14%)	0 (0%)	14	13 (45%)	15 (51%)	1 (4%)	29
Non-homophonic non-words	6 (15%)	32 (82%)	1 (3%)	39	7 (17%)	33 (83%)	0 (0%)	40

TABLE 16.12
Suggested and Non-suggested Visual Strategy—Reading Errors

	Errors			
	Words	*Non-words*	*No Response*	*Total*
Suggested strategy	5 (33%)	10 (67%)	0 (0%)	15
Non-suggested strategy	6 (32%)	12 (63%)	1 (5%)	19

LEVEL OF THE IMPAIRMENT

An attempt was made to specify at what level of processing there was a dysfunction that was responsible for the impairment of non-lexical reading. Two points were considered. The first one was whether the phonological dysfunction in L.B. was specific to reading or whether it involved a more global phonological kind of processing. The second one concerned the level of the disturbance occurring in this patient in the phonological reading process, in particular whether grapheme–phoneme conversion was preserved intact, even for those non-words that were extremely difficult for the patient so that he could hardly read them.

Was the Phonological Impairment Specific to Reading?

The impairment of two kinds of processing that are both very peripheral and general can be rejected immediately. First, it was very unlikely that the impairment for reading non-words was due to a deficit of auditory short-term memory: L.B.'s auditory span was five for letters and four for phonemes, whereas the non-words used in the experiments involved three to five letters and the impairment for reading non-words was observed even with three-letter syllables; it was also checked that the patient could repeat the three letters of the non-words that he had most difficulty in reading, after he had read them aloud incorrectly (see next section). Second, it appeared that the impairment was not due to a dysfunction of the response buffer because the patient's spontaneous speech and naming were normal; it was also checked that he could repeat seven- to ten-phoneme non-words correctly (37/40). However, two points required more attention and therefore needed more testing. Indeed, one needs to consider whether L.B. could carry out other kinds of phonological processing, such as those involved in auditory comprehension and in spelling.

Was a Phonological Impairment Observed in the Processing of Auditory Stimuli?

Four tests were designed to check this point. In the first one, L.B. listened to a non-word (e.g. /dʀyp/) pronounced by the examiner, then had to produce the last phoneme of the non-word (/pə/); his score was perfect (40/40). In the second test the patient was presented auditorily with three phonemes such as /ʒə/, /ʀə/, /a/ and was asked to pronounce the corresponding syllable /ʒʀa/; he performed very well (27/30) despite the fact that the test involved the kind of non-words that were the most difficult for him to read. In the third test, L.B., while being presented with a printed letter, listened to a non-word pronounced by the examiner and had to decide whether or not the printed letter corresponded to a phoneme of the spoken stimulus; his score was good although not perfect (36/40). Finally, he was presented with a written non-word in which one letter was missing (e.g. *pal.te*) together with the complete spoken form of this non-word (e.g. /palst/) and was asked to write down the missing letter; his score was 17/20.

It seems, therefore, that L.B. was perfectly able to carry out a phonological analysis of the stimuli when they were presented auditorily.

Was a Phonological Impairment Observed in Spelling and Writing?

Three tasks involving written language were constructed with some of the stimuli used in the study of reading and were administered to L.B. (see Table 16.13): writing to dictation, spelling aloud, and pronouncing a stimulus orally spelled out to the patient. Writing to dictation was very impaired for syllables, non-words, and regular and irregular words. On the whole, spelling aloud seemed to parallel writing to dictation. Pronouncing a word or a non-word orally spelled out by the examiner was also very bad, especially for non-words of four or five letters. In writing to dictation the longer the stimulus, the worse it was spelled, whatever the kind of stimulus: non-words (the percentage of correct responses was 65% for two-letter syllables↔33% for four- or five-letter syllables), regular words (five letters: 73%↔eight or nine letters: 39%), or irregular words (four letters: 100%↔eight or nine letters: 0%). Errors were similar for words and non-words. They were mainly errors of serial order (e.g. " idéal"→*idale*, "refa"→*reaf*), letter omissions ("sécurité"→*surité*, "puco"→*pco*), letter duplications ("rival"→*rivral*), and letter substitutions ("cabri"→*cabli*, "bémol"→*démol*, "tiba"→*tima*).

L.B's writing therefore differed from his reading to a considerable extent: (1) both words and non-words were very badly spelled; (2) for both words and non-words the crucial variable was the length of the target to be written; (3) the errors were similar in kind for words and non-words. It would therefore be very implausible to assign the writing impairment to phonological or deep agraphia (Bub & Kertesz, 1982; Shallice, 1981). It is more likely

TABLE 16.13
Correct Responses on Certain Tasks Involving the Processing of Written Language

	Syllables (2 Letters)	Non-words (4–5 Letters)	Regular Content Words (5–9 Letters)	Irregular Content Words (4–9 Letters)
Writing to dictation	65% (26/40)	33% (13/40)	55% (43/78)	29% (11/38)
Spelling aloud	85% (34/40)	50% (20/40)	50% (20/40)	
Pronouncing a stimulus orally spelled to him	70% (28/40)	5% (1/20)	43% (17/40)	
Reading aloud	85% (34/40)	48% (19/40)	95% (417/440)	98% (59/60)

that thc phonological writing proccss was preserved intact, whereas the graphemic buffer was impaired (Miceli et al., 1983).

What Was Impaired in Non-lexical Reading?

The results of the main experiment showed that both homophony and graphemic complexity affected L.B.'s performance in reading non-words, whereas no interaction was found between the effect of the two variables. It had been presupposed (Derouesné & Beauvois, 1979) that such effects are evidence that at least two different levels of processing would be impaired in non-lexical reading, that is, the graphemic processing stage and the phonemic processing stage. Then, it appeared (Beauvois et al., 1980) that the effect of graphemic complexity could be due to an impairment either of graphemic processing (which includes graphemic parsing but cannot be reduced to it) or of grapheme–phoneme conversion. Even though the main purpose of the present chapter is to study the effect of homophony and therefore to focus on what was called the "phonemic processing stage in non-lexical reading," it appeared important to specify the possible impairment of the three kinds of processing in L.B. This was the reason why the following tests were designed.

Graphemic Processing

If the patient suffered from an impairment of graphemic processing without impairment of grapheme-phoneme conversion, he would be unable to convert a string of letters into a string of functional graphemic units, whereas he would be able to convert these graphemic units, if they were given to him, into phonemes. This would produce, in particular, the following pattern of results: (1) his performance on a test involving the detection of functional graphemic units without involving grapheme–phoneme conversion would be poor; (2) on a test where he does not have to carry out by himself the detection of functional graphemic units, but only to convert these units into phonemes, his performance would be normal (if he does not suffer from other disturbances) or similar to what he could do when the detection of such units is not involved, that is, with graphemically simple stimuli (if he suffers from other disturbances, such as an impairment of the phonemic processing stage).

Tests.   Forty four-letter non-words were constructed in such a way that two vowels were surrounded by two consonants. In 20 of them the two vowels corresponded to a functional graphemic unit, that is, they had to be processed together before being translated into a single phoneme (e.g. *teul* pronounced /tœl/); in the other 20 the two vowels corresponded to two functional graphemic units, that is, they had to be processed separately to be converted into two different phonemes (e.g. *tael* pronounced /tael/). In a first test the 40 non-words were mixed in a list. The patient had to decide whether the two vowels corresponded to one or two phonemes. His performance was very poor (27/40). In a second test L.B. was asked to read aloud the 40 non-words without having received any kind of help. His score on this test was also very poor (3/40, 7%). Finally, the two kinds of non-words were presented to L.B. in two different lists and he was told whether the two vowels corresponded to one or two phonemes. Under this condition his reading performance (20/40) increased up to the mean level of his reading of non-words. No significant difference was observed between his reading on the two lists.

L.B.'s performance in reading aloud non-words with digraphs was therefore significantly better when he was told whether the two letters of the digraphs corresponded to one or two phonemes, that is, when the parsing of the letter string was given to him by the examiner. This can be accounted for if, at the graphemic stage, L.B. suffered from an impairment of the parsing mechanism. However, if he had had only a parsing deficit, the help given to him would have allowed him to obtain normal performance, which was not the case. The residual abnormality under this condition should be assigned to an impairment of the phonemic stage, of print-to-sound conversion, and/or to another impairment of the graphemic processing such as a lack of knowledge of abstract graphemes.

Grapheme–Phoneme Conversion

As the tests designed to investigate grapheme–phoneme conversion generally involve some operation of graphemic processing (with the exception of those involving single letters), which was impaired in L.B., they cannot be expected to be performed perfectly. However, if one can imagine tests which involve little graphemic processing, these should be performed fairly well, if no additional impairment of grapheme–phoneme conversion is involved.

Sounding Graphemes. As was noted before, letters could be sounded virtually without any mistakes (38/40). Strings of letters that corresponded to a single functional graphemic unit (e.g. *ain* pronounced /ɛ̃/) were also sounded fairly well, if not perfectly (35/40). This, in addition, seems to be an evidence that L.B.'s knowledge of abstract graphemes was pretty good and that his graphemic impairment was on the whole attributable to the deficit of the parsing mechanism.

Detection of Homophony Between Two Syllables. One hundred couples of syllables were constructed in order to investigate L.B.'s ability to detect whether a syllable was or not homophonic with another one. The test was composed of two lists involving two kinds of graphemic processing. List 1 (60

items) investigated the conversion of single complex graphemes into phonemes; it was made up of digraphs that were either homophonic (*en*, *an* both
pronounced /ɑ̃/) or not (*en* and *in*, respectively pronounced /ɑ̃/ and /ɛ̃/). List
2 (40 items) investigated the context-sensitive rules involved in graphemic
processing and the conversion of these written items into syllables; it included
pairs of CV syllables that differed only by their initial consonant. In 20 pairs
the syllables were homophonic (e.g. *ci* and *si* both pronounced /si/); in the
other 20 the syllables were not homophonic (e.g. *cu* and *su*, respectively
pronounced /ky/ and /sy/. The two lists were presented to L.B. on two
different occasions. He had to decide whether the two syllables corresponded
to the same sound or not, without being allowed to pronounce them. He
performed fairly well (86/100) but not perfectly. No difference was observed
between the two lists.

Phonological Lexical Decision Task.   On this task the patient was presented with non-words and had to decide whether or not each of them
sounded like a word. If the patient could carry out grapheme–phoneme
conversion correctly one should expect to find, unlike what was observed in
reading aloud, no effect of homophony or of visual similarity with a word.
The test involved the 120 non-words of the main experiment that were
graphemically simple (which reduced the possible effect of the impairment of
the graphemic processing stage). These non-words therefore allowed the
systematic manipulation in a factorial design of homophony and of visual
similarity with a word. The patient scored 100/120. There was no significant
effect of homophony or of visual similarity.

It seems reasonable to think that these results can be accounted for
without assuming the existence of an additional impairment in L.B., that is,
one of grapheme–phoneme conversion. Indeed the errors that were observed
could result only from the impairment of the graphemic processing stage.

Ability to Carry Out Phonological Segmentation

In the framework of theories that presuppose that non-word reading is
performed by means of lexical analogy, it has sometimes been argued
(Marcel, 1980) that an impaired ability to read non-words could result from
the fact that the patient cannot segment the whole phonological form of a
word into syllabic or subsyllabic units. The following tests were designed to
test L.B.'s ability to carry out a phonological segmentation of words.

*Segmentation of the Phonological Word-form Obtained from Implicit
Reading.*   The patient was presented simultaneously with two words in
which a graphemic unit had been underlined and had to decide whether these
graphemic units corresponded to the same phoneme or not, without being
allowed to pronounce the words. In 30 pairs the graphemic units were

different in their written form but corresponded to the same sound (e.g. *doyen* and *copain*, respectively pronounced /dwajɛ̃/ and /kɔpɛ̃/). In 30 pairs the graphemic units differed both in their written and in their phonological form (e.g. *fourgon* and *enjeu*, respectively pronounced /fuʀgɔ̃/ and /ãjø/). The patient performed fairly well (53/60, 88%).

This test had been constructed because it had been assumed that to carry out the task correctly it was necessary to read the words implicitly, that is, to access their phonological forms, then to segment them in order to be able to compare each of the phonemes of the two words. However, in principle it was possible to apply another strategy, that is, to avoid reading the whole words and to compare only the underlined graphemic units. This would have changed the task into a test of graphemic processing. Therefore, even though the use of the last strategy was very implausible with L.B., given that he performed so badly in graphemic tests, another test was constructed so that it avoided the possible recourse to direct comparison between graphemic units.

Segmentation of the Phonological Word-form. Because the explicit recourse both to the written form and to explicit reading aloud had to be avoided, and as it was necessary at the same time to control the targets on which the patient was working, the test could use only words. The patient was presented with a pair of pictures and had to decide whether the spoken name of the first one was part of the name of the second one, without being allowed to name the pictures before having decided. In 20 pairs the spoken name of the first picture was part of the spoken name of the second one. For instance the spoken form /li/ corresponding to the word *lit* was part of the spoken form /kɔklico/ of the word *coquelicot*; in the same way the spoken form /si/ corresponding to the word *scie* was part of the spoken form /sigaʀɛt/ corresponding to the word *cigarette*. In the other 20 pairs the spoken form of the first word was not included in the spoken form of the second word. However, in order to make the task sufficiently difficult, the phonemes which existed in the first word were also present in the second word, but in a different order. For instance, the two phonemes /pɔ̃/ of the word *pont* existed also in the second word of the pair, *poisson* pronounced /pwasɔ̃/. L.B. was correct for 36/40 pairs (90%). One can therefore consider that he did not suffer from an inability to segment the phonological form of the word.

THE BUILDING OF THE PHONOLOGICAL FORM

Introduction

With pseudohomophones the patient could have recourse to the phonological form of a word, that is, to a whole phonological form that had been stored previously and could therefore be retrieved in its entirety. This was obviously not the case with ordinary non-words for which the whole phonological form had to be built from the phonological information, which had been obtained by means of print-to-sound conversion. As pseudohomophones were better read aloud by L.B. than ordinary non-words, it can be assumed that one of his difficulties was integrating the phonological units into a whole phonological form. Pseudohomophony would have allowed him to avoid the kind of processing involved in this phonological integration process.

The following experiment was conceived to specify what is involved in the building of the whole phonological form of a non-word and, more specifically, the kind of units it is based on: only phonemes obtained from single graphemes or also subsyllabic units.

In theories that presuppose that reading aloud of non-words involves grapheme-by-grapheme conversion into phonemes (e.g. Coltheart, 1978), the building of the whole phonological form is conceived as resulting from the integration of the phonemes that correspond to each graphemic unit of the non-word. As a consequence, whatever the kind of non-word, reading aloud involves the building of the whole phonological form to the same extent. No difference should therefore be observed with L.B. if one manipulates the level of units likely to be involved in non-lexical print-to-sound conversion and to be integrated afterwards into a whole phonological form. In particular subsyllabic units should not be better processed in reading than phonemic units.

Other theories presuppose that the whole phonological form can be obtained directly for syllabic or subsyllabic units that exist in written and spoken words. One is the lexical analogy theory (e.g. Marcel, 1980), which presupposes that reading of non-words involves their segmentation on the basis of the units that exist in written and spoken words. Another one, the multiple-level theory (Shallice & Warrington, 1980; Shallice et al., 1983), presupposes the existence of different levels of print-to-sound conversion, one of them corresponding to subsyllabic units. According to these last two theories there would be a hierarchy in the conversion process, so that the processing of units of the lower level (e.g. grapheme/phoneme units) would occur only if the units of the upper level (e.g. subsyllabic units) have not been processed.

If one considers two categories of written non-words made of subsyllabic units that either exist or do not exist in written words, the two groups of theory would predict different patterns of results with L.B. The first one would predict that both kinds of non-words would be read aloud in the same way; the second group would predict that non-words made of subsyllabic units that exist in written and spoken words would be better read than the others.

Experiment

Two sets of 30 CCV syllables were constructed. In the syllables of set 1, like *bre* (which, from this example, will be called BRE syllables), the consonant clusters CC were selected so that they belonged to the consonant clusters present in French written words. These clusters were taken from a corpus of 5070 written syllables analysed by Meissonier (personal communication). In the syllables of set 2, like *jra* (which, from this example, will be called JRA syllables), the consonant clusters were selected so that it was very unlikely that they existed in French written words. Concretely, they were selected among syllables which did not belong to the corpus analysed by Meissonier.

In order to assure that JRA syllables were as easily pronounceable as BRE syllables, the frequency of the spoken form of the consonant clusters CC was matched in the two lists. This frequency was determined by using a corpus of 13,500 oral syllables recorded in spontaneous speech by Pécaut and Darmstadter (1977).[1] In each set, the frequency of occurrence of the consonant clusters in the corpus of 13,500 syllables was : $F \geqslant 20$ for 17 items, $6 \leqslant F \geqslant 19$ for 8 items, and $F \leqslant 5$ for 5 items.

Thus, consonant clusters of BRE syllables exist both in French written and spoken words, whereas consonant clusters of JRA syllables do not exist in French written or spoken words. However, consonant clusters of JRA syllables also appear quite frequently in spoken language, as they are pronounced as the combination of phonemes belonging to two different words. For instance, *je ramène* is often pronounced /ʒramɛn/ in spontaneous speech, whereas it would be pronounced /ʒə/ /ramɛn/ in reading aloud.

The syllables of the two types were presented to L.B. in the same list, in a pseudo-random order. He was asked to read them, one at a time. No particular instruction was given.

Results

L.B. read significantly much better ($\chi^2 = 32.40$, $P < .001$) BRE syllables (25/30 correct) than JRA syllables (3/30 correct). The 27 errors on JRA syllables all involved at least an error on the consonant cluster. Most of the errors on these consonant clusters (78%) consisted in the replacement of the original cluster, which did not exist in French words, by a consonant cluster that did exist in French words (four of these errors were words and 16 were syllables present in French words).

---

[1]In analysing the JRA syllables, it appeared that 8/30 of these stimuli included consonant clusters which, although absent from Meissonier's corpus, in fact did exist in French written words. However, their frequency was very low, since none of them occurred more than once in the corpus of 13,500 syllables analysed by Pécaut and Darmstadter.

The criterion of whether or not a consonant cluster existed in French words seemed really to be the most important one. In particular, the 23 erroneous non-words did not systematically consist of syllables that were phonetically more simple: 14 of them had also a CCV structure that existed in French words, whereas only 9 had a CV or CVCV structure. Even though the last ones appear to be more simple, it should be underlined that they are also more frequent in French words than CCV syllables.

Visual similarity between the stimulus and the error was roughly the same as the one observed in the main experiment: in 81% (26/32) at least 50% of the letters of the stimulus appeared in the response and in 59% (19/32) these letters appeared in addition in the same order as in the stimulus.

Control Test

It was checked that L.B.'s difficulty in reading aloud JRA syllables could not be due to his short-term memory deficit. On a control test he was presented with the 30 JRA syllables again. He was first asked to read aloud a syllable. Then the printed syllable was removed and L.B. was asked to give the three phonemes contained in it. He read only 20% (8/40) of the syllables correctly whereas he repeated the three phonemes in the correct order for 90% (36/40) of the stimuli.

DISCUSSION

L.B.'s reading disturbance can be considered as typical of phonological alexia. In other words his pattern of results seems compatible with good functioning of lexical reading (irregular words were read aloud almost perfectly) with impairment of non-lexical or phonological reading. As far as phonological reading is concerned three points should be considered: (1) L.B. suffered from an impairment of the graphemic processing stage, character-ised in particular by a disturbance of the parsing mechanism; (2) given this impairment, print-to-sound conversion itself seemed preserved rather well (L.B. was able to sound single graphemes, to decide whether a syllable was homophonic to another one or to a word in most of the examples, if not all of them); (3) L.B. also had an impairment of the phonemic stage, which is discussed at length in the following subsections. Furthermore, his difficulty in reading non-words is very likely to be due to a dysfunction in the reading process itself, and not to an external artefact such as an impairment of short-term memory (he could sound out almost perfectly and in the correct order the three phonemes of a non-word after he had failed to pronounce it) or an impairment of the response buffer (in particular he could pronounce non-words when they were presented to him auditorily).

Effect of Pseudohomophony and Visual Similarity: Visual and/or Non-lexical Access?

As soon as an experiment is carried out, a particular strategy is induced by experimental conditions in two different ways: by the kind of material the subject has to process and by the instructions that he receives. The analysis of the results will therefore not allow one to answer questions such as: how did L.B. *spontaneously* read non-words? It will allow one to assess whether under certain circumstances the patient was able to use a particular strategy to read non-words. In this chapter we are concerned with the following kinds of strategy: (1) approximate visual access; (2) reading by non-lexical processing up to print-to-sound conversion included, then retrieval of a word that sounds like the printed non-word; (3) possible combination of these two strategies. It will be considered first whether the instruction of using a particular strategy (pseudohomophony or approximate visual access) affected L.B.'s performance in reading non-words. Then the significance of the main results will be examined to attempt to assess whether L.B. was able to use a particular strategy under certain conditions.

Effect of the Induction of a Particular Strategy

Strategy of Pseudohomophony.   Pseudohomophones were read significantly better than non-homophonic non-words only when L.B. was told that pseudohomophones sounded like words. It seems therefore that in order for pseudohomophony to improve his reading aloud of non-words, L.B. had to be aware of the strategy he was supposed to use and to make a deliberate effort to use it. However, it is possible that pseudohomophony produced some unconscious effect on L.B.'s performance because when the use of pseudohomophony was not suggested there was a tendency ($P<.10$) for pseudohomophones to be better read than non-homophonic non-words; in addition some words were produced as errors. Comparing L.B.'s performance for pseudohomophones when pseudohomophony was suggested and when it was not suggested, it appears that the number of erroneous words is similar, whereas the number of correct words is significantly higher when pseudohomophony is suggested. The deliberate use of pseudohomophony seems, therefore, very efficient; it never induces wrong production of words.

Strategy of Approximate Visual Access.   An attempt to induce a strategy of approximate visual access did not produce any change in L.B.'s performance. It might be that, unlike the strategy of pseudohomophony, the one of approximate visual access cannot be manipulated voluntarily by the patient, because it would operate automatically, without awareness. However, this is not certain, for two reasons. First, the suggestion of using the strategy of approximate visual access was tried with non-homophonic non-words only, whereas when no suggestion was used it was with pseudohomophones that the effect of visual similarity was the most efficient. Second, a suggestion of using a particular strategy is something difficult to bring into play; it is therefore possible that if the suggestion had been tried more or in a different way, it would have been efficient.

What Kinds of Strategy Were Used by L.B. While He Read Different Types of Non-words?

It has been shown that both pseudohomophony and visual similarity with a word did affect L.B.'s reading of non-words. In addition there was a significant interaction between the effect of these two variables. Given the interaction, one has to consider first the effect of each variable when the other did not come into play, then the interaction itself.

L.B.'s Reading of Pseudohomophones Visually Distant From a Word Reflects Non-lexical Print-to-Sound Conversion Then Recourse to Pseudohomophony

Pseudohomophones were read significantly better than non-homophonic non-words. Moreover, it is noticeable that the effect of pseudohomophony was significant even when pseudohomophones were visually distant from a word, which shows that this effect can be independent of any visual proximity between non-words and words. This is predicted if one assumes that L.B. carried out print-to-sound conversion and then had recourse to a lexical output; it is not predicted if one assumes that he read pseudohomophones by means of approximate visual lexical access. Indeed, it is obviously difficult to imagine how it would be possible to use approximate visual access when non-words are visually distant from a word. This would require a very strong tendency to use approximate visual access, together with a total lack of utilisation of the non-lexical reading process. Other data support the idea that, on the whole, L.B. read pseudohomophones visually distant from a word by means of non-lexical print-to-sound conversion. First, if L.B. had tried to use lexical access with pseudohomophones visually distant from a word, he would probably also have tried with non-homophonic non-words visually distant from a word, which would have produced a large number of erroneous words; this was obviously not the case as under the last conditions he produced mainly non-words as responses (93%). Second, with pseudohomophones visually distant from a word, when errors were words, virtually no errors bore mainly an orthographic relationship with the stimulus whereas a relatively large number of errors had mainly a phonological relationship with the stimulus. Finally, if the erroneous words resulted from approximate visual access, L.B. would have produced less erroneous words for pseudohomophones visually distant from a word than for pseudohomophones visually similar to a word, whereas the reverse pattern of results was observed.

It seems, therefore, that most often L.B.'s reading of non-words visually distant from a word was carried out by means of phonological print-to-sound conversion, then, for pseudohomophones by having recourse to the sound form of a word that sounds like the non-word.

Does the Effect of Visual Similarity Alone Reflect Minimal Approximate Visual Access?

It could be assumed that when a non-word is visually similar to a word, a lexical entry is activated. This activation might result either from an automatic process, so that the activated word has to be rejected afterwards (in case of proof correction for instance), or from a change of strategy, whatever is the reason (e.g. lack of attention, deliberate decrease of threshold, etc.). If carried out up to the output, this would produce a large number of word responses, which, if the stimuli are non-homophonic non-words, would be errors. Therefore if approximate visual lexical access is the only strategy used to read this kind of non-words, one should expect a drastic decrease of the performance together with the production of errors that are words. However, phonological information resulting from approximate visual access might be combined with the one obtained by means of non-lexical reading. For non-homophonic non-words visually similar to a word, the combinations of these two sources of phonological information might have helped L.B. to produce the correct response. By means of approximate visual access it is possible to retrieve one to several words that look like the non-word. L.B. knew that he had to produce non-words. Because the non-word had been constructed so that it differs from a word by one phoneme only, if one gets this phoneme correctly by means of non-lexical reading, then computes this information with the one obtained from approximate visual access, this should sometimes allow one to produce the correct response. However, this is a somewhat complicated process. Several words might be activated by means of approximate visual access; for instance from the printed non-word *bralé* it is possible to have approximate visual access at least to *bravé, bradé, bramé, brulé*.

On the other hand the letter/phoneme, which in the non-word is different from one of those included in one of the possible words, has to be detected by means of non-lexical reading, then integrated in a particular word to produce a non-word. Concerning the last point, one has to consider that L.B. suffered from an impairment of non-lexical reading, in particular at the level of the parsing mechanism, which might make the detection of the appropriate letter/phoneme more difficult. Given the difficulty of the task, if L.B. read non-homophonic non-words visually similar to a word by combining the two sources of phonological information, one should therefore expect his chance of producing the correct response for non-homophonic non-words visually similar to a word to be slightly higher than for non-homophonic non-words visually distant from a word.

Visual similarity significantly improved L.B.'s performance in reading aloud non-words. However, the effect of visual similarity alone (that is, independently of its interaction with pseudohomophony) was weak. Indeed for non-homophonic non-words, those which were visually similar to a word were read only marginally better than those that were visually dissimilar to a word (the tendency was far from being significant). The slight improvement in the performance, instead of a decrease, favours the idea that at least both approximate visual access and non-lexical reading processes were used in combination to read this kind of non-words. It would even be possible to assume that only the non-lexical process was used. This is questioned by the analysis of the responses because L.B., who did produce a large majority of non-words (48/60), happened to produce some erroneous words (11) too, which could be considered as resulting from approximate visual access. However, there is an alternative explanation. As non-homophonic non-words visually similar to a word are also phonologically close to these words, L.B. might have produced erroneous words "by chance," that is, by making an error while he was using the non-lexical reading process (the error word brizé/brize/ given for the non-word blizé/blize/ can be interpreted in this way).

From this analysis it appears, therefore, that approximate visual access was not the main strategy used to read non-homophonic non-words visually similar to a word.

Significance of the Interaction Between Pseudohomophony and Visual Similarity

Two kinds of explanation could be proposed to account for an interaction between pseudohomophony and visual similarity with a word. Which one is appropriate to L.B.?

The first one is the approximate visual access theory. It presupposes that when a pseudohomophone is visually similar to a word, the patient can have access to a word, which sometimes happens to have the same sound as the non-word; he would therefore produce the correct response without using non-lexical print-to-sound conversion at all. For instance, if, when presented with the non-word céché, the patient accesses the visual lexical entry séché, he would be able to pronounce /seʃe/, which corresponds to the sound of both the word and the non-word, and would therefore improve his performance. Obviously, to be efficient, this would require a particular pseudohomophone to be visually similar to one word only. This is rare for pseudohomophones.

In any case in our material numerous non-words were similar to several words. For instance from the printed non-word *céché*, it is possible to have approximate visual access to *séché*, but also at least to *léché*, *bêché*, *péché*, *caché*, *coché*, *couché*. If. L.B. had used only the approximate visual access strategy, it is therefore very unlikely that he would have produced 51/60 (85%) correct responses.

The most plausible account of the interaction is therefore to assume that L.B. used phonological information coming from both lexical and non-lexical reading processes, and obtained the correct response by combining these two kinds of information. He was told that he had to produce a word. He therefore had to select among the phonological forms of a few words the one that better corresponded to the phonological code that he obtained. This is obviously more efficient than to use approximate visual lexical access information only, and can account for the high rate of correct responses. It is easy to understand that this strategy is much more efficient for pseudohomophones visually similar to a word than for pseudohomophones visually distant from a word on the one hand, and for non-homophonic non-words visually similar to a word on the other. For pseudohomophones visually distant from a word, the process of retrieving a word sounding like the non-word is obviously much more difficult because the only lexical information that can be used then is that the response should sound like *a* word. For non-homophonic non-words visually close to a word, because a non-word has to be produced, the non-lexical reading process is more involved, in particular the parsing mechanism that is impaired in this patient.

Conclusions

From the preceding analysis it is obvious that L.B. very often tried to read non-words by means of non-lexical processing alone, or in combination with approximate visual access. It is unlikely that he often used only approximate visual access. This is confirmed by other-data. On the whole, L.B. produced virtually as many non-words as words; in addition, two-thirds of his errors in the main experiment were non-words. When non-words were neither pseudo-homophonic nor visually similar to a real word, that is, when no relationship with a word was experimentally induced, he produced virtually no word as erroneous responses (2/60); almost all his responses were non-words. Finally, when errors were words there were virtually no errors (8%) that bore a clear, mainly orthographic relationship with the stimulus, whereas there was a considerable number of errors (32%) that had a mainly phonological relationship with the stimulus.

L.B.'s reading of pseudohomophones clearly supports the idea that he read them by means of print-to-sound conversion, then retrieval of the phonological form of a word that sounded like the non-word.

What Is Involved in the Building of the Whole Phonological Form?

The effect of pseudohomophony on L.B.'s reading of non-words was ascribed to the fact that it allowed him to get over his difficulty to build the whole phonological form. Instead of constructing the whole phonological form of the non-word from phonological information obtained by means of print-to-sound conversion (the phonological code), he would have retrieved the phonological form of a word that shares the same phonological code with it (a word sounding like the non-word). If so, the effect of pseudohomophony in L.B. constitutes evidence supporting the existence of what was defined as the "phonemic" stage in the non-lexical reading process, that is, the stage at which the phonological whole form is constructed.

From which kind of units is the phonological whole form built? In the present experiment syllables, including subsyllabic segments that exist in French words (BRE syllables), were almost perfectly read aloud by L.B. (25/30), whereas syllables that did not include such segments (JRA syllables) were virtually never read correctly (3/30). Subsyllabic segments seem therefore to be a crucial variable in non-lexical reading. In L.B.'s reading of non-words their effect parallels that of pseudohomophony, but is much stronger. If one considers that with BRE syllables the building of the whole phonological form is avoided whereas it cannot be avoided with JRA syllables, the above results constitute evidence that one kind of unit involved in non-lexical print-to-sound conversion and from which the whole phonological form is built are subsyllabic segments.

Such results are not predicted by theories that presuppose that reading aloud of non-words involves only grapheme-to-phoneme conversion (e.g. Coltheart, 1978). Indeed, from this point of view BRE and JRA syllables are strictly equivalent: whatever the type of syllable, one grapheme has to be converted into one phoneme, each grapheme–phoneme correspondence is familiar to a French reader, each syllable can be pronounced easily. According to such theories the building of the whole phonological form would be involved to the same extent with JRA syllables and with BRE syllables.

The difference observed between these two types of syllables would be predicted by two other kinds of theory. According to Marcel's (1980) point of view, *bre*, which is a syllable existing in a word, will not be segmented and will be retrieved at the phonological level as a syllable; whereas *jra*, which does not exist in a French word, will be segmented into three graphemes corresponding to three phonemes, which will have to be retrieved separately, then combined into a whole phonological form. According to the multiple-level theory (Shallice et al., 1983; Shallice & McCarthy, Chapter 15 in this book), print-to-sound conversion is carried out in parallel at different levels: morphemic, syllabic, subsyllabic, and graphemic. It can therefore be predicted that the performance for JRA syllables will be worse than the one for BRE syllables, because for the latter a subsyllabic unit can be retrieved as such, which is not possible for the former.

ACKNOWLEDGEMENTS

We particularly acknowledge the editors of this book, especially K.E. Patterson whose numerous comments were very helpful. We are grateful to T. Shallice for his helpful criticisms. We thank Professor C. Derouesné who permitted us to examine his patient. We are grateful to N. Smith who provided the multi-variate analysis. We acknowledge the assistance of D. Marinolli and H. Delisle in building some of the tests. We thank Professor J. Borie and Dr E. Turrell who provided the CT scans. We also wish to thank V. Meissonnier who provided us with personal data on the frequencies of French written syllables.

REFERENCES

Beauvois, M. F., & Derouesné, J. (1979a). Phonological alexia: Three dissociations. *Journal of Neurology, Neurosurgery and Psychiatry, 42*, 1115–1124.

Beauvois, M. F., & Derouesné, J. (1979b). Reading without phonology. Data from phonological alexia without expressive or receptive aphasia. Paper presented at the International Neuropsychological Society, Holland, June 1979.

Beauvois, M. F., Derouesné, J., & Saillant, B. (1980). Syndromes neuropsychologiques et psychologie cognitive. Trois exemples: aphasie tactile, alexie phonologique et agraphie lexicale. *Cahiers de Psychologie, 23*, 211–245.

Bender, L. (1967). *Test moteur de structuration visuelle*. Paris: Editions du Centre de Psychologie Appliquée.

Binois, R., & Pichot, P. (1958). *Test de vocabulaire*. Paris: Editions du Centre de Psychologie Appliquée.

Bub, D. (1983). Phonological processes in reading. Paper presented at the meeting on Cognitive Neuropsychology of Language, Venice, 1983.

Bub, D., & Kertesz, A. (1982). Deep agraphia. *Brain and Language, 17*, 146–165.

Coltheart, M. (1978). Lexical access in simple reading tasks. In G. Underwood (ed.), *Strategies of Information Processing*, London: Academic Press.

Coltheart, M. (1980). Reading, phonological encoding and deep dyslexia. In M. Coltheart, K. E. Patterson, & J. C. Marshall (eds.), *Deep Dyslexia*, London: Routledge & Kegan Paul.

Coltheart, M., Besner, D., Jonasson, J. T., & Davelaar, E. (1979). Phonological encoding in the lexical decision task. *Quarterly Journal of Experimental Psychology, 31*, 489-507.

Cox, D. R. (1970). *The Analysis of Binary Data*. London: Methuen.

de Renzi, E., & Vignolo, L.A. (1962). The token test: A sensitive test to detect receptive disturbances in aphasics. *Brain, 85*, 665–678.

Derouesné, J., & Beauvois, M. F. (1979). Phonological processing in reading: Data from alexia. *Journal of Neurology, Neurosurgery and Psychiatry, 42*, 1125–1132.

Ducarne de Ribaucourt, B. (1976). *Test pour l'examen de l'aphasie*. Paris: Editions du Centre de Psychologie Appliquée.

Funnell, E. (1983). Phonological processes in reading: New evidence from acquired dyslexia. *British Journal of Psychology, 74*, 159–180.

Henderson, L. (1982). *Orthography and Word Recognition in Reading*. London: Academic Press.

Juilland, A., Broding, D., & Davidovitch, C. (1970). Frequency of French words. In A. Juilland (ed.), *The Romance Languages and Their Structures*, The Hague: Mouton.

Lefavrais, P. (1963). *Test de l'alouette*. Paris: Editions du Centre de Psychologie Appliquée.

Légé, Y., & Dague, P. (1976). *Test de vocabulaire en images*. Paris: Editions du Centre de Psychologie Appliquée.

Marcel, A. (1980). Surface dyslexia and beginning reading: A revised version of the pronunciation of print and its impairments. In M. Coltheart, K. E. Patterson, & J. C. Marshall (eds.), *Deep Dyslexia*, London: Routledge & Kegan Paul.

Marshall, J. C., & Newcombe, F. (1973). Pattern of paralexia: A psycholinguistic approach. *Journal of Psycholinguistic Research, 2*, 175–200.

Martin, R. C. (1982). The pseudohomophone effect: The role of visual similarity in non-word decisions. *Quarterly Journal of Experimental Psychology, 34A*, 395–409.

Miceli, G., Silveri, C., & Caramazza, A. (1983). The role of the graphemic output buffer and the phoneme–grapheme conversion system in writing: Evidence of a case of pure dysgraphia. Paper presented at the Conference on Cognitive Neuropsychology of Language, Venice, 1983.

Morton, J., & Patterson, K. E. (1980). A new attempt at an interpretation, or, an attempt at a new interpretation. In M. Coltheart, K. E. Patterson, & J. C. Marshall (eds.), *Deep Dyslexia*. London: Routledge & Kegan Paul.

Oldfield, R. C. (1971). The assessment and analysis of handedness: The Edinburgh Inventory. *Neuropsychologia, 9*, 97–113.

Parkin, A. J., & Underwood, G. (1983). Orthographic versus phonological irregularity in lexical decision. *Memory and Cognition, 11*, 351–355.

Patterson, K. E. (1982). The relation between reading and phonological coding: Further neuropsychological observations. In A. W. Ellis (ed.), *Normality and Pathology in Cognitive Functions*, London: Academic Press.

Patterson, K. E., & Marcel, A. J. (1977). Aphasia, dyslexia and the phonological coding of written words. *Quarterly Journal of Experimental Psychology, 29*, 307–318.

Pécaut, N., & Darmstadter, D. (1977). Verbalisation des groupes consonantiques chez des aphasiques présentant des troubles articulatoires et chez des alexiques. Mémoire pour le certificat de capacité d'orthophoniste. Université Paris VI, Paris, 1977.

Saffran, E. M., & Marin, O. S. M. (1977). Reading without phonology: Evidence from aphasia. *Quarterly Journal of Experimental Psychology, 29*, 515–525.

Shallice, T. (1981). Phonological agraphia and the lexical route in writing. *Brain, 104*, 413–429.

Shallice, T., & Warrington, E. K. (1975). Word recognition in a phonemic dyslexic patient. *Quarterly Journal of Experimental Psychology, 27*, 187–199.

Shallice, T., & Warrington, E. K. (1980). Single and multiple component central dyslexic syndromes. In M. Coltheart, K. E. Patterson, & J. C. Marshall (eds.), *Deep Dyslexia*, London: Routledge & Kegan Paul.

Shallice, T., Warrington, E. K., & McCarthy, R. (1983). Reading without semantics. *Quarterly Journal of Experimental Psychology, 35A*, 111–138.

Temple, C. M., & Marshall, J. C. (1983). A case study of developmental phonological dyslexia. *British Journal of Psychology, 74*, 517–533.

Warrington, E. K. (1984). *Recognition Memory Tests*. Windsor: NFER Nelson.

APPENDIX I

Main Experiment: Suggested Homophonic Strategy

TABLE 1
Pseudohomophones: Visually Dissimilar—Graphemically Simple

Stimulus			L.B.'s Response	
Written Non-Word	*Spoken Non-Word*	*Word base[a] of Non-Word*	*Spoken[b]*	*Written[c]*
INCORRECT RESPONSES (WORDS)				
koké	/kɔke/	coquet	/kafe/	café
kozé	/koze/	causé	/eko/	écho
afécé	/afese/	affaissé	/ɛfase/	effacé
kasyé	/kɑzje/	casier	/kafe/	café
açajy	/asaʒi/	assagi	/akaʒu/	acajou
serso	/sɛʀso/	cerceau	/sɛʀvo/	cerveau
syvyl	/sivil/	civil	/silvɛstʀə/	sylvestre
préry	/pʀeʀi/	prairie	/pʀesi/	précis
fisik	/fizik/	physique	/finiʃ/	finish
INCORRECT RESPONSE (NON-WORD)				
ocito	/osito/	aussitôt	/kɔʒito/	cojito
CORRECT RESPONSES				
tono	/tɔno/	tonneau		
siso	/sizo/	ciseaux		
kacé	/kɑse/	cassé		
kavo	/kavo/	caveau		
moné	/mɔne/	monnaie		
tyçu	/tisy/	tissu		
sécé	/sese/	cessé		
mové	/mɔve/	mauvais		
cénié	/seɲe/	saigné		
abécé	/abese/	abaissé		
acéni	/aseni/	assaini		
cinié	/siɲe/	signé		
kolyé	/kɔlje/	collier		
ocito	/osito/	aussitôt		
berso	/bɛʀso/	berceau		
aplyk	/aplik/	applique		
komik	/kɔmik/	comique		
krapo	/kʀapo/	crapaud		
servo	/sɛʀvo/	cerveau		
morso	/mɔʀso/	morceau		

Note: The following footnotes apply throughout Appendices 1–5.
[a]: Spelling of the word from which the written non-word has been built.
[b]: Spoken response given by L.B.
[c]: One possible spelling of the incorrect response given by L.B.

TABLE 2
Pseudohomophones: Visually Similar—Graphemically Simple

Stimulus			L.B.'s Response	
Written Non-Word	Spoken Non-Word	Word base[a] of Non-Word	Spoken[b]	Written[c]
INCORRECT RESPONSES (WORDS)				
cévi	/sevi/	sévi	/sevɛʀ/	sévère
sakré	/sakʀe/	sacré	/sake/	saqué
ésité	/ezite/	hésité	/ɔbezite/	obésité
INCORRECT RESPONSE (NON-WORD)				
baklé	/bɑkle/	baclé	/kave/	kavé
CORRECT RESPONSES				
ruzé	/ʀyze/	rusé		
cano	/kano/	canot		
najé	/naʒe/	nagé		
vizé	/vize/	visé		
galo	/galo/	galop		
nomé	/nɔme/	nommé		
tapi	/tapi/	tapis		
salu	/saly/	salut		
kafé	/kafe/	café		
alumé	/alyme/	allumé		
abité	/abite/	habité		
éfacé	/efase/	effacé		
ydéal	/ideal/	idéal		
citué	/sitɥe/	situé		
panié	/panje/	panier		
ocupé	/ɔkype/	occupé		
arivé	/aʀive/	arrivé		
papié	/papje/	papier		
jiclé	/ʒikle/	giclé		
cofré	/kɔfʀe/	coffré		
ordur	/ɔʀdyʀ/	ordure		
brizé	/bʀize/	brisé		
forsé	/fɔʀse/	forcé		
ostil	/ɔstil/	hostile		
alcol	/alkɔl/	alcool		
parol	/paʀɔl/	parole		

TABLE 3
Pseudohomophones: Visually Dissimilar—Graphemically Complex

Stimulus			L.B.'s Response	
Written Non-Word	Spoken Non-Word	Word base[a] of Non-Word	Spoken[b]	Written[c]
INCORRECT RESPONSES (WORDS)				
aigo	/ego/	égaux	/aʒjo/	agio
airo	/ero/	héros	/aeʀɔ/	aéro
ydai	/ide/	idée	/dɛ/	dais
syman	/simã/	ciment	/sɛ̃patik/	sympathique
rauzé	/ʀoze/	rosé	/ʀɑze/	rasé
pholy	/fɔli/	folie	/filo/	philo
angré	/ãgʀe/	engrais	/agʀɛ/	agrès
phryr	/fʀiʀ/	frire	/faʀɛ̃ks/	pharynx
englé	/ãgle/	anglais	/ãgl/	angle
aksan	/aksã/	accent	/astʀakã/	astrakan
INCORRECT RESPONSES (NON-WORD)				
ylau	/ilo/	îlot	/igʀɛk, lo/	y, lau
auzé	/oze/	osé	/zote/	zauté
ajan	/aʒã/	agent	/alʒã/	aljan
lauké	/lɔke/	loquet	/lɔte/	lauté
déphé	/defe/	défait	/defʀe/	déphré
phuzi	/fyzi/	fusil	/fizi/	phizi
cèzon	/sɛzɔ̃/	saison	/sɛtɔ̃/	cèton
akrau	/akʀo/	accroc	/kakʀo/	kakrau
klyan	/klijã/	client	/kleã/	kléan
CORRECT RESPONSES				
aphu	/afy/	affût		
aimo	/emo/	émaux		
insy	/ɛ̃si/	ainsi		
ékau	/eko/	écho		
phécé	/fese/	fessée		
kaulé	/kɔle/	collé		
raizo	/ʀezo/	réseau		
sfair	/sfɛʀ/	sphère		
entik	/ãtik/	antique		
oprai	/opʀɛ/	auprès		
yvair	/ivɛʀ/	hiver		

TABLE 4
Pseudohomophones: Visually Similar—Graphemically Complex

Stimulus			L.B.'s Response	
Written Non-Word	Spoken Non-Word	Word base[a] of Non-Word	Spoken[b]	Written[c]
INCORRECT RESPONSES (WORDS)				
élen	/elã/	élan	/elemãtɛʀ/	élémentaire
augur	/ɔgyʀ/	augure	/agʀym/	agrume
INCORRECT RESPONSES (NON-WORD)				
ibou	/ibu/	hibou	/idu/	idou
anté	/ãte/	hanté	/ɔ̃te/	onté
NO RESPONSE				
angar	/ãgaʀ/	hangar		
CORRECT RESPONSES				
biai	/bjɛ/	biais		
céché	/seʃe/	séché		
valon	/valɔ̃/	vallon		
néan	/neã/	néant		
outi	/uti/	outil		
aizé	/eze/	aisé		
aman	/amã/	amant		
badau	/bado/	badaud		
balei	/balɛ/	balai		
nouri	/nuʀi/	nourri		
jenou	/ʒənu/	genou		
vandu	/vãdy/	vendu		
vagon	/vagɔ̃/	wagon		
debou	/dəbu/	debout		
nivau	/nivo/	niveau		
défau	/defo/	défaut		
genti	/ʒãti/	gentil		
intru	/ẽtʀy/	intrus		
ékrin	/ekʀẽ/	écrin		
ékrou	/ekʀu/	écrou		
antré	/ãtʀe/	entré		
parfin	/paʀfẽ/	parfum		
oubly	/ubli/	oubli		
auror	/oʀɔʀ/	aurore		
cleir	/klɛʀ/	clair		

TABLE 5
Non-words: Visually Dissimilar—Graphemically Simple

Stimulus		L.B.'s Response	
Written Non-Word	Spoken Non-Word	Spoken[b]	Written[c]
INCORRECT RESPONSES (NON-WORDS)			
guzé	/gyze/	/dyze/	duzé
tiko	/tiko/	/kiko/	kiko
jazu	/ʒazy/	/ʒyla/	jula
zida	/zida/	/zila/	zila
ilogu	/ilogy/	/igoly/	igolu
agoza	/agoza/	/gagola/	gagola
jofyé	/ʒɔfje/	/eʒɔkse/	éjoksé
ukobi	/ykobi/	/yʀydi/	urudi
ézida	/ezida/	/edida/	édida
refyé	/ʀəfje/	/ʀife/	ryfé
nolié	/nolje/	/golje/	golié
ozajo	/ozaʒo/	/zanak/	zanac
pilko	/pilko/	/pʀilko/	prilko
sojid	/soʒid/	/kolid/	colid
fisaf	/fisaf/	/fita/	fita
sfapi	/sfapi/	/pagi/	pagui
pruso	/pʀyzo/	/pʀyso/	prusso
tersa	/tɛʀsa/	/tesa/	tessa
kurpa	/kyʀpa/	/pyʀda/	purda
kubol	/kybol/	/tʀybol/	trubol
CORRECT RESPONSES			
béto	/beto/		
jéra	/ʒeʀa/		
févi	/fevi/		
vifo	/vifo/		
zoka	/zoka/		
péfu	/pefy/		
zinié	/zinje/		
izéco	/izeko/		
fulvo	/fylvo/		
ibluk	/iblyk/		

TABLE 6
Non-Words: Visually Similar—Graphemically Simple

Stimulus			L.B.'s Response	
Written Non-Word	Spoken Non-Word	Word base[a] of Non-Word	Spoken[b]	Written[c]
INCORRECT RESPONSES (WORDS)				
denu	/dəny/	tenu	/deni/	déni
vemu	/vəmy/	velu	/vety/	vêtu
bâvi	/bɑvi/	bâti	/bɑ/	bas
abovi	/abɔvi/	aboli	/abɔli/	aboli
aclif	/aklif/	actif	/aktiv/	active
blisé	/blize/	brisé	/bʀize/	brisé
INCORRECT RESPONSES (NON-WORDS)				
pami	/pami/	pari	/pani/	pani
jôté	/ʒote/	côté	/dole/	dolé
sepé	/səpe/	semé	/ɛspe/	espé
solé	/sole/	salé	/solʀe/	solré
rôpi	/ʀopi/	rôti	/dʀʀopi/	dropi
épevé	/epəve/	élevé	/epʀəve/	éprevé
avité	/avite/	agité	/navite/	navité
opéla	/ɔpela/	opéra	/ɔbela/	obéla
idoal	/idoal/	idéal	/odual/	odoual
terçu	/tɛʀsy/	perçu	/tʀɛke/	trèké
banul	/banyl/	banal	/bany/	banu
capmé	/kapme/	calmé	/kamne/	camné
NO RESPONSE				
alusé	/alyze/	amusé		
CORRECT RESPONSES				
goli	/gɔli/	poli		
rébé	/ʀebe/	bébé		
ivadé	/ivade/	évadé		
épité	/epite/	évité		
azimé	/azime/	animé		
itolé	/itɔle/	isolé		
birné	/biʀne/	borné		
bralé	/bʀɑle/	brûlé		
zadré	/zɑdʀe/	cadré		
pivil	/pivil/	civil		
varil	/vaʀril/	baril		

TABLE 7
Non-Words: Visually Dissimilar—Graphemically Complex

Stimulus		L.B.'s Response	
Written Non-Word	Spoken Non-Word	Spoken[b]	Written[c]
INCORRECT RESPONSES (WORDS)			
phiko	/fiko/	/piko/	picot
dazon	/dazɔ̃/	/dra/	drap
INCORRECT RESPONSES (NON-WORDS)			
yzin	/izɛ̃/	/yzy/	uzu
eulo	/ølo/	/yzo/	uzo
anru	/ɑ̃ʀy/	/ɑ̃kry/	ancʀu
inzé	/ɛ̃ze/	/ize/	izé
onzu	/ɔ̃zy/	/yzɔn/	uzone
eiri	/ɛʀi/	/iʀi/	iri
yché	/iʃe/	/sve/	své
zaiga	/zɛga/	/zaiga/	zaïga
phajo	/faʒo/	/pago/	pago
zinbi	/zɛ̃bi/	/zinby/	zinebu
zikai	/zikɛ/	/zinkɛ/	zinekai
zungu	/zœ̃gy/	/zygy/	zugu
kinti	/kɛ̃ti/	/inti/	ineti
nanlo	/nɑ̃lo/	/mɑ̃go/	mango
igron	/igʀɔ̃/	/igɔ̃/	igon
inlur	/ɛ̃lyʀ/	/inedyʀ/	inédur
spour	/spuʀ/	/spʀud/	sproud
enblo	/ɑ̃blo/	/ɔnblo/	oneblo
blyan	/blijɑ̃/	/bʀigan/	brygane
iksau	/ikso/	/iʀko/	irkau
usfon	/ysfɔ̃/	/yfɔn/	ufone
NO RESPONSE			
oubru	/ubʀy/		
abair	/abɛʀ/		
CORRECT RESPONSES			
agau	/ago/		
aicy	/ɛsi/		
ujau	/yʒo/		
zaché	/zaʃe/		
ansul	/ɑ̃syl/		

TABLE 8
Non-Words: Visually Similar—Graphemically Complex

Stimulus			L.B.'s Response	
Written Non-Word	Spoken Non-Word	Word base[a] of Non-Word	Spoken[b]	Written[c]
INCORRECT RESPONSES (WORDS)				
toué	/twe/	loué	/tRue/	troué
ilan	/ilã/	élan	/alɛ̃/	alain
moué	/mwe/	noué	/nwe/	noué
paidi	/pedi/	raidi	/pRedi/	prédit
coubé	/kube/	coupé	/kuRbe/	courbé
INCORRECT RESPONSES (NON-WORDS)				
aufo	/ofo/	auto	/ofwa/	aufoi
poué	/pwe/	doué	/pRue/	proué
aifu	/efy/	aigu	/wafy/	oifu
falon	/falɔ̃/	talon	/fatɔ̃/	faton
vombé	/vɔ̃be/	tombé	/vRɔ̃be/	vrombé
mouju	/muʒy/	moulu	/Rufy/	roufu
jalin	/ʒalɛ̃/	malin	/ʒaRlɛ̃/	jarlin
phito	/fito/	photo	/fido/	phido
méchu	/meʃu/	déchu	/efy/	éphu
ronté	/Rɔ̃te/	bonté	/Ruté/	routé
épran	/epRã/	écran	/etRã/	étran
édrou	/edRu/	écrou	/edRy/	édru
aumel	/omɛl/	autel	/amɛl/	amel
échac	/eʃak/	échec	/ekak/	écac
évrin	/evRɛ̃/	écrin	/evRi/	évri
CORRECT RESPONSES				
aijé	/eʒe/	aisé		
aiké	/eke/	aimé		
aimi	/emi/	aimé		
aivé	/eve/	ailé		
lovin	/lɔvɛ̃/	bovin		
abour	/abuR/	amour		
agour	/aguR/	atour		
impar	/ɛ̃paR/	impur		
enfur	/ãfyR/	enfer		
engol	/ãgɔl/	envol		

APPENDIX II

Control Experiment 1: Homophonic Strategy Not Suggested

TABLE 1
Pseudohomophones: Visually Dissimilar—Graphemically Simple

Stimulus			*L.B.'s Response*	
Written Non-Word	*Spoken Non-Word*	*Word base[a] of Non-Word*	*Spoken[b]*	*Written[c]*
INCORRECT RESPONSES (WORDS)				
koké	/kɔke/	coquet	/kɔle/	collé
kacé	/kɑse/	cassé	/tʀase/	tracé
kavo	/kavo/	caveau	/kaʀo/	carreau
cénié	/seɲe/	saigné	/denje/	dénié
kasyé	/kɑzje/	casier	/kaje/	cahier
kolyé	/kɔlje/	collier	/kɔle/	collé
serso	/sɛʀso/	cerceau	/sɛʀvo/	cerveau
fisik	/fizik/	physique	/finiʃ/	finish
INCORRECT RESPONSES (NON-WORDS)				
siso	/sizo/	ciseaux	/siko/	sico
moné	/mɔne/	monnaie	/nɔne/	noné
mové	/mɔve/	mauvais	/nɔve/	nové
ocito	/osito/	aussitôt	/osiko/	ocico
aplyk	/aplik/	applique	/kaʀpit/	karpite
syvyl	/sivil/	civil	/silvil/	sylvyl
komik	/kɔmik/	comique	/kʀəmy/	kremu
krapo	/kʀapo/	crapaud	/kaʀpo/	karpo
CORRECT RESPONSES				
tono	/tɔno/	tonneau		
kozé	/koze/	causé		
tyçu	/tisy/	tissu		
sécé	/sese/	cessé		
afécé	/afese/	affaissé		
abécé	/abese/	abaissé		
açajy	/asaʒi/	assagi		
acéni	/aseni/	assaini		
cinié	/siɲe/	signé		
ocito	/osito/	aussitôt		
berso	/bɛʀso/	berceau		
préry	/pʀeʀi/	prairie		
servo	/sɛʀvo/	cerveau		
morso	/mɔʀso/	morceau		

TABLE 2
Pseudohomophones: Visually Similar—Graphemically Simple

	Stimulus		L.B.'s Response	
Written Non-Word	Spoken Non-Word	Word base[a] of Non-Word	Spoken[b]	Written[c]
INCORRECT RESPONSES (WORDS)				
cévi	/sevi/	sévi	/sivɛ/	civet
panié	/panje/	panier	/pane/	pané
baklé	/bɑkle/	baclé	/bakɛ/	baquet
cofré	/kɔfʀe/	coffré	/kabʀe/	cabré
forsé	/fɔʀse/	forcé	/fɔʀʒe/	forgé
INCORRECT RESPONSES (NON-WORDS)				
najé	/naʒe/	nagé	/nale/	nalé
ésité	/ezite/	hésité	/edise/	édicé
ocupé	/ɔkype/	occupé	/ɔkɥe/	ocué
jiclé	/ʒikle/	giclé	/sikle/	ciclé
ordur	/ɔʀdyʀ/	ordure	/ɔʀdy/	ordu
brizé	/bʀize/	brisé	/bʀizje/	brizié
sakré	/sakʀe/	sacré	/saʀe/	saré
parol	/paʀɔl/	parole	/paʀsɔl/	parsol
NO RESPONSE				
ruzé	/ʀyze/	rusé		
CORRECT RESPONSE				
cano	/kano/	canot		
vizé	/vize/	visé		
galo	/galo/	galop		
nomé	/nɔme/	nommé		
tapi	/tapi/	tapis		
salu	/saly/	salut		
kafé	/kafe/	café		
alumé	/alyme/	allumé		
abité	/abite/	habité		
éfacé	/efase/	effacé		
ydéal	/ideal/	idéal		
citué	/sitɥe/	situé		
arivé	/aʀive/	arrivé		
papié	/papje/	papier		
ostil	/ɔstil/	hostile		
alcol	/alkɔl/	alcool		

TABLE 3
Non-Words: Visually Dissimilar—Graphemically Simple

Stimulus		L.B.'s Response	
Written Non-Word	Spoken Non-Word	Spoken[b]	Written[c]
INCORRECT RESPONSES (WORDS)			
béto	/beto/	/eto/	étau
refyé	/Rəfje/	/Rəleje/	relayé
INCORRECT RESPONSES (NON-WORDS)			
jéra	/ʒeRa/	/ʒipa/	jipa
févi	/fevi/	/feli/	féli
vifo	/vifo/	/sivo/	sivo
zoka	/zoka/	/zola/	zola
péfu	/pefy/	/fely/	félu
zinié	/zinje/	/zinənje/	zinenié
agoza	/agoza/	/akoza/	akoza
jofyé	/ʒofje/	/doflje/	doflyé
ukobi	/ykobi/	/ditobi/	ditobi
ézida	/ezida/	/ezja/	ézia
ozajo	/ozaʒo/	/azoʃo/	azocho
izéco	/izeko/	/ezeko/	ézéco
fulvo	/fylvo/	/fylfo/	fulfo
pilko	/pilko/	/pRilko/	prilko
ibluk	/iblyk/	/iblo/	iblo
sojid	/soʒid/	/ʃolid/	cholid
fisaf	/fisaf/	/fidal/	fidal
sfapi	/sfapi/	/sRapi/	srapi
pruso	/pRyzo/	/pRono/	prono
kurpa	/kyRpa/	/tyRpa/	turpa
kubov	/kybov/	/tRybov/	trubov
tersa	/tɛRsa/	/taRsa/	tarsa
CORRECT RESPONSES			
guzé	/gyze/		
tiko	/tiko/		
jazu	/ʒazy/		
zida	/zida/		
ilogu	/ilogy/		
nolié	/nolje/		

TABLE 4
Non-Words: Visually Similar—Graphemically Simple

Stimulus			L.B.'s Response	
Written Non-Word	Spoken Non-Word	Word base[a] of Non-Word	Spoken[b]	Written[c]
INCORRECT RESPONSES (WORDS)				
avité	/avite/	agité	/gʀavite/	gravité
terçu	/tɛʀsy/	perçu	/ʀəsy/	reçu
blisé	/blize/	brisé	/bʀize/	brisé
pami	/pami/	pari	/paʀmi/	parmi
vemu	/vəmy/	velu	/vety/	vêtu
INCORRECT RESPONSES (NON-WORDS)				
jôté	/ʒote/	côté	/ʒobe/	jobé
rébé	/ʀebe/	bébé	/ebe/	ébé
rôpi	/ʀopi/	rôti	/ʀypi/	rupi
épevé	/epəve/	élevé	/epʀəve/	éprevé
opéla	/ɔpela/	opéra	/ɔbela/	obéla
idoal	/idoal/	idéal	/idolal/	idolal
aclif	/aklif/	actif	/aktil/	actil
bralé	/bʀale/	brûlé	/pʀabe/	prabé
zadré	/zɑdʀe/	cadré	/dʀe/	dré
capmé	/kapme/	calmé	/kamne/	camné
pivil	/pivil/	civil	/ivil/	ivil
CORRECT RESPONSES				
goli	/gɔli/	poli		
denu	/dəny/	tenu		
sepé	/səpe/	semé		
solé	/sole/	salé		
bâvi	/bɑvi/	bâti		
ivadé	/ivade/	évadé		
épité	/epite/	évité		
alusé	/alyze/	amusé		
azimé	/azime/	animé		
itolé	/itɔle/	isolé		
abovi	/abɔvi/	aboli		
banul	/banyl/	banal		
birné	/biʀne/	borné		
varil	/vaʀil/	baril		

APPENDIX III

Control Experiment 2: Suggested Visual Strategy

	Stimulus		L.B.'s Response	
Written Non-Word	Spoken Non-Word	Word base[a] of Non-Word	Spoken[b]	Written[c]
INCORRECT RESPONSES (WORDS)				
rébé	/ʀebe/	bébé	/ʀeve/	rêvé
vemu	/vəmy/	velu	/vety/	vêtu
abovi	/abɔvi/	aboli	/abɔli/	aboli
aclif	/aklif/	actif	/aktif/	actif
zadré	/zɑdʀe/	cadré	/kɑdʀe/	cadré
INCORRECT RESPONSES (NON-WORDS)				
denu	/dəny/	tenu	/dany/	danu
sepé	/səpe/	semé	/sœlpe/	seulpé
bâvi	/bɑvi/	bâti	/vali/	vali
épevé	/epəve/	élevé	/epəne/	épené
idoal	/idoal/	idéal	/idolal/	idolal
itolé	/itɔle/	isolé	/lizɔle/	lisolé
terçu	/tɛʀsy/	perçu	/tʀesy/	tréçu
bralé	/bʀale/	brûlé	/bʀəle/	brelé
capmé	/kapme/	calmé	/kɑ̃pme/	campmé
pivil	/pivil/	civil	/pival/	pival
CORRECT RESPONSES				
pami	/pamì/	pari		
goli	/gɔli/	poli		
jôté	/ʒote/	côté		
solé	/sɔle/	salé		
rôpi	/ʀopi/	rôti		
ivadé	/ivade/	évadé		
épité	/epite/	évité		
alusé	/alyze/	amusé		
avité	/avite/	agité		
azimé	/azime/	animé		
opéla	/ɔpela/	opéra		
banul	/banyl/	banal		
birné	/biʀne/	borné		
blisé	/blize/	brisé		
varil	/vaʀil/	baril		

APPENDIX IV

The Building of the Phonological Form

TABLE 1
Consonant Clusters (CC) That Exist in French Written Words

Stimulus		L.B.'s Response	
Written Non-Word	*Spoken Non-Word*	*Spoken[b]*	*Written[c]*
INCORRECT RESPONSES (WORDS)			
fra	/fʀa/	/bʀa/	bras
vro	/vʀo/	/bʀo/	broc
INCORRECT RESPONSES (NON-WORDS)			
vra	/vʀa/	/fʀa/	fra
dre	/dʀə/	/gʀə/	gre
psa	/psa/	/das/	dasse
CORRECT RESPONSES			
fru	/fʀy/		
psi	/psi/		
gre	/gʀə/		
spe	/spə/		
spi	/spi/		
fle	/flə/		
spa	/spa/		
blu	/bly/		
fla	/fla/		
dri	/dʀi/		
pso	/pso/		
fli	/fli/		
pso	/pso/		
gre	/gʀə/		
bli	/bli/		
fro	/fʀo/		
glo	/glo/		
bre	/bʀə/		
dro	/dʀo/		
bre	/bʀə/		
gli	/gli/		
bla	/bla/		
spé	/spe/		
flé	/fle/		
pse	/psə/		

TABLE 2
Consonant Clusters (CC) That Do Not Exist in French Written Words

Stimulus		L.B.'s Response	
Written Non-Word	Spoken Non-Word	Spoken[b]	Written[c]
INCORRECT RESPONSES (WORDS)			
dso	/dso/	/do/	dos
kja	/kʒa/	/kaʒ/	cage
kdé	/kde/	/delɛ/	délai
jmo	/ʒmo/	/mo/	mot
INCORRECT RESPONSES (NON-WORDS)			
dli	/dli/	/dili/	dili
jsa	/ʒsa/	/ʒa/	ja
jpe	/ʒpə/	/dʒe/	djé
jpo	/ʒpo/	/dʒa/	dja
kjo	/kʒo/	/dʒo/	djo
dsi	/dsi/	/ksi/	ksi
jsi	/ʒsi/	/psi/	psi
dle	/dlə/	/dvə/	dve
dsé	/dse/	/gne/	guené
dlu	/dly/	/gny/	guenu
kju	/kʒy/	/kny/	knu
jpi	/ʒpi/	/silpi/	silpi
jko	/ʒko/	/dʒo/	djo
jré	/ʒʀe/	/dʒe/	djé
nsa	/nsa/	/na/	na
jto	/ʒto/	/ʒdo/	jdo
lru	/lʀy/	/ʀyly/	rulu
jku	/ʒky/	/ʒiky/	jiku
jra	/ʒra/	/dʒena/	djéna
jla	/ʒla/	/ʒela/	jéla
zlu	/zly/	/zy/	zu
jta	/ʒta/	/ita/	ita
jlu	/ʒly/	/dʒily/	djilu
CORRECT RESPONSES			
kji	/kʒi/		
dsa	/dsa/		
jso	/ʒso/		

17

Issues in the Modelling of Pronunciation Assembly in Normal Reading

L. Henderson

In what follows, I have attempted to chart the linguistic and behavioural data that might be expected to constrain models of the translation of print into sound in the unimpaired reading of English words. The chapter is divided into three sections. The first section sets out a memorandum of the pertinent characteristics of English orthography. The second section reviews the literature on the speeded naming of isolated English words. The third section introduces and evaluates the main theoretical options that have been considered in constructing models of orthographic translation for English.

ENGLISH ORTHOGRAPHY

English orthography has been described in a number of linguistic works (Albrow, 1972; Haas, 1970; Venezky, 1970; Wijk, 1966). My purpose here is simply to remind the reader of the difficulties that the orthography poses for a translation device. My general approach to this task is to consider the orthography from the viewpoint of the designer of a reading machine. We can then ask what sorts of knowledge it is necessary or useful to possess in order to solve the translation problem.

Of course, there are various ways in which reading machines may differ in design from reading brains. Extant machines have usually been designed so as to economise on storage. They have not had to learn to read. They are uncomprehending; hence the mappings between writing, speech, and *meaning* have not entered their design. Nor do they have the benefit of an education in the classics.

Reading Machines

One of the most highly developed reading machines is the MITalk-79 system, described by Allen (1980). Although this system is not intended to mimic human information-processing strategies, its design reflects aspects of English orthography in an interesting way. The system applies three strategies in a fixed order. First, an attempt is made to find a match for the input word among the representations of word spellings that are stored in the lexicon. With high-frequency monomorphemic words this attempt will succeed because they possess entries in the lexical store. By this means, the pronunciation is retrieved for many common words that exhibit "exceptional" spelling–sound correspondences.

If the first strategy fails, an attempt is made to analyse the word into constituent morphemes that are known to the lexicon. Morphological decomposition is achieved by the recursive application of an algorithm that generates an exhaustive listing of the possible parsings of the word. This analysis is based on a set of orthographically specified affixation rules, e.g. scarcity—scarc(e)+ity. The parsing solutions that result are tested against the 12,000 morpheme entries contained in the system's lexicon. For each such morpheme, the lexicon contains information about its spelling, sound, and part of speech, together with a tabulation of the other morphemes with which it may combine. Taken together, these two lexical retrieval procedures are claimed to analyse correctly 95% of words.

A third, backup, procedure is reserved for uncommon words not found in the system's lexicon. By the time that a word is subjected to this procedure, any potential affixes will have been detected and removed. The stem that remains, having no matching entry in the lexicon, has to be translated by letter–sound rules. Consonant pronunciations are assigned first, without reference to context. Then the vowels are translated using grapheme-context and phoneme-context constraints. Four hundred rules are required in order to yield adequate performance on these residual items.

For all polymorphemic words, the phonetic description obtained thus far is only provisional. Whether the specification has been retrieved from the morphemic entries in the lexicon or assembled by the application of letter–sound rules, a number of final adjustments are required. Morphophonemic rules are used to modify the phonetic specification as a result of certain types of concatenation. For example, the prefix *pre* is reduced before a bound morpheme (*prefer* vs. *pretest*).

Another set of decisions is required in order to deal with stress assignment. For words handled by the morpheme lexicon, stress assignment is retrieved from the lexicon and modified, if necessary, in accord with suffixation rules. However, those polysyllabic words translated by letter–sound rules require the application of a complex set of rules for the assignment of lexical stress.

Such rules often require knowledge of form class, which may be inferred from affixation or from syntactic context.

Finally, syllabic and morphemic boundaries are taken into account in order to select among allophones, where necessary. The need for this stage serves as a reminder that a translation process that terminates in a phonemic description of a word requires to be supplemented by further processing in order to yield an articulatory code. (For example, the sounds corresponding to *eap* have a different timing quality in *cheaply* from *teapot*, due to the difference in location of the morpheme boundary.) It is interesting to note that even when the MITalk-79 system cannot retrieve the stem of a polymorphemic word from its lexicon and is obliged to translate it by letter–sound rules, lexical/syntactic processing nevertheless enters into several stages of the computation of an articulatory code. The initial morphological decomposition is checked against syntactic context. All affixes are handled lexically and only stems are translated by non-lexical rules. Morphophonemic adjustments are then made and lexical stress rules applied. Finally, the transcription is marked for syllabic and morphemic boundaries and a number of phonetic adjustments are made in the environment of these boundaries.

Grapheme–Phoneme Correspondences[1]

The limiting case of mechanical translation would be exhibited by a device that translates each letter into a speech sound without use of any contextual information. I know of no estimate of how well such a *singular translator* would perform on English. In the first 10 words of the previous sentence it might assign correct pronunciations to *a* and *well* (spoken in isolation) but make at least one error on each of the other eight words.

We can regard the spelling–sound translation difficulties as falling roughly into two classes: *segmentation* problems and *translation* problems. The segmentation problems arise because there is not a one-to-one mapping of graphemes into phonemes. Convergent and divergent mappings exist: *ch* in *chop* is translated into a single phoneme; *x* in *ox* is translated into two phonemes. Moreover, two letters may sometimes function as a digraphic unit and sometimes as separate units. Compare *ea* in *react* and *reach*, *ph* in *uphill* and *morpheme*.

Translation problems are most common in English vowel spellings, especially in vowel digraphs (compare *ea* in *breach*, *break*, *bread*). Consonant

---

[1] I adhere to the definition of *grapheme* employed by Scragg (1974) among others, viz. "a group of symbols which collectively contrast (lexically) with other symbols in a writing system." I am grateful to Max Coltheart for pointing out that this usage conflicts with that given in the *Oxford English Dictionary*. See Henderson (in press) for a fuller treatment of *grapheme*.

digraphs may also present the reader with a range of options (compare *ch* in *yacht, ache, cache, arch*).

Polysyllabic words introduce further problems, notably the assignment of lexical stress. Decisions about what syllable to stress carry implications for vowel quality. Unstressed vowels tend, albeit unreliably, to converge on the schwa. Consider, for instance, the second syllable of *honour, martyr, actor, baker, altar, tapir, measure*, in which the same reduced vowel is spelled in seven different ways. Eighteen percent of words in conversation are polysyllabic (Gimson, 1980) and presumably the proportion is larger in printed text.

We can improve upon the performance of our singular translation device by allowing segmentation, translation, and stress assignment to be guided by various kinds of contextual constraint. Words that can be translated accurately by the appropriate use of contextual constraints are often spoken of loosely as "regular" (see later). Given the great range of factors that can be said to influence the translation of a grapheme, it is clearly unsatisfactory to speak of "regularity" as if there existed an agreed set of translation rules, which permitted the unambiguous classification of all words as regular or irregular. Let us turn, therefore, to a brief review of these contextual influences.

Contextual Influences on Grapheme–Phoneme Translation

A large number of constraints can be described in terms of the immediate graphemic environment of the to-be-translated grapheme. It may be worth distinguishing the fact that a rule can be described in terms of a graphemic context from the wider question of what motivates the rule.

Compare, for example, the "rule" that *a* following *w* is pronounced /ɒ/, except when the vowel precedes any of /k/g/ŋ/ (e.g. *wad, wasp, wand*, but *wag*). This is a curious rule not only because it is so limited, describing the influence of one consonant on one vowel, but because it appears to lack any principled motivation. One incidental consequence of such a local rule is that it can create an orthographic neighbourhood, in Glushko's (1979) sense, wherein there is inconsistency between two "regular" words (e.g. *wand/ hand*).

In any case, the *wa* rule can be formulated more powerfully as a phonemic context rule, without reference to spelling. Thus, following Venezky (1970), we may say that *a* is to be pronounced /æ/ after /w/, save when followed by a velar consonant. Hence we have the /ɒ/ translation in *wand* and *quad* but /æ/ in *wag* and *quack*. This raises the possibility that such a rule could be realised by translating *a* as /æ/ and subsequently making an adjustment /æ/→/ɒ/, determined by the phonemic environment.

It should not be thought that such limited rules are very rare. Venezky (1970) describes a considerable number. These include influences on vowel translation of preceding and succeeding consonants (e.g. *a* after *w* = /ɒ/; *i* before *nd* = /aɪ/), influences on consonant translation exerted by a following vowel (e.g. *c* before *e* = /s/), and influences of word position on the translation of consonants (*gh* = /g/ in word-initial positions) and vowels (*ie* = /i/ in medial position, /aɪ/ in final position of monosyllabics). Contextual influences on vowel translation in English tend to operate in a right-to-left direction and may skip a consonant, as in the final-*e* rule. Clearly such rules differ greatly in power. In interpreting the power of a rule we need to have regard to the number of instances to which the rule applies, as well as the proportion of exceptions. For example, the marking of vowels by a word-final *e* applies to a very large number of words so it is powerful, despite the existence of several exceptions (e.g. *have, none*).

In yet another sort of rule we can see a dissociation between having power and being principled. Phonotactic constraints in English are indubitably principled, in the sense that they can be formulated as universal prohibitions on certain phonemic sequences. However, their effect in rendering silent certain consonants (e.g. in *knee, bomb*) is restricted to relatively few instances, so they are not powerful constraints on orthographic translation.

All the constraints discussed thus far have been capable of description in terms of grapheme sequences and word position, even if, as is the case with phonotaxis, their motivation stems from some other level of linguistic description. Elsewhere (Henderson, 1982), I have thought it worth distinguishing these *same-level constraints* on grapheme translation from *higher-level constraints*, on the grounds that the former can be incorporated into a translation device of altogether simpler design. As we see later, it is just this sort of lower-level grapheme translator that is postulated in recent psychological models that include a non-lexical path to pronunciation.

In general, higher-level constraints have to do with morphology and syntax. I know of no systematic treatment of the morphological influences on English orthographic translation, though brief discussions have been offered by Venezky (1970), Klima (1972), Henderson (1982), and Smith et al. (1983).

Morpheme boundaries determine segmentation where the possible occurrence of a digraphic unit creates ambiguity. Consider the *ea* in *reach* and *react*, the *gn* in *signer* and *ignore*, the ph in *uphill* and *aphid*.

Morphological factors also influence translation. In final consonant clusters where there is a silent grapheme (e.g. *sign, bomb*), inflectional suffixes leave the grapheme silent (*signed, bombing*) whereas derivational suffixes usually lead to it being sounded (*signature, bombard*). Another example of the influence of morphemic boundaries is to be found in the different translations of *g* in *finger, singer*, and *singed*.

Form class exercises a number of important influences on translation. An often-cited example is the pronunciation of initial *th*, which is voiced in functors (*the, this*) and unvoiced in contentives (*thick, thin*). This particular rule has received experimental attention from Campbell and Besner (1981).

The single-grapheme vowels of English have two major pronunciations, a long or "free" form (*sane*, *cone*) and a shorter "checked" form (*sanity*, *conical*). In monomorphemic words the appropriate form is usually predictable from graphemic context, such as the final-*e* marker rule, though there are many exceptions (e.g. *have*, *love*). In polymorphemic words, vowel translation tends to be influenced by the morphemic rather than the graphemic environment. Suffixation, in particular, leads to complex adjustments in phoneme assignment. Frequently vowels that were free in the monomorphemic form become checked when it is suffixed (*athlete*, *athletic*; *induce*, *induction*), but this depends in complex ways on the particular suffix.

Morphophonemic adjustment in vowel values and shifts in lexical stress are parallel but largely independent processes that depend on suffixation. In the foregoing examples, in which suffixation leads to checking of a free vowel, the primary stress does not shift in one case (*induce*, *induction*) but does in the other (*athlete*, *athletic*).

The best known attempt to formulate stress assignment rules occurs in the phonological theory of Chomsky and Halle (1968). These rules are based upon the number of syllables in the word, its form class, and structural aspects of the final syllable. (In stress assignment as in many of the effects of graphemic environment the flow of constraint is right to left.) As Venezky's (1970) analysis of grapheme–phoneme correspondences has served as the authority for most attempts by experimental psychologists to manipulate orthographic "regularity," it is worth observing that he deliberately avoids discussion of unstressed vowels and the complexities of suffixation as it affects vowel checking and stress assignment.

Phonemic and Articulatory Codes

Discussions of spelling–sound translation have usually been confined to the question of grapheme–phoneme correspondences (GPCs). This restriction poses a number of problems. First, it is sometimes difficult to relate such discussion to phonological theories in linguistics, some of which do not have recourse to the concept of phonemes. Second, the GPC approach seems to predicate all discussion of spelling–sound translation on the psychological reality of phonemes. It seems to be taken for granted that at some stage of translation, the reader's mental representation of the word resembles a broad, phonemic transcription. A third, and perhaps more substantial, problem is that a phonemic description is an abstract one that does not pretend to specify the actual articulatory realisation of a spoken word. Even if when reading aloud we do rely at some stage of processing on a phonemic representation, this requires further processing to eventuate in speech. Now, here, the crucial question is whether we can simply assume that some relatively low-level output machinery routinely converts the phonemic code into one suitable for articulation, taking into account coarticulatory constraints, etc.

It seems to me that phonological theory is of little help in deciding this question because it has generally assumed that the phonemic transcription is marked for syllabic, morphemic, and word boundaries, as well as for patterns of lexical stress. Yet of these markings, only word boundaries are directly and unambiguously available in English orthography.

Variation of articulation at word boundaries is considerable and the larger context may determine many kinds of allophonic variation and even sometimes a change of phoneme. Variations within a word are much less common, but they pose more of a problem for spelling–sound translation. The most often cited are presence versus absence of syllabic /l/ and /n/ at morphemic boundaries, and the phonetic treatment of /tr/ junctures. Jones (1956) illustrates the former by the pairs *coddling/codling* and *lightening/lightning*. The first (verbal) member of each pair displays long, syllabic /l/ and /n/, respectively, at the morphemic boundary, whereas the second does not. The juncture of /t/ and /r/ is discussed by Gimson (1980). In most speakers, the pronunciation of *nitrate* is distinguishable from *night-rate* because the former involves a juncture of the close type, with devoiced /r/.

Non-lexical Spelling–Sound Translation

In the foregoing discussion of orthographic segmentation, grapheme–phoneme translation, stress assignment, and allophonic variation, I have placed considerable emphasis on higher-level (usually morphological) determinants. It is time now to introduce the reason for this emphasis, which lies in the reliance of many psychological models on a theoretical distinction between "lexical" and "non-lexical" pathways from print to speech.

Later in this chapter I consider the somewhat neglected question of what it might mean to assert that a process is "non-lexical." For the moment it must suffice to say that there are three original reasons for postulating a non-lexical pathway: (1) to provide a mechanism for translating into speech printed forms that have not previously been encountered; (2) to explain why words that are "regular" in their spelling–sound correspondences are sometimes handled faster in oral reading; (3) to explain the reading errors that characterise surface dyslexia.

It can be seen, therefore, that the definitions offered for "non-lexical" and "regular" are likely to be tied to each other. I have assumed that predictabilities of pronunciation that can only be derived from syntactic and morphemic information about a word have no place in this. Hence, these predictabilities do not contribute to "regularity" and cannot be part of a "non-lexical" process.

Regularity

Because the concept of low-level grapheme–phoneme translation has become part of the standard theoretical luggage of psychological models of reading and because, by extension, the classification of stimulus words as "regular" or "irregular" has become a common experimental manipulation, invested with a standard diagnostic significance, it is surprising to find so little explicit discussion of what rules the reader is supposed to employ.

There are several aspects of this. The classification of words as *regular* or *irregular* should be taken as a psychological working hypothesis rather than the expression of an established linguistic fact. Two issues can be discerned here. First is the question of what regularities to count. When asserting that *regular* words can be processed by application of some particular cognitive strategy, theorists need to be explicit about what sort of regularities they have in mind, with particular regard to the level of linguistic knowledge on which the translation rule is based. Second, the treatment of regularity as a strictly dichotomous variable should not be regarded as a linguistic truth flowing ineluctably from the Wijk–Venezky GPC tabulations (see Henderson, 1984). The inspiration of the dichotomous interpretation is psychological and not linguistic, and stems from the supposed privileged status of regular words with respect to non-lexical translation. The important point here is that non-lexical translation is, by definition, a "one-pass" process. Recursive testing of possible correspondences is ruled out for two reasons, one of principle and one of feasibility. The principle is that translations, being supposedly non-lexical, cannot be checked against lexical information. The practical consideration is that a purely phonological check would result in false confirmations of regular translations of some irregular words. For example, *bread*, when translated by the highest frequency GPCs, would have a candidate pronunciation that would match the phonological entry for *breed* in the lexicon.

It is not difficult to find examples in the experimental literature of inconsistencies and contradictions in the classification of stimuli occasioned by the adoption (usually tacitly) of quite different definitions of regularity. Much of this confusion is due to disagreement about the size of the orthographic units that are available in the translation tables, or in other words, the question of the extent of graphemic environment that can be considered in translation.

For example, Glushko (1979) allows the regular correspondence for a vowel to be determined by its consonantal environment, as tabulated by Venezky (1970). Thus, he lists both *posh* and *cold* as regular (*ld* vowel lengthening rule). Other experimenters have tended not to admit consonantal environment as a determinant of regularity, though this practice has not been adhered to consistently. For example, Andrews (1982) and Seidenberg et al.

(1984) ignore Venezky's *all* rule (regular in *fall*); Coltheart et al. (1979) ignore the *ign* rule (regular in *sign*), and Baron and Strawson (1976) and Parkin (1982) ignore the *wa* rule (regular in *watch*). On the other hand, all experimenters concede the retroactive, vowel-lengthening effect of final *e*.

Not only has the rationale for admitting some but not other graphemic environment constraints been left inexplicit, but other sources of ambiguity exist. Most experimenters have avoided the problems posed by polysyllabic and polymorphemic words. However, Baron and Strawson (1976) cite *joker* as regular. So it may be, but we need to know the nature of the rule applied here to give $er \rightarrow /\partial/$. Other problems of classification are introduced by the considerable variations of pronunciation in different dialects and by variation of pronunciation of words in isolation as opposed to sentential context. Let us consider, for example, *been*. Glushko (1979) classified this as an exception, presumably because in Southern California it is pronounced like the word *bin*. In standard English the word is pronounced like *bean* and is therefore regular. However, most standard users of English will pronounce *been* like *bin* in natural speech when saying "we've been going away ...".

Some idea of the confusion existing in this realm can be gathered from the following list of words. On the basis, I assume, of the correspondence assigned to the letter *a*, half have been employed experimentally as "regular" words and half as "exceptions".

gang, dance, cart, lass, chant, ankle, cask, shack,
caste, shall, fall, fast, watch, water, wad, warp.[2]

It follows that experiments purporting to demonstrate the psychological reality of *regularity*, can at best only be said to do so in some general sense that leaves unanswered questions about which particular rules the reader is equipped with, or what the general form and nature of the rules are.

The lack of any systematic attempt to gain a direct estimate of the pronunciation rules available to the reader seems a curious omission. How might this lacuna be filled? It avails us little to ask subjects to classify words as regular and exceptional. In my experience this causes them much hesitation and such a deliberated decision does not appear to recruit whatever rules are implicit in fluent and effortless reading. The most obvious alternative is to determine the nature of the pronunciations assigned to pseudowords. How, for example, should *ciny* be pronounced? On what basis are we to reach a decision?

At least two questions can be addressed in such investigations. The first concerns the size of unit that seems to be taken into account in translation.

---

[2]The words are drawn in pairs from the following studies, in order: Coltheart et al. (1979), Andrews (1982), Baron and Strawson (1976), Parkin (1982), Seidenberg et al. (1984), Andrews (1982), Baron and Strawson (1976), Parkin (1982). The first row of eight was classified as *regular* and the second row as *exceptions*.

The second concerns the proportion of responses that are regular (by whatever reckoning).

Many methodological difficulties attend such studies. Long lists of nonsense words may evoke special-purpose strategies in the reader. On the other hand, embedding the test items in a context of real words may give rise to priming artefacts (cf. Seidenberg et al., 1984). Another difficulty lies in deciding whether, in a particular instance, rules or analogies were applied. If *wamp* is pronounced regularly, is it by application of the rule that *w* influences a subsequent *a*, or is it by analogy with the word *warp*? Clearly, in testing a pure rule-based theory we should set the analogies against the rules (*damp* vs. *wa*→/wɔ/). This has only been done, to my knowledge, in studies of phonological theory, such as Steinberg and Krohn's (1975) work on vowel-alternation rules and Baker and Smith's (1976) work on stress-assignment rules.

Patterson and Morton (this volume) have reported some data for the *ook* and *ind* clusters, suggesting that the consonant environment in these cases very rarely influences vowel translation. (Curiously, Venezky, 1970, treats *ind/ild* as an admissible unit but not *ook*.) An unpublished study by Kelliher (1983) offers some further support for this view. For both *ook* and *ind/ild* pseudowords, only 14% of readers assigned the vowel pronunciation that is usual when followed by that consonant pattern. However, other consonant environments were more influential. At the top of the range, *old* pseudowords were pronounced as in *bold* by 72% of subjects, and *igh* pseudowords were pronounced as in *sigh* by 92% of subjects.

Kelliher found, as had Glushko (1979), that on some occasions pronunciations were assigned that were irregular by any reckoning. Glushko (1979) found "regular" pronunciations on 94–95% with stimuli, all of whose orthographic neighbours were regular and only 78–88% when the pseudoword had at least one irregular neighbour. Kay and Marcel (1981) found what they considered to be regular pronunciations on 84–90% of occasions in the conditions of their experiment when priming would not be expected to induce major biases.

The interpretation of these complexities is not an easy matter. Nevertheless, the approach is an important one and it promises to yield more detailed information about the reader's translation rules than can be gleaned from the gross comparison of performance on groups of words, classified as either regular or exceptional on the basis of some a priori and frequently inexplicit linguistic criteria. Moreover, the fact that normal subjects disagree, often to a substantial extent, on how a pseudoword should be pronounced has practical implications for the interpretation of reading disorders, because it suggests that one should not expect 100% performance on oral reading of regular words when access to their particular lexical representation is lost.

EVIDENCE FROM SPEEDED NAMING

In the previous section I argued that an important source of information about the mechanisms for assembling phonology lay in the nature of the pronunciations assigned to pseudowords. Because, for the most part, we lack this information, I have turned to the speeded naming task as the most directly pertinent source of existing evidence.

Tasks

In the interests of simplicity and brevity I have focused on the speeded naming task at the expense of other candidates for consideration, notably the lexical decision task. At risk of oversimplification, it might be said that experimenters have turned to the lexical decision task in hope of determining *whether* phonological recoding plays a role in lexical access, whereas the naming latency task has seemed to offer a more direct means of investigating the *mechanisms* of phonological recoding.

The virtue of the naming latency task is that it *compels* phonological recoding by some means or other. It has the following limitations: (1) the latencies may include a component due to articulatory programming (cf. Sternberg et al., 1978)—such effects are likely to be very small; (2) there is the logical possibility that subjects can stop the clock with the initial articulation before assembling the whole of a word's phonology (cf. Henderson, 1982, for an evaluation); (3) the inferences linking latency effects to particular processing mechanisms are highly indirect.

Effects

I have organised this review into seven parts. The first five have to do with latency effects associated with:

1. Repetition, word frequency, lexicality.
2. Letter and syllabic length.
3. Predictability of sound from spelling.
4. Priming.
5. Morphological, semantic, and syntactic effects.

The next part deals with the determinants of:

6. Errors.

The last part deals with:

7. Interactions with reading ability.

Repetition, Word Frequency, and Lexicality

Repetition of a word facilitates naming (Durso & Johnson, 1979; Scarborough et al., 1977). The magnitude of this effect is considerably greater in

TABLE 17.1
Results From Three Studies of Lexical Decision Latency and
Naming Latency

Study	Frequency Effect in		
	Naming	Lexical Decision	Frequency Contrast
Frederiksen & Kroll (1976)	36 msec	89 msec	Hi > 30 p.m.
			Lo < 2 p.m.
Forster & Chambers (1973)	71 msec	196 msec	Hi > 50 p.m.
			Lo < 3 p.m.
Seidenberg et al. (1984)			
Regular words	22 msec	68 msec	Hi $\bar{X}$ = 9514
			Lo $\bar{X}$ = 97
Exception words	49 msec	74 msec	Hi $\bar{X}$ = 9213
			Lo $\bar{X}$ = 97

Each study used the same word set for both tasks. In both tasks the subject was confronted with a random mixture of words and non-words. Frequency was estimated from the Thorndike Lorge word count in the first two studies and from the Carroll, Davies, and Richman count in the third.

the lexical decision task than in the naming task (Scarborough et al., 1977). However, this task difference only holds for words. Pseudowords show a repetition effect in naming that is much larger and is comparable in magnitude to the effect found in lexical decision (Scarborough et al., 1977).

Familiarity, in terms of the frequency of occurrence of a word, also facilitates performance on both tasks. Frequency effects, like repetition effects, are of much greater magnitude in lexical decision as compared to naming. This is clearly evident in Table 17.1, which summarises the results of three studies in which naming latencies and lexical decision latencies were determined for the same set of words. In similar vein, Richardson (1976) found a reliable frequency effect for lexical decision but not for naming in a *post-hoc* regression analysis of his data.

With regard to lexicality, both Forster and Chambers (1973) and Frederiksen and Kroll (1976) found that their low-frequency words were named slightly faster (c. 18 msec) than their pseudowords.

Letter and Syllabic Length

Word-length effects have been reviewed in some detail in Henderson (1982, Chapter 7). The general conclusion reached there was that in unskilled readers naming latencies increase with both the number of letters and the number of syllables in a word. When the reader is relatively skilled, syllabic effects in word reading are negligible but letter length usually continues to exercise an effect, albeit much smaller than in unskilled readers. However, even skilled readers show syllabic effects in naming pseudowords. At this stage we shall confine our attention to skilled reading.

Effects of syllabic length on word naming have been reported in a number of studies by Klapp and his colleagues (see Klapp & Wyatt, 1976, for a review). In the present context it is worth noting that Klapp's evidence comes from picture naming, Arabic numeral naming, and visual comparison tasks, as well as word naming, so it is unlikely to have a direct bearing on orthographic translation. Failures to obtain reliable effects of number of syllables have been reported by Forster and Chambers (1973), Frederiksen and Kroll (1976), Richardson (1976), Mason (1978), and Cosky (1980). This failure to obtain syllabic effects contrasts, in several of these studies, with the findings of reliable letter-length effects.

Many studies report an increase of word-naming latency as the number of letters in the word is increased. Henderson (1982) reviews eight studies, all of which show effects. These range, in skilled readers, from about 6 to 63 msec/ letter. Occasional failures to find length effects have, however, been reported. Ellis (1982) found a reliable effect in only one out of three experiments. Letter-length effects have generally only been pursued in words of four to six letters. This limitation is well founded, because outside of that range lexical and morphological factors are difficult to control.

The number of letters in a word is quite likely to be correlated with other factors. We have already seen that the apparent effect of letter length is not mediated by syllabic length. Cosky (1980) and Henderson (1982) also present data to show that phonemic length is not the active factor. Attempts to increase letter length while holding syllabic length constant usually result in larger consonant clusters in the longer words, but there is no evidence to suggest that this causes the effect (see Frederiksen & Kroll, 1976, Table 2).

One last possible contaminating factor must be considered. Jastrzembski (1981) has shown that lexical decisions are made more rapidly to words that have more meanings and, furthermore, letter length is often confounded with number of meanings (e.g. in Cosky's, 1976, study of naming latencies). Ellis (1982) controlled number of meanings and found no length effect. However, there are three reasons for doubting Ellis's claim that no length effect obtains when number of meanings is controlled. First, Ellis obtained a significant length effect in his experiment 1 with a fairly close matching of number of meanings. Second, neither Jastrzembski nor Ellis actually demonstrates that naming latencies (as distinct from lexical decision latencies) are influenced by number of meanings. Third, meaningless pseudowords exhibit a length effect in naming latency.

Predictability of Sound From Spelling

The linguistic variable that has attracted most interest in the study of naming latencies is spelling–sound predictability. A large number of investigations since the mid-1970s have been devoted to the question of whether latencies are affected by the predictability of a word's pronunciation. More recently the question has been posed with greater refinement as it has become evident that at least some forms of predictability influence latencies under some circumstances. The question therefore becomes *what form of predictability* and *in what circumstances*.

Two general conceptions of predictability have been advanced. A word is held to be *regular* if its graphic elements are pronounced in the way that is most common for that graphic element, taking a census of the language in general. As we have seen in the preceding section, considerable ambiguity attaches to the notion of a functional graphic element. In order to decide whether or not *sigh* is a regular word, we need to know whether the *i* is treated as an independent graphic element or whether the functional element is *igh*. In other words, we need to know what size of segment to enter into our frequency count. (*Sigh* is irregular on the former basis, but regular on the latter.) Moreover, we need to know *how* to count. Is it a "type" count or a "token" count that matters? Coltheart (1978) is one of the few theorists to be explicit on this and has based his notion of regularity on a type count (i.e. one that ignores the natural frequency of occurrence of words containing a particular graphic element). By adopting Venezky's (1970) type-count tabulation, others have implicitly made the same commitment.

The alternative conception of predictability is that of *consistency* with a word's orthographic neighbours. The notion of a word's orthographic neighbourhood remains largely intuitive, although some empirical work has been done to define it (Glushko, 1981). Circularity has been avoided by adopting a working definition in which the neighbourhood of a monosyllabic word consists of those words that differ in spelling only in the initial consonant or consonantal cluster (Glushko, 1979).

Concerning the classification of words as predictable or unpredictable in pronunciation, these various schemata agree in many cases, though the actual grounds for the decision differ according to the schema. On almost any reckoning *haze* is predictable (assuming only that final-*e* marking of the preceding vowel is admitted into the notion of regularity). Similarly, *have* is unpredictable within regularity schemata whether the unit of translation is taken as (*a* + consonant + *e* marker) or as -*ave*. From the standpoint of the consistency schema, *have* finds itself in a uniformly hostile neighbourhood (*gave, cave, nave*, etc.) with which its pronunciation is inconsistent. From these examples it can be seen that a notion of regularity applied to large graphic elements such as *ave* is bound to yield much the same sort of classification as the consistency notion. Whether the classifications are identical depends largely on the precise formulation of the schemata with respect to the relevant frequency count. Most regularity schemata have been formulated to meet the needs of "single-pass" models (see the discussion of *regularity* in the first section). Accordingly, they do not allow degrees of irregularity. If a graphic element is not assigned its most common pronunciation then it is simply *irregular*, whether its pronunciation is unique, or quite common but not the most common. (The pronunciation of *oo* in *brooch* is, I think, unique. That in *foot* is quite common, but "irregular" in many dialects because not as common as in *broom*.) Glushko (1979) formulated his view of inconsistency with similar absoluteness. Thus, *have* and *wave* were both simply classed as inconsistent, with no account taken of the fact that *wave* has only *have* in opposition, with all its other neighbours consistent with itself. Contrast between large-segment views of translation (whether formulated in terms of consistency or regularity) and small-segment views can be achieved in limited areas of the lexical inventory. Glushko (1979) exploited this in his analysis of *regular* (small-segment definition) *but inconsistent* words. *Bead*, for example, employs the most common pronunciation of *ea*. However, the most common vowel pronunciation among its *ead* neighbours is actually that assigned in *dead*. *Bead* is therefore regular within the small-segment definition but highly inconsistent with its neighbours. A converse case is that of words that are *irregular but consistent* (such as *cold*, see Andrews, 1982).

One final stimulus classification concerns non-words. One cannot speak of regularity in non-words because, by definition, they have no lexically specified pronunciation to enter into a classification. Non-words can, however, be classified as consistent (e.g. *pold*) or inconsistent (e.g. *jull*), though of course one cannot decide how inconsistent (because one cannot say whether *jull* should be sounded like the majority, *dull*, etc., or the minority, *bull*, etc.).

We can now turn to the data. In doing this I wish first to dismiss from further consideration data derived from the time taken to complete reading of lists of words. Using such a task, Baron and Strawson (1976) and Coltheart et al. (1979) found faster reading of lists consisting of entirely predictable words. Parkin (1982) found a time cost only for lists of highly unpredictable words.

Concerning this task, my contention is brutally simple. The list reading task provides such an obscure view of the process of deciding on pronunciation that it should be ignored. By far the greatest contribution to the time measure is the production process itself, and studies of list reading have not permitted the separation of decision time from production time. Moreover, there are other complications in the task. Subjects often "trip up" and correct errors and it is difficult to know how to treat these aspects of the data.

Turning to studies of naming latencies for isolated words, we find a large body of evidence to suggest that spelling–sound predictability influences decision time, at least under some circumstances. As an index of the gross effect of predictability we may take the traditional comparison of regular with irregular words. Most of these experiments were designed around a small-segment definition of regularity and most of them took no account of consistency. Nevertheless, as regular words tend to have few or no inconsistent neighbours and irregular words tend to have a preponderance of inconsistent neighbours, the traditional contrast gives almost any sort of predictability a chance to manifest itself.

Reliable effects of predictability have emerged from this contrast in studies by Gough and Cosky (1977), Stanovich and Bauer (1978), Glushko (1979, experiments 1 and 3), Parkin (1983, experiments 1 and 3), and Seidenberg et al. (1984, experiments 1 and 2). The largest of all these effects was a mere 36 msec in magnitude, so it would not be surprising for this reason alone to find some studies with negative outcomes. To such studies we shortly turn. However, in addition to sampling fluctuations in the measurement of barely detectable effects, there are two possible systematic sources of variance in the predictability effect. The first arises from any interaction of the effect with other factors and the second arises out of the grossness of the predictability manipulation, with the confounding of small- and large-segment factors.

Several studies report interactions in which the predictability effect is abolished when combined with some other factor. Underwood and Bargh (1982) found predictability effect for uppercase but not lowercase words. As Parkin (1983) and Seidenberg et al. (1984) did obtain predictability effects using lowercase format, I shall dismiss this variable from further consideration.

Word frequency seems to act as an important qualifying variable. In some studies predictability has been partially confounded with word frequency due to the difficulty in finding enough low-frequency exception words. The exception words were of higher frequency in Glushko's (1979) experiments, in which a reliable regularity effect was nevertheless obtained, but also in four experiments in which no effect was obtained (Mason, 1978, experiments 1 and 2; Wallis, 1982, experiments 3 and 4). Given the relative insensitivity of naming latency to word frequency and the very small imbalance of frequency in the Mason and Wallis stimuli, it would be unwise to set aside these negative findings entirely.

A more important aspect of word frequency has been uncovered by Seidenberg et al. (1984). The predictability effect that they obtained was severely reduced or abolished in very high-frequency words (experiments 1 and 3). It is also notable that the negative results of Wallis (1982) were obtained with very high-frequency words, all chosen so as to be familiar to 6-year-olds. Moreover, in the study by Andrews (1982), the only condition in which a regularity effect was obtained was that of low-frequency words.

The other qualifying factor that has been explored is that of priming, arising through recurrences of spelling patterns within a stimulus series. Because such priming seems to qualify consistency effects rather than regularity effects, discussion is deferred to a later point.

So far, we have seen that the contrast of regular with exception words generally yields a small but reliable latency effect, though there have been several failures to obtain the effect. Some of these failures, at least, seem to be due to the absence of predictability effects for high-frequency words. I have referred to the traditional regular versus exception contrast as the *gross* test of predictability effects because it has usually confounded various measures of predictability. For example, exception words have tended to be irregular on both small-segment and large-segment counts and to be higher in counts of inconsistent neighbours. For this reason, it is crucial that we turn now to examine those few studies in which an attempt has been made to partition the effects of various types of predictability.

The first class of word that concerns us is that which Glushko (1979) has described as *regular and inconsistent*. Such words vary greatly in how large a proportion of hostile neighbours they may have. At one extreme there are words like *wave*, possessed of only a single inconsistent neighbour (*have*) but with many consistent neighbours (*cave, gave*, etc.). Towards the other extreme lie words like *hove* with almost as many inconsistent as consistent neighbours (e.g. *dove, love, move*). Exception words, of course, tend to have an even greater proportion of inconsistent neighbours.

Glushko (1979, experiment 3) reported that regular but inconsistent words suffered a penalty in naming latency that was almost as great as that for exception words, when compared to regular words that were also consistent. This finding was confirmed by Andrews (1982, experiment 2). Seidenberg et al. (1984) showed that Glushko's effect was likely to have been artificially magnified by priming. The matching of words in Glushko's study was done in such a way that a subject encountered pairs of words that shared a tail segment differing in pronunciation (e.g. *give, five*). Seidenberg et al. found that this priming selectively penalised regular but inconsistent words. However, they also found that when such priming was precluded (experiment 4), a consistency effect was obtained for regular words if and only if they were of low frequency. As with their regular versus exception contrast, no effect was detectable among high-frequency words. This interaction of consistency with frequency was also obtained by Andrews (1982).

Glushko (1979), Andrews (1982), and Seidenberg et al. (1984) had all been able to detect consistency effects that were reliable across stimulus material as well as subjects (with the proviso in the last study that the effect could only be obtained with words of lower frequency). More recently, however, Parkin (1983) has reported consistency effects that could be generalised across subjects in two out of three experiments, but not across words.

One other combination of word properties that has been explored in an attempt to tease apart regularity and consistency effects occurs in the case of words that are irregular but consistent.[3] Such words are not easy to find. Examples include *cold, book,* and *ball.* For the most part, these are words governed by Venezky's (1970) graphemic environment rules wherein vowel translation is influenced by a following consonantal context. Andrews (1982) reported latencies for such items in the only study to explore all combinations of regularity with consistency. She found that irregular words that were nevertheless consistent were named faster than irregular inconsistent words. There are, however, numerous defects in the classification of stimuli in this experiment, although it might be argued that these would merely tend to dilute the consistency effects obtained. (For example, *hind* and *bind* are classified as consistent despite the noun *wind. Mild* is likewise classified, despite *gild.*)

The last realm in which an attempt has been made to partition consistency effects from regularity effects is the naming of unfamiliar pseudowords. The conventional interpretation of regularity, whatever the size of segment considered, cannot be applied to the classification of pseudowords. Because there is no authority for how a pseudoword is pronounced, one cannot decide whether its pronunciation conforms to frequency-based rules. In contrast, Glushko's (1979) view of inconsistency is such that a stimulus can be classified as inconsistent on the basis of conflict within its orthographic neighbourhood, irrespective of how the item itself is pronounced. Hence, *tave* is inconsistent because, however it is pronounced, its pronunciation will conflict with that of at least one orthographic neighbour (*gave* or *have*).

Glushko (1979) has reported two experiments in which a consistency effect obtains for pseudowords. This effect is similar in magnitude to that obtained for real words. Parkin (1983) has subsequently reported results that appear to qualify Glushko's claim in an important way. The essence of Parkin's finding is that inconsistency only leads to slower pronunciation

---

[3] In calling these words "irregular but consistent," I adopt the terminological convention of Glushko, Andrews, and others. They might equally be called "regular" if a large-segment definition of regularity were adopted, namely one that admits units of translations like *old*. This brings out the close taxonomic relationship between large-segment definitions of regularity and consistency. That these taxonomies are not *identical*, however, can be illustrated by the different type-count criteria. Consider *cold*: on a large-segment view it is "regular" because it conforms to the *most common* pronunciation of *old*. The requirement for "consistency" is more severe. In Glushko's (1979) formulation, *cold* is consistent because the *entire* -*old* neighbourhood is unanimous. Thus, although there is no necessary logical difference between these two taxonomic principles when conceived of as continuous measures, a difference emerges in practice because the dimensions have in fact been treated strictly dichotomously, with quantitatively different criteria applied to dichotomisation.

decisions when it exceeds some critical amount. Pseudowords like *yint* that have inconsistent neighbourhoods in which one pronunciation clearly predominates, seem to suffer no disadvantage (*pint* is an unique exception). A disadvantage is, however, suffered by pseudowords like *frow* that have inconsistent neighbourhoods containing several examples of each type of pronunciation (e.g. the ambiguous *bow* and *row*).

The possibility that inconsistency is only an effective variable when it exceeds some critical amount was first suggested by Kay (1982). It has several important implications. In practical terms, it requires to be considered when choosing or evaluating experimental stimuli. Conceptually, it suggests that consistency is not a dichotomous matter, or at least that Glushko's dichotomy was not the appropriate one.

In a number of recent studies, the effects of regularity and consistency have been investigated using the lexical decision task. The interpretation of such investigations presents several problems. The primary difficulty is that the task does not logically require phonological recoding. Indeed, the purpose of these studies has often been to determine *whether* phonological recoding plays a role in lexical access. Accordingly, a simple failure to obtain an effect of spelling–sound predictability is likely to be unilluminating. However, even when an effect is obtained, its interpretation need not be straightforward. For example, Andrews (1982) obtained a consistency effect under conditions designed to eliminate phonological recoding and was forced to the puzzling conclusion that consistency effects arose in the process of identifying words rather than assembling their pronunciation. Finally, lexical decision and naming are not directly comparable due to the possibility that orthographic translation might yield up an abstract phonological code that could serve lexical access, yet was insufficiently specified (e.g. in stress or in morphological information) to support articulation.

Coltheart et al. (1979) used their finding of the presence of a regularity effect in list reading, together with its absence in lexical decision, as a basis for their claim that phonological recoding plays at most a subsidiary role in lexical access. Other failures to obtain a regularity effect in lexical decisions have been reported by Andrews (1982) and Seidenberg et al. (1984). Waters and Seidenberg (1983) could only find regularity effects for slow subjects and low-frequency words. This is broadly in agreement with Stanovich and Bauer's (1978) finding of a regularity effect that was abolished by forcing subjects into faster decisions.

Parkin (1982) has reported a series of experiments in which regular words were compared with mildly and extremely irregular words. No difference was found between regular and mildly irregular words. However, extremely irregular words yielded slower lexical decision even when subjects were given speeded-response instructions. This is potentially interesting as an indication that irregularity admits of degrees (see also Shallice et al., 1983) but there are several problems with the selection of stimuli in this study.[4]

Other studies of lexical decisions in which a regularity effect is obtained have been conducted by Parkin (1984) using much the same highly irregular words as Parkin (1982) and by Bauer and Stanovich (1980)

Of greatest interest in the present context are studies of lexical decision performance that have searched for both regularity and consistency effects. Three such studies have been published. Seidenberg et al. (1984) found no reliable regularity or consistency effects even under circumstances where an effect had been found on naming latencies. Bauer and Stanovich (1980, experiment 2) found an effect of consistency and a marginal effect of regularity. Andrews (1982) found an effect of consistency but no effect of regularity, save when it was combined with consistency.

In summary, then, effects of spelling–sound predictability are common but not universal in studies of naming latency and somewhat less common in lexical decision studies. In lexical decisions, effects are most likely to obtain when performance is slow. In naming, predictability effects are most likely to be obtained for low-frequency words.

Attempts to partition effects due to regularity from those due to consistency encounter a number of problems. The gross comparison of regular with exception words will not suffice as exception words are usually also highly inconsistent. Only Andrews (1982) has attempted to investigate *consistent* exception words; in her study consistency effects were much larger than regularity effects. Another approach has been to compare, within regular words, those that are consistent and those that are inconsistent. Unfortunately, most of the latter are only mildly inconsistent. Nevertheless, Glushko (1979), Bauer and Stanovich (1980), Andrews (1982), and Seidenberg et al. (1984) have been able to detect consistency effects in such comparisons, whereas Parkin (1983) has not.

None of these studies allows us to distinguish the consistency notion from a regularity interpretation that is based upon translation units as large as those that define orthographic neighbourhoods. To some extent the terms *regularity* and *consistency* differ in their implications due to their attachment

---

[4]Drastically summarised the problems are these: (1) Highly irregular stimuli are classified as such on the grounds that their pronunciation is listed in the *Oxford Paperback Dictionary*. The basis of this inscrutable lexicographic convention is unclear. (2) Over a third of the words used are polysyllabic and it is peculiarly difficult to classify these as to regularity. (3) A high proportion of the highly irregular words are French borrowings (e.g. *biscuit, regime, colonel, cafe, litre, corps, debris, meringue*). It is not evident that irregularity of pronunciation is their only distinctive lexical characteristic. (4) As Seidenberg et al. (1984) have pointed out, Parkin's highly irregular words have markedly lower average bigram frequencies than the other sets. Such items incidentally tend to have few orthographic neighbours. (See also Seidenberg et al.'s comment (1984, footnote 6) on Parkin and Underwood's (1983) study.)

to different conceptions of how predictabilities are stored, retrieved, and assembled to yield a pronunciation. Consideration of these vague but important issues is deferred until the concluding section. The data reviewed earlier do, however, bear upon features of regularity or consistency that have become more or less fortuitously associated with one or other view, though not of its essence. For example, such evidence as favours a large-segment view on translation tends also to favour the notion that monosyllabic words are usually segmented into a head, consisting of any initial consonants, and a tail consisting of the remainder. There is some slight indication to the effect that consistency/regularity exercises a continuous effect, or at least that the conventional cut-points defining an exceptional or inconsistent form are incorrect.

Finally, there is the question of predictability effects in naming latencies for non-words. Glushko (1979) was able to obtain such an effect. In unpublished work from our laboratory, Wallis (1982) has had difficulty in replicating the effect. Parkin's (1983) finding may therefore be crucial, because he found a deleterious effect confined to highly inconsistent non-words.

Predictability effects for non-words are crucial for several reasons, First, although they could, in principle, be accomodated in a regularity view, this would require a radical reformation of the traditional conception of how regularity works (for a hint in this direction, see Shallice et al., 1983). Second, consistency effects that obtained only for familiar words are vulnerable to dismissal as interference epiphenomena that arise somehow in the course of lexical access but do not reflect the workings of the mechanism for assembling pronunciations for unfamiliar forms.

Priming

Contextual priming is a fashionable paradigm and it is not surprising to find a large number of recent demonstrations that the speed of naming or the nature of the pronunciation assigned can be influenced by a variety of types of priming. As my concern here is with the light that such studies may be able to shed upon the mechanisms of pronunciation assembly, I shall commence with a *caveat*.

Studies of priming tend to involve sequences of stimuli that are peculiarly artificial, even by the standards of cognitive experimentation. Such sequences, with their inbuilt, teasing relationships between items, are rather likely to engage special strategies and there is a wealth of evidence available that subjects do tailor their strategies to fit the nature of the stimulus series, at least in some tasks. For these reasons, we require to be satisfied on one or other of the following points. Either it has to be shown that priming of the sort in question is inherent in the context of normal reading, or it has to be shown that the sort of process that is activated by the structural relationship of primer and target is also spontaneously activated by an unprimed target. These points can be illustrated by the example of semantic priming that we are about to consider. Suppose we wanted to argue that the fact that word naming can be speeded by semantic priming serves to establish a lexical component in the process of word naming. For this argument to have force, we would either have to support our case by showing that a lexical strategy was not specially recruited by the availability of a semantically related primer, or we would have to show the semantic relatedness of the sort introduced in the experiment is inherent in natural text.

Meyer et al. (1975) have indeed shown that semantic relatedness between successive words facilitates naming latency to about the same extent as lexical decision latency. Rosson (1983) has attempted to apply this priming technique to the question of whether lexical processing plays a role in pronunciation assembly for non-words. She was able to confirm Meyer et al.'s result for word–word priming and extend it also to non-word–word priming. That is, *lamb–sheep* priming was matched in magnitude by *famb–sheep* priming. However, when the lexically suggestive non-word was the target, no facilitation obtained: *sheep–famb* was no faster than *lure–famb*.

Considering this outcome in isolation one might be inclined to conclude that the lexical processing of *famb* was not intrinsic to pronunciation assembly but merely, as it were, an afterthought, capable of influencing the next decision (*famb–sheep*) but not the concurrent decision (*sheep–famb*). However, Rosson (1983) goes on to show that when a non-word target is ambiguous, in the sense of having alternative, plausible pronunciations, the probability of one or other pronunciation can be biased by a lexical primer. Priming with *sofa* increases the probability that *louch* will be pronounced to rhyme with *couch*, as compared to priming with *feel* (*touch*).

This is indeed a valiant attempt at establishing a role of lexical process in the oral reading of non-words. However, I believe it is indecisive, because the crucial extension to unprimed processing is insecure.

A rather more subtle form of context is employed in some elegant experiments reported by Campbell and Besner (1981). They capitalised upon the fact that initial *th* is usually voiced only in function words, and go on to show that subjects' decisions about whether to voice the initial *th* of a non-word, are strongly determined by whether it is embedded in a syntactic context that leads them to expect a functor or a contentive. This certainly shows that quite refined lexical/syntactic expectations may influence non-word pronunciation. However, it stops short of establishing that such mechanisms are an inevitable part of the assembly of pronunciations even when no expectations have been induced.

The remainder of this discussion of priming is directed towards conditions where there is an orthographic relationship between primer and target. In some of the earliest experiments of this sort, Meyer et al. (1974) used the lexical decision task to show that words sharing the same orthographic and phonological segments primed each other in a facilitatory way when compared to unrelated controls. Words sharing an orthographic pattern that is translated differently into phonology were responded to more slowly than unrelated controls (e.g. RT for *bribe/tribe* < *fence/tribe*; *couch/touch* > *freak/touch*). They interpreted these priming effects as being due to priming of GPCs. Bradshaw and Nettleton (1974) also found inhibitory effects of divergent orthographic mappings (*mown/down*) in a pronunciation task.

To make any progress in this area we must take care to distinguish between three possible types of priming: (1) *orthographic priming*, which is mediated by shared spelling patterns, regardless of their pronunciation; (2) *translation priming*, which is mediated by shared mappings between spelling and sound; and (3) *phonological priming*, which is mediated by shared sound, irrespective of spelling. A case can be made for the existence of each of these forms of priming. As priming between pairs of the *bribe/tribe* sort could be attributed to any of the three types of process, clearly we must look beyond such examples to stimulus conditions that permit a more discriminating analysis.

Evidence for the existence of purerly phonological priming with visual presentation has been provided by Hillinger (1980). He found facilitation of lexical decisions to the second member of a pair of words that rhymed but possess very different spelling (e.g. *late/eight*). This finding has been confirmed by Humphreys et al. (1982).

There seems little doubt that purely orthographic priming may also occur. Evett and Humphreys (1981) have demonstrated orthographic priming within the somewhat different demands of the tachistoscopic recognition task. Circumstantial evidence is also available in the lexical decision task: Shulman et al. (1978) have shown that the inhibitory priming that Meyer et al. found between pairs of the *couch/touch* type could be converted into facilitatory priming by the simple expedient of converting the non-words used in the task into consonant strings, or other orthographically illegal patterns. Such non-words have the effect of speeding up lexical decisions considerably, and there are good reasons to assume that this is because the subject is able to use an orthographic criterion to decide whether a stimulus is wordlike. This criterion renders irrelevant the conflicting mappings into phonology of *couch/touch* pairs. Their residual orthographic similarity allows them to enjoy the facilitatory orthographic priming that was peculiar to pairs of the *bribe/tribe* sort, when words had to be distinguished from plausible non-words.

The inhibitory effect of divergent mappings (*couch/touch*) cannot readily be explained in purely phonological terms and there is a strong case for treating this effect as one of translation.

An aspect of the divergent mapping (*couch/touch*) stimuli that has not been remarked upon is that the very properties that lead to their selection guarantee that at least half of them will be orthographically irregular and all of them inconsistent, in Glushko's sense. It would be interesting to know whether irregular words prime regular words to the same extent as the converse priming. Moreover, if it is elementary GPCs that are primed, then *veal* should inhibit *break* as much as *freak* does. Were it to be found that priming increased in magnitude with increases in the number of graphemes shared by primer and target, then this would have an important bearing on the nature of the translation units. Venezky's GPC rules only take into account graphemic strings of up to three letters. If priming is influenced by larger strings then this would suggest that either a very large number of translation units of varying size is codified, or that the translation mechanism involves orthographic neighbourhoods in the lexicon.

The answer to the empirical question about size of priming units is not known but some further information about characteristics of translation priming is available. Glushko (1981) conducted a naming latency study in which target words were preceded by a potential priming word. This priming word either had to be named or it was the subject of a lexical decision.

As the results turned out, the pattern and magnitude of the priming effects did not differ between naming and lexical decision conditions. (Targets were always named, whatever the task applied to the primers.) Glushko interprets this result as showing that (post-lexical) phonological activation takes place automatically, even when, as in this lexical decision task, the resultant phonological code is distracting.

Another manipulation was built into Glushko's experiment. Primer and target could share various different orthographic properties. These are illustrated in Table 17.2. The results can be summarised by saying that the largest priming effect was obtained with identical primer and targets and the magnitude of the effect declined monotonically as we move towards the right through the conditions listed in Table 17.2. Monosyllabic words that share

TABLE 17.2
Types of Orthographic Relatedness Between Primer and Target Words in
Glushko's (1981) Experiment

| | Differing Segment | | | Shared | Unrelated |
Identical	Initial	Medial	Final	GPC Rule	Control
dice	fire	dome	daze	mole	trap
dice	dire	dime	date	duke	dine

Where stimuli shared the same GPC rule (vowel free in VC*e* context), they had no pronounced letters in common.

all but the initial consonant yield a larger priming effect than those that differ medially or finally. Priming of abstract GPC rules, rather than particular letter sequences, was ineffective. However, this purported attempt at GPC priming extends to only one of many possible ways of writing GPC rules. As a refutation of the general principle of GPC-based translation it does not deserve to be taken seriously.

A priming study that focused on the nature rather than the speed of pronunciation was reported by Kay and Marcel (1981). Their targets were invariably pseudowords, preceded by a number of different types of priming stimuli. For the sake of simplicity, I shall only descibe the most important of these. They were priming by an irregular word that shared the same medial and final spelling (*head/yead*), by a regular word (*bead/yead*), and by an irregular word with unrelated orthography (*hood/yead*). We shall consider this last as the control condition, although various other controls were included.

In the control condition, the non-word was given the regular pronunciation on 84% of occasions. When primed by a word that exhibited the regular translation, the pseudoword was assigned the regular pronunciation on 96% of occasions. When the irregular translation was primed, then the incidence of regular pronunciations declined to 60%. This finding was confirmed using a different technique in the Rosson (1983) study, already discussed.

There are two points of interest in Kay and Marcel's results. First, the response decision could be biased both in the regular and the irregular direction. Second, in the control condition, where no priming is believed to operate, the incidence of regular pronunciation was only 84%. This suggests that if subjects consult a frequency tabulation to make pronunciation decisions about orthographic segments, they do not invariably restrict their attention to the highest-frequency translation, as is supposed in the traditional dual-process model.

Most of these foregoing priming experiments have involved interactions that take place between rapidly successive words. The study by Seidenberg et al. (1984) is exeptional in that the potential targets appear in a second block of trials. It will be remembered that the main thrust of their experiment was methodological. They were able to show that priming occurred over such lags and that its effect was to exaggerate the cost of inconsistency. This claim has wide implications. Its main focus was Glushko's (1979) study in which such priming was inadvertently designed into the experiments due to matching of regular inconsistent and exeption words; for example, *leaf* would be matched with *deaf*. However, most studies have included opportunities for such long-term priming.

What Seidenberg et al. found was that exception words like *deaf* were named slower than regular consistent controls, and this effect was uninfluenced by whether or not the exception word had been preceded by a regular inconsistent word sharing the same spelling pattern (e.g. *leaf*). In contrast, regular inconsistent words, themselves, were only slower than regular consistent controls when they had been preceded by the matched exception word.[5]

Note first that if this priming over long delays were of the same species as Meyer et al.'s (1974) and Bradshaw and Nettleton's (1974) *couch/touch* translation priming, then we should have an answer to one of the questions I posed earlier. The inhibitory effect in immediately successive priming would reside exclusively in the condition where the target was the regular form. Concerning this prediction I freely advertise my pessimism.

Whether the selective inhibitory priming of regular inconsistent words is peculiar to long lags or not, I suggest it might be fruitful to view the inhibitory priming effect alongside the question about whether a critical amount of inconsistency is required before consistency effects become evident. Activating the exception in an orthographic neighbourhood may temporarily increase the saliency of the inconsistency that obtains in that neighbourhood.[6]

Morphological, Semantic, and Syntactic Effects

There are several reasons why it would be desirable to know whether pronunciation decisions are influenced by the morphological, semantic, or syntactic characteristics of isolated words. First, this information is important for the design of controlled experiments. Second, many patients with acquired dyslexias are acutely sensitive in their oral reading to these factors. (Unfortunately, however, the lack of any detectable effect in normal readers would not allow us to draw any firm conclusion about whether they arrived at pronunciations by some quite different means.) Third, a number of models of reading ascribe some measure of independence to the storage of semantic and phonological information in the lexical system, allowing the possibility that phonology might be retrieved without semantic influences. Fourth, some models of lexical access treat the lexicon as a morpheme dictionary with

---

[5] Inexplicably this effect reverses in the lexical decision task. Seidenberg et al. found that task regular inconsistent words were unaffected by priming with matched exceptions, whereas decisions about exception words were slowed when preceded by matched regular words. In view of this puzzle, it would be useful to have a replication of the study.

[6] It remains a problem how this could work if magnitude of inconsistency is determined by a type-count of pronunciations in the neighbourhood. How could such an index be modified by temporary activation of one of the words already entered into the count? One way to resolve this is to think of activation as temporarily duplicating the entry for the primer, such temporary duplications being eventually weeded out by a continuous but slow-acting supervisory process.

words having to be decomposed into their constituent morphemes as a preliminary to lexical access.

Some authors have suggested that the semantic system may be consulted in the course of lexical decisions. The evidence for this view is not over-whelming, although James (1975), for example, found a small disadvantage attaching to abstract words. Richardson (1976), on the other hand, reported that neither lexical decisions nor naming latencies were influenced by abstractness. No other tests of semantic influences on naming seem to have been performed.

Syntactic factors have been equally neglected, the only study being that of Campbell and Besner (1981) on the determinants of voicing of initial *th* in pseudowords.

With regard to morphological factors, Richardson (1976) found no difference in lexical decision latency or naming latency between nouns derived by the suffixation of root form (e.g. *pollution*) and simple nouns (*charlatan*). On the other hand, Taft (1981) reported that pseudo-prefixed words took longer to name than either prefixed or non-prefixed words. Neither of these studies permits any general conclusion about morphological influences. It would perhaps be interesting to study the speed and nature of pronunciations assigned to pseudowords that had been invested with various sorts of quasi-morphological structure, but this has not been done. One problem confronting any investigation of morphological complexity is that affixation has complex repercussions in pronunciation. For example, a spelling pattern often has a different pronunciation when it functions as a true prefix as opposed to a pseudo-prefix.

Errors

The error rate obtained for words in the speeded naming task is usually very low. For skilled readers, the overall error rate is under 5% in all published studies known to me. Error rate appears to vary inversely with word frequency (Forster & Chambers, 1973; Frederiksen, 1976). Error rate increased from 2% for regular words to 4% for irregular words in Mason (1978, experiments 1 and 2). The study by Glushko (1979) produced particularly high error rates for irregular words. In his experiment 1 the rates were: regular 2%, irregular 12%; and in experiment 3: regular 1%, irregular 8%. Seidenberg et al. (1984) found error rates that were negligible in all conditions except for low-frequency exception words, where the error rate approached 10%.

Clearly, we cannot speak of errors in pseudoword naming in quite the same sense as with real words. However, some have designated irregularisations in this way. In the Kay and Marcel (1981) study, 84–90% of unprimed pseudowords were given a regular pronunciation. In that of Glushko (1979), 94–95% of consistent pseudowords were pronounced regularly, but only 78–

88% of inconsistent pseudowords were assigned a regular pronunciation.

One question that has been insufficiently pursued is whether changes in error rate can be used to detect strategy shifts in pronunciation decisions. I have previously suggested in another context (Henderson, 1980) that words may tend to lose their familiar identity when embedded in a mixture with pseudowords. Others have argued that word-specific recognition machinery is automatically engaged when a word occurs, whatever the expectation (Carr et al., 1978). On the former premise, one might expect to induce an increased proportion of errors on low-frequency exception words by camouflaging them against a background of pseudowords. There is slight but inconclusive evidence of such an effect in the comparison of Glushko's (1979) experiments 1 and 3.

Interactions With Reading Ability

A number of studies have pursued the interaction of those factors reviewed in the previous subsection with reading ability. The main focus of attention has been word frequency and lexicality (word vs. non-word) effects (Frederiksen, 1976; Mason, 1978; Wallis, 1982), length effects (Frederiksen, 1976; Mason, 1978, Seymour & Porpodas, 1980), and regularity effects (Mason, 1978; Stanovich & Bauer, 1978; Wallis, 1982).

One general problem attends the interpretation of these interactions. Most of the effects increase in absolute magnitude at lower reading-ability levels. This results in fan interactions such that effects magnify as the absolute magnitude of reaction time increases. In cases of this sort, the interaction can often be abolished by appropriate transformation of the scale on one axis. However, this probably does not allow us to discard all such interactions as unworthy of attention, if only because the various interactions would require radically different transformations for their removal.

Length effects are very sensitive to reader ability. Frederiksen (1976) dichotomised a sample of high-school children on the basis of their scores on the Nelson–Denny Reading Test. The less proficient readers showed larger increases in naming latency with increased letter length and syllabic length of the stimulus word. Furthermore, whereas the better readers' length effect was negligibly affected by word frequency, the less good readers showed increased effects of length as word frequency diminished. The difference between the length effects shown by the two ability groups was particularly marked on non-words.

This finding was confirmed for letter length by Mason (1978), who dichotomised a group of college freshmen on the Nelson-Denny Test. The more skilled readers showed a length effect on words of 23 msec/letter. The effect for the less skilled readers was 50 msec/letter. With non-words the effect. was more striking, being 34 msec/letter for more skilled readers and 72 msec/letter for less skilled.

Seymour and Porpodas (1980) also studied letter-length effects in non-word naming. In children with a reading age of 12.1 the length effect was 63 msec/letter, whereas a younger group, with a reading age of 7.9, showed an effect of 308 msec/letter. A group classed as developmental dyslexics showed an effect of 721 msec/letter.

Word frequency and lexicality effects are also magnified at lower levels of reading ability, though the interaction is less striking than that involving word length. Frederiksen (1976) found a difference in RT for pseudowords and high-frequency words of 59 msec in his highest reading-ability school-children. For the lowest-ability group the difference was 142 msec. Mason's (1978) more skilled group showed an effect of 113 msec and the less skilled 211 msec. Similarly, Wallis (1982), in a number of experiments on primary schoolchildren, found an interaction between lexicality and reading age with the less-able children showing a larger lexicality effect.

The error rate in naming high-frequency words has usually been negligible in all but the very lowest levels of reading skill. Differences do, however, emerge with low-frequency words. Forster and Chambers (1973), studying skilled adults, found error rates for high- and low-frequency words of only 0% and 2% respectively. In his study of schoolchildren, Frederiksen (1976) found that the error rate on high-frequency words did not reliably distinguish between the ability-level groups. Overall, the error rate on high-frequency words was about 4%. However, on low-frequency words a reliable difference emerged. The highest-ability group showed an error rate of 8% compared to 17% in the lowest-ability group.

In contrast to the substantial interactions between reading ability and both length effects and frequency effects, the effects of orthographic regularity on naming latency do not seem to depend very noticeably on reading ability. In Mason's (1978) study of college freshmen, the more and less skilled reading groups differed by about 70 msec in naming latency yet neither group showed any evidence of a regularity effect. More errors were made on exception words, though this effect was not reliable across stimuli and it did not interact with reader ability.

In a number of unpublished experiments from our laboratory, Wallis (1982) has measured regularity and consistency effects in the word naming of primary schoolchildren and undergraduates. Over 350 schoolchildren were studied across a 4-year age band. Small but generally reliable effects of both regularity and consistency were found, usually in the 10–40 msec range. However, there was no evidence that these effects increased in magnitude as age or reading level diminished, despite substantial changes in overall RT. In these same experiments, the advantage of words over pseudowords markedly declined with increasing reader ability. In Wallis's experiments on skilled undergraduate readers, the effect of regularity and consistency was very small and generally unreliable.

Wallis's study appears to be the only investigation of regularity effects in the naming latencies of children, but Barron (1980, 1981) has investigated regularity effects in the lexical decision latencies of children. In Barron's (1980) study of 11–12-year-olds, the 5-msec advantage of regular words was unreliable. The error rate did, however, increase from 6.7% to 11.5% with irregularity. Barron (1981) replicated his previous study with the major difference that he employed illegal non-words (e.g. *imxk*). This time there was a reliable 60 msec regularity effect on latencies as well as an error effect. In both of these studies, the better readers tended to show the *larger* regularity effects.

THEORETICAL ISSUES

When children first learn to read English, they often acquire an initial "sight" vocabulary of words that can be named when visually presented. A bright and enquiring child may learn these print–sound correspondences incidentally and without formal tuition. If reading is to progress, however, then there comes a stage at which general procedures have to be learned. This is required in order to free the child from the necessity of having experienced the conjunction of the written and spoken forms of a word. Translation of print into sound that is based on *recognition* of particular orthographic forms needs to be supplemented by a process that is *transformational*, a process that can accept a printed form presented for the first time and decompose it into familiar segments to which a pronunciation can be assigned. For most beginning readers this procedure alone is not adequate. The resultant phonology remains segmental, halting, and shapeless. If the pronunciation is to be assembled properly then it has to be "recognised" as a known word sound. Fortunately, the child with normal hearing usually has the target word in his or her speech vocabulary. Nevertheless, the inability to recognise his or her segmental translations represents a major practical difficulty. It also constitutes a theoretical puzzle. Why cannot the child's speech recognition system accept an approximation that is perfectly recognisable by most adults? The same question can be posed about the oral reading, especially the neologisms, produced by surface dyslexics.

At this stage, then, the child's fluent productions are to a great extent limited by what he or she can lexically recognise either immediately, and presumably visually, or via his or her own hesitant segmental translations into a sound pattern that can be lexically interpreted by the child's speech recognition system.

Progress beyond this stage cannot simply depend upon improvement in recognising the translations that are generated, because the child may eventually learn to pronounce forms never previously encountered in either language modality. Thus, there is a sense in which oral reading is no longer limited by the lexicon. Yet, this does not mean that reading of familiar words is achieved by the same means as pseudowords are read. Even the child of reading age 11–12 who can initiate naming of a familiar word in about 550 msec takes a further 100 msec to decide the pronunciation of a matched pseudoword (Wallis, 1982).

The emergent ability to assign a pronunciation to printed pseudowords has been widely accepted as evidence of some sort of segmental translation process that stands in contrast to the retrieval of a familiar word's pronunciation as a whole from the lexicon. In theoretical treatments, this contrast has been heightened by appeal to logical considerations. Hence, in Baron and Strawson's (1976) terminology, we are told that: "we *must* use the orthographic mechanism in pronouncing words we have never seen before, such as names, and the lexical mechanism for words for which no rules are available, such as lb ... (p. 391)."

Similarly, Coltheart (1980) has argued that the ability to read non-words establishes the existence of a non-lexical translation mechanism, because presumably non-words lack lexical entries. In Coltheart's version of the argument, logographs are joined by irregular words as forms that cannot be correctly translated by non-lexical rules and so require the existence of a lexical route to phonology. Finally, he argues that this non-lexical translation process must result in a phonological code that can be used to address the lexicon, as most readers can understand to what animal *phocks* refers.

The core of these arguments seems to me incontrovertible. Nevertheless, the distance they carry us forward can easily be overestimated. Much hinges on the interpretation of surprisingly ambiguous terms like "lexical", "non-lexical," and "route." Accordingly, I attempt to show that behind each of these seemingly innocent terms lies a set of fundamental theoretical choices.

"Lexical"

At least two questions arise about the lexical retrieval of phonology: (1) What is the relationship between lexical phonology and lexical semantics? (2) What form is taken by the lexical representation of phonology? We consider these in turn.

Lexical Phonology and Lexical Semantics

Much of the early concern with access to lexical information in reading was directed towards the question of how we gain access to word meanings. As a consequence, the term "lexical" has come to be implicity associated with the process of retrieving semantic information. Perhaps the dictionary metaphor has also been at work, with its implication that orthographic and phonetic forms and meanings are all immediately available together. This consolidation of the semantic and phonological aspects of lexical functioning has been strengthened further by the tendency to equate the dual-process theory of semantic access with the dual-process theory of access to phonology. Hence when we speak of a direct, lexical route from print to meaning, in contrast to a route via non-lexical translation rules, and of a direct, lexical route to phonology, in contrast to a route via non-lexical rules, it has been easy to fall into the unquestioning assumption that the lexical route referred to is the same in both cases. Recently, however, a number of reasons for re-examining this issue have emerged.

Much of the evidence on the relationship between the semantic and phonological lexical systems has been neuropsychological in provenance. In deep dyslexia, the retrieval of a printed word's pronunciation seems to involve semantic processing to an extent that is not obvious in normal reading. It might be that a certain breakdown of reading competence is able to reveal a contingency between retrieval of phonological and semantic information from the lexical system that is simply not detectable in normal reading. Alternatively, deep dyslexia may be characterised by an abnormal strategy for oral reading. Both sorts of theory have found persuasive advocates, so we must turn to some other realm for decisive evidence.

Perhaps the most frequently cited evidence of a dissociation between access to sound and meaning in reading is that of Schwartz, Marin, and Saffran (1979), who described a case of pre-senile dementia. This patient had greatly impaired semantic functioning but could read aloud words that she could neither comprehend nor produce in object naming. The crucial factor was her ability to read aloud orthographically irregular words, such as *do*, *come*, and *bury*. Schwartz et al. argued that their patient could not have been reading such irregular words by means of non-lexical translation rules, because the rules are not supposed to work for irregular words. They concluded, therefore, that it must be possible in reading to retrieve pronunciation from the lexicon independently from semantic information. They concentrated on the fact that their patient was able to read many irregular words. However, it is also clear that performance on irregular words was considerably worse than on regular words, a finding also obtained by Warrington (1975) for the demented patient E.M.

Two general theoretical strategies have been employed to deal with the Schwartz et al. finding. Morton and Patterson (1980) have postulated three routes to the phonology of printed words. One goes via lexical semantics and is required to account for the surviving competence in the reading of deep dyslexics. Another route is entirely non-lexical and utilises spelling–sound rules. This route is postulated to accommodate effects of orthographic regularity in normal and impaired reading. The last route gives orthographic access to whole-word phonology while bypassing semantics and is required to account for oral reading of irregular words in the absence of comprehension, such as was displayed in Schwartz et al.'s patient.

Shallice and Warrington (1980) concur in postulating a route via semantics, but they differ from Morton and Patterson (1980) in assuming but a single non-semantic route. The key attribute of this route, and indeed the only one that they explicitly described, is that as it becomes increasingly impaired, competence with highly irregular then mildly irregular words is lost.

A different sort of evidence for word-specific links between orthography and phonology has been provided by Coltheart et al. (1983). Their evidence also rests on instances of irregular words being assigned the correct phonology without receiving the appropriate semantic interpretation, but the circumstances were quite different from the Schwartz et al. case. Their subjects were two surface dyslexic readers who occasionally exhibited the following confusion. When asked the meaning of an irregular homophone such as *route* they would supply the meaning of the homophonous word *root*. From such systematic errors Coltheart et al. concluded that their surface dyslexic readers could not on these occasions gain direct visual access to the meaning of the printed word. However, as the meaning supplied was appropriate to an identically pronounced but differently spelled word, their subjects must have succeeded in arriving at the correct phonology for an irregular word and had then been able to use that phonology to gain access to lexical semantics. This conjunction of correct phonology with lack of direct semantic access could only be detected in the case of homophones.

Yet another line of evidence for this word-specific access to phonology independent of semantics has been provided by Funnell (1983). In some ways her evidence is stronger because it does not rest on the assumption that irregular words can only be pronounced by lexical (word-specific) means. Funnell's patient exhibited phonological dyslexia, in which there is an almost total inability to read aloud non-words. This disability seems to imply that any oral reading of words must have been achieved lexically. But her subject could read aloud words that he could not understand, so his word-specific access to phonology must have been independent of semantics.

The converse dissociation has been reported in studies of surface dyslexia, that is, a written word can be comprehended but cannot be pronounced (e.g. Deloche et al., 1982, and the chapters in Part II of this book).[7]

The Structure of Lexical Representations of Phonology

One problem that is too important to pass without mention, but too extensive to treat here in detail, is that of the relationship between input and

---

[7] It would be interesting to know whether this also occurs in normal beginning readers. And if not, as I suspect, why not?

output phonology. This has been something of a classic question in the study of speech recognition. It becomes a question also for students of reading as soon as the case is made for an independent phonological lexicon that can be directly addressed at a word-specific level by means of an orthographic code. It has generally been assumed that it is output phonology that is addressed directly by the orthographic input code. Thus, in the notation of *logogens*, Morton and Patterson (1980) represent this competence by a processing pathway from the *visual input logogens* to the (articulatory) *output logogens*, bypassing semantics. Since Coltheart et al. (1983) have shown that lexical phonology that has been obtained without semantic mediation can be used to gain access to lexical semantics, the Morton and Patterson model must be supplemented with a connection leading from the output logogen back into semantics, perhaps via the *auditory* input logogens.

In an alternative approach (Allport & Funnell, 1981), the phonological functions of the lexicon are consolidated in one structure that serves input and output. It is sometimes difficult to decide to what extent these alternative formulations differ substantively rather than in mere notational conventions. This difficulty is increased by a certain vagueness about the precise nature of the codes that are implied in the flow diagrams. For example, Morton and Patterson (1980) do not discuss the level of code that is supplied by the output logogens or by grapheme–phoneme conversion and it is unclear how closely these codes resemble each other and how removed they are from an articulatory realisation, or from a speech recognition code.

A different, though possibly related, set of questions is raised by theories that attribute a major role to morphological structure in the organisation and access of the lexicon. For example, the contrast that is often made between the retrieval of whole-word phonology from the lexicon and the assembly of phonology from translated segments might seem to imply that the former, "lexical," process is direct and immediate. That this need not be the case is most clearly evident in theories that hold the lexicon to be constructed from morphemic elements (e.g. Taft & Forster, 1975). In order to gain access to a morpheme-based lexicon the orthographic pattern has to be decomposed into morphemic segments. This poses two problems in English: the orthographic form taken by a root morpheme is not invariant (*crux/crucial, hang/hung*, etc.) and many words are subject to alternative, plausible decompositions (*fully* is suffixed but *bully* is not).

Theories that treat the lexical representation of words as having to be derived from a morphemic base tend to blur the wholistic/segmental distinction otherwise made between the retrieval of whole-word phonology from the lexicon and the assembly of segmental phonology, derived from non-lexical spelling–sound translation. In morphological decomposition theories, both the lexical and the non-lexical processes involve parsing of the orthographic pattern into segments (albeit of quite different composition). Similarly, pronunciation of an entire word has to be assembled from morphemic segments, at least in the case of polymorphemic words. In pronunciation tasks, these complex procedures might give rise to a number of effects due to the internal structure of words, effects that arise due to the workings of the input decomposition procedure (Taft, 1981), or the stage of pronunciation assembly (MacKay, 1978).

Morpheme-based models of the lexicon owe part of their inspiration to the desire to achieve economy of storage. Accordingly, no phonological information is stored in the lexicon if it is predictable from linguistic rules. Thus the abstract morphemic elements retrieved from the lexicon are concatenated and given articulatory shape by the application of phonological rules, such as the vowel-checking and stress-assignment rules that govern suffixation. From such a perspective, the direct word-specific connection between orthography and output phonology begins to appear somewhat less direct.

One interesting aspect of English morphology is that the meaning of derived forms is not reliably predictable from the meaning of their morphemic constituents (Henderson, Wallis, & Knight, 1983). However, as soon as we confront the possibility of an independent phonological lexicon, we are able to contemplate the notion that the morphemic structure of words plays more of a role in the organisation of lexical phonology than lexical semantics. This may seem a surprising idea, given the definition of a morpheme as a unit of meaning and given the historical relationship between morphology and etymology, but if we take an ahistorical view of the regularities currently to be found in the language then it seems evident that morphology is reflected more predictably in the workings of syntax and phonology than in lexical semantics. This is in accord with the close association between morphology and phonology in generative linguistic theories.

"Non-lexical" Mechanisms

Here we come to the heart of the debate about the nature of the mechanism responsible for translation of segments and assembly of a pronunciation. Under this heading I intend to treat all the proposals that have been advanced concerning the mechanisms of pronunciation assembly, despite the fact that the label "non-lexical" incorporates the theoretical commitments of the dual-process account.

In the dual-process account, the concept of a non-lexical mechanism owes its inspiration to a number of diverse ideas. Three of these can be encapsulated in the terms "non-word reading," "GPC tabulations," and "pre-lexical phonology." Thus, for example, Coltheart (1980) writes:

... phonological coding is a process which can be carried out whether or not a letter string is a word, and hence is a nonlexical process. It is also nonlexical in the sense that it is prelexical, because it is carried out so as to produce a phonological representation which is *subsequently* used to access the internal lexicon (p. 203).

One difficulty with the characterisation of the mechanism of pronunciation assembly as "non-lexical" and "pre-lexical" is that it seems to preclude from the start, by terminological *fiat*, the possibility that pronunciation assembly might be "lexical" in the restricted sense of drawing on a lexical data base, as in the proposals advanced by Glushko (1979), Marcel (1980), and Henderson (1982).

We have already rehearsed the non-word argument. It is essentially definitional rather than substantive. It reminds us that non-words are non-lexical. More generally, pseudoword reading reminds us that orthographic translation has to become generative for us to learn to read. The fact that our oral reading can be creative rules out certain possibilities but it does not, in itself, tell us anything more about the mechanism for translating non-lexical forms.

The notion of "pre-lexical" phonology has been historically associated with the concept of non-lexical translation by GPCs, but its essential function is to express the idea of phonological recoding as a preliminary of access to the semantic lexicon. Unfortunately the term can easily lead to the confusion of two distinct concepts, *assembled* phonology (in contrast to *retrieved* phonology, see Patterson, 1981) and phonology used to address lexical semantics. Phonology derived from print and used to address lexical semantics is often, but not inevitably, assembled phonology. In the case of Coltheart et al.'s (1983) surface dyslexic who identified *bury* as "a fruit on a tree," the phonology is assumed to be pre-semantic but not assembled. Instead, it is assumed to be retrieved from an independent phonological lexicon that can be used to address semantics. Where a pseudohomophone such as *brane* or *phocks* addresses its semantic referent, the mediating phonology is presumably assembled. Whether such phonology is assembled from tabulated segmental translations or from lexical analogies remains to be decided.

In sum, then, the bald facts that we can assign a (more or less agreed) pronunciation to non-words and that we can transform print into a phonological code that can subsequently be used to address semantics have to be reckoned with. However, they do not, in themselves, identify the nature of the mechanisms of pronunciation assembly.

Let us turn now to the fundamental questions that separate existing theoretical approaches. In my view, the issues are best described as follows: (1) What is the size of translation units from which pronunciations are assembled? (2) How are translations stored? In other words, what sort of mental representation is addressd in translation? (3) What factors delay pronunciation decisions? Each of these issues is discussed in turn.

Concerning the size of translation unit, I believe that the recent accumulation of evidence points incontrovertibly to a broad range of size. Although the issue has been insufficiently explored, this conclusion seems to stem from two sources; the nature of pronunciations assigned to pseudowords and the so-called consistency effect.

Where large and small segments provide divergent clues to pseudoword pronunciation, large segments often seem to be taken into account but do not overwhelm the decision process (Kelliher, 1983; Patterson & Morton, this volume). My informal impression is that large unit translations are most influential when unequivocal, as in *old* and *igh*. Concerning priming studies, I have urged caution in generalising to unprimed pronunciation decisions. However, the studies by Kay and Marcel (1981) and Rosson (1983) support the view that large units, such as the medial and final portion of a syllable, influence but do not wholly determine pronunciation.

Effects on naming latency attributable to consistency within an orthographic neighbourhood seem to argue also for the importance of the larger orthographic context in pronunciation decisions. Although such effects seem to be more limited than was first claimed by Glushko (see Parkin, 1983; Seidenberg et al., 1984), the balance of evidence suggests that they do reliably occur under some circumstances.

The question as to what form of data base yields up the candidate translations for segments is most clearly posed in the opposition of Coltheart's (1978) and Glushko's (1979) views. Coltheart's view of the nature of the store consulted in deciding pronunciations is that it is a precodified translation table in which orthographic segments are listed together with their appropriate translation. Appropriateness is determined by the frequency with which a translation occurs. The translation of an orthographic segment that occurs in the greatest number of words is held to be "regular."

Whereas Coltheart's GPC theory supposes a frequency-based tabulation that exists independently from the lexicon, in Glushko's analogy theory information about correspondences is inherent in the connections between orthographic and phonological entries in the lexicon and has no separate existence. In order to speak of correspondences, however, it is necessary to assume that orthographic entries are structured into segments of various sizes that can be related to segments in the phonological lexicon (Henderson, 1982; Marcel, 1980).

This, then, is the fundamental difference between regularity theories such as Coltheart's (1978) GPC theory and consistency theories such as Glushko's (1979) analogy theory. Unfortunately, however, the theories differ in a number of other important respects and these other differing assumptions have proved easier to test experimentally than the fundamental difference in the way that spelling–sound correspondences are supposed to be stored.

I have already alluded to one of these differences. The typical unit of translation is larger in analogy theory than in GPC theory. Glushko (1979) was rather equivocal about the size of unit that could lead to lexical analogies. His discussion of orthographic neighbourhoods focused on stimuli that share all but the initial consonant cluster. However, this leaves open the question of how the initial consonants become translated. Moreover, the size of the unit of translation is logically constrained by the nature of a stimulus's orthographic neighbourhood: *tead* has many close neighbours and analogies may involve large overlapping segments (*tear, lead*, etc.); *kwub*, in contrast, has only remote lexical neighbours.

At least one regularity tabulation theory, on the other hand, includes large segments. Shallice et al. (1983) assume that units as large as the morpheme are tabulated by their "phonological system."

Another incidental difference between Coltheart's GPC theory and Glushko's analogy theory lies in what I call the *decision process*, though neither theorist has been very explicit about the process. By the decision process I mean the way in which the translation data base is used to arrive at a pronunciation decision, and, by extension, the factors that complicate and retard that decision.

Coltheart (1978) implied that in his GPC procedure, the regular (most frequent) translation was invariably chosen. There now seem to be grounds for contesting that assumption. First, the evidence from pseudoword reading and from errors in reading words shows that less frequent translations are sometimes assigned. This, in turn, seems to imply that the process of reading off the most frequent correspondences is subject to noise, or else that the decision rule is not a straightforward frequency discrimination. Second, evidence of effects apparently due to some sort of competition between the alternative translations of a segment suggests a more complex decision process. Such effects include consistency effects and magnitude of irregularity effects.

Glushko (1979) was even less explicit about the decision process that operated upon analogies to produce a pronunciation. He merely states two assumptions: (1) assembly will take longer the smaller the segments that have to be assembled (this appears to be a gesture towards explaining the lexicality effect: non-words *must* be assembled from segments); (2) inconsistency somehow slows decisions.

In summary, we have seen that Glushko's theory differs from Coltheart's in several respects: the nature of the data base in which correspondences are stored (lexical connections vs. non-lexical segment tabulations), the size of translation units (typically large vs. GPC), and the decision process (under-specified but sensitive to inconsistency vs. frequency algorithm). I have somewhat perversely held the least testable question, the nature of the data base, to be the fundamental one. On size of the translation unit, Coltheart's position is not essential to the non-lexical tabulation view (cf. Shallice et al., 1983).

Before leaving the question of segment size, it is worth pointing out that *at the limit*, frequency tabulation approaches become difficult to distinguish even in principle from lexical analogy approaches. Suppose, for example, that we found that subjects were inclined to pronounce *slood* to rhyme with *thud*. Our frequency tabulation theorist interprets this as showing that the tabulations list /ʌ/ as the regular correspondence for *oo* in the environment *lood*. The analogy theorist asserts, to the contrary, that the response is evidence that *slood* activated information about the lexical items *blood* and *flood*. The analogy theorist might go on to deride the GPC theorist's bloated tabulation. Why not suppose, then, a rule that *olo* is pronounced /ə/ in the graphemic environment *colone* (hence *colonel* but *colonial*)? The point is that by allowing a segment so large that there is only one entry in the tabulation, we have, in effect, a lexicon.

Let us now turn our attention to the decision process that operates upon the translation data base, whatever its form, to supply the phonology for assembly. Whereas I have previously argued that consistency effects would constitute conclusive evidence favouring the analogy view over the correspondence tabulation view (Henderson, 1982), I wish here instead to suggest that the analogies versus tabulations issue bears on the nature of the data base, whereas consistency effects have implications for the nature of the decision process. An alternative way to express this is to say that the analogy hypothesis and the consistency hypothesis are fortuitously combined in Glushko's (1979) seminal work. If we can show that correspondence tabulation models can be constructed so as to predict consistency effects, then we shall have blunted the apparently incisive adjudication in favour of the analogy hypothesis.[8]

Consider the following first approximation to a model. The lexical retrieval process supplies its word-specific solution. Within the limits of the

---

[8] My initial attempts to devise tabulation models that could yield consistency effects were made in collaboration with my colleague Julie Wallis. The model briefly mentioned in the conference paper on which this chapter is based was designed specifically to yield consistency effects for words but not pseudowords. This strong assumption about the empirical state of affairs now seems to be premature. Although the balance of evidence seems clearly to indicate that consistency effects quite often obtain, it is not yet securely evident what circumstances govern their appearance. Rather than base a detailed model on more or less arbitrary assumptions about the form taken by consistency effects, I have preferred to consider a few of the general questions that arise in constructing such models. Others have been exercised by similar questions (Funnell, 1983; Patterson & Morton, this volume).

reader's competence, this will be the appropriate pronunciation. At the same time a non-lexical process sets about supplying a translation based upon correspondence tabulations of whatever sort. The outputs of both processes are compared. When they agree, this agreed response is chosen. When they disagree, greater weight is attached to the lexical solution and that candidate is generally chosen. Disagreement costs decision time, however.

A model along these lines has been entertained by Funnell (1983). Patterson & Morton, this volume, on the other hand, seem inclined to reject such a mechanism on common-sense grounds, because there seems no good reason to check the pronunciation assembled from the tabulations if the lexical output is invariably correct.

I dispute this reasoning. If it cannot be determined in advance that lexical search will supply a candidate then work must always commence immediately on an assembled translation. Where such an alternative solution is available, therefore, and conflicts with the lexical solution, it may well prove impossible to ignore. A large body of evidence testifies to our limited ability to ignore codes that we may "know" to be irrelevant, whether in card sorting or Stroop interference tasks. Moreover, lexical retrieval may be fallible, especially for low-frequency words, so some sort of recursive checking may make sense.

What is most interesting about this first approximation is that it gives an account of the classic regularity effect on latencies. For this purpose I believe it is superior to the traditional horse-race model (cf. Henderson, 1982). However, as a piece of predictive machinery it is inadequate to our purpose. It gives no account of the disadvantage suffered by regular but inconsistent words, because in such cases the two outputs agree. Nor does it provide an explanation of consistency effects in pseudowords, as *ex hypothesi* they do not activate a lexical solution at all.

It is instructive to consider the failure of the first approximation model. What it seems to lack is a source of decision difficulty internal to the non-lexical process. Only by this means does it appear that we can explain consistency effects. It is not a difficult matter to postulate appropriate difficulties that might arise within the non-lexical procedure. For illustrative purpose I consider but two contrasting examples.

Suppose that selection from the tabulations is based upon a straightforward frequency rule but that even though the rule is unambiguous, the tabulation itself is not. I call this the *frequency discrimination* problem. When we look up the tabulation for *ee*, say, it is readily evident that the dominant translation is /i/ as in *eel*. Only a tiny minority of exceptions exist, such as *mêlée*. In contrast, the tabulations for *ea* contain three distinct correspondences, all of them quite common, with the most frequent (as in *each*) barely discriminably so from the next most (as in *deaf*).

The importance of this sort of difficulty has scarcely been investigated.[9] However, we know that this simple story will not suffice as an account of consistency effects anyway, because the intrinsic ambiguity of *ea* does not allow us to distinguish between the cases of, for example, *breach* and *bread*. Yet if end-segment consistency effects are real then the tabulations should list /i/ as the almost universal vowel translation in *each* (*each*, *reach*, *teach*, etc.) but for *ead* the tabular entries are finely balanced, with a slight bias favouring /ɛ/ over /i/. Thus for *bread* there are two possible sources of difficulty in reading off the correspondence from the tabulations: (1) even if attention is restricted to the largest segment listed (say, *ead*), frequency discrimination is difficult; (2) if appropriate segments of all sizes are considered, there is conflict between the majority solution for *ea* and for *ead*. (Notice, in passing, that Glushko (1979) does not consider this distinction between conflicting correspondences within a segment and between segments of different size.)

The sort of frequency discrimination hypothesis just sketched fits Glushko's (1979) latency data in one respect that is of particular interest. Glushko found no reliable difference between naming RT for regular inconsistent words like *gave* and exception words like *have*. This prediction is obligatory for any model that locates ambiguity effects entirely within the non-lexical process. The difference between *gave* and *have* in the difficulties that they might present to the decision process arise out of the relationship between the lexical solution and the tabulation data. This does not mean, however, that the *frequency discrimination* mechanism is insensitive to the magnitude of inconsistency. To be sure, *have* cannot differ from *gave* in difficulty, but both *have* and *gave* would be expected to be easier than, say, *move* and *cove*, as the selection of the commonest translation from the *ove* table is less easy than the *ave* table. Thus, magnitude of inconsistency is effective in one sense but not the other.

An alternative to the *frequency discrimination* notion is one in which the decision difficulty inheres in the number of possible translations supplied by the tabulations for a given segment. Let us call this the *search set* difficulty. Search set difficulty might slow consultation of the tabulations. Alternatively, if the tabulations supply all possible candidates and choice is made not by frequency determination but by lexical checking (as in the Wallis/ Henderson model referred to in footnote 8) then the checking process might be sensitive to number of alternatives.

---

[9]Seidenberg et al. (1984, experiment 1) failed to find an effect of such ambiguity. Unfortunately, however, their stimuli fell in a high-frequency band in which they were also unable to detect consistency effects, so their result is not decisive.

Routes

The hypothetical lexical and non-lexical processes are sometimes spoken of as "routes." The idea that each may serve as an independent route sufficient, at least for some type of stimulus, to convert an orthographic stimulus into a final spoken response constitutes a fundamental tenet of *dual-route* theory. This theory has been most explicitly applied to lexical decisions (e.g. Coltheart et al., 1977), where it has been assumed that stimuli are automatically entered into both routes and a "horse-race" determines which route will trigger the response decision. The model has been generalised, at least implicitly, to the naming task. Under this final heading I consider the question of whether the distinction between assembled and word-specific processes requires us to postulate that each serves as the basis of an independent route.

It is worth remarking from the start that the *independent route* postulate is a much stronger assertion than the *distinguishable process* one. Acceptance of the weaker assertion certainly does not entail the stronger proposition.

One source of inspiration for the dual-process account has undoubtedly been the purported double dissociation between the lexical and non-lexical routes in the acquired dyslexias. Considerable dispute attaches to the question of how clearly this dissociation has been demonstrated and how relevant such a demonstration might be to our understanding of normal reading. Suffice it to say here that I know of no data capable of sustaining the strong assertion of independence, though, of course, it is always possible that such data might in future be found.

A number of tests of the independent-route, horse-race model are possible on normal word-naming data. The first of these is based on the convergent estimates of the relative completion time of the two routes. The fact that words can be named faster on average than pseudowords entails the conclusion that the lexical route is faster on some occasions. On the other hand, effects of spelling–sound predictability on naming latency must lead to the conclusion that the non-lexical route sometimes yields its product first. It follows, therefore, that the two routes must have overlapping response time distributions. Now, because exception words can supposedly only be read by the lexical route and pseudowords by the non-lexical route, the overlap of the naming latency distributions for these two classes of item should allow us to estimate the proportion of trials on which the non-lexical route was the faster. However, when the non-lexical route is faster for an exception word, and presuming that the routes are independent, the response must be a regularisation error. We should be able, therefore, to predict the error rate from the latency distribution overlap, provided we have matched the exceptions and pseudowords carefully.[10]

---

[10] My conjecture is that there will turn out to be fewer errors than predicted. The overlap of distributions, even with high-frequency words, is usually substantial (e.g. Glushko, 1979, experiment 1).

A different sort of test concerns the interaction between word frequency and spelling–sound predictability. This test becomes available if we grant the assumption that word frequency affects the lexical route but not the non-lexical route. As a preliminary, recall that the magnitude of the word frequency effect is only half as great in the naming task as in the lexical decision task. This *might* be due to the involvement of the non-lexical route in the naming task, thus diluting the frequency effect. However, it might equally be due to any of: (1) a pre-lexical global familiarity effect in lexical decisions; (2) a post-lexical, semantic effect in lexical decisions; (3) differences in frequency effects between the semantic and phonological lexicons.

What should be the case, however, is that frequency effects should be larger for exception words than regular words on occasions when regular words enjoy a latency advantage. This is so because this advantage stems from the fact that the non-lexical route terminated faster than the lexical route on a proportion of trials, giving an edge to the regular words. Such an effect has recently been reported by Andrews (1982) and by Seidenberg et al. (1984). The question therefore arises whether this finding can be accommodated in alternative models, in which the routes interact.

If we assume that length effects, notably number of letters, are due to the operation of the non-lexical route, then we can devise further tests. Frederiksen and Kroll (1976) have endorsed this assumption, because they found length effects in naming but not in lexical decision, and Seymour and Porpodas (1980) have also adopted it, but it amounts to no more than a plausible conjecture. Granting the assumption, we should find larger length effects for lower-frequency words (less lexical involvement) and largest of all length effects for pseudowords (no lexical involvement to dilute the length effect). The length × frequency interaction has been tested by Cosky (1976) and by Ellis (1982). Both reported effects of length and of frequency with no reliable tendency for the length effect to increase at lower frequencies. The length × lexicality effect was investigated by Frederiksen and Kroll (1976), who found roughly equal length effects for words and pseudowords. On the other hand, less skilled readers show much larger frequency, lexicality, and length effects as well as an interaction between frequency (or lexicality) and length.

There is another possible approach to the search for independent lexical and non-lexical routes. We may search for strategies in which one route is favoured over the other. In one version of the approach through strategies, individual differences in the disposition towards one or other strategy are investigated. This is the approach taken by Baron (1977) and by Barron (1980). An alternative method, which is, in principle, more robust, is to attempt to manipulate strategies. This is often done by investigating the consequences of guaranteeing that stimulus items will belong to a particular class, for which one strategy is especially appropriate (or inappropriate). In this vein, Frederiksen and Kroll (1976) compared a condition in which words and pseudowords were blocked with one in which they were randomly intermingled. Non-word naming appeared to be unaffected by this manipulation but words were named faster when lexicality was blocked and the word-frequency effect seemed larger. This is actually something of a puzzle from the viewpoint of dual-process theory as it is unclear why the subjects should employ the lexical route more in one condition than the other. (*Ex hypothesi* it won't work for non-words, but it won't interfere either.)

The last test of the horse-race model to be considered is a somewhat indirect one that appeals to developmental considerations. It is well established that the advantage for real words over pseudowords in children's naming latencies diminishes greatly with increasing reading age (Frederiksen, 1976; Mason, 1978; Wallis, 1982). Even taking account of the increased variance of their latency distributions, this implies that very unskilled readers should show negligible effects of spelling–sound predictability, as such effects can only be manifest on occasions when the non-lexical route is completed first. This prediction is not fulfilled. Wallis (1982) found no tendency whatsoever for regularity or consistency effects to change over reading age in young children, despite a substantial age trend in the magnitude of the lexicality effect. A lack of interaction between regularity and reading ability was also reported by Briggs and Underwood (1982).

Indeed, further reflection on beginning readers seems to suggest the conclusion that initially, at least, there must be considerable interaction between the routes. As Funnell (1983) has pointed out, for words first encountered in print the non-lexical route must be capable of creating a new phonological entry in the lexicon. Moreover, my own suspicion is that improvement in the word-specific strategy *depends* on progress in segmental translation. It is often remarked in the pedagogical literature that the child may rapidly acquire a small "sight vocabulary" but then further progress will depend on the acquisition of some skill in segmental translation. The adherent of a horse-race theory would presumably have to maintain that the routes develop into independence.

The difficulties encountered by the horse-race model suggest that it is worth exploring models in which the lexical and non-lexical processes interact. One possible locus of convergence occurs after non-lexical translation. I argued in the first section of this chapter, as others have previously done, that the products of non-lexical translation would require considerable further processing in order to yield a code suitable for articulation. Polysyllabic items, in particular, require stress assignment, morphophonemic adjustment of vowels, and, if pronunciation is to be correct, various phonetic markings of morpheme boundaries. For these reasons it may be expedient to attempt to use the assembled translation to access the phonological component of the lexicon rather than transform the translation directly into an articulatory code. This, I surmised earlier, is what beginning readers are attempting to do when they struggle to recognise the faltering products of segmental translation. Somehow success at this venture may increase the likelihood of progressing to the successful access of lexical phonology by means of a purely orthographic word code, though it is very difficult to see how this might actually work.

This line of thought is highly speculative and it would be helpful if we could find some relevant evidence or at least indicate where evidence might be sought. One possible resort lies concealed in a footnote to Coltheart et al. (1979, p. 495). They point out that for certain irregular words a regular translation will match a real but inappropriate entry in the phonological lexicon (e.g. *bread→breed, move→mauve, come→comb*). Whether such words pose any special problems for the reader remains to be determined.

Fragments of evidence do, however, exist in the literature on two different types of acquired dyslexia. Derouesné and Beauvois (Chapter 16 in this book) have shown that a patient whose primary difficulty lay in the oral reading of non-words was much more successful when the non-word was a pseudohomophone, that is, when its likely translation matched an entry in the phonological lexicon. Unfortunately, this advantage depended on instructing the patient in the use of a lexical strategy. Hence the strategy might be peculiar to the impairment.

It is well established that lexicalisation plays a role in the reading errors of most surface dyslexic readers. Where such errors occur on non-words they seem to imply a degree of lexical involvement in non-word reading. This is especially puzzling in light of the prevailing assumption that the primary deficit in surface dyslexia is in the lexical process. This finding does not, in itself, serve to establish what form this lexical involvement takes. However, recent evidence presented by Saffran (this volume) sheds some light on the problem. She analysed a corpus of errors from a patient, L.L., who exhibited a difficulty, not uncommon in surface dyslexia, with choice of the appropriate checked or free form of vowel pronunciation (*mat* is read as "mate" and vice versa). Saffran seems to have succeeded in showing that the probability of misapplying the translation rule was greatly augmented when the mistranslation matched another phonological entry in the lexicon, and this applied equally to words and non-words (e.g. *rat→*"rate," *dipe→*"dip"). Because such errors did not appear to arise through purely visual confusions, they seem to imply a role for the phonological lexicon in the patient's reading of non-words. Whether this role is purely one of interference or is a part of the strategy for reading non-words is not clear.

The crucial question with regard to normal reading is whether a model in which the two processes converge or interact can be made to give an account of word frequency and spelling–sound predictability effects. Certainly the foregoing discussion of decision processes in non-lexical translation suggests that predictability effects might arise in models where the lexical and non-lexical codes are compared. However, the apparent diminution of predictability effects for very high-frequency words (Andrews, 1982; Seidenberg et al., 1984) suggests that the lexical process may sometimes support naming without consultation of assembled phonology. Moreover, if the time cost of inconsistency in lower-frequency words arises through decision difficulty confined within the non-lexical process, it is difficult to understand why the system "waits" for the non-lexical output, as it does not appear to do so for high-frequency words. This problem may be more easily handled by an *activation* model than a *comparator* model. Suppose that entries in the phonological lexicon can be activated by both the orthographic lexicon and the translation process, the former in a lexical code, the latter in a segmental phonological code. For a high-frequency word the lexical activation may build up sufficiently rapidly to trigger an output. For lower-frequency words the translation mechanism will generally contribute some activation, more rapidly in the case of regular, consistent words. Presumably the translation process must be able to drive pronunciation directly for non-words. Otherwise we are left with a lexical analogy theory.

ACKNOWLEDGEMENTS

I am grateful to D. Besner, S. E. Henderson, A. Parkin, and the editors for their comments on a first draft and to J. Monaghan for advice on phonetic matters.

REFERENCES

Albrow, K. H. (1972). *The English Writing System: Notes toward a description*. London: Longmans.
Allen, J. (1980). Speech synthesis from text. In J. C. Simon (ed.), *Spoken Language Generation and Understanding*. Dortrecht: D. Reidel.
Allport, D. A., & Funnell, E. (1981). Components of the mental lexicon. *Philosophical Transactions of the Royal Society of London, B295*, 397–410.
Andrews, S. (1982). Phonological recoding: Is the regularity effect consistent? *Memory and Cognition, 10*, 565–575.
Baker, R. G., & Smith, P. T. (1976). A psycholinguistic study of English stress assignment rules. *Language and Speech, 19*, 9–27.
Baron, J. (1977). Mechanisms for pronouncing printed words: Use and acquisition. In D. LaBerge, & S. J. Samuels (eds.), *Basic Processes in Reading: Perception and comprehension*. Hillsdale, NJ: Lawrence Erlbaum Associates Inc.
Baron, J., & Strawson, C. (1976). Use of orthographic and word-specific knowledge in reading words aloud. *Journal of Experimental Psychology: Human Perception and Performance, 2*, 386–393.
Barron, R. W. (1980). Visual and phonological strategies in reading and spelling. In U. Frith (ed.), *Cognitive Processes in Spelling*. London: Academic Press.
Barron, R. W. (1981). Reading skill and reading strategies. In A. M. Lesgold, & C. A. Perfetti (eds.), *Interactive Processes in Reading*. Hillsdale, NJ: Lawrence Erlbaum Associates Inc.

Bauer, D. W., & Stanovich, K. E. (1980). Lexical access and the spelling-to-sound regularity effect. *Memory and Cognition, 8*, 424–432.

Bradshaw, J. L., & Nettleton, N. C. (1974). Articulatory interference and the mown-down heterophone effect. *Journal of Experimental Psychology, 102*, 88–94.

Briggs, P., & Underwood, G. (1982). Phonological coding in good and poor readers. *Journal of Experimental Child Psychology, 34*, 93–112.

Campbell, R., & Besner, D. (1981). This and thap—constraints on the pronunciation of new written words. *Quarterly Journal of Experimental Psychology, 33A*, 375–396.

Carr, T. H., Davidson, B. J., & Hawkins, H. L. (1978). Perceptual flexibility in word recognition: Strategies affect orthographic computation but not lexical access. *Journal of Experimental Psychology: Human Perception and Performance, 4*, 674–690.

Chomsky, N., & Halle, M. (1968). *The Sound Pattern of English.* New York: Harper & Row.

Coltheart, M. (1978). Lexical access in simple reading tasks. In G. Underwood (ed.), *Strategies of Information Processing.* London: Academic Press.

Coltheart, M. (1980). Reading, phonological recoding and deep dyslexia. In M. Coltheart, K. Patterson, & J. C. Marshall (eds.), *Deep Dyslexia.* London: Routledge & Kegan Paul.

Coltheart, M., Besner, D., Jonasson, J. T., & Davelaar, E. (1979). Phonological encoding in the lexical decision task. *Quarterly Journal of Experimental Psychology, 31*, 489–507.

Coltheart, M., Davelaar, E., Jonasson, J. T., & Besner, D. (1977). Access to the internal lexicon. In S. Dornic (ed.), *Attention and Performance VI.* London: Academic Press.

Coltheart, M., Masterson, J., Byng, S., Prior, M., & Riddoch J. (1983). Surface dyslexia. *Quarterly Journal of Experimental Psychology, 35A*, 469–495.

Cosky, M. J. (1976). The role of letter recognition in word recognition. *Memory and Cognition, 4*, 207–214.

Cosky, M. J. (1980). Word length effects in word recognition: Evidence from word naming latency data. Unpublished manuscript, St. Olaf's College, Maine.

Deloche, G., Andreewsky, E., & Desai, M. (1982). Surface dyslexia: A case report and some theoretical implications to reading models. *Brain and Language, 15*, 12–31.

Durso, F. T., & Johnson, M. K. (1979). Facilitation in naming and categorizing repeated pictures and words. *Journal of Verbal Learning and Verbal Behaviour, 5*, 449–459.

Ellis, A. W. (1982). Letter length, orthographic regularity, number of meanings and word naming latency. Paper presented to the Tenth International Conference on Attention & Performance. Venlo, Holland, 1982.

Evett, L. J., & Humphreys, G. W. (1981). The use of abstract graphemic information in lexical access. *Quarterly Journal of Experimental Psychology, 33A*, 325–350.

Forster, K. I., & Chambers, S. M. (1973). Lexical access and naming time. *Journal of Verbal Learning and Verbal Behaviour, 12*, 627–635.

Frederiksen, J. R. (1976). Decoding skills and lexical retrieval. Presented at Psychonomic Society Conference, St Louis, 1976.

Frederiksen, J. R., & Kroll, J. F. (1976). Spelling and sound: Approaches to the internal lexicon. *Journal of Experimental Psychology: Human Perception and Performance, 2*, 361–379.

Funnell, E. (1983). Phonological processes in reading: New evidence from acquired dyslexia. *British Journal of Psychology, 74*, 159–180.

Gimson, A. C. (1980). *An Introduction to the Pronunciation of English,* 3rd ed. London: Edward Arnold.

Glushko, R. J. (1979). The organization and activation of orthographic knowledge in reading aloud. *Journal of Experimental Psychology: Human Perception and Performance, 5*, 674–691.

Glushko, R. J. (1981). Principles for pronouncing print: The psychology of phonography. In A. M. Lesgold, & C. A. Perfetti (eds.), *Interactive Processes in Reading.* Hillsdale, NJ: Lawrence Erlbaum Associates Inc.

Gough, P. B., & Cosky, M. J. (1977). One second of reading again. In N. J. Castellan, D. B.

Pisoni, & G. R. Potts (eds.), *Cognitive Theory*, Vol. 2. Hillsdale, NJ: Lawrence Erlbaum Associates Inc.

Haas, W. (1970). *Phonographic Translation*. Manchester: Manchester University Press.

Henderson, L. (1980). Is there a lexicality component in the word superiority effect? *Perception & Psychophysics, 28,* 179–184.

Henderson, L. (1982). *Orthography and Word Recognition in Reading*. London: Academic Press.

Henderson, L. (1984). Introduction. In L. Henderson (ed.), *Orthographies and Reading*. London: Lawrence Erlbaum Associates Ltd.

Henderson, L. (In press). On the use of the term *grapheme. Language and Cognitive Processes*.

Henderson, L., Wallis, J., & Knight, D. (1983). Morphemic structure and lexical access. In H. Bouma, & D. Bouhuis (eds.), *Attention and Performance X*. London: Lawrence Erlbaum Associates Ltd.

Hillinger, M. L. (1980). Priming effects with phonemically similar words: The encoding-bias hypothesis reconsidered. *Memory and Cognition, 8,* 115–123.

Humphreys, G. W., Evett, L. J., & Taylor, D. E. (1982). Automatic phonological priming in visual word recognition. *Memory and Cognition, 10,* 576–590.

James, C. T. (1975). The role of semantic information in lexical decisions. *Journal of Experimental Psychology: Human Perception and Performance, 1,* 130–136.

Jastrzembski, J. E. (1981). Multiple meanings, number of related meanings, frequency of occurrence, and the lexicon. *Cognitive Psychology, 13,* 278–305.

Jones, D. (1956). *The Pronunciation of English*. Cambridge: Cambridge University Press.

Kay, J. (1982). Psychological mechanisms of oral reading of single words. Unpublished PhD. thesis, Cambridge University.

Kay, J., & Marcel, A. J. (1981). One process, not two, in reading aloud: Lexical analogies do the work of nonlexical rules. *Quarterly Journal of Experimental Psychology, 33A,* 397–413.

Kelliher, S. (1983). Orthographic rules in relation to print-to-pronunciation processes in oral reading. Unpublished BSc project dissertation, Psychology Division, The Hatfield Polytechnic.

Klapp, S. T., & Wyatt, E. T. (1976). Motor programming within a sequence of responses. *Journal of Motor Behavior, 8,* 19–26.

Klima, E. S. (1972). How alphabets might reflect language. In J. F. Kavanagh, & I. G. Mattingly (eds.), *Language by Eye and by Ear*. Cambridge, Mass.: MIT Press.

MacKay, D. G. (1978). Derivational rules and the internal lexicon. *Journal of Verbal Learning and Verbal Behavior, 17,* 61–71.

Marcel, A. J. (1980). Surface dyslexia and beginning reading. In M. Coltheart, K. Patterson, & J. C. Marshall (eds.), *Deep Dyslexia*. London: Routledge & Kegan Paul.

Mason, M. (1978). From print to sound in mature readers as a function of reader ability and two forms of orthographic regularity. *Memory and Cognition, 6,* 568–581.

Meyer, D. E., Schvaneveldt, R. W., & Ruddy, M. G. (1974). Functions of graphemic and phonemic codes in visual word recognition. *Memory and Cognition, 2,* 309–321.

Meyer, D. E., Schvaneveldt, R. W., & Ruddy, M. G. (1975). Foci of contextual effects in word recognition. In P. Rabbitt, & S. Dornic (eds.), *Attention & Performance V*. New York: Academic Press.

Morton, J., & Patterson, K. (1980). A new attempt at an interpretation, or, an attempt at a new interpretation. In M. Coltheart, K. Patterson, & J. C. Marshall (eds.), *Deep Dyslexia*. London: Routledge & Kegan Paul.

Parkin, A. J. (1982). Phonological recoding in lexical decision: Effects of spelling to sound regularity depend on how regularity is defined. *Memory and Cognition, 10,* 43–53.

Parkin, A. J. (1983). Two processes not one in reading aloud. Paper presented to the Experimental Psychology Society Meeting, Oxford, July 1983.

Parkin, A. J. (1984). Phonological recoding and context. *Current Psychological Research, 2*, 187–194.

Parkin, A. J., & Underwood, G. (1983). Orthographic versus phonological regularity in lexical decision. *Memory and Cognition, 11*, 351–355.

Patterson, K. (1981). Neuropsychological approaches to the study of reading. *British Journal of Psychology, 72*, 151–174.

Richardson, J. T. E. (1976). The effects of stimulus attributes upon latency of word recognition. *British Journal of Psychology, 67*, 315–325.

Rosson, M. B. (1983). From SOFA to LOUCH: Lexical contributions to pseudoword pronunciation. *Memory and Cognition, 11*, 152–160.

Scarborough, D. L., Cortese, C., & Scarborough, H. S. (1977). Frequency and repetition effects in lexical memory. *Journal of Experimental Psychology: Human Perception and Performance, 3*, 1–17.

Schwartz, M. F., Marin, O. S. M., & Saffran, E. M. (1979). Dissociation of language function in dementia: A case study. *Brain and Language, 7*, 277–306.

Scragg, D. G. (1974). *A History of English Spelling*. Manchester: Manchester University Press.

Seidenberg, M. S., Waters, G. S., Barnes, M. A., & Tanenhaus, M. K. (1984). When does irregular spelling or pronunciation influence word recognition? *Journal of Verbal Learning and Verbal Behavior, 23*, 383–404.

Seymour, P. H. K., & Porpodas, C. D. (1980). Lexical and non-lexical processing of spelling in developmental dyslexia. In U. Frith (ed.), *Cognitive Processes in Spelling*. London: Academic Press.

Shallice, T., & Warrington, E. K. (1980). Single and multiple component central dyslexic syndromes. In M. Coltheart, K. Patterson, & J. C. Marshall (eds.), *Deep Dyslexia*. London: Routledge & Kegan Paul.

Shallice, T., Warrington, E. K., & McCarthy, R. (1983). Reading without semantics. *Quarterly Journal of Experimental Psychology, 35A*, 111–138.

Shulman, H. G., Hornack, R., & Sanders, E. (1978). The effects of graphemic, phonetic and semantic relationships on access to lexical structures. *Memory and Cognition, 6*, 115–123.

Smith, P. T., Meredith, T., Pattison, H. M., & Sterling, C. (1983). The representation of internal word structure in English. In L. Henderson (ed.), *Orthographies and Reading*, London: Lawrence Erlbaum Associates Ltd.

Stanovich, K. E., & Bauer, D. W. (1978). Experiments on the spelling-to-sound regularity effect in word recognition. *Memory and Cognition, 6*, 410–415.

Steinberg, D., & Krohn, R. (1975). The psychological validity of Chomsky and Halle's vowel shift rule. In E. Koerner, J. Odmark, & J. Shaw (eds.), *The Transformational-Generative Paradigm and Modern Linguistic Theory*. Amsterdam: John Benjamin.

Sternberg, S., Monsell, S., Knoll, R. L., & Wright, C. E. (1978). The latency and duration of rapid movement sequences: Comparisions of speech and typewriting. In G. Stelmach (ed.), *Information Processing in Motor Control and Learning*. New York: Academic Press.

Taft, M. (1981). Prefix stripping revisited. *Journal of Verbal Learning and Verbal Behavior, 20*, 284–297.

Taft, M., & Forster, K. I. (1975). Lexical storage and retrieval of prefixed words. *Journal of Verbal Learning and Verbal Behavior, 14*, 638–647.

Underwood, G., & Bargh, K. (1982). Word shape, orthographic regularity and contextual interactions in a reading task. *Cognition, 12*, 197–209.

Venezky, R. L. (1970). *The Structure of English Orthography*. The Hague: Mouton.

Wallis, J. (1982). Strategies used by beginning readers in the processing of written words. Unpublished progress report, Psychology Division, The Hatfield Polytechnic.

Warrington, E. K. (1975). The selective impairment of semantic memory. *Quarterly Journal of Experimental Psychology*, *27*, 635–657.

Waters, E. S., & Seidenberg, M. S. (1983). Children and adults' use of spelling–sound correspondences in three reading tasks. Paper presented to Society for Research in Child Development Meeting, 1983.

Wijk, A. (1966). *Rules of Pronunciation for the English Language*. Oxford: Oxford University Press.

VI NEUROLOGICAL APPENDIX

18 CT Scan Correlates of Surface Dyslexia

M. Vanier and D. Caplan

We report nine CT scans of seven cases presented in this book. We have presented enough data on each scan for the interested reader to form his or her own opinion of the scan. We include cuts that we think represent the lesion. For most cuts, we present a diagram of the brain on which we indicate the extent of the lesion. When CT cuts are along orbitomeatal (or cantho-meatal) lines, we use Dejerine's atlas for these diagrams (Dejerine, 1895, 1901). When the cuts are made at other angles, in the case of M.P. and B.F., we use other appropriate atlases (Gonzalcs ct al., 1976). When possible, we provide a reconstruction of the lateral surface of the lesion on a diagram taken from Dejerine.

We wish to stress that the localisations presented here are approximate, due to individual variations in brain anatomy and size, partial CT studies in some cases, and other factors. Two additional points regarding the analyses presented here should be noted. First, all reconstructions of lesions on the diagrams taken from Dejerine's atlas are depicted on diagrams of the right hemisphere. This is because the diagrams in that atlas are of the right hemisphere. The CT reproductions themselves of course illustrate the lesions in the appropriate hemisphere, and we trust the accompanying text is clear with respect to the hemisphere involved.[1] We do not restate this feature of the reconstruction of lesions on the Dejerine diagrams for each such analysis.

---

[1] There is, however, a further complication that should be explained for readers unfamiliar with CT scans. In some laboratories, the left hemisphere appears on the left side of the CT photograph, but in other laboratories, the photographs are mirror-imaged. For the seven patients included in this report, the following conventions apply: M.P. (L=L); B.F. (L=L); H.A.M. (L=R); R.F. (L=R); L.B. (L=R); E.S.T. (L=L); S.U. (L=R).

511

Second, in some cases, it is impossible to make a complete estimate of the extent of a lesion, because scans are missing or because certain cerebral areas are not well visualised on available scans (as happens with lower cuts on some occasions). This is most apparent in our reconstruction of lesions on the lateral surface of the brain. In these cases, we simply do not indicate the extent of the lesion in the direction where there is insufficient information; we leave some portion of the reconstruction "open" in these cases (as in Fig. 18.6).

PATIENT M.P. (Bub, Cancelliere, & Kertesz, Chapter 1)

The clinical history is one of head trauma. Scans are made without contrast enhancement; each cut represents 8 mm of brain thickness.

Scan Made on Day 1 (11 April 1979)

The scan is made at an angle of approximately 15° beneath the orbitomeatal (OM) line. We have no reference atlas with cortical identification for horizontal sections made at 15° below the OM line. The anatomical interpretation of this scan is thus made by reference to an atlas made parallel to the orbitomeatal line and to a lateral diagram of the brain (with ventricular, ocular, and osseous landmarks) showing anatomical relationships when cuts are made at an angle approximately 10-15° under the OM line (Fig. 18.1).

Cut 1A (Fig. 18.2) shows an area of hyperdensity, irregular in shape, in the anterior part of the superior and middle temporal gyri; there is an area of hypodensity on its internal border. Cut 1B (Fig. 18.2) shows more pronounced involvement of the middle temporal gyrus, the hyperdensity extending to its posterior part. Cut 2A (Fig. 18.2) corresponds to a level slightly inferior to level B indicated on the lateral diagram of Fig. 18.1. The hyperdensity still predominantly affects the middle temporal gyrus but the superior temporal gyrus is also involved.

On cut 2B (Fig. 18.2) the hyperdensity seems concentrated along the sylvian fissure, suggesting accumulation of blood in that space; there is also some hyperdensity on the external surface of the superior temporal gyrus. On cut 3A (Fig. 18.2) there is hyperdensity in the sylvian fissure and in the posterior part of the superior temporal gyrus at the level of the planum temporale. The inferior part of the supramarginal gyrus is probably also involved.

Scan Made on Day 20 (1 May 1979)

This scan is made more parallel to the orbitomeatal line. There is a unilateral hypodensity in cuts 2A, 2B, and 3A.

On cuts 2A and 2B (Fig. 18.3) there is an area of hypodensity in the anterior half of the middle temporal gyrus. There is also some dilatation of the temporal horn of the left lateral ventricle.

Cut 3A (Fig. 18.3) corresponds approximately to the level indicated at Fig. 229 of Dejerine's atlas (Fig. 18.4). The hypodensity is seen mainly in the cortex and white matter of the middle temporal gyrus but may also involve part of the adjacent superior temporal gyrus. There are hyperdense areas on cut 3B (Fig. 18.3) (Fig. 226 of Dejerine, Fig. 18.5) that may correspond to residual blood; these areas are seen in the sylvian fissure, at the level of Heschl's gyrus, and probably in the superior temporal sulcus. Some hypodensity is seen in the white matter bordering the external surface of the ventricular trigone.

Summary

On day 20 (1 May 1979), the CT examination shows an area of hypodensity mainly localised in the cortex and white matter of the middle temporal gyrus. Some extension to the superior temporal gyrus is possible. A diagram of the lateral extent of the lesion is presented in Fig. 18.6.

PATIENT B.F. (Goldblum, Chapter 7)

The scan is made at an angle of 15° inferior to the orbitomeatal line. Cuts are made at 1-cm intervals. As for case M.P., the anatomical interpretation will be made by reference to an atlas made parallel to the OM line, and to a lateral diagram of the brain showing anatomical relationships when cuts are made at an angle of approximately 10-15° under the OM line. There is an area of hypodensity in the left hemisphere on the cuts at 3, 4 and 5 cm.

The cut at 3 cm (Fig. 18.8) corresponds approximately to level 3 on Fig. 18.7. A hypodensity affects the middle part of the superior temporal gyrus and the middle temporal gyrus. The cut at 4 cm (Fig. 18.9) corresponds approximately to level 4 on Fig. 18.7. The hypodensity affects the cortex bordering the superior temporal sulcus, that is, the posterior part of the superior and middle temporal gyri. The cut at 5 cm (Fig. 18.10) corresponds to level 5 on Fig. 18.7. The hypodensity seems to involve the inferior part of the angular gyrus or the cortex immediately anterior to it.

Impression

The scan is in keeping with a stroke involving the superior and middle temporal gyri and part of the angular gyrus (Fig. 18.11).

PATIENT H.A.M. (Kremin, Chapter 5)

Scans are made parallel to the orbitomeatal line. Cuts are made approximately every 10–12 mm.

Scan Made on 14 April 1980

The scan is made without contrast enhancement. On cuts 3 and 4 there is an area of hyperdensity surrounded by a zone of hypodensity in the left hemisphere. The median line is displaced 5 mm to the right.

Cut 3 (Fig. 18.12) corresponds approximately to the level illustrated in Dejerine's Fig. 229 (Fig. 18.13). The hyperdensity is mainly in the cortex and white matter of the middle temporal gyrus but extends anteriorly to the superior temporal gyrus where hypodensity is more prominent. Fibres from the thalamic radiations and from the inferior longitudinal fasciculus (occipito-temporal fibres) are involved in this area of the pathology.

Cut 4 (Fig. 18.12) corresponds approximately to Fig. 225 of Dejerine (Fig. 18.14). The area of hyperdensity involves the cortex and white matter of the superior and middle temporal gyri as well as fibres from the thalamus and of the inferior longitudinal fasciculus. There is a hypodensity in the superior temporal gyrus including Heschl's gyrus and in part of the occipital lobe (part of visual cortex).

Scan Made on 28 April 1980

In the left hemisphere, there is a large area of hypodensity surrounding a small hyperdense area (which may be residual blood from a haemorrhagic stroke).

Cut 5 (Fig. 18.15) corresponds to the level illustrated in Fig. 226 of Dejerine's atlas (Fig. 18.16). There is hypodensity in the posterior part of the insula, the putamen and globus pallidus, the cortex and white matter of Heschl's gyrus, and the superior and middle temporal gyri. The white matter of the occipital lobe at the level of the occipito-temporal fasciculus is involved.

Cut 6 (Fig. 18.15) corresponds approximately to Dejerine's Fig. 222 (Fig. 18.17). A hypodensity is seen in the insula, the arcuate fasciculus, the internal capsule (mainly its posterior limb), the cortex, and the white matter of the inferior parietal lobule and of the external surface of the occipital lobe. Thalamic radiations and occipito-temporal fibres are involved.

Cut 7 (Fig. 18.15) corresponds to a level slightly inferior to the one illustrated in Dejerine's Fig. 219 (Fig. 18.18). The hypodensity seems to affect mainly the white matter of the post-central, inferior parietal, and lateral occipital lobe. Cut 8 (Fig. 18.15) shows some hypodensity in the white matter of the posterior parietal region, probably of the angular gyrus.

Impression

The sequence of scans is consistent with a haemorrhagic stroke, with residual necrosis in the temporo-parietal cortex and adjacent white matter (Fig. 18.19). The lesion extends inferiorly to the cuts presented.

PATIENT R.F. (Margolin, Marcel, & Carlson, Chapter 6)

The scan is said to be a long-term follow-up study of a case of an intracerebral haematoma. The scan is made parallel to the orbitomeatal line. Cuts are made at 1-cm intervals. There is an area of decreased density in the left hemisphere on the cuts at 30-60 mm and probably on the cut at 20 mm. There is evidence of a ventricular shunt.

On cut 20 (Fig. 18.20) there seems to be a hypodensity in the temporal pole. Cut 30 (Fig. 18.20) corresponds approximately to the level illustrated in Dejerine's Fig. 232 (Fig. 18.21). The hypodensity mainly affects the cortex and white matter of the superior and middle temporal gyri but may extend posteriorly to the inferior temporal gyrus. Fibres from the uncinate fasciculus are involved. In the right hemisphere, there are two small areas of hypodensity, one in the white matter of the orbital part of the inferior frontal gyrus, and the other in the white matter of the superior temporal gyrus; these hypodense areas may be artefacts or they may suggest some atrophy of the uncinate fasciculus joining these two cortical regions. If this is the case, it is valid to consider the small hypodense area in the left orbital cortex and that in the inferior frontal gyrus as non-artefactual.

Cut 40 (Fig. 18.20) corresponds to Dejerine's Fig. 229 (Fig. 18.22). A hypodensity is seen in the cortex and white matter of the middle temporal gyrus with a discrete extension to the white matter of the superior temporal gyrus.

Cut 50 (Fig. 18.20) corresponds approximately to Dejerine's Fig. 225 (Fig. 18.23). As in cut 40, a hypodensity affects the posterior third of the middle temporal gyrus with a discrete extension to the white matter of the superior temporal gyrus. Posteriorly, the hypodensity probably affects the occipito-temporal fasciculus.

Cut 60 (Fig. 18.20) corresponds to Dejerine's Fig. 222 (Fig. 18.24). The area of hypodensity is limited to the inferior part of the angular gyrus.

Summary

The lesion occupies essentially all of the second temporal gyrus and a small portion of the first temporal gyrus (Fig. 18.25).

PATIENT L.B. (Derouesné & Beauvois, Chapter 16)

L.B. suffered a right hemisphere stroke on 7 July 1971, with a left hemipare-sis, left hemianaesthesia, left homonymous hemianopsia, and neglect. The hemiparesis improved quickly in the leg and the hemianopsia was not detectable one year after the stroke. Eye movements were impaired for commands to look to the left at one stage of the illness. Arteriography in July 1971 showed occlusion of the ascending parietal branches of the right middle cerebral artery with a normal internal carotid. An EEG done in July 1971 showed right sided slowing, particularly noticeable in the parietal and occipital lobes. In 1981 and 1983, when he was examined with respect to his reading abilities, L.B. remained hemiparetic and hemianaesthetic.

The scan was made 12 years after the stroke. It was made parallel to the orbitomeatal line. Each cut represents a brain thickness of 6 mm. On cuts 4–18 there is an area of hypodensity in the right hemisphere.

On the lower cuts (4–8), the hypodensity affects the inferior frontal gyrus (cortex and white matter of the pars orbitalis and triangularis), the white matter of the middle frontal gyrus, the limen of insula, the temporal pole, the anterior third of the superior temporal gyrus, the anterior two-thirds of the middle temporal gyrus, the white matter of these temporal gyri, as well as uncinate fibres and possibly the external portion of the putamen.

Cut 9 (Fig. 18.26) corresponds approximately to the level shown in Dejerine's Fig. 228 (Fig. 18.27). In the frontal lobe, there is involvement of the white matter of the superior middle and inferior frontal gyri (including occipito-frontal fibres) and of the cortex of the triangular part of the inferior frontal gyrus. More posteriorly, the insula, the putamen (and probably the globus pallidus), the cortex, and the white matter of the superior and of the middle temporal gyri, the occipito-temporal fibres and the thalamic radia-tions are involved.

Cut 10 (Fig. 18.28) corresponds to the level shown in Dejerine's Fig. 226 (Fig. 18.29). A hypodensity affects the white matter of the frontal lobe, mainly that of the middle and inferior frontal gyri, and the interhemispheric fibres at this level. The cortex of the pars triangularis and opercularis, parts of the inferior frontal gyrus, the insula, the putamen, and probably the globus pallidus are involved. The cortex and white matter of the superior temporal gyrus including Heschl's gyrus, part of the middle temporal gyrus, and occipito-temporal fibres are affected.

Cut 11 (Fig. 18.30) corresponds to Dejerine's Fig. 224 (Fig. 18.31). Structures affected are the white matter of the middle and inferior frontal gyri, including interhemispheric fibres, the cortex of the opercular part of the inferior frontal gyrus and rolandic operculum, the insula, the putamen, the globus pallidus, possibly the head of the caudate nucleus, the internal capsule, and the thalamus. The hypodensity also affects the superior temporal gyrus and planum temporale, part of the middle temporal gyrus, the white matter of these temporal gyri, the thalamic radiations, and occipito-temporal fibres.

Cut 12 (Fig. 18.32) corresponds to the level shown in Dejerine's Fig. 222 (Fig. 18.33). In the frontal lobe, the hypodensity is mainly seen in the white matter of the three frontal gyri although some cortical atrophy is also apparent; more posteriorly, the inferior part of the pre-central and post-central gyri and the inferior parietal lobule (mainly the supramarginal gyrus) are involved. Medially, the hypodensity affects the higher part of insula, the arcuate fasciculus, the internal capsule where it becomes the corona radiata, the thalamic radiations, and occipito-temporal fibres. Involvement of the caudate nucleus and of the thalamus is possible.

Cut 13 (Fig. 18.34) corresponds to the level shown in Dejerine's Fig. 220 (Fig. 18.35). In the frontal lobe, the hypodensity is mainly seen in the white matter of the middle and inferior frontal gyri; posteriorly, the cortex and the white matter of the pre-central, post-central, and supramarginal gyri, and possibly of the anterior part of the angular gyrus, the corona radiata, and arcuate fasciculus are affected. The body of the caudate nucleus may be spared.

Cut 14 (Fig. 18.36) is shown in Dejerine's Fig. 219 (Fig. 18.37). The white matter of the frontal gyri is hypodense, as well as the arcuate fasciculus and corona radiata; the cortex and white matter of the pre-central and post-central gyri and of the inferior parietal lobule including, probably, the anterior part of the angular gyrus are involved.

On cut 15 (Fig. 18.36), the hypodensity is present in the white matter of the middle frontal gyrus, the corona radiata, the cortex and white matter of the pre-central and mainly post-central gyri, the supramarginal gyrus, and part of the angular gyrus. On cut 16 (Fig. 18.36), the cortex and white matter of the post-central gyrus and the superior part of the supramarginal gyrus are hypodense. On cuts 17 and 18 (Fig. 18.36), the hypodensity is limited to the superior part of the inferior parietal lobule.

Summary

There is a very large area of hypodensity in the right hemisphere affecting all the peri-sylvian cortex and white matter, as well as parts of more distant cortical regions: the white matter of the superior and middle frontal gyri, the white matter of the middle temporal and angular gyri. Cortical involvement in these latter areas seems to be more limited. Projection fibres from the thalamus, intrahemispheric fibres, as well as subcortical nuclei are very much affected. Interhemispheric fibres of the frontal lobe may be partly affected (Fig. 18.38).

PATIENT E.S.T. (Kay & Patterson, Chapter 4)

E.S.T. came to medical attention in early 1968 after a single seizure. In the ensuing nine months he had several more attacks, without obvious focal onset. Investigations in December 1968 revealed an essentially normal neurological examination, but left hemisphere EEG slowing, left temporo-parietal isotope uptake, elevation and displacement of branches of the left middle cerebral artery, and enlargement and depression of the anterior choroidal artery all suggested a cerebral tumour. He was treated with anticonvulsants until he developed a right homonymous hemianopsia and speech difficulties in 1976. EMI scanning and repeat angiography confirmed the growth of the lesion, and strongly suggested meningioma of the tentorium or a choroid plexus tumour. The latter diagnosis was confirmed in August 1977, when a large temporal meningioma originating in the choroid plexus was removed.

The CT scans are made parallel to the orbitomeatal line. Each cut represents 13 mm of brain thickness; cuts overlap. The first scan is made without infusion: cuts 2B, 3A, and 3B show an area of increased density on the left. After Conray injection (cuts 12B and 13B), the hyperdensity increases markedly.

Cut 2B (Fig. 18.39) corresponds approximately to the level illustrated in Dejerine's Fig. 229 (Fig. 18.40). The scan shows a rectangular area of increased density in the posterior half of the insula, the putamen, the globus pallidus, the superior temporal gyrus; there is possible extension of the abnormal hyperdensity to the white matter of the middle and inferior temporal gyri and of the occipito-temporal gyrus. Areas of decreased density around the hyperdense area may correspond to oedema.

Cut 3A (Fig. 18.41) corresponds approximately to the level illustrated in Dejerine's Fig. 225 (Fig. 18.42). The area of hyperdensity is located in the region of the rolandic operculum, the posterior half of the insula, the putamen, the globus pallidus, and the posterior limb of the internal capsule. It is also seen in the superior temporal gyrus, at the level of Heschl's gyrus and in the white matter of the superior and middle temporal gyri. Projection fibres (thalamic fibres, including optic radiations) and association fibres such as the occipito-temporal fasciculus are normally located in this posterior region. There is a questionable hyperdensity in the white matter of the occipital lobe.

In the right hemisphere, there is an area of hypodensity posterior to the occipital horn: this may be an artefact or could reflect retrograde degeneration of interhemispheric fibres.

Cut 3B (Fig. 18.43) corresponds approximately to the level shown in Dejerine's Fig. 221 (Fig. 18.44). The hyperdensity is in the cortex and the white matter of the inferior part of the pre-central and post-central gyri. It affects intrahemispheric and interhemispheric fibres (including fibres from the splenium of the corpus callosum) and projection fibres (posterior limb of the internal capsule). There is questionable involvement of the cortex of the angular gyrus and of the external surface of the occipital lobe but the white matter of these regions is affected. On the internal surface of the hemisphere, the hyperdensity affects the precuneus and the posterior cingulate gyrus. There is hypodensity in the cortex of the supramarginal gyrus (which may represent oedema). There is dilatation of the right ventricular body and possibly hypodensity in the white matter of the occipital lobe.

After Conray injection, the mass shows considerable enhancement (cuts 12B and 13B). Cut 12B (Fig. 18.45) seems to be a few millimetres below cut 3A, and thus at the level of the pineal body (Fig. 226 of Dejerine) (Fig. 18.46). On this cut, the hyperdense mass does not seem to affect the cortex of the middle temporal gyrus nor to extend to the occipital lobe. However, it does involve the rolandic operculum, the posterior half of the insula, the putamen and the globus pallidus, and the posterior limb of the internal capsule, pushing the (left) thalamus towards the right hemisphere. It involves the superior temporal gyrus and Heschl's gyrus, the white matter of these gyri and of the middle temporal gyrus, and the occipito-temporal fasciculus.

On cut 13B (Fig. 18.47), which is at the same level as cut 3B (Fig. 221 of Dejerine, Fig. 18.44), the hyperdensity does not seem to affect the cortex of the supramarginal, angular, and occipital regions of the convexity of the hemisphere, although a hypodensity is present in the supramarginal gyrus. On the internal surface, the cuneus is of normal density but the precuneus and posterior cingulate gyrus are affected. For white matter involvement, see the description of cut 3B.

Summary

On the cuts shown, the hyperdensity, known to be a meningioma arising from the choroid plexus of the temporal horn of the left ventricle, occupies the superior temporal gyrus, including Heschl's gyrus and the posterior planum temporale (not shown), the posterior half of the insula, the putamen, the globus pallidus, and the internal capsule, and the white matter of the superior and middle temporal gyri and possibly that of the inferior temporal and occipito-temporal gyri.

On higher cuts, the tumour occupies the lower part of the pre-central and post-central gyri and possibly the anterior part of the supramarginal gyrus, and the white matter of the angular and occipital gyri. On the internal surface, the tumour extends to the precuneus and limbic lobe.

In the right hemisphere, there is dilatation of the lateral ventricle and a hypodensity in the white matter of the occipital lobe at the level of the inferior longitudinal fasciculus (occipito-temporal fibres) and of the thalamic radiations. The significance of this hypodensity is not known. We have not provided a lateral reconstruction because of the paucity of cuts available.

PATIENT S.U. (Sasanuma, Chapter 9)

The clinical history available is of stroke, with removal of an intracerebral haematoma. The scan is made parallel to the orbitomeatal line. Cuts are 1 cm apart.

There is an area of hypodensity in the temporo-parieto-occipital region of the left hemisphere that involves the posterior horn of the lateral ventricle; there are also areas of hypodensity in the left and right frontal poles and in the right temporal cortex. The scan also shows ventricular dilatation and diffuse cortical atrophy.

On cut 40 (Fig. 18.48) a large area of hypodensity is seen on the left, affecting the cortex and white matter of the middle temporal gyrus with some extension to the superior temporal gyrus. Anteriorly, the inferior parts of the superior frontal gyrus of both hemispheres show hypodensity (mainly of the white matter); the white matter of the inferior frontal gyrus (orbital part) is also hypodense.

Cut 50 (Fig. 18.48) corresponds approximately to the level shown in Dejerine's Fig. 230 (Fig. 18.49). In the left posterior region, the hypodensity affects mainly the white matter of the middle temporal gyrus but extends to the white matter of the superior temporal gyrus; fibres from the occipito-temporal fasciculus and from the thalamic radiations are involved in this area. There is also a small and well-delimited area of hypodensity in the white matter of the superior temporal gyrus. In the frontal lobes, the hypodensity seems to be restricted to the white matter of both superior frontal gyri.

Cut 60 (Fig. 18.48) corresponds approximately to Dejerine's Fig. 226 (Fig. 18.50). In the left hemisphere, a large hypodense area affects the white matter of the superior temporal gyrus, the cortex and white matter of the middle temporal gyrus, and mainly the white matter of the occipital pole. Occipito-temporal and thalamic fibres are involved.

The small area of decreased density in the white matter of the superior temporal gyrus seen on cut 50 is also present here: it may correspond to the white matter of Heschl's gyrus.

Anteriorly, a hypodensity in the white matter of the superior frontal gyrus is limited to the left hemisphere but there is some cortical atrophy of the polar region in both hemispheres. In the right hemisphere, there is an area of decreased density in the cortex of the superior temporal gyrus next to Heschl's gyrus; this and the next cut (cut 70) suggest that the hypodensity affects the planum temporale.

Cut 70 (Fig. 18.48) corresponds approximately to Dejerine's Fig. 223 (Figs. 18.52 and 18.53). In the left hemisphere, the large hypodense area involves the cortex and white matter of the superior temporal gyrus (including the planum temporale), mainly the white matter of the inferior part of the inferior parietal lobule, and the white matter of the occipital lobe.

Thalamic occipito-temporal and probably some callosal fibres are involved.

In both hemispheres, there is cortical atrophy of the frontal poles with involvement of the white matter of the superior frontal gyrus in the left hemisphere. In the right hemisphere, there is atrophy of the posterior part of the superior temporal gyrus (including the planum temporale) and of the inferior part of the inferior parietal lobule.

Cut 80 (Fig. 18.48) is approximately at the level illustrated in Dejerine's Fig. 231 (Fig. 18.54). The hypodensity in the posterior part of the left hemisphere is limited to the white matter of the supramarginal and angular gyri and that of the occipital lobe. Anteriorly, there is a hypodensity in the cortex and white matter of the left superior frontal gyrus and in the cortex of the right frontal gyrus.

Cut 90 (Fig. 18.48) corresponds approximately to Dejerine's Fig. 219 (Fig. 18.55). A hypodensity in the left posterior region seems to be restricted to the white matter of the inferior parietal lobule.

Impression

The large area of hypodensity in the left temporo-parieto-occipital region may be due to the presence of cerebrospinal fluid in cerebral parenchyma due to communication with the ventricle. The areas of hypodensity in frontal poles may be due to head trauma. The area of hypodensity in the right temporo-parietal cortex may be due to a cerebrovascular accident (CVA). We have not presented a lateral reconstruction of this complex case.

GENERAL CONCLUSIONS

Surface dyslexia occurs with a wide variety of lesion types and lesion sites. The lesions seen on these scans include tumour, head trauma, stroke, and probably degenerative disease (leading to cortical atrophy). The lesion sites include one case with unilateral right hemisphere lesion (a stroke, L.B.), one or possibly two cases with bilateral lesions (probably head trauma or stroke and degenerative disease, S.U.; and possibly E.S.T. with transsynaptic degeneration). In the cases with lesions restricted to the left hemisphere, the lesion sites tend to include temporal lobe structures, and in three cases are largely restricted to the temporal lobe (B.F., M.P., and R.F.). The insula is usually involved, as is the putamen. Several lesions are quite extensive and involve frontal, parietal, and occipital structures as well. It is impossible to generalise with confidence from these scans, but we suggest that the involvement of posterior structures, especially temporal lobe structures, is necessary for the occurrence of acquired surface dyslexic symptoms.

ACKNOWLEDGEMENTS

We wish to acknowledge the assistance of Dr R. Ethier, Radiologist-in-chief, Montreal Neurological Hospital. The preparation of this manuscript was partially supported by an Establishment Grant from the F.R.S.Q. to the second author. The first author is supported by an M.R.C. Fellowship.

REFERENCES

Dejerine, J. (1895). *Anatomie des centres nerveux*. Paris: Rueff et Cie. (Reprinted by Masson, Paris, 1980.)

Gonzalez, C. F., Grossman, C. B., Palacios, E. (1976). *Computed Brain and Orbital Tomography — Technique and Interpretation*. New York: John Wiley & Sons.

APPENDIX
Dejerine's Diagrams: Abbreviations of Anatomical Structures

Al	anse lenticulaire (ansa lenticularis)
AM	avant-mur (claustrum)
Aq	aqueduc de Sylvius (cerebral aqueduct)
Arc	faisceau arqué (arcuate fasciculus)
BrQa	bras du tubercule quadrijumeau antérieur
C	cuneus
CA	corne d'Ammon (Ammon's horn)
CB	carrefour olfactif
Cc	corps calleux (corpus callosum)
Cc (g)	genu du corps calleux (genu of corpus callosum)
Cc (sp)	bourrelet du corps calleux (splenium of corpus callosum)
Ce	capsule externe (external capsule)
Cex	capsule extrême (extreme capsule)
Cg	circonvolution godronnée (dentate gyrus)
Cge	corps genouillé externe (lateral geniculate body)
Cgi	corps genouillé interne (medial geniculate body)
Cia, Cip	segments antérieur et postérieur de la capsule interne (anterior and posterior limbs of internal capsule)
Ci (g)	genou de la capsule interne (genu of internal capsule)
Cing (a), (p)	faisceaux antérieur et postérieur du cingulum (anterior and posterior fasciculi of cingulum)
Cirl	segment rétrolenticulaire de la capsule interne (retrolenticular limb of internal capsule)
CL	corps de Luys (Luys body)
cm	sillon calloso-marginal (cingulate sulcus)
CM	commissure de Meynert
CO	centre ovale (centrum ovale)

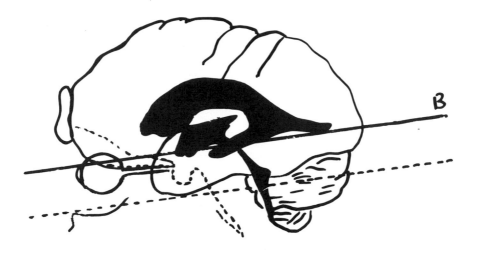

FIG. 18.1.   Diagram showing the angle of CT cuts in M.P.

1A

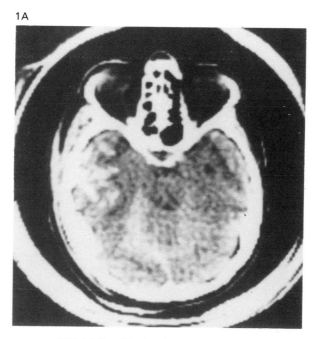

FIG. 18.2.   CT of Patient M.P. (11/4/79)

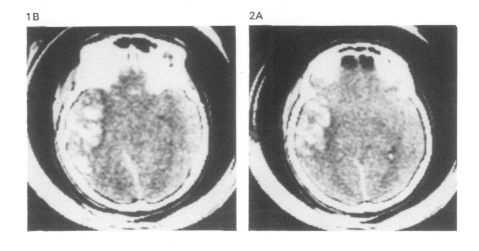

1B

2A

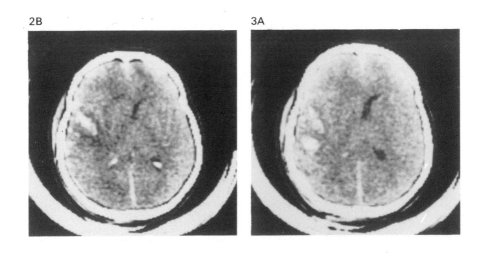

2B

3A

FIG. 18.2. Continued

2A 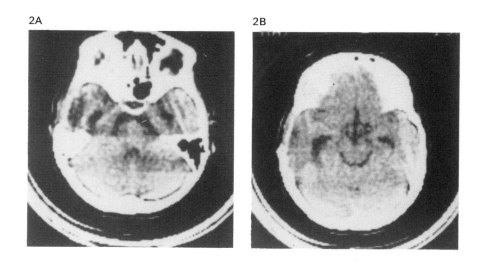 2B

3A 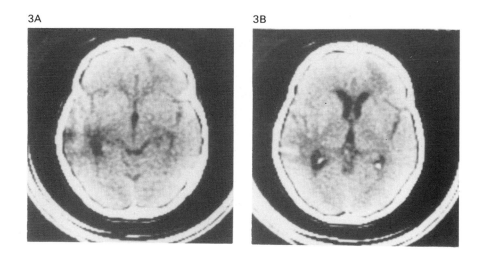 3B

FIG. 18.3. CT of Patient M.P. (1/5/79)

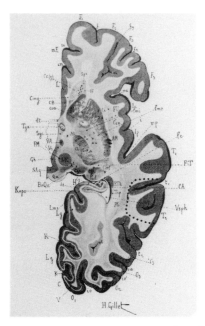

FIG. 18.4. Horizontal reconstruction of lesion in M.P. (1/5/79)

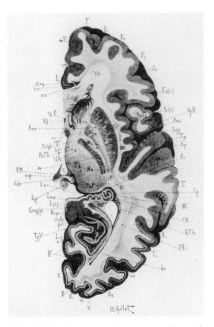

FIG. 18.5. Horizontal reconstruction of lesion in M.P. (1/5/79)

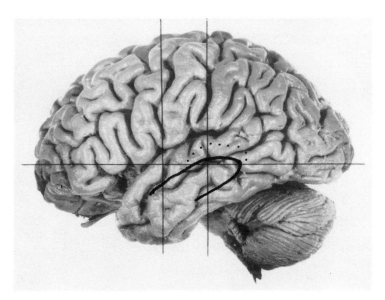

FIG. 18.6. Reconstruction of lateral extent of lesion in M.P. (1/5/79). The inferior border of the lesion cannot be determined from the scan, and is left unspecified. Solid lines indicate a cortical lesion; dotted lines indicate a purely subcortical aspect of the lesion

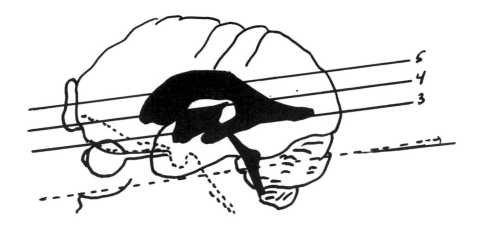

FIG. 18.7. Location of CT cuts in B.F.

3

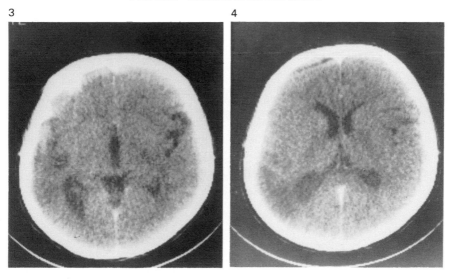

4

FIG. 18.8. CT of Patient B.F.   FIG. 18.9. CT of Patient B.F.

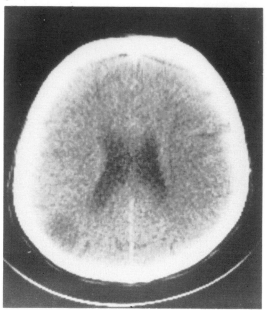

FIG. 18.10.   CT of Patient B.F.

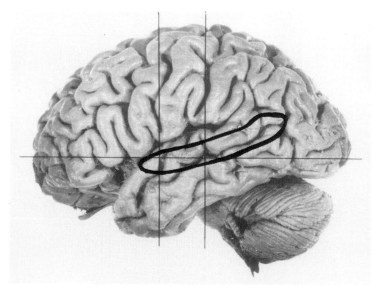

FIG. 18.11.   Lateral extent of lesion in B.F.

3

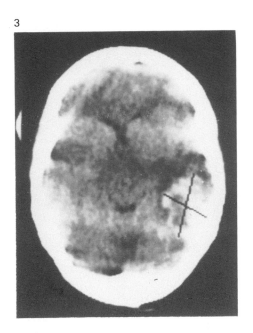

4

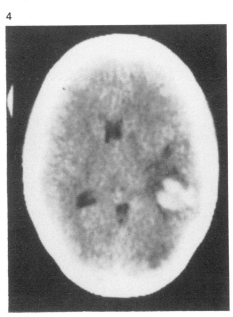

FIG. 18.12.   Scan of Patient H.A.M. (14/4/80)

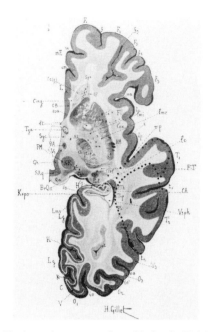

FIG. 18.13.   Horizontal reconstruction of lesion in H.A.M. (14/4/80)

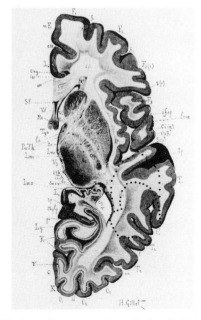

FIG. 18.14.   Horizontal reconstruction of lesion in H.A.M. (14/4/80)

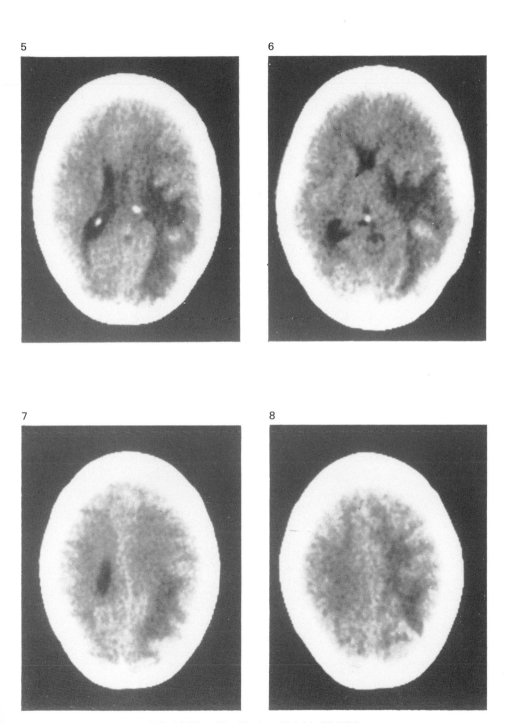

FIG. 18.15.   CT of Patient H.A.M. (28/4/80)

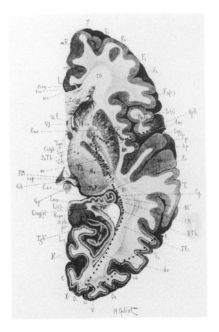

FIG. 18.16.   Horizontal reconstruction of lesion in H.A.M. (28/4/80)

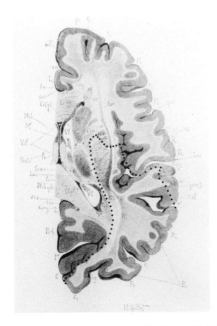

FIG. 18.17.   Horizontal reconstruction of lesion in H.A.M. (28/4/80)

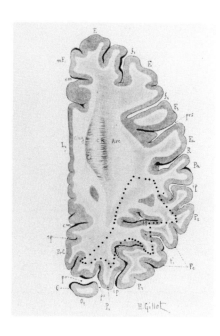

FIG. 18.18.   Horizontal reconstruction of lesion in H.A.M. (28/4/80)

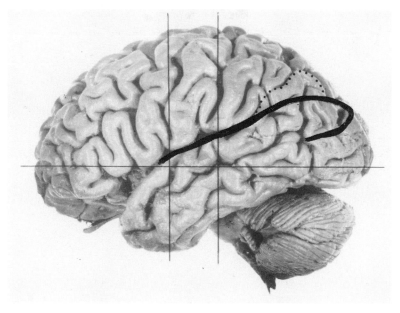

FIG. 18.19.   Lateral extent of lesion in H.A.M. (28/4/80)

20

30

40

50

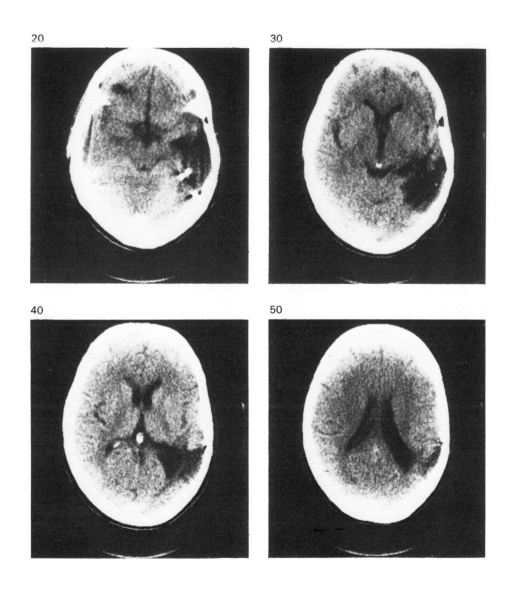

FIG. 18.20.   CT of Patient R.F.

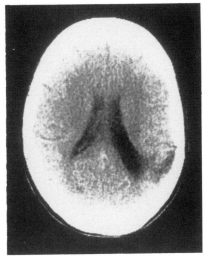

FIG. 18.20. Continued

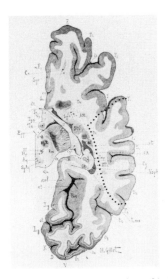

FIG. 18.21. Horizontal reconstruction of lesion in R.F.

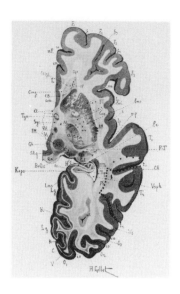

FIG. 18.22.   Horizontal reconstruction of lesion in R.F.

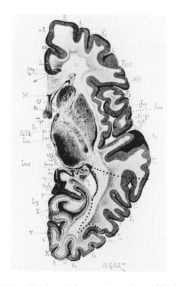

FIG. 18.23.   Horizontal reconstruction of lesion in R.F.

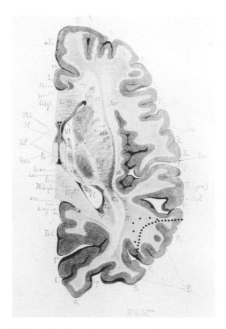

FIG. 18.24.   Horizontal reconstruction of lesion in R.F.

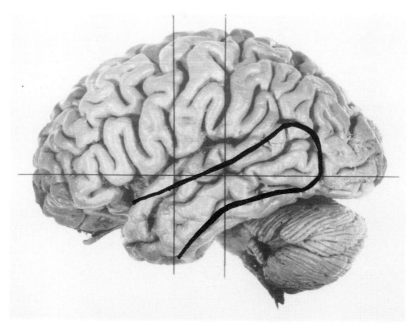

FIG. 18.25.   Lateral extent of lesion in R.F.

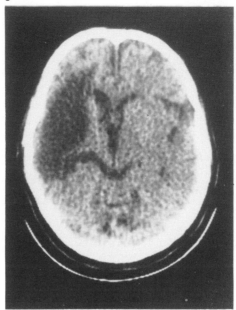

FIG. 18.26.   CT of Patient L.B.

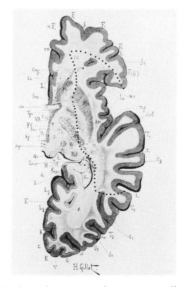

FIG. 18.27.   Horizontal reconstruction corresponding to Fig. 18.26

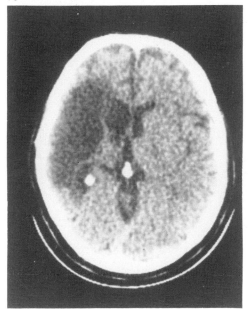

FIG. 18.28.   CT of Patient L.B.

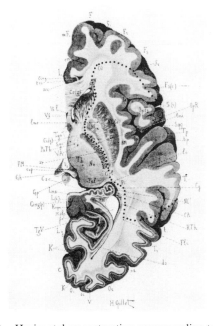

FIG. 18.29.   Horizontal reconstruction corresponding to Fig. 18.28

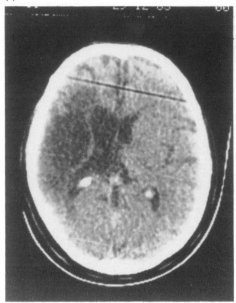

FIG. 18.30.   CT of Patient L.B.

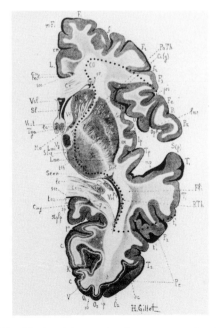

FIG. 18.31.   Horizontal reconstruction corresponding to Fig 18.30

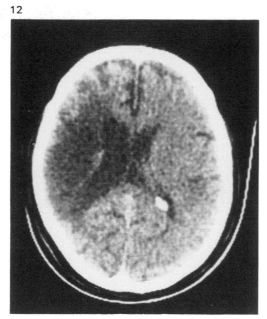

FIG. 18.32.   CT of Patient L.B.

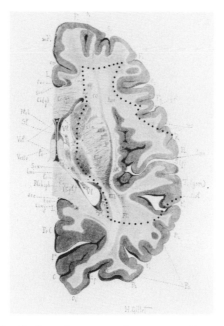

FIG. 18.33.   Horizontal reconstruction corresponding to Fig. 18.32

13

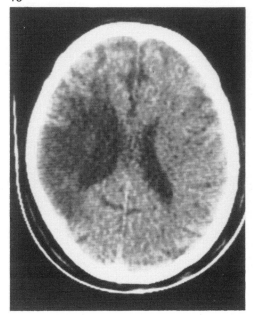

FIG. 18.34.   CT of Patient L.B.

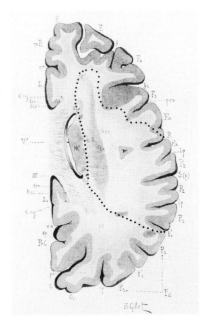

FIG. 18.35.   Horizontal reconstruction corresponding to Fig. 18.34

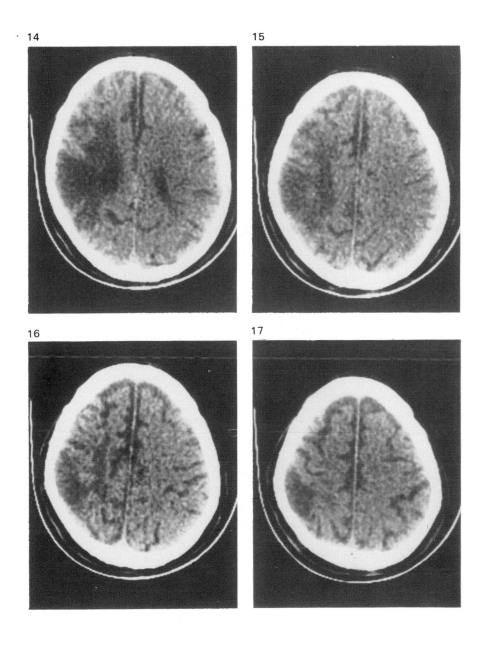

FIG. 18.36.   CT of Patient L.B.

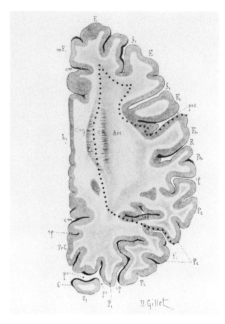

FIG. 18.37.   Horizontal reconstruction corresponding to Fig 18.36, Cut 14

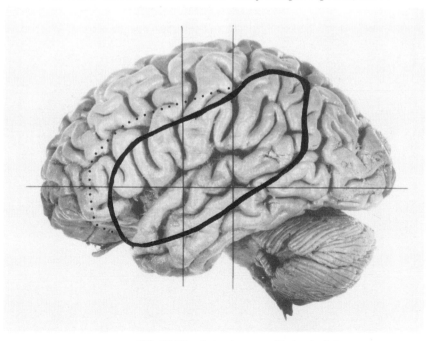

FIG. 18.38.   Lateral extent of lesion in L.B.

2B

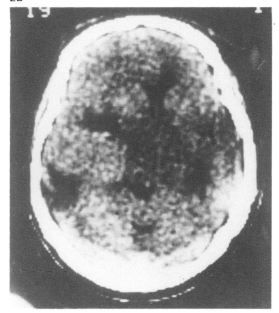

FIG. 18.39.   CT of Patient E.S.T.

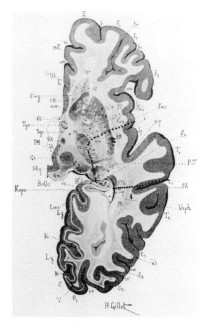

FIG. 18.40.   Horizontal reconstruction of lesion in Fig. 18.39

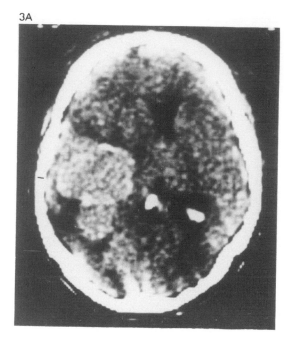

FIG. 18.41. CT of Patient E.S.T.

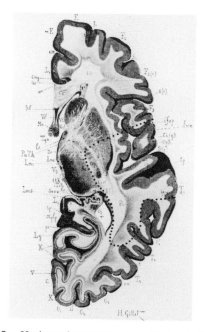

FIG. 18.42. Horizontal reconstruction of lesion in Fig. 18.41

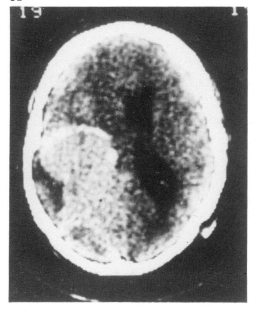

FIG. 18.43.   CT of Patient E.S.T.

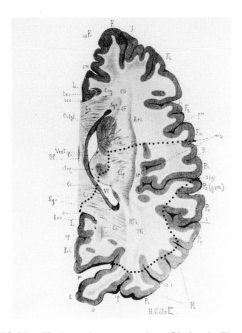

FIG. 18.44.   Horizontal reconstruction of lesion in Fig. 18.43

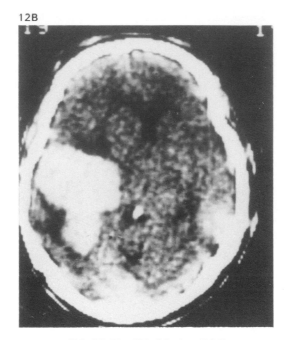

FIG. 18.45.   CT of Patient E.S.T.

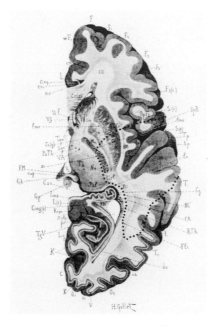

FIG. 18.46.   Horizontal reconstruction of lesion in Fig. 18.45

13B

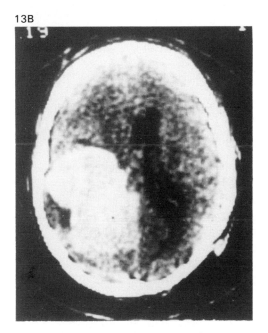

FIG. 18.47.   CT of Patient E.S.T.

40

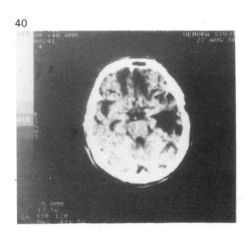

50   **60**

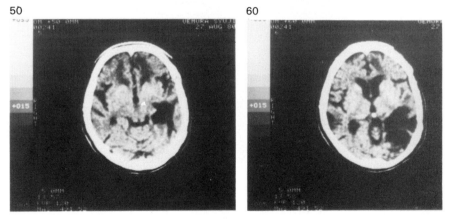

FIG. 18.48.   CT of Patient S.U.

70

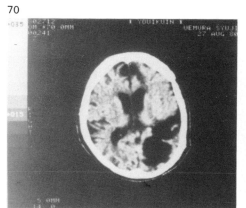

80

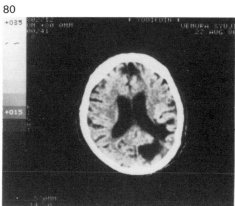

90

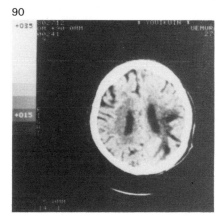

FIG. 18.48. Continued

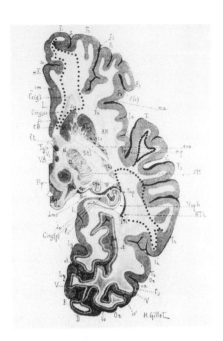

FIG. 18.49.   Horizontal reconstruction of lesion in Fig. 18.48, Cut 50

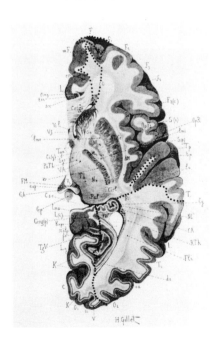

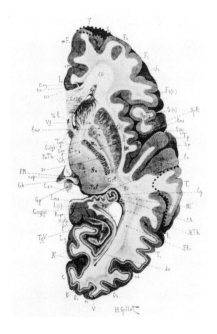

FIG. 18.50.   Horizontal reconstruction of lesion in Fig. 18.48, Cut 60. Left hemisphere lesion drawn on right hemisphere region

FIG. 18.51.   Horizontal reconstruction of lesion in Fig. 18.48, Cut 60. Right hemisphere lesion

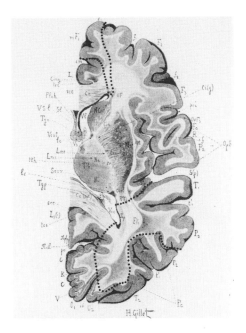

FIG. 18.52. Horizonal reconstruction of lesion in Fig. 18.48, Cut 70. Left hemisphere lesion drawn on right hemisphere diagram

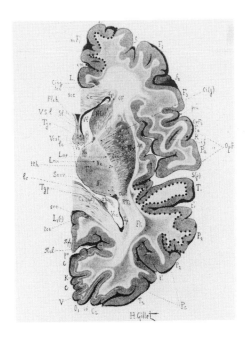

FIG. 18.53. Horizontal reconstruction of lesion in Fig. 18.48, Cut 70. Right hemisphere lesion

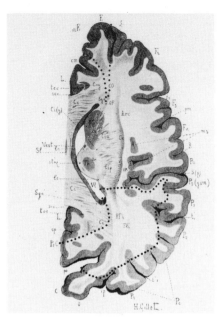

FIG. 18.54.   Horizontal reconstruction of lesion in Fig. 18.48, Cut 80. Left hemisphere lesion

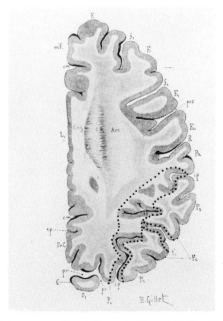

FIG. 18.55.   Horizontal reconstruction of lesion in Fig. 18.48, Cut 90. Left hemisphere lesion

coa, cop	commissures antérieure et postérieure (anterior and posterior commissures)
CR	couronne rayonnante (corona radiata)
Csc	circonvolutions sous-calleuses (subcallosal gyri)
D	gyrus descendens d'Ecker
do	diverticule occipital
ds	diverticule du subiculum (prosubiculum)
dsp	diverticule sous-pineal (sub-pineal diverticulum)
Epp	espace perforé postérieur (posterior perforated space)
F_1, F_2, F_3	première, deuxième et troisième circonvolutions frontales (superior, middle and inferior frontal gyri)
F_3 (c)	cap de la troisième circonvolution frontale (pars triangularis of the third frontal convolution)
f_2, f_3	deuxième et troisième sillons frontaux (middle and inferior frontal sulci)
F	champ de Forel (Forel's field)
Fa	circonvolution frontale ascendante (pre central gyrus)
Fl	faisceau lenticulaire de Forel (lenticular fasciculus of Forel)
Fli	faisceau longitudinal inférieur (inferior longitudinal fasciculus)
Flp	faisceau longitudinal postérieur (posterior longitudinal fasciculus)
Fm, Fm'	forceps major et minor
FM	faisceau de Meynert
Ft	faisceau de Türck
Fu	faisceau uncinatus (uncinate fasciculus)
FV	fibres visuelles
Fus	lobule fusiforme (occipito-temporal gyrus)
Gh	habénula
Gp	glande pinéale (pineal gland)
H	hippocampe (hippocampus)
h	sillon de l'hippocampe (hippocampal sulcus)
I	insula
i	sillon de l'insula (insular sulcus)
Ia, p	insula antérieur et postérieur (anterior and posterior insula)
io	sillon inter-occipital (inter-occipital sulcus)
ip	sillon interpariétal (intra parietal sulcus)
K	scissure calcarine (calcarine sulcus)
K + po	union des scissures calcarine et pariéto-occipitale (junction of calcarine and parieto-occipital sulcus)
L_1	circonvolution limbique (cingulate gyrus)
L_1 (i)	isthme du lobe limbique (isthmus of gyrus cinguli)
lc	lame cornée
lg	lobule lingual (gyrus lingula)
Lme, Lmi	lames médullaires externe et interne du noyau lenticulaire (external and internal medullary laminae of lenticular nucleus)
Lms	lame médullaire superficielle
Ln	locus niger
lt	lame terminale embryonnaire (lamina terminale)

ma	sillon marginal antérieur (anterior limiting sulcus of insula)
mF$_1$	face interne de la première circonvolution frontale (medial surface of superior frontal gyrus)
Mo	trou de Monro (Foramen of Monro)
mp	sillon marginal postérieur (posterior limiting sulcus of insula)
ms	sillon marginal supérieur (superior limiting sulcus of insula)
NA	noyau amygdalien (amygdala)
Na	noyau antérieur du thalamus (anterior nucleus of thalamus)
NC	noyau caudé (caudate nucleus)
NC'	queue du noyau caudé (tail of caudate nucleus)
Ne, Ni, Nm	noyaux externe, interne et médian du thalamus
NL	noyau lenticulaire (lenticular nucleus)
NR	noyau rouge (red nucleus)
O$_1$, O$_2$, O$_3$	1ère, 2e et 3e circonvolutions occipitales (superior, middle and inferior occipital gyri)
o$_2$	deuxième sillon occipitale (middle occipital sulcus)
oa	sillon occipital antérieur (anterior occipital sulcus)
OF	faisceau occipito-frontal (occipito-frontal fasciculus)
OpF$_3$	opercule de la troisième circonvolution frontale (opercular part of inferior frontal gyrus)
OpF	opercule rolandique (rolandic operculum)
ot	sillon collatéral (collateral sulcus)
P	pied du pédoncule cérébral (foot of cerebral peduncle)
P$_1$	lobule pariétal supérieur (superior parietal lobule)
P$_2$	lobule pariétal inférieur (inferior parietal lobule)
po	scissure pariéto-occipitale (parieto-occipital solcus)
PrC	precuneus
pri, prs	sillon prérolandique inférieur et supérieur (inferior and superior parts of pre-central sulcus)
P$_2$ (gsm)	gyrus supramarginal (supramarginal gyrus)
Pa	circonvolution pariétale ascendante (precentral gyrus)
Pul	Pulvinar
Qa	tubercule quadrijumeau antérieur (superior colliculus)
R	scissure de Rolando (central sulcus)
Rm	ruban de Reil médian
Rth	radiations thalamiques (thalamic radiations)
S(a), (p), (v)	branches antérieure, postérieure et verticale de la scissure de sylvius (anterior, posterior and vertical branches of sylvian fissure)
scc	sinus du corps calleux
SgAq	substance grise de l'aqueduc de sylvius (grey matter of cerebral aqueduct)
Sgc	substance grise centrale
Sge	substance grise sous-épendymaire
Sl	septum lucidum
Sih	scissure inter-hémisphérique
so	sillon sus-orbitaire
sp	scissure sous-pariétale

Spa	substance perforée antérieure (anterior perforated substance)
Spp	substance perforée postérieure (posterior perforated substance)
SR	substance réticulée
Sti	substance innominée
STrz	stratum zonale
T_1, T_2, T_3	première, deuxième et troisième circonvolutions temporales (superior, middle and inferior temporal gyri)
t_1, t_2	premier et deuxième sillons temporaux (superior and middle temporal sulci)
T_1 (gsm)	première circonvolution temporale au niveau du gyrus supramarginal (superior temporal gyrus at the level of the supramarginal gyrus)
Tap	tapetum
Tc	tuber cinercum
tec	taenia tecta
Tga, Tgp	piliers antérieur et postérieur du trigone (column and posterior part of fornix)
TgV	trigone ou carrefour ventriculaire (collateral trigone of lateral ventricle)
Th	thalamus
Tm	tubercule mamillaire (mamillary body)
Tp	circonvolution temporale profonde (Heschl's gyrus)
tp	sillon temporal profond
tth	taenia thalami
V_3	troisième ventricule (third ventricle)
V	ruban de Vicq d'Azyr
VA	faisceau de Vicq d'Azyr
Vf	corne frontale du ventricule latéral (frontal horn of lateral ventricle)

Author Index

Subject Index

Abstract letter identities, assigning of, 35

Abstractness/concreteness of words, influence of, 180, 182–186, 209, 227, 229

Acalculia, 107

Agnosia, associative, 9, 84, 107, 256

Agraphia, 5, 121, 131, 365
  Lexical or orthographic, 9, 368

Alexia, 5, 177, 178, 202
  Phonological, 399–441
  Pure, 209, 213, 365

Anomia, 16, 84, 96, 130, 157, 158, 214

Analogy Theory, 353–357

Aphasia, 5, 8, 18, 39, 94, 116, 131–3, 137, 142, 159, 178, 226, 246, 247, 251, 256
  Anomic, 140, 142, 156

Apraxia, 107, 256

Associative loss, 3

Auditory checking procedures, 105, 111–3, 124, 125, 128, 134

Auditory input logogen system, 120, 121, 198, 492

"b/d" confusion, 40, 48, 85, 278

Biscriptal patients, 7

Bishop's Test of the Reception of Grammar, 279

Blending, 35, 48, 273, 274, 276, 280, 282, 285, 286, 334

Boston Diagnostic Aphasia Examination (BDAE), 54, 83, 142, 143

Chinese, dsylexias in, 198, 209, 210, 212, 223

Chunking, 281, 282, 284
  Errors, 276

Circumlocutions, 152–4, 158, 160–3, 161–4, 226, 228, 230, 238, 239, 245

Comprehension:
  & accessing phonological words, 158
  Auditory, 80, 84–5, 89, 93–4, 107, 128, 131–4, 143, 158, 226, 247, 257
  Homophone, 115–6, 122–3, 128, 137, 210–1, 219–20
  In surface dyslexia, 75–7, 81, 92, 93
  Of given responses vs. target words, 79, 81, 157, 232–4
  Of inconsistent words, 190–5
  Reading, 15–20, 47, 76, 99, 116, 123, 126–8, 130, 132, 133, 134, 139, 141, 145, 189, 190, 201, 221, 222

DATE DUE